Biomedical Science
Lecture Notes

Biomedical Science
Lecture Notes

Ian Lyons

Oxford University Medical School *and*
St Edmund Hall, Oxford University

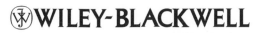

WILEY-BLACKWELL

A John Wiley & Sons, Ltd., Publication

This edition first published 2011, © 2011 by Ian Lyons

Blackwell Publishing was acquired by John Wiley & Sons in February 2007. Blackwell's publishing program has been merged with Wiley's global Scientific, Technical and Medical business to form Wiley-Blackwell.

Registered office: John Wiley & Sons Ltd, The Atrium, Southern Gate, Chichester, West Sussex, PO19 8SQ, UK

Editorial offices: 9600 Garsington Road, Oxford, OX4 2DQ, UK
      The Atrium, Southern Gate, Chichester, West Sussex, PO19 8SQ, UK
      111 River Street, Hoboken, NJ 07030-5774, USA

For details of our global editorial offices, for customer services and for information about how to apply for permission to reuse the copyright material in this book please see our website at www.wiley.com/wiley-blackwell

Library of Congress Cataloging-in-Publication Data

Lyons, Ian, author.
  Lecture notes. Biomedical science / Ian Lyons, Oxford Clinical Medical School and St Edmund Hall, Oxford University.
     p. ; cm.
  Biomedical science
  Includes bibliographical references and index.
    ISBN 978-1-4051-5711-7 (pbk. : alk. paper)   1.   Medical sciences–Outlines, syllabi, etc.   I.   Title.
  II.   Title: Biomedical science.
  [DNLM: 1. Clinical Medicine. WB 102]
  R740.L96 2011
  610–dc22

                              2010052267

A catalogue record for this book is available from the British Library.

Set in 8.5pt/11pt Utopia by Thomson Digital, Noida, India.
Printed and bound in Malaysia by Vivar Printing Sdn Bhd

1 2011

Contents

Preface

The medical curriculum has undergone significant change in recent years. Most noticeably, it has broadened, even since we started at medical school early in the twenty-first century. As students we noticed that the vast majority of textbooks for medical sciences focused on a very narrow area, often at a level of detail far beyond what we required. We have endeavoured to provide a resource of the essential facts, without too much additional detail.

The book follows the areas of medical science in which tomorrow's doctors are examined. It follows the *Lecture Notes* format of short prose and bullet points. Many of the illustrations have been kept intentionally concise so that they can be reproduced by the students in an exam or as an *aide memoire*.

The book helps draw together the various areas of medical science. We hope that this will help the consolidation of knowledge gained from more detailed works, thus drawing together the knowledge we are all required to understand as medical students and as doctors.

First, I would like to thank my four co-authors who wrote significant portions of particular chapters in this book: Sarah Cook (Endocrinology and Reproduction), Catherine Hildyard (Neuroscience), David McCartney (Physiology and Pharmacology) and Imogen Staveley (Anatomy). In addition to their skills and expertise as applied to those chapters, their comments on the book as a whole have been instrumental in shaping it. Furthermore, their support and persistent endeavour in this project has been greatly appreciated.

Second, I would like to acknowledge the senior editorial team: Profs. Christopher Lote, Paola Domizio and Donal McNally. The other student authors and I had little idea of the task we were undertaking when we began this project; their insight and advice has been enormously helpful.

Third, I am grateful for the input and support of Miss Rebecca Anderson, Mr Jonathan Best, Mr David Grant, Miss Rachel Humphreys, Dr Michael Lyons, Mr Stuart Lyons, Mrs Young-Ja Lyons, Mr Samuel Offer, Mr Jack Pottle, Miss Charlotte Seymour, Miss Claire Strauss, Miss Rebecca Ting, Miss Laura Watts and Sub-Lt Dr Timothy Wills, and (though they were unaware of their assistance) all the members of 2009 Tingewick Firm. They have all helped in some way with the preparation of this manuscript.

Finally, it has been a pleasure to work with Laura Quigley, Beth Bishop and all the staff at Wiley-Blackwell who have aided and assisted us through what has been a long creative process. Special thanks must be reserved for Karen Moore – she has been directly involved in both the development and production of this project since its inception. Her advice and cooperation have been truly invaluable.

Ian Lyons

Acknowledgements

We wish to thank the following people from medical schools around the country for their help when, as medical students, they provided useful feedback on chapter content: John Bainton, Laura Barraclough, Ian Buchanan, Andy Carson-Stephens, Sarah Cowey, Paul Dent, Anahita Dua, Raquel Duarte, Antonia Edge, Mohammed Faraaz, Carl Fernandes, Gulnaz Gill, Remi Guillochan, Caroline Heelas, Becky Johnson, Bernice Knight, Nicki Linscott, David Miranda, Alice Myers, Vinay Parmar, Donna Pilkington, Richard Pinder, Sarah Shore, Shinan Sivakumar, Robert Stellman, Sabrina Talukdar, Christopher Thexton, Jillian Wall and Caryn Wujanto.

Abbreviations

ACE	angiotensin-converting enzyme	DMD	Duchenne muscular dystrophy
ACh	acetylcholine	DNA	deoxyribonucleic acid
ACTH	adrenocorticotrophic hormone	2,3-DPG	2,3-diphosphoglycerate
ADH	antidiuretic hormone	DPPC	dipalmitoylphosphatidylcholine
ADP	adenosine diphosphate	DVT	deep vein thrombosis
AGN	acute glomerulonephritis	DZ	dizygotic
AIDS	acquired immune deficiency disease	EBV	Epstein–Barr virus
AMH	anti-müllerian hormone	ECF	extracellular fluid
AMP	adenosine monophosphate	ECG	electrocardiogram
AMPA	α-amino-3-hydroxy-5-methyl-4-	ECL	enterochromaffin-like
	isoxazolepropionic acid	EEG	electroencephalogram
ANP	atrial natriuretic peptide	EGF	epidermal growth factor
APC	antigen-presenting cell	EJV	external jugular vein
Apo	apoliprotein	ELISA	enzyme-linked immunosorbent assay
APP	amyloid precursor protein	ENS	enteric nervous system
ASD	atrial septal defect	EPO	erythropoietin
ATP	adenosine triphosphate	EPP	end-plate potential
AV	atrioventricular	ER	endoplasmic reticulum
AVP	arginine vasopressin	EPSP	excitatory postsynaptic potential
BCG	Bacillus Camille–Guérin	FAD	flavin adenine dinucleotide
BCR	B-cell receptor	FEV_1	forced expiratory volume in 1 second
BMR	basal metabolic rate	FGF	fibroblast growth factor
CABG	coronary artery bypass graft	FGFR	fibroblast growth factor receptor
CAM	cell surface adhesion molecule	FH	familial hypercholesterolaemia
cAMP	3′-5′-cyclic adenosine monophosphate	FRC	functional residual capacity
CBT	cognitive–behavioural therapy	FSH	follicle-stimulating hormone
CCK	cholecystokinin	GABA	γ-aminobutyric acid
CF	cystic fibrosis	GFR	glomerular filtration rate
CFTCR	cystic fibrosis transmembrane	GHRH	growth hormone-releasing hormone
	conductance regulator	GI	gastrointestinal
cGMP	3′-5′-cyclic guanosine monophosphate	GIP	gastric inhibitory polypeptide or
CN	cranial nerve		glucose-dependent insulinotropic
CNS	central nervous systems		peptide
CO	cardiac output	GLP	glucagon-like peptide
CoA	coenzyme A	GnRH	gonadotrophin-releasing hormone
COC	combined oral contraceptive	GPCR	G-protein-coupled receptor
COMT	catechol-O-methyltransferase	GPe	globus pallidus pars externa
COX	cyclooxygenase	GPi	globus pallidus pars interna
CRH	corticotrophin or cortisol-releasing	GSH	glutathione
	hormone	GTP	guanosine triphosphate
CSF	cerebrospinal fluid	HAART	highly active antiretroviral therapy
CT	computed tomography	Hb	haemoglobin
CTL	cytoxic T-lymphocyte	HBsAg	hepatitis B surface antigen
CVP	central venous pressure	HBV	hepatitis B virus
CYP	cytochrome P450	hCG	human chorionic gonadotrophin
DAG	diacylglycerol	HDL	high-density lipoprotein
DCT	distal convoluted tubule	hGH	human growth hormone
DHEA	dehydroepiandrosterone	HIV	human immunodeficiency virus
DHT	dihydrotestosterone	HLA	human leukocyte antigen

HMG	hydroxymethylglutaryl	NSAID	non-steroidal anti-inflammatory drug
HONK	hyperosmolar non-ketotic state	NTS	nucleus tractus solitarius
hPL	human placental lactogen	NYHA	New York Heart Association
HPV	human papillomavirus	PAG	periaqueductal grey area
5-HT	5-hydroxytryptamine or serotonin	PAH	*para*-aminohippuric acid
Ig	immunoglobulin	PAMP	pathogen-associated molecular pattern
IGF-1	insulin-like growth factor 1	PCR	polymerase chain reaction
LGN	lateral geniculate nucleus of the thalamus	PCT	proximal convoluted tubule
		PDA	patent ductus arteriosus
IFN	interferon	PDGF	platelet-derived growth factor
IJV	internal jugular vein	PECAM-1	platelet endothelial cell adhesion molecule 1
IL	interleukin		
IMA	inferior mesenteric artery	PEF	peak expiratory flow
IP_3	inositol 1,4,5-trisphosphate	PG	prostaglandin
IPSP	inhibitory postsynaptic potential	PICA	posterior inferior cerebellar artery
IUD	intrauterine device	PIP_2	phosphatidylinositol 4,5-bisphosphate
IUS	intrauterine system	PFK	phosphofructokinase
IVF	in vitro fertilisation	PKA	protein kinase A (also known as cAMP-dependent protein kinase)
JGA	juxtaglomerular apparatus		
LCA	left coronary artery	PKC	protein kinase C
LDL	low-density lipoprotein	PKG	protein kinase G (also known as cGMP-dependent protein kinase)
LH	luteinising hormone		
LPS	lipopolysaccharide	PLC	phospholipase C
LOS	lipo-oligosaccharide	PNS	peripheral nervous system
LTD	long-term depression	POMC	pro-opiomelanocortin
LTP	long-term potentiation	PPARγ	peroxisome proliferator-activated receptor-γ
MALT	mucosa-associated lymphoid tissue		
MAOI	monoamine oxidase inhibitor	PPP	pentose phosphate pathway
MBL	mannan-binding lectin	PRL	prolactin
MDR	multidrug resistance	PTH	parathyroid hormone
MER	milk ejection reflex	PVR	poliovirus receptor
MERRF	myoclonic epilepsy with ragged red fibres	PYY	peptide YY
		RAG	recombination activity genes
MG	myasthenia gravis	RCA	right coronary artery
MGN	medial geniculate nucleus of the thalamus	REM	rapid eye movement
		RFLP	restriction fragment length polymorphism
MHC	major histocompatibility complex		
MI	myocardial infarction	RNA	ribonucleic acid
MLCK	myosin light chain kinase	RQ	respiratory quotient
MRI	magnetic resonance imaging	RV	residual volume
MRSA	methicillin-resistant *Staphylococcus aureus*	SA	sinoatrial
		SCM	sternocleidomastoid
MS	multiple sclerosis	SD	standard deviation
α-MSH	α-melanocyte-stimulating hormone	SMA	superior mesenteric artery
MZ	monozygotic	SNP	single nucleotide polymorphism
NAD	nicotinamide adenine dinucleotide	SNpc	substantia nigra pars compacta
NADP	nicotinamide adenine dinucleotide phosphate	SNpr	substantia nigra pars reticulata
		SR	sarcoplasmic reticulum
NK	natural killer	SSB	single-stranded DNA-binding
NKCC	$Na^+/K^+/2Cl^-$ co-transporter	SSRI	selective serotonin reuptake inhibitor
NMDA	*N*-methyl-D-aspartate	STN	subthalamic nucleus
NMJ	neuromuscular junction	T_3	triiodothyronine
NO	nitric oxide	T_4	thyroxine
NOS	nitric oxide synthase	TB	tuberculosis
NPY	neuropeptide Y	TCA	tricarboxylic acid

TCR	T-cell receptor
TENS	transcutaneous electrical stimulation
TGF-β	transforming growth factor β
THC	tetrahydrocannabinol
TLC	total lung capacity
TNF	tumour necrosis factor
TRE	thyroid response element
TRH	thyrotrophin-releasing hormone
TSH	thyroid-stimulating hormone
TxA	thromboxane A
UDP	uridine diphosphate

UTI	urinary tract infection
UV	ultraviolet
VC	vital capacity
vCJD	variant Creutzfeldt–Jakob disease
VIP	vasoactive intestinal peptide
VLDL	very-low-density lipoprotein
vWF	von Willebrand factor
VNTR	variable number tandem repeat
VPN	ventroposterior nucleus
VSD	ventricular septal defect
ZPA	zone of polarising activity

Cell biology

The cell is the basic unit of living organisms; while some organisms are made up of a single cell (e.g. protozoa and bacteria), others are made up of many cells, organised into tissues and organs, that perform specific functions.

Individual cells in humans and other eukaryotic organisms are organised into functional areas – organelles – that perform a specific function. Cells usually divide by mitosis to produce identical daughter cells to allow the development of tissue or the replacement of dying cells. However, for the purpose of reproduction, they divide by meiosis in which the daughter cells each possess half a full set of chromosomes. In developed tissues, mitosis occurs to replace those cells that have become damaged; if such cell division occurs in an unregulated fashion, cancer may result.

Organelles: structure and function

A cell contains specialised regions that take on specific functions. These organelles are discussed below; however, the biochemical interactions that occur are discussed in more detail in Chapter 3.

The cell membrane

The cell membrane is a **phospholipid bilayer** that surrounds the cell, defining its boundaries. The membrane contains many specialised molecules embedded within it, for the transport of molecules across it, as well as regulating the properties and behaviour of the membrane itself (Fig. 1.1).

Structure

The formation of the bilayer relies on the properties of the constituent phospholipids. They are made up of two parts:

1 A **polar head** region, which is soluble in water (**hydrophilic**). This region often contains a charged group which mediates its hydrophilic nature.
2 A **non-polar tail** region, which is insoluble in water (**hydrophobic**). This hydrophobic property results from the long uncharged fatty acyl chains.

These properties promote phospholipids to form a bilayer, in which the hydrophilic head regions are in contact with water while the hydrophobic tail regions accumulate in the middle of the bilayer. The fluidity of the membrane is regulated by the presence of **cholesterol**.

The cell membrane is a dynamic structure, with the various **protein** components free to rotate and diffuse laterally around the lipids, allowing their aggregation, which is often required for signalling. These proteins can be grouped into two types:

1 **Integral proteins** are embedded in the membrane.
2 **Peripheral proteins** are associated with the surface of the membrane as a result of non-covalent interactions.

Biomedical Science Lecture Notes, First Edition. Ian Lyons.
© 2011 by Ian Lyons. Published 2011 by Blackwell Publishing Ltd.

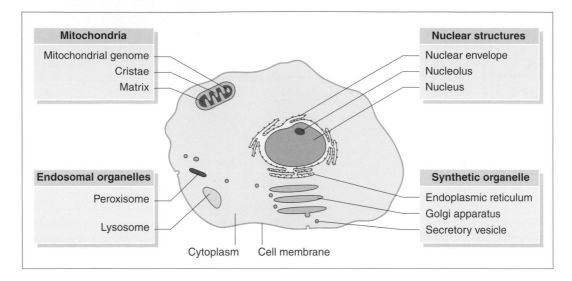

Figure 1.1 The organelles in a eukaryotic cell. There are various organelles within the cell that are specialised to perform specific functions, as can be reflected by their features. Many of the components shown – such as the mitochondria – are found in several copies within the cell, although they have been represented only a single time, for ease.

The precise proteins associated with the membrane differ depending on the cell specialisation, other external signals that have been received and the specific state of the individual cell.

Both proteins and lipids in the membrane may be **glycosylated**, whereby carbohydrates are added to the molecule. These carbohydrates may be involved in the interaction between the cell and the environment or other cells.

The cytoplasm

The organelles are contained in the cytoplasm, which is made up of a wide variety of ions and solutes, as well as a complex cytoskeletal structure. This structure maintains the cell shape and regulates various transport and trafficking pathways in the cell. The cytoplasm is also the site of most cellular metabolic reactions.

The nucleus

The nucleus contains almost all the genetic information necessary to produce any cell in the human body; this genetic information is densely packed as **chromatin**. The nucleus is separated from the rest of the cell by a **nuclear envelope**, which is made up of two lipid bilayers – the outer membrane being

continuous with the **endoplasmic reticulum**. Transport of molecules across the nuclear membrane is tightly regulated by many **nuclear pores** in the nuclear envelope.

Despite its important function, the nucleus usually occupies a relatively small volume, often around 5% of the total cell volume.

The **nucleolus**, which is the site of synthesis of **ribosomal RNA** and the assembly of **ribosomes**, is one of the few structures visible in the nucleus (by light microscopy).

The endoplasmic reticulum

The endoplasmic reticulum (ER) is a network of tubes continuous with the outer membrane of the nuclear envelopes. It produces lipids and protein for secretion or use in cellular organelles. There are two types of ER:

1 **Rough ER** is the site of protein production. Its 'rough' appearance under an electron microscope comes from the presence of protein-synthesising **ribosomes** on its surface. The resulting proteins are secreted into the ER lumen, from where they are transported for further modification

2 The **smooth ER** lacks ribosomes and is responsible for the production of lipids, which

contribute to the cellular membranes, and *also* the production of steroids. Smooth ER is associated with detoxifying reactions, particularly in the liver, and is also the site from which components are transported to other organelles by **vesicular transport**.

The proportions of rough and smooth ER may reflect the specialisation of the cell, e.g. in the adrenal cortex, which is responsible for the production of steroid hormones, the smooth ER accounts for most of the cell volume.

The Golgi apparatus

The Golgi apparatus modifies many cellular proteins, through the addition of carbohydrates.

It resembles a series of sac-like structures – **cisternae** – which receive proteins from the rough ER by **vesicular transport**. As proteins are transported between the different cisternae, they receive carbohydrate modifications; transport may be forwards or backwards between compartments, before the proteins are packaged into vesicles for secretion or transport to specific organelles. This process, **trafficking**, relies on the presence of specific signals in the proteins themselves, which target them to their final destination.

Mitochondria

Mitochondria synthesise ATP and other phosphate compounds that power cellular reactions through the catabolism of a variety of metabolic compounds.

Structure

Mitochondria are double-membrane organelles. The outer membrane is smooth whereas the inner membrane possesses a series of projections – **cristae** – that impinge on the interior of the mitochondria, known as the **matrix**.

Mitochondria contain a primitive genome that encodes some of the proteins not found in the nuclear genome that are necessary for their function. This, and their replication independently of the nucleus of the cell, may reflect their **endosymbiotic origin**. However, many of the proteins that mitochondria require are solely encoded in the main genome in the nucleus of the cell.

Unlike the main human genome, the mitochondrial genome is always inherited entirely from the mother; mitochondria in sperm do not contribute to the zygote.

 DEFINITION **Endosymbiotic theory of the origin of mitochondria**

The mitochondrial genome has been sequenced and has many features consistent with a bacterial genome. It has been suggested that, at some point in the past, a bacterium became engulfed by a primitive cell and remained within it, resulting in a symbiosis between the two organisms. It is thought that this symbiotic bacterium evolved into the mitochondria of today.

Function

Mitochondria meet the energy needs of the cell. In the matrix the **TCA** (tricarboxylic acid) cycle occurs, which supplies the **electron transport chain** with the reduced co-factors necessary to generate **ATP**, the main energy currency of the cell.

The number of mitochondria present in the cell reflects its energy need; muscle cells and neurons have high energy demands and frequently have many mitochondria, whereas cells with lower energy requirements may possess very few.

 CLINICAL **Myoclonic epilepsy with ragged red fibres**

Myoclonic epilepsy with ragged red fibres (MERRF) is a rare condition characterised by myoclonus, epilepsy and ataxia, usually manifesting in the teens or student age. Further symptoms include muscle weakness, deafness, dementia and seizure. The cause has been traced to a decrease in the function of the electron transport chain resulting from mutation in a mitochondrially-encoded protein. As such, the condition is maternally inherited, although the mother may express a weaker phenotype than her child.

Ribosomes

Ribosomes are minute organelles, around 20 nm in diameter, that synthesise amino acids. They are found free floating in the cytosol, or on the rough ER, where the proteins produced are destined for secretion or transport to another organelle.

Lysosomes and the endosomal compartment

The endosomal compartment consists of many membrane-bound compartments in the cytoplasm that package and transport molecules to other regions of the cell or to the external environment. They can also isolate reactions that may be damaging to the cell as a whole – often involving degradative enzymes.

Lysosomes

Lysosomes are membrane-enclosed compartments, involved in the degradation of some molecules and old organelles, so that the components can be broken down and reused to synthesise new macromolecules. They contain a variety of **acid hydrolases**, potent degradative enzymes that act in an acid environment. Consequently, the interior of the lysosome is acidic, typically pH 5.

In phagocytic cells, lysosomes have developed a more specific role. The enzymes can degrade bacteria and other pathogens that have been ingested to control infection.

Cellular processes

The cell survives and performs its role through the function of the various macromolecules within it. The synthesis and chemical properties of these macromolecules are discussed in Chapter 3, although the following major processes are discussed below:

- Transport across a membrane
- Enzymes – catalysis of the chemical reactions
- Trafficking of proteins to their site of action.

> **DEFINITION Osmosis**
>
> Osmosis can be defined as 'the flow of water across a semi-permeable membrane'. The cell membrane is permeable to water, though not to many of the solutes found within it. The presence of different solutes in different concentrations on either side of the membrane contributes to a concentration gradient. This gradient must be equilibrated by movement of water across the membrane. As such, the volume of a compartment is altered due to the flow of water down the concentration gradient.

Membrane transport

Membranes can regulate the movement of molecules across them. Although the phospholipid bilayer is insoluble to most polar molecules, non-polar molecules and small polar molecules can traverse the membrane by diffusion. This diffusion is crucial for the regulation of the cellular volume by **osmosis**.

Diffusion

Diffusion is the movement of molecules down a concentration gradient (osmosis is diffusion of water). Diffusion continues until the concentration gradient has been abolished and a dynamic equilibrium established, where the flow across the membrane in each direction is the same. There are a number of factors that govern the rate of diffusion:

- The rate of diffusion is proportional to the square of the **distance**.
- The **size** – small particles diffuse faster.
- The rate of diffusion is proportional to the **concentration gradient**.
- A **thicker membrane** will slow the rate of diffusion.

Non-polar molecules (e.g. steroid hormones) can dissolve within the bilayer and are capable of diffusing across the membrane, as are small particles such as H_2O and O_2. Polar molecules (and large molecules in general) cannot pass unaided through the lipid bilayer.

Mechanisms of membrane transport

Large or charged molecules cannot diffuse across the lipid bilayer and must be helped by specific transport proteins; some molecules must be transported against the concentration gradient, through **active transport**. Membrane transport is achieved through the presence of channels and carrier proteins in the bilayer.

Channels are pores that let specific water-soluble molecules across the membrane while in solution. Channels may be gated to restrict the flow of their target molecule to specific periods. Gating may be in response to a ligand (e.g. acetylcholine), voltage or another stimulus.

Carrier proteins bind their target molecule and transport it across the bilayer by a conformational shift. Three different types of transport can be distinguished:

1 **Facilitated diffusion** allows the movement of molecules that cannot diffuse directly through the lipid bilayer to move down their concentration gradient. The binding of the ligand to its carrier protein is sufficient to induce a conformation change so that it can move the molecule(s) across the membrane without using the cell's energy. Alternatively, the transporter may 'flip' between two states, allowing the movement of molecules across the lipid bilayer if they are bound at the moment of conformational change. Facilitated diffusion is used by many ion exchangers (e.g. Cl^-, HCO_3^- exchanger) and by transporters of larger molecules (e.g. the glucose transporters)

2 **Primary active transport** is the transport of molecules against their concentration gradient, directly using ATP to power the process. This generates a large concentration gradient that can power other cellular processes. It can also allow the compartmentalisation of harmful molecules and their removal from the cell. The **Na^+/K^+ATPase** works through primary active transport.

3 **Secondary active transport** is the movement of a molecule against its concentration gradient that is powered by a different concentration gradient generated by primary active transport, e.g. the Na^+/Ca^{2+} exchanger transports Ca^{2+} against its concentration gradient due to the flow of Na^+ down the gradient, which was previously generated through the action of the Na^+/K^+ ATPase.

Enzymes and catalysis

Enzymes are **proteins** that catalyse a chemical reaction. All enzymes contain an **active site** in which catalysis of the reaction takes place. This active site is defined by the amino acid residues in the molecule and the folding patterns that emerge. Two distinct types of region can be identified in the active site:

1 The **binding sites** hold the substrate on the active site.
2 The **catalytic site** is the region of the active site where the reaction takes place.

Two distinct theories of how the active site contributes to catalysis have been put forward:

1 The 'lock-and-key' hypothesis
2 The induced fit hypothesis

The 'lock-and-key' hypothesis

This hypothesis suggests that there is a high complementarity between the enzyme and its substrate – similar to a lock and key. The specificity is determined by the amino acid residues in the active site that are not involved in binding or catalysis of the substrate. These interactions may be the result of complementary shape, the presence of chemically complementary charges, or a combination of both.

The induced fit hypothesis

The induced fit hypothesis suggests that interactions between an enzyme and its substrate result in a conformational change, 'steric strain' that promotes the catalysis of the reaction. In multisubunit proteins, the binding of a ligand to one subunit may induce a conformational change in the other subunits to promote binding further, e.g. in haemoglobin.

Multienzymes

Enzymes are often found in large multimeric complexes. These **multienzymes** consist of several copies of each subunit and co-factors that are required. **Pyruvate dehydrogenase** is an example of a multienzyme.

Multienzymes may also express different subunits in a tissue-specific manner. These **isoenzymes** may have different kinetic properties or slightly different kinetic functions. **Lactate dehydrogenase** is a tetramer made up of two different types of subunit: 'H' form subunits are found predominantly in the heart, whereas 'M' form subunits are found in the muscles. The different subunits have different properties – 'H' subunits catalyse the conversion of lactate to pyruvate, whereas the 'M' forms are required for anaerobic glycolysis and catalyse the conversion of pyruvate to lactate. As a result of these two subunit types, five different proteins may be produced: H_4, H_3M, H_2M_2, HM_3, M_4.

Co-factors

Co-factors are non-protein molecules that aid the function of an enzyme:

- **Metal ions** are frequently used as electron donors/acceptors because they can exist in a variety of oxidation states.
- **Organic molecules** are referred to as **coenzymes** and bind a substrate required for the reaction, or may be reduced or oxidised during the enzymatic reaction. NAD^+ and $NADP^+$ are examples of co-factors that become reduced, and can be used in other reactions.

Protein trafficking

Proteins must be targeted to the correct sites in the cell to perform a function. This information is contained in the amino acid sequence of the protein. The following are two broad methods by which this information is encoded:

1 **The signal peptide** results from a chain of around 15–60 amino acids typically located at one end of the polypeptide. This signal sequence encodes the destination of the protein and is recognised by various proteins to trigger the transport of the protein. After targeting of the protein, the signal peptide is be cleaved from the polypeptides by enzymes known as **signal peptidases**.
2 **Signal patches** are a less well-understood method of targeting. The fully folded protein encodes a region in its structure that is recognised and targets the protein to a specific location. Signal patches are difficult to identify, because they rely on the folded nature of the protein, and are not identifiable solely from the amino acid sequence.

Targeting of protein to the endoplasmic reticulum

All protein synthesis is initiated on free-floating ribosomes, yet the protein synthesis must be targeted to the correct location as a result of a signal peptide encoded at the start of the amino acid chain. This ER-targeting sequence produces a series of changes:

- The signal peptide rapidly folds around the ribosome such that it pauses in translation.
- The signal peptide allows the binding of the ribosome to specific pores in the ER.
- Cleavage of the signal peptide permits the continuation of translation, with the protein product being secreted into the ER lumen.

Targeting of proteins to other compartments

Many different signals have been identified that target proteins to different compartments. Often, these rely on signals in the protein sequence; however, the protein may promote an additional modification that targets the protein. This can be seen in lysosomal targeting, where the addition of the sugar mannose 6-phosphate is responsible for the targeting of the protein to the lysosome. Deficiencies in protein targeting may contribute to serious diseases.

Cellular transport and secretion

 CLINICAL I-cell disease

I-cell disease is a very rare inherited disease that results from the presence of non-functioning lyso-somes. These become engorged because they are unable to break down their contents. The cells become non-viable, which is manifested grossly in skeletal deformities, restricted joint movements and hepatosplenomegaly. The condition is currently untreatable and therapy focuses on limiting symptoms. Nevertheless, death results early in infancy.

I-cell disease results from a deficiency in the enzyme *N*-acetylglucosamine-1-phosphotransfer-ase, which is involved in the carbohydrate modifications targeting a protein to the lysosomes. Instead the enzymes are secreted from the cell and unable to perform their essential function in the lysosome.

Vesicular transport

Transport of molecules to their target in the cell often requires the passage of a molecule through a lipid bilayer. Vesicular transport allows the transport of a molecule from the interior of one membrane-bound organelle to the interior of another in a lipid capsule.

The future contents of a vesicle are often aggregated together on the lipid bilayer and the vesicle is formed around them. The newly formed vesicle is then transported to the target, where the lipid bilayer of the vesicle fuses with the membrane, releasing its contents.

Vesicular transport is important in the **maintenance of cellular membranes**; fusion of a vesicle to a membrane contributes to the lipid bilayer. Fusion of a vesicle with the cell membrane also results in release of the vesicular contents – as is seen in the **constitutive** and **regulatory** secretory pathways.

Exocytosis and endocytosis

Vesicular transport to and from the cell membrane is required for the release or accumulation of molecules by the cell, as well as the redistribution of the lipid bilayer:

- **Exocytosis** is the process by which vesicles fuse with the cell membrane releasing their contents into the external environment. Exocytosis is also important for the contribution of a vesicle-derived bilayer and membrane-associated protein to the cell membrane.
- **Endocytosis** is the reverse of exocytosis, whereby vesicles are generated on the surface of the cell. This allows the recovery of membrane or cell-surface proteins from the cell surface or, through the aggregation of receptor-bound molecules, the transport of specific molecules into the cell. Two distinct forms of receptor-mediated endocytosis exist:
  - **pinocytosis** results from the ingestion of small vesicles, typically 100 nm in diameter; pinocytosis can occur in all cell types
  - **phagocytosis** is the ingestion of large particles into specialised vesicles, known as **phagosomes**; this process is restricted to a few specialised cell types and allows the uptake of particles that may be over 1 µm in size.

> ✓ **DEFINITION Clathrin-mediated transport**
>
> Clathrin is a protein associated with the formation of endocytic vesicles. It binds to the membrane proteins via a series of specific adapter proteins. The clathrin molecules interact with each other to form a lattice structure that progressively deforms the membrane into a vesicle. Formation of the vesicle allows it to bud from the membrane, at which point the clathrin coat dissociates and the vesicle travels to the endosomal compartment.

Transcytosis

Epithelial cells are found at barriers between the body and the environment. There is often a necessity to transport molecules from one side of the cell to the other. This process is mediated by specific receptors that trigger receptor-mediated endocytosis of the target molecules and their transport to the endosomal compartment. Molecules are then transported to the other side of the cell by exocytosis.

Secretion

Two major secretory pathways have evolved to regulate the secretion of proteins from the cell:

1 The **constitutive secretory pathway** is present in all cells. This is the default secretory pathway that targets proteins to the cell membrane, if they do not possess a signal that targets them elsewhere.
2 The **regulated secretory pathway** is seen only in cells specialised for secretion – such as in neurons or hormone-secreting cells. Such cells tend to produce large amounts of their secretory product and store them in **secretory granules**.

Cell division and the cell cycle

Everyone develops from a single zygote as a result of cell division, differentiation and cell death. During the proliferation required for this development, cells divide to produce two daughter cells that contain the full complement of chromosomes – **diploid** cells. This form of cell division is named **mitosis**.

During reproduction, a sperm and an ovum, which express only one copy of each chromosome, must fuse to produce a **zygote** that bears a full complement of 46 chromosomes. The production of the **haploid** cells that contain only one copy of each chromosome is essential for reproduction, and occurs by **meiosis**.

Some cells are constantly replenished throughout an individual's life as a result of cell division, e.g. epithelial cells are constantly sloughed off as a result of wear and tear and must be replenished by the division of stem cells and their differentiation.

The cell cycle

The life of the cell can be described in the cell cycle, which is split into four stages: **G1**, **M**, **G2** and **S**. Cells may also leave the cell cycle and become

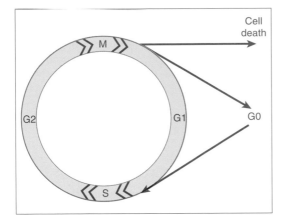

Figure 1.2 **The cell cycle**. The cell cycle consists of four phases that occur in sequence. Mitosis occurs in the M phase and is followed by the G1 phase. The cell spends most of its time in this phase, although the length of the phase may vary depending on the cell. The S phase is the point at which the synthesis of DNA occurs, so that each chromosome is made up of two identical chromatids and is followed by a short G2 phase before the cell division. This cycle can continue, or the cell may exit the cycle into G0 when it is fully differentiated and not considered part of the cell cycle. However, rarely, cells may re-enter the cycle from G0. Cells may also leave the cell cycle through cell death.

non-dividing differentiated cells, **G0**, or through cell death (Fig. 1.2):

- G1 and G2 reflect the parts of the cell cycle where the cells are not dividing and there is no synthesis of DNA. This is the period in which cells spend the most time.
- The S stage of the cycle is the period during which DNA is synthesised.
- The M stage of the cycle is the point at which cell division occurs.

Cell division

There are structures and features of meiosis and mitosis that are common to both, and reflect key processes in cell division:

- The **aggregation of chromosomes** must occur after DNA replication. The DNA becomes tightly packaged so that each chromosome becomes easily distinguishable.
- **Migration of the centrioles** to opposite ends of the cell is essential to form the **spindle**. These structures are made up of microtubules and

exhibit a nine plus two arrangement: nine pairs of microtubules arranged in a circle around an additional two microtubules.

> **DEFINITION The spindle**
>
> The spindle is a microtubule structure associated with cell division. The microtubules are organised by two centrioles, which are positioned at either end of the cell and form a network of microtubules between them. This spindle becomes associated with the chromosomes and regulates their movement to the opposite poles of the cell, ensuring that the correct chromosome complement occurs with both mitotic and meiotic cell division.

Mitosis

Mitosis occurs as a series of stages. As mitosis is a dynamic process the determination of when one stage becomes the next is difficult; however, there are certain key features that can be identified at each stage of mitosis (Fig. 1.3):

- **Interphase** – the period during which the cell is not dividing. During this period the chromosomes exist in their normal disaggregated state.
- **Prophase** – the first stage of replication. The centrioles migrate to the poles and the spindle begins to form. The nuclear envelope begins to break down and the DNA condenses such that the individual chromosomes are visible.
- **Metaphase** – the chromosomes align along the centre of the cell, where they attach to the spindle.
- **Anaphase** – the spindle pulls the chromosome, such that one **chromatid** from each chromosome migrates to each pole. The cytoplasm begins to contract as the cells start to divide.
- **Telophase** – the cells become two separate daughter cells, as cleavage of the cytoplasm is completed.

After mitosis the cells return to the G1 phase of the cell cycle.

Meiosis

Meiosis generates **haploid** cells, which contain only one of each pair of chromosomes. This process occurs through two special cell divisions that produce four haploid ($1n$) cells from a single parent diploid cell ($2n$).

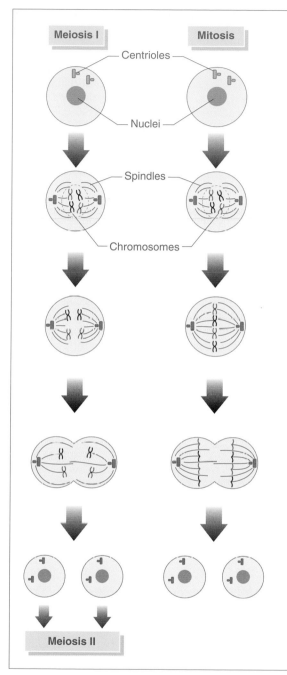

Interphase

During interphase, the cells are at rest. For ease only two pairs of chromosome are represented within the cells.

Prophase

During prophase, the processes that occur during meiosis and mitosis are very similar. The spindle starts to form, following the migration of the centrioles, and the nuclear envelope starts to degrade. The chromosomes start to aggregate.

Metaphase

The crucial difference between the two forms of cell division is that within mitosis the chromosomes align on the equator of the cell. During meiosis the chromosomes match up in their homologous pairs, such that one of each chromosome pair is situated either side of the equator.

Anaphase

The spindle pulls the chromosomes to the poles. In mitosis, one chromatid from each chromosome is pulled to either pole, whereas, in meiosis, one chromosome from each chromosome pair is pulled, halving the number of chromosomes in the daughter cells. Contraction of the cytoplasm occurs during anaphase.

Telophase

Separation of the cells is completed and the nuclear structures start to reform. In meiosis, however, a second round of cell division occurs immediately; meiosis II is similar to mitosis and completes the production of four haploid cells from a single diploid cell.

Figure 1.3 Mitosis and Meiosis. The two different forms of cell division have similar steps. Whilst mitosis produces two identical daughter cells, meiosis produces two cells with half the number of chromosomes of its parent cell.

Meiosis I

The first division in meiosis results in the separation of homologous chromosomes after the replication of the DNA to produce chromosomes that have two chromatids, as for mitosis. The resultant division is referred to as 'reduction division' because it reduces the number of chromosomes in the cell from 46 to 23:

- **Prophase I** – the chromosomes condense and then pair up with their homologous chromosomes such that one chromosome of each homologous pair lies on either side of the midline of the cell. At this stage recombination between the homologous chromosomes may occur as a result of '**crossing over**'.
- **Anaphase I** – as a result of the random division of maternal and paternal chromosomes one either side of the midline, the separation of the chromosomes leads to each daughter cell possessing one chromosome from each pair, although it is random whether each chromosome is maternally or paternally derived.

Meiosis II

The second division in meiosis closely resembles mitosis. Each of the chromosomes aligns on the midline of the cell, and the chromatids separate to the poles. The result of the two divisions of meiosis is the formation of four daughter cells, each with half the chromosome complement of their parent cells.

 DEFINITION Chromosome structure

For most of the cell cycle, chromosomes are diffusely distributed in the nucleus; however, during cell division they become tightly condensed. Although the molecular mechanisms underlying this packaging are covered in detail in Chapter 2, the gross structure is important to the process of cell division. The tightly packaged chromosome consists of two identical **chromatids**. These are joined together at a region known as the **centromere**. During the anaphase of mitosis and meiosis the chromosomes or chromatids are pulled to the poles by the spindle:

- Separation of chromatids results in the production of two identical daughter cells.
- Separation of chromosome pairs results in the movement of both chromatids to the same pole. This occurs in meiosis I to generate a haploid cells.

Cell differentiation

Cells may leave the cell cycle and become differentiated, expressing specific patterns of genes such that the cells can perform a particular function. The genes expressed result in specific protein complements, e.g. in nerve cells, they will be very different from those in a muscle cell.

The zygote is **totipotent** and has the potential to become any cell in the body or placenta. The potency of a cell decreases as it becomes **pluripotent**, capable of generating a wide variety of cell types, although not all (e.g. a haematopoietic stem cell can generate all types of blood cell, but is unable to generate other tissues, such as epithelium or nervous tissue). Finally, a cell becomes **unipotent** when it is irreversibly committed to a single fate.

Regulation of differentiation

Differentiation is regulated by various developmental signals received by the cell from its surrounding environment (e.g. signalling molecules such as transforming growth factor β (TGF-β)) which interact with the existing pattern of gene expression in the cell.

Cell growth

Cells in the body, and the tissues that contain them, may grow and shrink in response to stimuli, while remaining at the same stage of differentiation. Both atrophy (the reduction in size of a tissue) and hypertrophy (the growth in size) are physiological occurrences, although they may also occur pathologically.

Atrophy

The progressive reduction in the size of a tissue or organ – atrophy – is an important process during development. Shortly after birth, the ductus arteriosus must decrease to prevent blood bypassing the lungs; the tissue then atrophies, forming the ligamentum arteriosum.

Many pathologies are associated with a decrease in size of an organ or tissue, which may represent a generalised effect or be specific to a tissue.

Generalised atrophy can occur as a result of chronic starvation and can also be seen in the advanced stages of malignant disease (e.g. cachexia).

CLINICAL Cachexia

Cachexia is associated with a variety of chronic diseases, and is characterised by loss of weight, weakness and a generalised deterioration of the condition of the body. The mechanism underlying cachexia is thought to be associated with the high levels of cytokines and hormones.

Tissue-specific atrophy reflects changes affecting a specific tissue or organ system in the body, and is due to changes directly affecting that organ, e.g. skeletal muscles atrophy if they are not used; the size of the individual myocytes (and therefore the force that the muscle can generate) reduces rapidly.

Atrophy restricted to a specific tissue or site can be the result of a variety of causes, including:

* Ischaemia – lack of blood flow and related nutrients to nourish the tissue
* Disuse
* Neuropathy – lack of nervous impulse to stimulate the tissue
* Idiopathic.

Increased growth

The increased growth of a tissue can be broken down into hyperplasia (increase in cell number) and hypertrophy (increase in cell size). Both occur physiologically in response to external stimuli and are usually reversible when the external stimulus is withdrawn.

Hypertrophy

Hypertrophy is commonly seen where there is relatively little cell turnover (e.g. muscle). It can also occur in response to a pathological change in another part of the body, e.g. in aortic stenosis the left ventricle is required to work harder to overcome the additional pressure cause by the constriction; as a result left ventricular hypertrophy occurs.

Hypertrophy may become a pathological process: in those who exercise, generalised cardiac hypertrophy is often seen. However, the coronary circulation may not develop sufficiently rapidly to respond to the additional tissue mass. Athletic heart syndrome may occur in young individuals, in whom there is a sudden failure of the coronary circulation to adequately supply the myocardium. Here what was initially a physiologically advantageous hypertrophy has developed into a pathological condition.

Hyperplasia

Increased growth through an increase in cell numbers is commonly seen in tissues that are constantly being renewed. This allows an increase in production of the required terminally differentiated cell, e.g. increased production of red blood cells in those exposed to chronic hypoxic conditions. Hyperplasia is often seen in endocrine tissues, when increased production of a hormone associated with that tissue is needed.

Cancer

There may be changes in a cell that contribute to its excessive multiplication. This change, **neoplasia**, is different to the changes seen in hyperplasia, because there is no useful function attributed to the cell growth – the cells involved will often have an abnormal histological appearance. The growth is rarely reversible. Cancerous growth is a serious cause of death – it is currently the second biggest killer in Britain – and can occur in almost every tissue in the body. Tumours may be defined as benign or malignant.

Benign tumours

Benign tumours are well defined from the surrounding tissue and often encapsulated. They are frequently harmless because they do not spread to other sites and in rare cases (e.g. skin warts) may regress. Benign tumours may cause illness as a result of local and systemic effects:

* **Local effects** may result from the occupation of space, generating pressure on a location (e.g. intracranial tumours pressing on the brain). Similarly, tumours may obstruct crucial vessels or ducts, restricting blood flow depending on their location.
* **Systemic effects** may occur in hormone-secreting tumours, e.g. a **phaeochromocytoma** is an adrenaline-secreting tumour that leads to severe hypertension.

Malignant tumours

Malignant tumours are distinguished from benign tumours because they directly invade the host tissue. They can spread rapidly, and may produce **metastases** in distant sites. The cells in malignant tumours are usually less well differentiated than benign tumours and are often made up of histologically abnormal cells, showing features of stem cells.

Spread of malignant tumours

Local invasion into the tissue surrounding the tumour may be aided by the de-differentiation of the cells:

- They express altered adhesion molecules; this has two effects to:
  - increase dissociation and release from the primary tumour
  - promote adherence to the seeding site in new tissue.
- They secrete enzymes to degrade the extracellular matrix.
- The reduced dependence of the tumour for growth factors (which are often tissue-specific) aid its survival and proliferation.

There are a variety of routes through which a malignant tumour may spread into local tissue:

- Direct invasion into tissue
- Growth into a body cavity
- Growth along a fascial plane
- Growth into blood or lymphatic vessels – this process can contribute to the formation of metastases.

Metastasis

Metastasis is the generation of secondary tumours at distant sites. This form of spread is found only in malignant tumours and is often associated with a very poor prognosis. There are three main routes through which metastases can occur:

1 Cells may enter the bloodstream and lodge in a remote tissue site.
2 Lymphatic involvement can lead to cells entering the lymph nodes and from there entering the bloodstream
3 Tumour cells may seed in body cavities; they may grow in suspension in fluid within the cavity and from there seed to a distant organ.

The distribution of metastases will often reflect the location of the primary tumour and the route of spread. Locations of metastatic growth also rely on specific interactions between the tumour and the tissue, which contributes to the specific locations favoured by particular tumours, e.g. melanomas typically form metastases in the liver or brain.

The liver is a common site of metastases for most tumours (except brain tumours); this is thought to be due to its rich blood supply to carry cells, and also due to the expression of many growth factors that aid the survival and promote the proliferation of metastatic tumour cells.

The local effects of metastases are similar to the local effect for other tumours, although, as they are disseminated and invasive, destruction of the host tissue as a result of the outgrowth of the metastases also occurs.

The genetic basis of malignancy

Tumours occur as a result of the accumulated genetic changes within a cell that lead to its de-differentiation and uncontrolled proliferation. These changes require the loss of **tumour-suppressor genes** and the activation of **oncogenes**. Tumours are generally the result of malignant changes in a single cell, reflecting the rarity of the events.

As a long period of time is required for such events to occur, most tumours become more common with age – as the pro-malignant changes develop. There are a variety of factors and stimuli that have been identified to increase the likelihood of cancer:

- **Chemical stimuli** can increased the risk of cancer by damaging DNA, e.g. smoking is linked with the occurrence of lung cancer.
- A variety of **physical stimuli** has been identified that promotes malignant changes:
  - **ionising radiation** (e.g. X-rays) causes single-stranded breaks in DNA; if such damage is incorrectly repaired by cellular mechanisms, it may contribute to cancer
  - **ultraviolet (UV) light** can promote base changes in the DNA; UV commonly leads to cytosine conversion to the RNA base uracil; DNA repair mechanisms, however, recognise the uracil as incorrect and will replace it with a thymine base. The exposure to UV light has been linked with an increased risk of developing skin cancer.

- **Trauma** has been implicated in cancer, because the increased cell growth may promote malignant changes. This is extremely rarely seen in the development of skin cancers at burn sites.

There are a number of tumours that are associated with childhood and for which the frequency decreases with age. These tumours are likely to affect young people for one of two main reasons:

- The tumour is **derived from a stem cell**, the number of which decrease as the individual ages.
- The individual has **inherited a mutation** associated with the development of the tumour (e.g. the Wilms' tumour gene is associated with the development of renal cancer in children).

Oncogenes

Oncogenes are genes that are often activated in cancerous cells. These genes have a physiological role during development; however, their inappropriate expression can lead to uncontrolled proliferation. Oncogenes may be activated as a result of a variety of changes:

- Mutations in the genes may **alter the nature or activity of the protein product**, which can contribute to malignant changes within the cell, e.g. the molecule CD117 is a receptor for cytokine stem cell factor and signalling through it stimulates cell survival and proliferation. Mutation of this protein so that it signals without binding its ligand is associated with the development of cancer, in particular leukaemia and some forms of testicular germ cell cancer.
- **Over-expression of a gene** can lead to cancerous changes. This may be seen as the result of a chromosomal translocation, leading the oncogene to become translocated to a site on a different chromosome that is highly expressed. The 'Philadelphia translocation' is associated with many leukaemias and results from a trans location between chromosome 9 and chromosome 22.

Tumour-suppressor genes

The activation of oncogenes in not sufficient to result in malignancy. In most cases tumorigenesis also requires loss of **tumour-suppressor genes**. These genes are often associated with DNA repair or regulation of the cell cycle, preventing damaged cells proliferating.

A commonly lost tumour-suppressor gene is *p53*, which is involved in regulating the entry of cells into the cell cycle. It acts to detect DNA damage, preventing damaged cells from entering the cell cycle.

Several changes are required in an individual cell for malignancy to result. Many oncogenes must be activated and several tumour-suppressor genes must be lost. This is known as the 'multi-step theory of malignancy'.

Infectious causes of cancer

There are specific viral infections that have been established as causing cancer – in particular, the **human papillomaviruses (HPVs)**. The production of viral proteins is aided by the proliferation of cells; HPVs inactivate a number of tumour-suppressor genes (e.g. *p53*) so increasing the entry of cells into the cell cycle to aid replication of HPV, although at the same time this can lead to tumour formation. Most HPV strains are associated with warts, although others are associated with more serious conditions such as cervical cancers – in particular HPV-16 and HPV-18.

Infectious diseases may cause an increased risk of cancer through repeated damage to a tissue – repeated replication of the tissue can increase the likelihood of errors occurring during DNA replication, and thus enhance the risk of malignant changes. This is illustrated by **hepatitis B** infection; chronic carriers are at an increased risk of primary hepatocellular carcinoma due to the constant damage and regeneration of the liver as a result of the immune response against the infection.

Treatment of cancer

Treatment of tumours focuses on destruction or removal of the neoplastic cells from the body. Three methods may be used:

1 **Surgical excision** of the tumour
2 **Radiotherapy** to destroy localised tumours
3 **Chemotherapy** to destroy tumour cells and treat metastases, because they cannot be removed adequately by surgical/radiotherapeutic means.

Mechanisms of chemotherapy

Chemotherapy targets features of the cells that are different from normal differentiated cells, primarily through targeting dividing cells. This contributes to the high toxicity, because many stem cells in the body are also affected. Despite the severe side effects, chemotherapy is the only method that can effectively target metastatic cancer. The drugs used in chemotherapy act in a variety of manners to promote the destruction of cancerous cells:

- **Alkylating agents** (e.g. cisplatin) bind to and cross-link DNA to prevent further replication of the tumour cells.
- **Antimetabolites** (e.g. methotrexate) replace key components in the synthesis of DNA or RNA. Methotrexate blocks the synthesis of purine bases. However, this action also contributes to the side effects of the drug, such as myelosuppression and nephrotoxicity.
- **Antitumour antibiotics** act primarily through binding to DNA to prevent its uncoiling, which leads to breakage of the helix and inhibits replication of the cells. Such drugs (e.g. doxorubicin) may also inhibit **topoisomerases**.

- **Spindle tubule inhibitors** (e.g. vincristine) destroy microtubules, preventing spindle formation that is required for the chromosome segregation in cell division. Similar to other chemotherapy agents, they are associated with severe side effects of nephrotoxicity and bone marrow suppression.

Monoclonal antibodies in cancer therapy

Owing to their de-differentiated state, many malignant cancers express molecules that are not seen commonly in adult individuals (although they may be expressed during embryonic development and early life). These molecules, if expressed on the cell surface, may be used to target the cancer specifically (e.g. Herceptin targets HER2 which is expressed on some breast cancers).

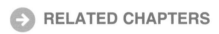 **RELATED CHAPTERS**

2

Molecular biology and genetics

The human genome contains all the information necessary to generate all the components of the human body; it is found in almost every cell in the body. This information is encoded through the four different nucleotide types in deoxyribonucleic acid (DNA). DNA contains functional units known as genes, which encode protein or nucleic acid molecules with a specific function.

The process by which a gene is converted into its product is well established, as are the mechanisms that regulate the expression of a gene. Changes to a gene, or deletions of parts of the genome, can result in disease, through changes to the proteins produced.

DNA and genes

The basic unit of genetic information is the **gene**. Genes are stretches of DNA that encode protein or RNA molecules with a specific function (or group of functions). The DNA in a cell (in almost every case) is the same as the DNA found in the **zygote** and possesses all the genetic information for creating a complete organism; the ability to reliably copy DNA to ensure accurate transmission of the genome is aided by the structure of DNA and its method of replication.

Structure of nucleic acids

DNA and RNA are made up of chains of nucleotides that are linked together to form a long continuous molecule. Each nucleotide base has common elements (Fig. 2.1):

- A phosphate group
- A deoxyribose (in DNA) or a ribose (in RNA) sugar
- A base group made up of carbon–nitrogen rings; there are two types of bases used in nucleic acids:
  – **purine bases** (adenine and guanine) are made up of two carbon–nitrogen rings. The bases differ in the side chains attached to the rings
  – **pyrimidine bases** (cytosine and thymine) are made up of a single carbon–nitrogen ring; the different pyrimidine bases also have different side chains.

The bases are the only part of the nucleotides that vary, and this variation stores information in the genetic code.

The precursors for DNA synthesis are the **deoxynucleotide triphosphates**. During DNA synthesis two phosphate groups are removed so that only a single phosphate group is incorporated into DNA. The phosphate group forms a covalent bond with the 3′-carbon atom on the next nucleotide,

Biomedical Science Lecture Notes, First Edition. Ian Lyons.
© 2011 by Ian Lyons. Published 2011 by Blackwell Publishing Ltd.

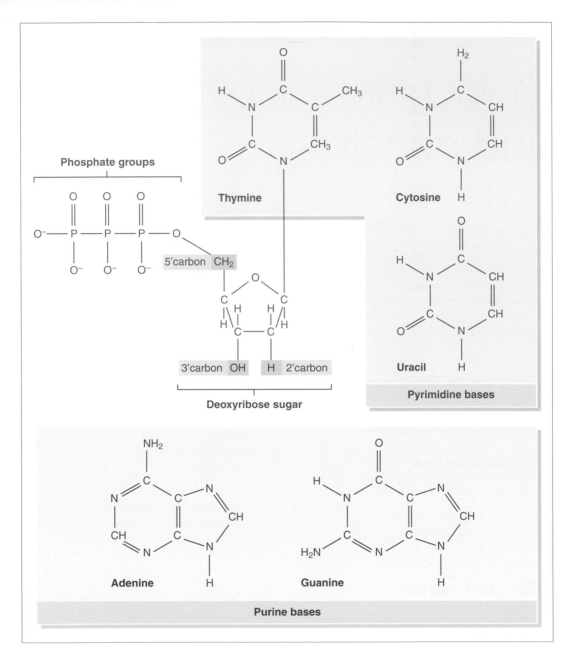

Figure 2.1 **The structure of nucleotides**. The nucleotides within DNA contain sugar (deoxyribose) and phosphate units. The nucleotide is distinguished by the base that is attached to the sugar. The body utilises adenine and guanine, purine bases, and thymine and cytosine, pyrimidine bases. Within RNA, the sugar (ribose) found in the nucleotides possesses a hydroxyl group on its 2′-carbon. In addition, uracil is used instead of thymine. Polymerisation of the bases is through the formation of a bond between a phosphate group on the 5′-carbon, and the hydroxyl group on the 3′-carbon of a different nucleotide.

resulting in a string of 3′,5′-phosphodiester bonds. This occurs throughout the DNA molecule, with the exception of the first and last bases; this allows distinction between the two ends of the DNA molecule:

1 The first base has a 5′-phosphate not bonded to any other nucleotide – the **5′ end** of the DNA.
2 The last base has a free 3′-hydroxyl group not bonded to a phosphate – the **3′ end** of the DNA.

A base can form different numbers of hydrogen bonds with one specific base on another 'complementary' nucleic acid strand. This process is known as 'base pairing':

- **Adenine** always pairs with **thymine** through two hydrogen bonds.
- **Guanine** and **cytosine** are always paired through three hydrogen bonds.

DNA is arranged in two strands that are complementary to each other. The two strands run in opposite directions – one runs from 5′ to 3′, whereas the other runs 3′ to 5′; the bases from the two strands form hydrogen bonds with each other's complementary bases.

The double-helical structure of DNA

The complete DNA molecule is twisted, forming a **double helix**, with around 10 nucleotides in each complete turn of the molecule. The double-helical structure has two grooves in which the bases are accessible from outside the molecule: a narrow minor groove and the wider major groove – an important site for the binding of proteins to specific sequences.

Genomic organisation

A complete copy of the human genome contains around 3×10^9 nucleotides. This DNA must be tightly packaged in the nucleus of the cell through the association of DNA with histones and other structural proteins. Most cells are haploid, possessing two complete copies of the genome, one from the mother and one from the father. There are three groups of cells that do not contain two complete copies of the human genome:

- Cells that lack a nucleus (e.g. red blood cells)
- The gametes, which possess a haploid nucleus with effectively a single copy of the genome
- Lymphocytes, which undergo a recombination of specific genes during their development.

Chromosomes

DNA is grouped into molecules known as **chromosomes**. In humans, there are 46 chromosomes. These chromosomes are arranged into 23 pairs, where one is maternally derived and the other paternally derived, which can be identified by **karyotyping**. Twenty-two pairs are the **autosomal** chromosomes, normally containing the same genes. The final pair of chromosomes is the **sex chromosomes**:

- Females have two X chromosomes, one from each parent.
- Males inherit one X and one Y chromosome – the Y chromosome is derived from the father and contains the genes required to regulate the development of a male child.

A single X chromosome is required by both sexes to be viable, whereas the Y chromosome encodes genes allowing the development of male characteristics.

The X and Y chromosomes possess a small region that is homologous (around 2.5 million bases (Mb)), which encodes those genes where both male and female individuals require two copies.

 DEFINITION Karyotyping

Chromosomes are identified in a process called karyotyping. Cells from an individual are isolated and drugs are used to halt the cell cycle during cell division, so that the highly condensed structures of the chromosomes are identifiable. Staining the chromosomes on the slides results in specific banding patterns, which are unique to a chromosome pair. The absence, or duplication in particular, of the pattern allows the identification of abnormalities and missing portions of chromosome, through abnormal patterns.

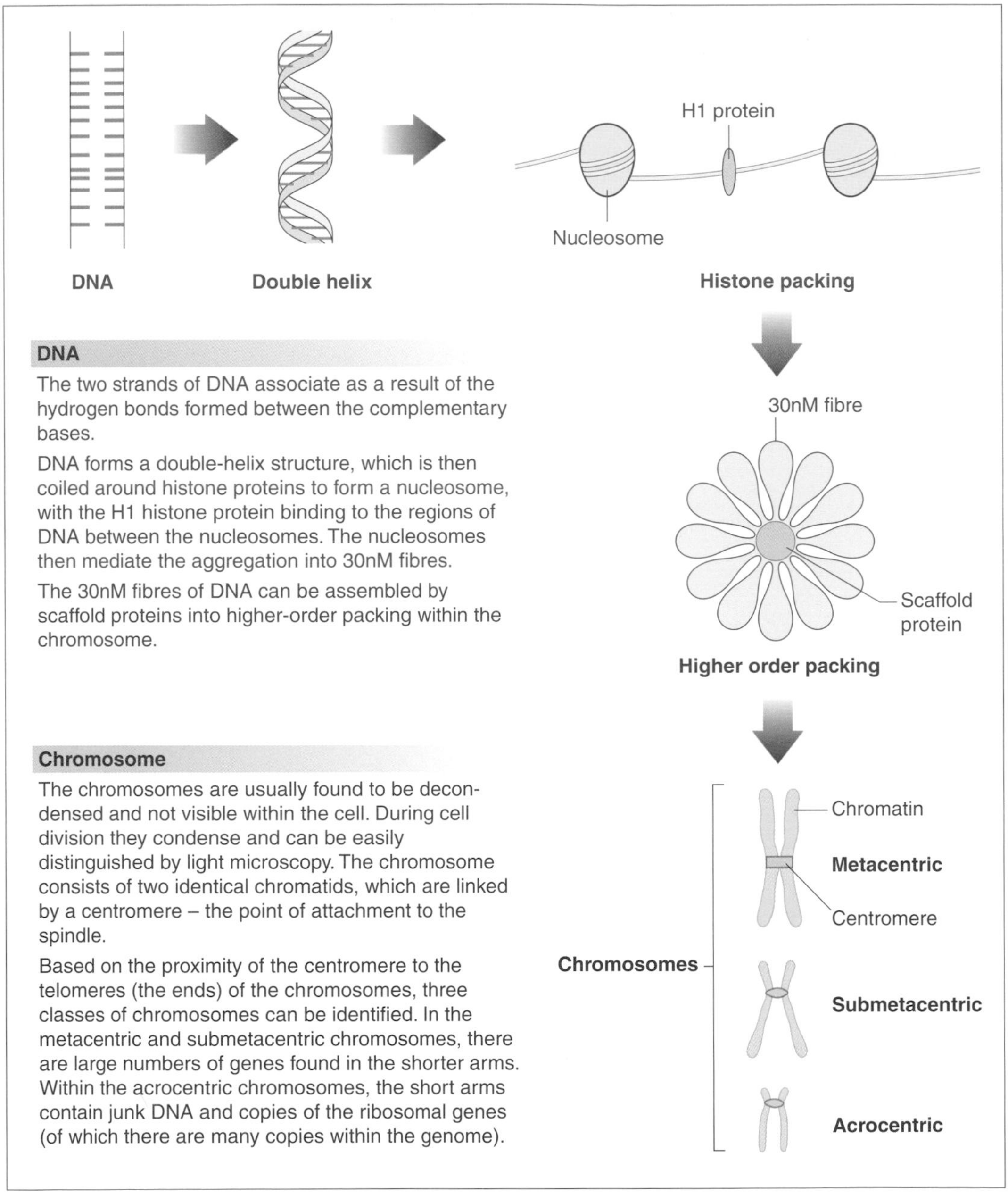
H1 protein
Nucleosome
DNA
Double helix
Histone packing
30nM fibre
Scaffold protein
Higher order packing
Chromatin
Metacentric
Centromere
Chromosomes
Submetacentric
Acrocentric
DNA
The two strands of DNA associate as a result of the hydrogen bonds formed between the complementary bases.
DNA forms a double-helix structure, which is then coiled around histone proteins to form a nucleosome, with the H1 histone protein binding to the regions of DNA between the nucleosomes. The nucleosomes then mediate the aggregation into 30nM fibres.
The 30nM fibres of DNA can be assembled by scaffold proteins into higher-order packing within the chromosome.
Chromosome
The chromosomes are usually found to be decondensed and not visible within the cell. During cell division they condense and can be easily distinguished by light microscopy. The chromosome consists of two identical chromatids, which are linked by a centromere – the point of attachment to the spindle.
Based on the proximity of the centromere to the telomeres (the ends) of the chromosomes, three classes of chromosomes can be identified. In the metacentric and submetacentric chromosomes, there are large numbers of genes found in the shorter arms. Within the acrocentric chromosomes, the short arms contain junk DNA and copies of the ribosomal genes (of which there are many copies within the genome).

Figure 2.2 Chromatin and chromosomes.

Structure of chromosomes

A single chromosome is made up of two identical **chromatids** joined by a centromere. The position of the centromere along the length of the chromosome creates two arms – one short and one long arm. Chromosomes can be classified based on the location of their centromere. Three such classes are defined (Fig. 2.2):

- **Metacentric**. The centromere is located close to the centre of the chromatids.
- **Submetacentric**. The centromere of the chromosomes is located off-centre.
- **Acrocentric**. The centromere of the chromosome is located near one end of the chromosome.

The location of specific regions in the chromosome is labelled in reference to morphological markers, e.g. the banding patterns produced in staining.

- Locations on the short arm are labelled 'p' (petit) and those on the long arm 'q' The chromosome arms are divided into smaller regions labelled p1, p2, q1, q2, etc. The numbers of the regions count outwards from the centromere.
- Regions are further subdivided into bands labelled p11, p12, p13, etc. (p one–one, etc.). Smaller resolution is then achieved through further subdivision, e.g. p11.1, p11.2, etc.

Chromosomes exist as a single chromatid for most of the cell cycle – the second chromatid is produced during the S phase of the cell cycle, and separation of the chromatids occurs during mitosis, and during meiosis II. The arms of the chromosome are only easily visible during the stages of cell division, where they are highly condensed. During the rest of the cell cycle, the chromosomes are in a more 'open', decondensed state, and are not distinguishable by microscopy.

Chromatin

DNA is tightly packaged around protein to form a condensed form of DNA known as **chromatin**. The modification of the packaging proteins, as well as the DNA, alters the packaging, which is an important mechanism to allow the regulation of the expression of genes (Fig. 2.2).

The best understood packaging mechanism is that of the **histone** proteins, which are the most numerous of DNA packing proteins. There are five distinct types of histone protein: H1, H2a, H2b, H3 and H4:

- Two molecules each of H2a, H2b, H3 and H4 form a **nucleosome** around which DNA can wind nearly two times.
- Between nucleosomes are regions of 'linker DNA' to which the H1 proteins bind. These H1 proteins are thought to be involved in higher level organisation of the chromatin.

The nucleosomes are not fixed to the DNA and their location can change. In addition, the histone proteins possess long tails, which can wrap around the DNA to reduce its accessibility. The histone tails can be modified by the covalent addition or removal of various groups, which can allow the histone tails to become more or less attached to the DNA. The enzyme **histone acetyltransferase** (HAT), which acetylates histone tails, has a well-understood mechanism. This promotes their association with the DNA, typically inhibiting expression of genes in that region.

Higher organisation of chromatin

A series of different levels of organisation of the DNA occur, following the packaging of DNA on to nucleosomes:

- Nucleosomes are packaged together to produce a series of **fibres** around 30 nm in size. It is thought that this package takes the form of a spiral, whereby H1 proteins form a rod-like structure down the centre of the spiral.
- The 30-nm fibres are packaged into **loops** by 'scaffold proteins'. These structures allow regions of DNA to be rapidly decondensed, allowing proteins to gain access to the DNA. The loops allow distant parts of the chromosome to interact, such that genes with similar functions and roles can be concentrated in a small spatial area of the cell, along with any protein factors that may modulate their expression.
- Specific regions of chromatin may be attached to structures within the nucleus, such as the nucleolus, which is associated with the production of ribosomal RNA.

The density of the packaging of chromatin in the cell can reflect the transcriptional activity of the DNA. Through their packaging, chromatin is classed into two broad categories: **euchromatin** and **heterochromatin**. In particular, one copy of the X chromosome is sufficient for the cell's transcriptional needs (as illustrated in males, who have only a single X chromosome); in females, one copy of the X chromosome is usually densely packaged, forming the **Barr body**.

 DEFINITION Euchromatin and heterochromatin

There are two broad classes of chromatin, in relation to how densely they are packaged:

- **Euchromatin** makes up most of the chromatin in a cell and is relatively loosely packaged.
- **Heterochromatin** is much more densely packaged, and is typically located close to the nuclear envelope. It is thought that transcription factors can less easily bind to the DNA in heterochromatin, reducing expression of the genes that it contains.

Other elements within the genome

Only 1–10% of the human genome has been identified as encoding genes. However, recent estimates suggest that around 70% of the human genome is transcribed. Extragenic DNA refers to those regions of DNA that are not part of genes. Some of these regions have been classified and, in some cases, a function has been found:

- **Satellite DNA** consists of large series of short repeated sequences of DNA and are clustered around the centromeres.
- **Minisatellite DNA** is made up of two types of element:
  – **telomeric DNA** is found at the telomeres and consists of the same repeating sequence of six base-pairs which aids the replication of chromosomes without the loss of genetic information.
  – **hypervariable minisatellite DNA** is made up of polymorphic repeating patterns of a short nucleotide sequence (typically around 10–100 base-pairs in length).
- **Microsatellite DNA** consists of repeats of one to six nucleotides. The number of repeats is highly variable between individuals, although it is often stable between parents and children, and forms the basis of DNA profiling

Microsatellite and minisatellite DNA are together referred to as variable nucleotide tandem repeats.

Highly repeated interspersed repetitive DNA sequences are found throughout the non-coding region of the genome, and make up around a third of the whole genome. The function of these elements is not well understood, although they have been suggested to have roles in disease. Two main classes of these elements have been identified:

1 **Short interspersed nuclear elements** (SINEs) make up around 5% of the human genome and are typically around 300 base-pairs (bp) in length. The most common are Alu repeats, which contain a repeat sequence that can be cut by the **restriction enzyme** *Alu I*.
2 **Long interspersed nuclear elements** (LINEs) are much longer regions of DNA – typically around 6000 bp per repeat. The most common example is the LINE-1 sequence, which resembles the sequence of a retrovirus and encodes a reverse transcriptase.

Genes may be found as single or multiple copies:

- **Single-copy genes** are the normal form of genes. They code for a specific polypeptide, such as enzymes, receptors.
- **Multiple-copy genes** usually encode products that must be expressed rapidly. This permits the rapid production of huge numbers of mRNA transcripts, thus allowing rapid generation of the protein product. This is particularly evident with the histone genes where many copies of the protein must be synthesised rapidly during DNA replication.

DNA replication

The replication of DNA in eukaryotes is mediated by **DNA polymerase**, which catalyses the stepwise addition of deoxyribonucleotides to the $3'$ end of the DNA chain. There are four requirements for replication:

- **A DNA template**, from which a copy can be made.
- The presence of all four precursor **nucleoside triphosphates**
- **A primer** (a small sequence of RNA complementary to the DNA template) to start the process, to which nucleotides can be added.
- Mg^{2+} ions are also required for the appropriate function of DNA polymerase.

The polymerase recognises the next base in the template strand and adds a complementary base to the $3'$ end of the nascent DNA molecule. In this process, two phosphates are released and a $3',5'$-phosphodiester bond is created. This stepwise process is repeated along the length of the molecule, to generate a new copy of the DNA template in a $5'$ to $3'$ direction.

RNA Primers

DNA polymerase requires a primer sequence to initiate DNA elongation. Each primer is a short stretch of RNA that is synthesised by the enzyme **primase**. The RNA primer is extended by DNA polymerase on both the leading and the lagging strands. After synthesis, the RNA primers are removed by the **exonuclease** activity of DNA polymerase I which then synthesises DNA to fill in the gaps that have been left. The DNA fragments are then joined by DNA ligase.

Okazaki fragments

Synthesis of DNA occurs in a 5′ to 3′ direction; it cannot occur in a 3′ to 5′ direction. As a result, one strand of DNA can be elongated as a single continuous piece of DNA; this is known as the **leading strand**. On the other strand (known as the **lagging strand**), the complementary DNA is synthesised as a series of short segments (around 1000 nucleotides in length). Each fragment requires its own separate primer and the resulting fragments of DNA are known as **Okazaki fragments.**

Other proteins involved in DNA replication

Proteins, in addition to DNA polymerase, are required in replication to unwind and unpackage the chromosome. This is achieved by three groups of proteins:

1 **DNA helicase** unwinds DNA to produce two single strands of DNA.
2 **Single-stranded DNA-binding (SSB) proteins** bind to single-stranded regions of unwound DNA to prevent them rebinding. This allows the DNA polymerases and other enzymes access to the base sequence.
3 **Topoisomerases**: unwinding DNA can cause other regions to become 'supercoiled' – overwound. To reduce this, **topoisomerase I** creates a single-stranded break in the DNA, to allow the DNA to rotate about the intact strand. Topoisomerase I can then reform the single-stranded break.

After synthesis of the DNA, the two strands of DNA may need to be separated. This is achieved by a double-stranded DNA break, made transiently by the enzyme **topoisomerase II**. Topoisomerase II then re-joins the ends of the chromosome.

Proofreading during DNA replication

Proofreading mechanisms are crucial to ensure that mistakes in the copying of the DNA do not occur; such changes are likely to affect the survival of the daughter cells – potentially leading to either cell death or malignancy. Three mechanisms work to reduce the error rate:

1 **DNA polymerase** ensures the fidelity of replication because it relies on the higher-affinity binding of a correct nucleotide to its complementary base. Between the binding of the nucleotide and the formation of the covalent bond, the DNA polymerase undergoes a conformational change that encourages the dissociation of an incorrect nucleotide pairing.
2 **Exonucleotide proofreading** occurs when an incorrect nucleotide is added during DNA synthesis. A separate catalytic site exists in the DNA polymerase that 'proofreads' the DNA sequence, and removes mismatched nucleotides in a 3′ to 5′ direction, until a correct match is reached. The section is then re-synthesised in a 5′ to 3′ manner.
3 **Strand-directed mismatch repair** relies on the semiconservative mode of DNA replication. The presence of incorrectly matched bases can be detected as distortions in the DNA helix, due to the incorrect hydrogen bonding between the non-complementary bases. The template strand can be distinguished from its daughter strand, due to the presence of nicks in the sugar–phosphate backbone of the daughter strand. The detection of an error triggers degradation of the DNA from the 'nick' back to the site of the error. The degraded region of DNA is then re-synthesised.

DNA replication in eukaryotes must occur before each cell division. In multicellular organisms, there are differences in the length of the cell cycle with different cell types. Some cells (e.g. nerve cells) may enter G0 and stop dividing.

The process of DNA replication can be split into a series of steps, similar to those in prokaryotic cells:

• The **initiation of replication** by the splitting of DNA strands.
• The **assembly of the DNA polymerase** complex which mediates the replication process and the production of RNA primers that allow the DNA polymerases to add DNA to start the elongation and replication of the DNA.
• The **elongation** of the new DNA strands through the action of the DNA polymerase.
• The **removal** of the RNA primer fragments, their replacement with DNA and the joining of the DNA fragments, to produce a full length.
• **Repackaging** of the new DNA molecules with histones and other associated proteins.

There are around 100 sites of initiation of replication on a single chromosome in eukaryotes, where the large replication complexes bind during the S phase of the cell cycle.

Elongation of DNA

DNA replication in eukaryotes is always from 5′ to 3′ and the two strands are synthesised in slightly different manners:

- The **leading strand** is synthesised as a complete molecule.
- The **lagging strand** is synthesised as a series of short 'Okazaki fragments', as sufficient template is exposed to 5′ to 3′ synthesis.

The DNA polymerase

DNA polymerase is an extremely error-free mechanism of copying, although initially it requires a small RNA primer to allow it to initiate transcription. Primers are around 10 nucleotides long and are produced by the enzyme **DNA primase** which is found as a subunit on DNA polymerase α. Although the leading strand requires only one such primer, several will be required on the lagging strand – one for each Okazaki fragment.

DNA polymerase recruits bases complementary to those in the template strands and then catalyses the formation of the sugar–phosphate bond to permit elongation. After generation of the DNA chain, the RNA primers are replaced by DNA through the action of the polymerase, and the DNA fragments then joined by **DNA ligase**. To ensure that the DNA polymerase remains attached to the template and is not impeded during replication, clamp proteins and topoisomerase enzymes ensure that the DNA polymerase is maintained attached to the DNA and that it is untangled.

Clamp proteins

The DNA polymerase tends to dissociate rapidly from the DNA molecule so that it can be recycled at a different site. During replication, it must be held on the strand by a 'clamp'. This protein is made up of two halves that assemble around the DNA molecule in an ATP-dependent process. This ring structure is then able to move freely with the polymerase.

Replication of telomeres

At the end of linear chromosomes there is no space for **primase** to produce an RNA primer for the lagging strand during replication – over the course of several cell divisions DNA is progressively lost from the chromosome ends. Telomeres, the regions at the end of chromosomes, contain a repeating six-nucleotide sequence **GGGTTA**, which may repeat for 10 000 nucleotides. The enzyme **telomerase** is capable of binding and synthesising new copies of the repeat using an RNA template that is part of the enzyme itself, preventing loss of the chromosome ends during DNA replication.

Telomeres ensure that the nucleotide sequences encoding genes or regulatory elements are not lost during cell divisions. However, in many tissues, the telomerases are inactivated resulting in loss of approximately 100 nucleotides with each cell division. In normal cells this leads to **cell senescence** where the cells withdraw from the cell cycle before there is loss of information in the genome.

Reformation of nucleosomes

During replication DNA is tightly packaged around histone proteins, however the DNA polymerase and associated machinery must pass through the histones to synthesise new DNA. How this is achieved is not clearly understood, though following synthesis the nucleosomes remain predominantly with the leading strand, which new nucleosomes are assembled on the DNA molecules derived from the lagging strand.

A huge number of histone proteins must be produced to package the DNA. Around 20 sets of histone-encoding genes, which encode for all five proteins, have been identified at different sites in the genome to enable rapid generation of RNA transcripts.

While the resulting protein products are very stable, the histone RNA itself is actually very unstable ensuring translation is rapidly stopped such that unneeded histone proteins are not produced, which would be a waste of the cell's resources.

RNA and transcription

RNA has a very similar structure to DNA. It is made up of a series of nucleotides joined by 3′,5′-phosphodiester bonds. There are two main differences with DNA:

- The bases in RNA are adenine, guanine, cytosine and uracil. Uracil has a very similar structure to thymine and forms base-pairs with adenine.

- The sugar in RNA is ribose rather than the deoxyribose seen in DNA.

RNA is typically single-stranded, but regions can form where the RNA loops back on itself. Here complementary base pairing can occur in the RNA molecule to produce 'hairpin' secondary structures. The resulting double-stranded regions form helices and may interact with each other to produce complex three-dimensional structures. The resulting RNA molecules can have specific functions themselves, and do not encode for protein. These include the ribosomal RNAs (rRNAs) and the transfer RNAs (tRNAs).

Transcription

The eukaryotic nucleus contains three distinct forms of RNA polymerase that have specific functions:

1 **RNA polymerase I** (RNA Pol I) is responsible for the synthesis of rRNA in the nucleolus.
2 **RNA polymerase II** (RNA Pol II) mediates mRNA synthesis.
3 **RNA polymerase III** (RNA Pol III) synthesises smaller RNAs, e.g. tRNA, and some rRNA.

The basic mechanism of transcription in eukaryotes is very similar to that in prokaryotes:

- Initiation is directed by a promoter site 5′ to the transcription initiation site.
- Transcription does not require a primer to start.
- Synthesis occurs 5′ to 3′.

Transcription of protein-encoding genes

Protein-encoding genes are transcribed into mRNA by RNA Pol II; the mechanisms by which transcription occurs are similar to those in prokaryotic cells. Other forms of RNA are transcribed by different polymerase complexes and are discussed later in the chapter.

Structure of protein-encoding genes

The protein-encoding genes of eukaryotes are made up of two distinct regions:

1 **Exons** encode amino acid sequences that will produce a protein product.
2 **Introns** are regions of the gene that do not code for proteins; they separate the exons and are removed in the post-transcriptional processing of the RNA.

During transcription a **pre-mRNA** contains all the introns and exons of the gene. This is processed by the removal of introns, and the addition of a 5′ cap and usually a poly(A) tail at the 3′ end. The roles of this and the mechanisms by which they are generated are discussed later.

Initiation of transcription

The promoter for RNA Pol II transcription classically contains a **TATA box** located around 25 nucleotides upstream of the transcription initiation site (-25 position). Many genes do not possess a TATA box and have an initiator element instead which is not well defined (Fig. 2.3).

The key process in transcription initiation is the assembly of the initiation complex. Crucial to this is the general transcription initiation factor, TFIID, which binds to the TATA box. After the binding of TFIID, other factors are recruited that contribute to the initiation of elongation:

- Many factors make up elements of the functional polymerase.
- Some factors alter the **chromatin structure** to improve the access to other factors.
- Factors may recruit **histone acetylase** proteins, which acetylate the histone tails, reducing their interaction with the DNA.

Elongation

Many factors involved in the assembly of the initiation complex are not directly required for the formation of the nucleotide chain. Many of these factors are released during elongation, allowing RNA Pol II to escape the promoter and transcribe the gene.

A subunit in the RNA Pol II possesses a long repeated region of amino acids containing many serine residues. This region can be phosphorylated and the resulting negative charge causes dissociation of some transcription factor subunits, which permits elongation. DNA is thought to move through the immobile transcription complex and is unwound by **topoisomerase enzymes**, as is the case in DNA replication.

The RNA polymerase does not require a primer to start transcription; it is capable of directly initiating transcription from the template. However, it is more error prone, typically making an error on **1 in 10^5 bases**. This high error rate is permissible, because RNA is not inherited.

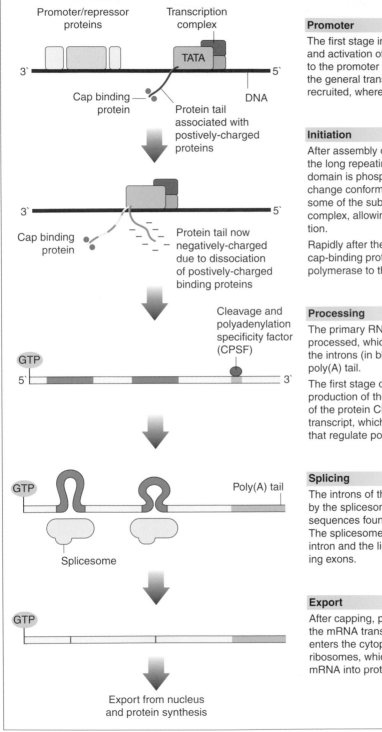

Promoter

The first stage in transcription is the binding and activation of specific transcription factors to the promoter region of a gene, such that the general transcription complex is recruited, where it binds to the TATA box.

Initiation

After assembly of the transcriptional complex, the long repeating tail of the C-terminal domain is phosphorylated, causing it to change conformation and trigger the loss of some of the subunits of the transcriptional complex, allowing the initiation of transcription.

Rapidly after the initiation of transcription, the cap-binding proteins are transferred from the polymerase to the primary transcript.

Processing

The primary RNA transcript must be processed, which requires the removal of the introns (in blue) and the production of a poly(A) tail.

The first stage of the process is the production of the poly(A) tail is the binding of the protein CPSF to the 3`?end of the transcript, which recruits the other proteins that regulate polyadenylation.

Splicing

The introns of the transcript are recognised by the splicesomes, through consensus sequences found at either end of the intron. The splicesome mediates the excision of the intron and the ligation of the two neighbouring exons.

Export

After capping, polyadenylation and splicing, the mRNA transcript is ready for export. It enters the cytoplasm where it can bind to ribosomes, which mediate translation of the mRNA into protein.

Figure 2.3 Prokaryotic transcription.

Termination

In RNA Pol (II) transcription, termination is associated with the addition of the poly(A) tail to the mRNA during processing. The other transcription enzymes have different mechanisms of termination.

Regulation of transcription by RNA Pol (II)

There are some protein-encoding genes that are required in all cells. These **housekeeping genes** perform essential functions, such as glycolysis, the tricarboxylic acid cycle and the electron transport chain. Other genes are expressed only in specific cells, e.g. the TCR (T-cell receptor) genes are expressed only in T cells.

Regulation of transcription is achieved through transcription factors, which are proteins that bind to specific regulatory sequences (**control sequences**) associated with the genes. The control factors can be classified into two types:

1 *Cis*-**acting elements** are thought to be located close to the gene on the same chromosome.
2 *Trans*-**acting elements** are more distantly acting regulatory sequences, which are often found far from the gene that it regulates. These *trans*-acting elements may be found on different chromosomes.

The binding of transcription factors may increase (promote or activate) or decrease (repress) the transcription of the target gene. A single gene in a eukaryotic cell typically has several control elements in its promoter. Transcription factors may interact on a single gene and also interact with each other to modulate transcription of the target gene.

Cis-*acting elements*

Many positive control elements are located immediately upstream of the transcriptional start site to increase the level of transcriptional activity. There are some elements that are in many genes:

- **SP1** is a transcription factor that interacts with a component of TFIID
- **CAAT box**.

Other elements are found in only very few genes, which may limit the expression of a gene to specific tissues (where the transcription factor is expressed) or to certain stimuli.

Enhancers

Long-distance positive control sequences are referred to as **enhancers**. These elements are made up of several sequences, often hundreds of base-pairs long. Enhancers work through the looping of DNA, which brings the enhancer sequence (and the factors that it has bound) into close proximity to the gene, allowing protein–protein interaction to occur between the transcription complex and the enhancer.

Repressors

Repressor proteins inhibit the genes that they target, by binding to specific sequences in the promoter. Those that have a long-distance action are referred to as **silencers**. Repression can be achieved in a variety of ways:

- **Blocking the binding site** of an activator protein
- **Masking the activation domain of a protein**, preventing the domain binding DNA or interacting with other transcription factors
- Forming a **non-DNA-binding complex** with the activator proteins
- **Inhibiting transcription directly**.

mRNA processing

The initial RNA transcript must be processed into functional mRNA for translation. Four major steps can be identified in this process:

1 5′ capping of the mRNA transcript
2 Splicing of pre-mRNA
3 RNA editing
4 Polyadenylation of the mRNA tail.

After transcription, the primary transcript rapidly associates with specific proteins found in the nucleus to form a **ribonucleoprotein**. These proteins regulate of many of the subsequent processing steps and ensure the stability of the transcript. After processing, the mature mRNA is exported from the nucleus to the cytoplasm.

5′ Capping

The 5′ end of a mature mRNA transcript possesses a methylated GTP residue covalently attached to it 'the wrong way round'. This 'capping' occurs during transcription, through a cap-binding complex which is associated with the RNA polymerase. In addition, the first two bases in the RNA must be methylated. The 5′-cap structure is a crucial signal to trigger the movement of mRNA out of the nucleus through the **nuclear pores**.

Splicing

The transcribed regions of genes can be divided into introns and exons. Although the introns are almost always absent from a mature mRNA transcript, the exons present within the transcript may vary. As a result, one gene can produce many different proteins.

The process of splicing removes introns from the mRNA transcript. It is regulated by a complex known as the **splicesome** which is made up of proteins and small nuclear RNAs (snRNAs). Splicing is initiated by consensus sequences at either side of the intron, although other protein factors may influence the splicing, contributing to the formation of alternative splice variants.

Alternative splicing explains the surprisingly small number of genes that have been found within the human genome in comparison to less complex organisms. It allows a single mRNA to potentially produce several different proteins with different functions. The mechanisms that regulate alternative splicing are not fully understood.

 DEFINITION The splicesome

The splicesome mediates the splicing reaction and is made up of both RNA and protein. The specificity of the splicing reaction is maintained through the complementarity of the splicing consensus sequences to a sequence found in one of the RNA components of the splicesome.

Splicing occurs through breaking the phosphate backbone of the RNA molecule at either end of the intron, to allow the joining of two exons, via re-annealing of the sugar–phosphate backbone of the RNA.

There are also rare **group II introns** which have self-splicing activity. The RNA in these introns is capable of mediating its own splicing from the primary RNA transcript. This process is seen in some protein-encoding genes, as well as rRNAs and tRNAs. Self-splicing requires the assistance of **maturase** enzymes, although this is a far less complex form of assistance than is seen from the splicesome.

RNA EDITING

There are other changes to the nucleotide sequence that result from mechanisms other than RNA splicing. In the liver, apolipoprotein B100 (Apo B100) is produced because the apolipoprotein B mRNA is not edited. However, in the small intestine, RNA editing causes the conversion of a cytosine in the mRNA to a uracil by deamination, and generates a premature **stop codon**, resulting in a smaller protein product, apolipoprotein B48, which lacks a low-density lipoprotein (LDL)-receptor-binding domain. Apo B100 is used to package LDL and high-density lipoprotein (HDL) which can be bound by LDL receptors, whereas Apo B48 is used to package chylomicrons, which are not taken up by the LDL receptor.

Polyadenylation

A crucial step in the processing of mRNA is the cleavage of the 3′ end of the RNA transcript and the addition of a poly(A) tail. The poly(A) tail allows the binding of a variety of proteins, which reduce its breakdown. The proteins that regulate polyadenylation are associated with the tail of the RNA polymerase, allowing their rapid transfer to the RNA on recognition of the relevant sequences in the transcript.

Polyadenylation is triggered by the binding of the cleavage-and-polyadenylation factor (CPSF) to a consensus sequence located upstream of the poly(A) site. Other protein factors are recruited to cleave the RNA transcript. Additional adenine residues are added to the end of the transcript, by a poly(A) polymerase – which does not require a template. The addition of the poly(A) tail allows the binding of many copies of the poly(A)-binding protein II (PABII), which stabilises the transcript.

In the cytosol, the poly(A) tail is gradually degraded by nucleases. Once the tail reaches a length of around 30 nucleotides, it triggers the removal of the 5′ cap, precipitating the rapid degradation of the mRNA. Degradation can also be mediated by factors that cleave off the poly(A) tail at specific sites. This mechanism permits rapid alterations in protein production through control of the rate and levels of translation.

Translation

Translation is the production of a polypeptide chain from an transcript mRNA by a ribosome, located in the cytoplasm. Translation is reliant on many forms of RNA:

- messenger RNA (mRNA)
- ribosomal RNA (rRNA)
- transfer RNA (tRNA).

Formation of ribosomes and tRNA

The ribosome is the site of translation. It consists of two subunits, each made up of protein and rRNA, which catalyse the formation of a polypeptide encoded by an mRNA transcript. The amino acids required for this process are supplied by tRNA molecules.

Ribosomal formation

The cell possesses many ribosomes – typically around 10 million – and many copies of the ribosome genes are required to allow sufficient synthesis. The rRNA molecules are produced in the nucleolus by RNA Pol I and Pol III. These RNAs are chemically modified and cleaved in processes regulated by a class of small nucleolar RNAs (snoRNAs). Many bases in rRNA are methylated and many of the uridine bases are converted to pseudouridine.

In a cell that synthesises large amounts of protein, the nucleolus may make up around 25% of the nuclear volume, reflecting the amount of ribosomal production required by the cell. The ribosomal proteins are produced in the cytoplasm and then transported back into the nucleus for assembly with the rRNA, to produce two subunits.

Formation of tRNA

Transfer RNA (tRNA) is produced by RNA Pol III and is highly processed before becoming functional. Around **25% of tRNA bases are modified**, either through conversion to inosine or pseudouridine or through methylation. The tRNAs are produced from a larger precursor molecule and must be spliced, trimmed and folded to generate a functional molecule.

The tRNAs are folded into a 'clover-leaf' structure. Most of the bases in tRNA are paired, although two important unpaired regions exist:

1 The **anticodon** consists of three unpaired bases on the tRNA, which bind to a complementary **codon**. The codon is a three-base sequence in the mRNA that is specific for an amino acid, and it is this interaction that is at the heart of the translational mechanism.
2 **Amino acid attachment site** is a short single-stranded region found at one end of the RNA molecule.

Amino acids are attached to tRNA by **aminacyl-tRNA synthetase** in an ATP-dependent reaction. A different synthetase exists for each amino acid.

The molecular mechanism of translation

The genetic code

The mRNA sequence of a gene encodes the order of the amino acids as they should be encoded in the protein; this is the **genetic code**. From 5′ to 3′ the mRNA sequence can be divided into blocks of three nucleotides, referred to as **codons**:

- Most codons specify an amino acid. There are 20 amino acids used in the human body, although there are 64 (4^3) potential codon sequences, so a single amino acid may be represented by more than one codon; however, a single codon encodes for only one amino acid.
- The codons UAG, UGA and UAA terminate protein synthesis, and do not encode an amino acid. They are referred to as **termination codons**.

The first codon, AUG, is referred to as the **initiation** or **start codon**; all polypeptides start with methionine (although in prokaryotes this is modified to *N*-formylmethionine), but this may be removed subsequently.

In the case of each codon, it is complementary to the anticodon located on the tRNA molecule. The specificity of the first two bases is strictly regulated, but the requirements of the third base are less well defined; this is known as the **wobble position** and allows some tRNAs to bind to more than one codon.

Initiation of translation

The initiation of translation is mediated by the small ribosomal subunit and always starts at a

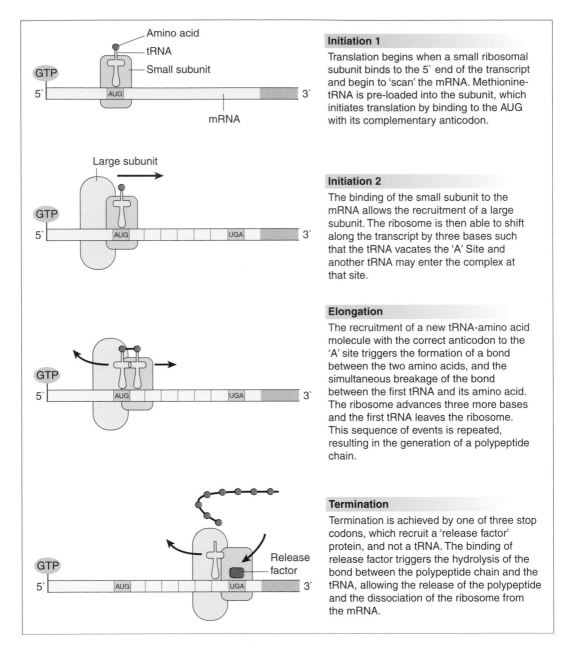

Initiation 1

Translation begins when a small ribosomal subunit binds to the 5` end of the transcript and begin to 'scan' the mRNA. Methionine-tRNA is pre-loaded into the subunit, which initiates translation by binding to the AUG with its complementary anticodon.

Initiation 2

The binding of the small subunit to the mRNA allows the recruitment of a large subunit. The ribosome is then able to shift along the transcript by three bases such that the tRNA vacates the 'A' Site and another tRNA may enter the complex at that site.

Elongation

The recruitment of a new tRNA-amino acid molecule with the correct anticodon to the 'A' site triggers the formation of a bond between the two amino acids, and the simultaneous breakage of the bond between the first tRNA and its amino acid. The ribosome advances three more bases and the first tRNA leaves the ribosome. This sequence of events is repeated, resulting in the generation of a polypeptide chain.

Termination

Termination is achieved by one of three stop codons, which recruit a 'release factor' protein, and not a tRNA. The binding of release factor triggers the hydrolysis of the bond between the polypeptide chain and the tRNA, allowing the release of the polypeptide and the dissociation of the ribosome from the mRNA.

Figure 2.4 Translation. The process of translation involves a series of repeating steps within the ribosome which sequentially add amino acids to the growing polypeptide change, as specified by the mRNA.

codon encoding **methionine.** The initial methionine is usually contained within a consensus sequence known as a **Kozak sequence**, which aids the initiation of translation (Fig. 2.4).

• An **initiator tRNA** (methionine) is loaded into the small subunit, which is associated with

translation initiation factors (eIFs). Methionyl-tRNA is the only tRNA capable of binding to the small ribosomal subunit without the presence of a complete ribosome.

• The small subunit **recognises the 5′ cap and binds to the mRNA.**

- The subunit **scans the mRNA**, its movement powered by ATP-hydrolysing initiation factors.
- The small subunit **stops** on encountering an AUG codon and its surrounding consensus sequence, and recruits the large ribosomal subunit.

If the sequence surrounding the initiation codon differs from the consensus ribosomal binding sequence, it may promote 'skipping' in the transcript, such that a subsequent AUG becomes the site of initiation of translation. This may allow the production of different proteins – and in particular **different leader sequences** – from a single mRNA. These different leader sequences may target one protein to two different cellular compartments.

As the base-pairing code is arranged in groups of three (the size of the codon), there are three potential sequences that can be produced from a string of nucleotides. Each of these is known as a **reading frame.** There is usually only a single functional reading frame because the others are likely to introduce premature stop codons to generate a very small protein product; however, in some viruses there are overlapping reading frames, as a result of the limits on genome size. *In vivo*, the correct reading frame is determined by the presence of the AUG initiation codon.

Elongation

After initiation of transcription, amino acids must be bound to together to produce a polypeptide chain. Three tRNA-binding sites are identifiable in the ribosome – **A**, **P** and **E**; the movement of tRNAs through these sites and the catalytic activity associated are responsible for the production of the polypeptide chain. The tRNA complementary to the mRNA is recruited to the A and P sites; a hydrolysis reaction then occurs to form the peptide link and the ribosome moves three bases down the mRNA, with the now empty tRNA exiting from the E site.

The **termination of translation** is signalled by one of the three termination codons (UAA, UAG, UGA) for which no tRNA is specific. Instead, 'release factor' proteins bind to the A site and induce the addition of H_2O to the polypeptide chain, mediating its release from the ribosomal complex. The ribosome then dissociates from the transcript.

As the 5′ and 3′ ends of mRNA are closely associated, the ribosome is able to rapidly reassociate with the 5′ end of the molecule to begin translation once again.

Polysomes

The synthesis of a single copy of a protein by a ribosome may take many minutes. To increase the production of protein, many ribosomes translate a single mRNA. As soon as one ribosome is sufficiently clear of the AUG, a second will start translation. Thus, mRNAs are found in polysomes – large clusters of many actively translating ribosomes, allowing the rapid production of many copies of a protein from a single mRNA transcript.

Post-translational modification

Proteins can be covalently modified by translation. These modifications may be crucial for the function of the protein or can modify its efficacy. The most common forms of modification are:

- The addition of **phosphate**, which is commonly used in second messenger pathways to activate or repress the performance of individual proteins.
- **Glycosylation** is commonly regulated through the recognition of specific amino acid sequences in the protein. The addition and removal of carbohydrates occurs in the rough endoplasmic reticulum (ER) and the Golgi apparatus.
- Other groups can also be added. For example, **ubiquitin** is often covalently added to a protein to signal targeting of the protein to the proteasome for degradation.

Protein targeting

Sequences in the polypeptide regulate whether translation occurs in the cytoplasm or the rough ER to produce a protein for secretion or trafficking to a subcellular compartment. The mechanisms of trafficking are discussed in detail in Chapter 1.

Regulation of gene expression

Differentiation results from long-term changes in gene expression. This is caused by modifications of the packaging of the genome, ensuring that a particular transcription pattern is achieved. It is this pattern that allows an individual cell to take on a distinct phenotype – despite containing exactly the same DNA, many different specialised cell types may result. Cells may also differentiate in response to specific stimuli (e.g. an immune response) as part of the body's response to a homoeostatic change.

The expression of specific genes may be altered in response to specific stimuli. Such modifications can occur through signals such as hormones. These modifications allow cells to respond to the changing environment, while still maintaining an overall pattern of gene expression that keeps them in the same differentiated state.

Mechanisms of gene expression

The expression of genes, and hence their protein product, can be regulated. It is this process that allows one genome to permit the development of many different types of differentiated cell.

Regulatory proteins bind to specific sequences through many weak interactions, which contribute to produce a strong binding. These proteins may bind several thousand bases from the promoter in the target gene and can act in many ways to influence the level of transcription:

- Transcription factors
- Promoter and repressor elements
- Modification of histones and structural genes
- Chromatin condensation.

Genetics of disease

The pathology of many diseases involves a genetic component: in some cases, mutations or abnormalities can occur spontaneously and may contribute to a disease, through the altered function or expression of proteins and their interaction with environmental factors. The nature of such a mutation can vary from chromosomal abnormalities to the change in a single nucleotide base. Many such mutations are inherited. There are some key terms related to genetic disease:

- **Allele** – different forms of the same gene, found at the same location on homologous chromosomes
- **Genotype** – the genetic constitution of an individual
- **Phenotype** – the appearance of an individual, which results from the interactions of the environment and the genotype.

Chromosomal abnormalities

It is possible that, through abnormal meiosis, large-scale abnormalities may occur. Chromosomal abnormalities are usually extremely severe. Fetuses carrying chromosomal abnormalities rarely survive to birth; they are thought to account for around half of all early miscarriages.

Polyploidy

Polyploidy is the most severe abnormality, when additional complete sets of chromosomes may be inherited. Triploid ($3n$) embryos are sometimes seen, as a result of the simultaneous fusion of two sperm with an egg. Polyploidy usually results in miscarriage or stillbirth. In some rare cases – particularly with a double maternal contribution – the infant may survive to birth. There is severe growth retardation and widespread developmental abnormalities, and the infant dies shortly after birth.

An abnormal diploid ($2n$) embryo may form from only one parental set of chromosomes. These embryos do not survive, because the **imprinting** on the chromosomes necessary for development requires one male and one female set. **Hydatidiform moles** may develop from these abnormal diploid embryos.

Numerical abnormalities

Abnormalities of the autosomal chromosomes

Single chromosome numerical abnormalities of the autosomal chromosomes occur when the wrong numbers of a specific chromosome are inherited, as a result of incorrect separation, usually during meiosis (they may very rarely occur in an early mitosis):

- All cases where there is only a single copy of an autosomal chromosome (**monosomy**) are embryonically lethal.
- There are three **trisomies** (where an extra copy of a chromosome is inherited) that survive until birth, although only **Down's syndrome** (trisomy of chromosome 21) permits survival into adulthood. In Patau's syndrome (trisomy 13) and Edwards' syndrome (trisomy 18) death usually occurs within a few weeks of birth. These chromosomes have the least number of genes,

accounting for their greater viability than other trisomies.

 CLINICAL Down's syndrome

Down's syndrome (trisomy of chromosome 21) occurs in around 1 in 600 births, and may be of varying severity. Typically, there is some degree of learning disability and abnormal facial features. Down's syndrome is also associated with congenital heart defects, a wide gap between the first and second toes, and flattened facial features. The occurrence of Down's syndrome is associated with increased age of the mother.

Numerical abnormalities within the sex chromosomes

These abnormalities are compatible with life into adulthood. This is reflected in the sufficiency of one X chromosome in men and that women do not have a Y chromosome. Turner's (XO) syndrome is the result of abnormal numbers of X chromosomes.

 CLINICAL Turner's syndrome

Turner's syndrome is **monosomy** of chromosome X in women – XO. It is relatively common at conception and usually leads to spontaneous abortion, although some cases survive to birth (around 1 in 3000 births). Patients with Turner's syndrome are infertile, not going through puberty, and are generally abnormally short. **Coarctation of the aorta** is often seen. If detected early, Turner's syndrome can be treated by hormone therapy and most problems associated with the condition can be corrected, except infertility.

 CLINICAL Cri-du-chat syndrome

Cri-du-chat syndrome is caused by deletion of the short arm of chromosome 5, and occurs in around 1 in 50 000 births.

The features of cri-du-chat syndrome appear early in life: a cat-like cry, from which the syndrome derives its name; short stature; and facial abnormalities. There are often breathing problems and congenital heart defects, and there may be some learning disability.

Structural abnormalities

Structural abnormalities are common in chromosomes. Four main sets of structural abnormalities of chromosomes may occur:

1 Translocations
2 Duplications
3 Deletions
4 Inversions.

Translocations

Translocations are the result of the exchange of segments between non-homologous chromosomes, which typically occurs between the long arms of the chromosomes. If the break point in the DNA does not disrupt a gene, carriers of a translocation are phenotypically normal – they express all genes normally because no genetic material has been lost. Some translocations may be unbalanced and result in gametes that do not express the correct complement of genetic material.

 DEFINITION Robertsonian translocations

The small acrocentric chromosomes may become fused, such that the long arms of one chromosome fuse with the long arms of another. The short arms of the chromosomes are lost, although do not produce a phenotype, because the short arms contain only the genes for rRNA, of which there are enough copies on other acrocentric chromosomes. Robertsonian translocations are relatively common and may be seen in around 1 in 800 live births, most without a phenotype.

Unbalanced gametes possess two or no copies of the chromosome which can lead to monosomies or trisomies.

Deletions

Deletions are the loss of part of a chromosome – there is effectively monosomy for a section of the chromosome. Large deletions are not compatible with life, although smaller deletions can lead to certain conditions. Some deletions are visible microscopically, e.g. **cri-du-chat syndrome**.

Small, submicroscopic deletions have been identified through the use of sequencing probes specific for a single locus. **Angelmann's** and **Prader–Willi syndromes** are both diseases that may result from submicroscopic deletions.

Inversions

An inversion is the reversal of a section of a chromosome, as a result of it becoming broken at two points. The inversions are balanced chromosome rearrangements, causing a disease phenotype only if one of the break points disrupts a gene. Inversions may be pericentric – involving the centromere – or paracentric, where only one arm of the chromosome is affected.

Ring chromosomes

Ring chromosomes may occur when there are breaks within each arm of a chromosome and the exposed ends then unite, forming a ring. The distal fragments are lost, which can lead to serious phenotypes in the autosomal chromosomes.

Ring chromosomes are quite unstable during mitosis, and may be found in a proportion of cells; other cells have lost the ring chromosome and are **monosomic**.

Imprinting and associated abnormalities

It is essential that, in each pair, one chromosome is derived from the mother and one from the father. The nature of covalent modification to the DNA and its associated proteins may differ. In particular, the methylation of some of the bases varies between chromosomes.

The importance of this imprinting can be illustrated by two syndromes: **Prader–Willi syndrome** and **Angelmann's syndrome**. Although the diseases have very distinct features, they are both the result of deletion of chromosome 15 – the difference in the conditions depends on whether the deletion occurs on the maternally derived or the paternally derived copy of chromosome 15. The precise roles that the deletions play in the development of the syndromes is not clear. These diseases show that paternal and maternal chromosomes may have different roles at different times, and may be preferentially expressed in different cell types, and at different points in development.

 CLINICAL **Prader–Willi syndrome**

Prader–Willi syndrome is associated with a deletion in the **paternally-derived** chromosome 15, and is associated with severe hypotonia shortly after birth. Short stature, obesity and learning disability are also features. People with Prader-Willi syndrome often develop type 2 diabetes.

 CLINICAL **Angelman's syndrome**

Angelman's syndrome results from a deletion in the **maternally-derived** chromosome 15. The symptoms of the syndrome are very different from those of Prader–Willi syndrome, featuring an apraxic gait, jerky movements, epilepsy and severe learning disability, and an inability to speak.

Single-gene abnormalities

Several thousand single-gene abnormalities have been identified; most are extremely rare, although together it is thought they may affect 1–2% of the population. Diseases that can be inherited as the result of changes associated with a single gene exhibit 'mendelian characteristics'. In relation to a trait that is governed by a single gene mutation, the trait may be referred to as dominant or recessive:

- **Dominant traits** are seen when a single copy of the mutated gene is inherited.
- **Recessive traits** require both alleles to contain the mutation for the trait to become apparent.

The inheritance of such diseases within a specific family can be illustrated diagrammatically, each type of disease showing a specific pattern of inheritance (Fig. 2.5).

Autosomal dominant traits

Autosomal dominant traits are those disorders where the inheritance of a single faulty copy of a gene is sufficient to induce a phenotype. In most cases, an individual with an autosomal dominant disorder has a 50% chance of passing the disorder on to their children, if the other parent is not affected.

Autosomal dominant disorders may arise from a spontaneous mutation, in which case the **relative risk** of siblings being affected is almost zero, although this varies between specific diseases.

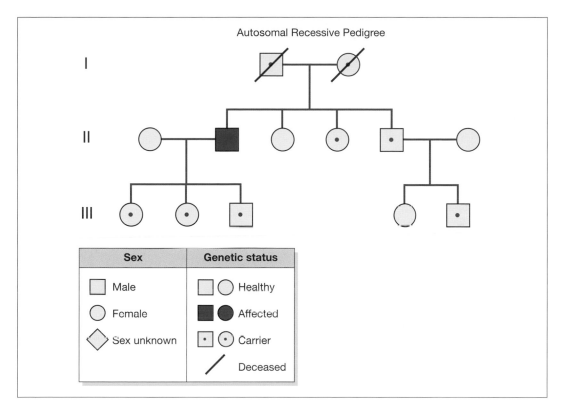

Autosomal Recessive Pedigree

Sex	Genetic status	
☐ Male	☐ ◯	Healthy
◯ Female	■ ●	Affected
◇ Sex unknown	⊡ ⊙	Carrier
	╱	Deceased

Figure 2.5 Genetic inheritance. The sex of an individual in a genetic pedigree is determined by shape. The genetic status is determined by shading – healthy individuals who do not carry the disease allele are hollow, whereas affected individuals are shaded. In recessive diseases, a carrier state may arise, which is indicated by a dot. If an individual within the pedigree has died, this is indicated by a diagonal line striking through the individual's marker. Different individuals are labelled by roman numerals, and individuals within that generation are labelled with Arabic numerals. The pedigree shown in the figure represents one that may be typical of an autosomal recessive disorder.

> ✔ **DEFINITION Homozygotes and heterozygotes**
>
> Individuals are referred to as **homozygous** with respect to a specific gene if they have inherited two alleles that are identical. In **heterozygotes** the alleles inherited are different.

Most individuals with these disorders are **heterozygous** for the relevant gene; however, in some cases individuals who are homozygous for an autosomal dominant trait have been reported (e.g. **familial hypercholesterolaemia**). The phenotype is more severe and often lethal, although such individuals are rare due to the low occurrence of autosomal dominant disorders in the general population. A typical autosomal dominant condition is **achondroplasia**.

> 🔍 **CLINICAL Achondroplasia**
>
> Achondroplasia is the result of an autosomal dominant mutation affecting the fibroblast growth factor receptor 3 (*FGFR3*) gene; it leads to abnormalities in the formation of cartilage, in particular, the growth plates, abnormally in the long bones, and accounts for the short stature characteristic of the condition. Achondroplastic individuals have a disproportionate stature as membranous bone forms normally, leading to the formation of a normally sized axial skeleton. Homozygous achondroplasia is lethal as the FGFR3 protein has some essential functions requiring at least a single copy of the gene.

Autosomal recessive

Autosomal recessive phenotypes are expressed by those homozygous for the disease allele. As a result, there are heterozygous carriers, who are phenotypically normal (or express a mild phenotype, as in sickle cell anaemia). The offspring of two carriers of a recessive trait have a 25% chance of developing the disease phenotype, through being homozygous for the recessive allele. Similarly, 25% are likely to be homozygous for the wild-type allele and 50% will become heterozygous carriers.

When one parent has an autosomal recessive disorder, all children are likely to be heterozygous carriers; they will all inherit one disease allele. In cases where the other parent is also a carrier for the same disease, **pseudodominance** will occur: 50% of the children will be homozygous for the mutation and the other 50% will be heterozygous carriers.

Often, recessive diseases result from mutations in genes, leading to a loss of function of the encoded protein. Many recessive mutations occur in genes encoding enzymes, where the functional 50% of the enzyme derived from the wild-type allele is sufficient to compensate for the non-functional allele.

There may be heterogeneity in the nature of the mutation causing autosomal recessive disorders:

- **Locus heterogeneity** refers to the fact that an inherited disorder can be caused by mutations in more than one gene. This occurs in deafness, which can be caused by mutation of one of many different genes. As a result of schooling and interactions in the deaf community, deaf people often have children with other deaf people. Their children may be phenotypically normal: they will be heterozygotes for two different genes, at different genomic locations.
- **Mutational heterogeneity** results from the fact that more than one mutation exists that can result in a non-functional protein product. A variety of alleles may be associated with a specific disease. Most autosomal recessive disorders are likely to result from compound heterozygous alleles – two different mutations at the same locus have been inherited. It is unlikely that an individual is truly heterozygous (where both alleles have the same mutation) unless there

is some **consanguinity** – the disease-causing allele having been inherited from a common ancestor.

 CLINICAL Cystic fibrosis

Cystic fibrosis (CF) is the most common autosomal recessive disorder in the western world. Around 5%of white people are estimated to be carriers of the disease. The cystic fibrosis transmembrane conductance regulator (*CFTCR*) gene is the site of mutation, and encodes a chloride transporter, although it may also have a role in regulating other membrane proteins. Depending on age of presentation, the main sites of pathology are the gastrointestinal tract and pancreas, or within the lungs.

In infants, CF may present as **meconium ileus**, where there is intestinal obstruction due to the hindered passage of meconium. Alternatively, pancreatic pathology can lead to the infant failing to gain weight despite an adequate diet. There is no detectable abnormality within the lungs at birth.

In later life, lung pathology is the predominant symptom of CF, due to the production of abnormal mucus, which can lead to pneumonia and other infections. Repeated damage can lead to destruction of the lungs.

X-LINKED DISORDERS

Disorders associated with mutations at loci on the X chromosome show a particular inheritance pattern. Only males are usually affected, because they possess a single X chromosome; the mutation cannot be masked by a wild-type allele. Females carrying the mutation are almost always heterozygous carriers with a normal phenotype.

Affected sons will have carrier mothers, unless the child represents a new mutation – there will never be father-to-son transmission of an X-linked trait (they must inherit the Y chromosome), although daughters of afflicted fathers are obligate carriers of the condition (they must inherit the affected X chromosome). Some X-linked conditions may be predominantly transmitted by the mother because affected males may not survive to reproductive age.

> ### CLINICAL **Duchenne muscular dystrophy**
>
> Duchenne muscular dystrophy (DMD) is the result of mutation the gene encoding dystrophin. The disease is usually identified in the third or fourth year, when the child encounters difficulty in walking and falls regularly. Affected individuals typically begin to walk relatively late (often later than 18 months). Contractures of muscles are particularly prominent in DMD; weakening of the anterior muscles of the leg leads to individuals walking on their toes. Intellectual impairment is also seen in some cases.
>
> A similar, although milder, condition – Becker muscular dystrophy – is also caused by mutations in the dystrophin gene; however, such mutations are usually **in-frame**, resulting in a protein with decreased function. Mutations causing DMD are commonly due to a deletion or substitution mutation, which produces a short, non-functional product, through the premature generation of a stop codon.

Expression of X-linked disorders within females can occur occasionally as a result of a variety of situations, often caused by inactivation of the healthy X chromosome:

- **Skewed X-chromosome inactivation** may result in carrier females expressing a mild phenotype of an X-linked disorder – a **manifesting carrier**. As X-chromosome inactivation is a random process, it can be that, by chance, most of the cells in the body express the mutant allele. Such cases have been reported in haemophilia and DMD.
- **Numerical X-chromosome abnormalities** can lead to the manifestation of an X-linked disease in females. Typically this occurs in Turner's syndrome, where the inheritance of a single mutant X chromosome will lead to a phenotype.
- **X-autosome translocation** occurs when there is the translocation of the X chromosome on to an autosomal chromosome. When the breakpoint of the X chromosome disrupts a gene, it may result in the female being afflicted with an X-linked disorder. Both copies of the autosomal chromosome must be transcriptionally active. As such, the non-translocated X chromosome may be preferentially inactivated, because there is a greater need to transcribe the autosomal genes translocated on the X chromosome (as a result it, and the X chromosome that contains it, must remain transcriptionally active). Such translocation has been observed in some females with DMD – where there has been translocation of the short arm of the X chromosome at the site of the DMD gene.

X-linked dominant inheritance is very rare. The sons and daughters of affected women both have a 50% chance of being affected. An affected father will transmit the trait to all his daughters, although to none of his sons. The inheritance of such traits leads to an excess of affected females. This can be seen in **vitamin D-resistant rickets**.

Mitochondrial inheritance

The mitochondria contain a limited genome that encodes proteins essential for the function of the mitochondria. Given the role of mitochondria in energy generation, if there is a mutation in the mitochondria, affected tissues are usually those with high-energy demands. A well-studied mitochondrial disease is **MERRF** (myoclonic epilepsy with ragged red fibres), which is associated with hearing loss, optic atrophy, dementia and respiratory failure. Mitochondrial DNA has a higher rate of spontaneous mutation, which is probably due to the oxidative damage resulting from higher exposure to oxidative species.

Mitochondria are maternally inherited. If the mother is affected, there is a 100% risk of inheritance by the offspring, although the age of onset and the severity of the phenotype may vary through interactions with other genes and the environment, and as a result of **heteroplasmy**. There are many mitochondria in the body and it is unlikely that all will contain the mutation – only cells with a high proportion (around 70–80% of mitochondria containing the mutation) are likely to exhibit a phenotype.

The symptoms can be different in different tissues as a result of portioning of the affected mitochondria in early cell division. In an early cell, the division will unevenly segregate mitochondria, and some cells may develop regions of tissue that have a high proportion of affected mitochondria, leading to severe phenotypes. Other regions may carry very few affected mitochondria and exhibit no phenotype.

Single-base mutations

The alteration of a single nucleotide base in a gene is sufficient to cause a distinct phenotype. These **substitution mutations** are classified depending on the type of change and its effects:

- **Missense** – the mutation leads to a different amino acid being encoded.

- **Silent** – the mutation has no effect on the final product, usually because it alters a nucleotide in a degenerate position.
- **Frame-shift** – the insertion or deletion of a nucleotide results in a shift in the entire reading frame during translation.
- **Nonsense** – the mutation leads to the formation of a stop codon.

These mutations show a **mendelian inheritance** pattern and can occur during DNA replication. Mispairing of bases during DNA replication can be categorised to two forms:

1 **Transition mutations** are purine-to-purine changes, i.e. A to G, or vice versa
2 **Transversion mutations** are purine-to-pyrimidine chances, e.g. A to T.

Substitution mutations may lead to changes in the amino acid code of the protein, which can be sufficient to cause a phenotype (e.g. sickle cell anaemia). Substitutions can cause more serious consequences if they lead to the production of a stop codon, e.g. β thalassaemia.

 DEFINITION Polymorphism

Polymorphism occurs when more than one version of a specific version exists within a species. Polymorphisms must also be heritable traits and not spontaneous mutations that subsequently disappear from a population. This is typically taken to mean that at least 1% of the population expresses the allele.

Deletion mutations

Deletion mutations are less common than substitutions, although frequently more severe. If the deletion is of a three-base-pair multiple, it will lead to the loss of one or more amino acids. However, if the amino acid is not a three-base-pair multiple, it will alter the reading frame downstream of the mutation, leading to the formation of a completely different C terminus to the amino acid, most rapidly containing a stop codon. This type of mutation is the basis for many cases (around 65%) of Duchenne Muscular Dystrophy, most of the rest (30%) being the result of point mutation.

Triplet repeat mutations

Although DNA polymerases are highly accurate, there are sequences that can increase the likelihood of copying errors. The occurrence of long regions of single-, di- or trinucleotide repeats can lead to mutations as a result of slippage of the DNA polymerase during copying. Two conditions resulting from triplet repeat mutations are **Huntington's disease** and **fragile X syndrome.**

 CLINICAL Fragile X syndrome

Fragile X syndrome accounts for a large proportion of developmental intellectual impairment. The name is derived from the 'fragmented' appearance of the X chromosome (under light microscopy) in these individuals – physically the chromosome does remain intact. This 'fragile site' is located in the *FMR1* gene on the X chromosome, which is involved in regulating the translation of RNA in neuronal cells; absence of *FMR1* leads to abnormal synapse formation, which accounts for the syndrome. The *FMR1* gene contains a number of CGG triplet repeats. In the normal gene 15–40 repeats are seen, although in afflicted individuals the number may be more than 200.

Although fragile X syndrome usually affects males, if a particularly high number of repeats are inherited there may be a mild phenotype seen in heterozygote females; this is also modulated by X-chromosome inactivation in females.

Learning disability is the most common symptom of fragile X syndrome. Large testes are also characteristic, as is an elongated face. A stutter is common and loss of muscle tone has been reported.

Polygenic diseases

Many traits result from the combined effects of more than one gene. Polygenic traits account for much of the variation seen in the population, such as hair colour and height. Polygenic traits often have a **continuous distribution** in the population and often rely on interactions of the individual's genotype with the environment.

The environmental and genetic component of polygenic traits can be investigated by looking at concordance within monozygotic (MZ) and dizygotic (DZ) twins. As MZ twins share an identical genome, whereas DZ twins are likely to share only 50% of genes – similar to siblings – traits where there is a large inherited component are likely to be much more frequent in MZ twins than in DZ twins. Traits where the heritable component is low are likely to show similar inheritance in MZ and DZ twins.

Susceptibility genes

It is possible to identify specific loci in polygenic diseases that increase the likelihood of developing the disease. Many diseases show a familial clustering of inheritance, although there is obviously no form of mendelian inheritance. Type 1 diabetes represents the prototypic polygenic disease, and many of the 'susceptibility loci' for the condition have been identified.

Population genetics

It is important to understand how a disease may occur and be sustained in a population.

The Hardy–Weinberg equilibrium

In a large, randomly mating population, where there are no outside influences, the relative proportions of individual who are heterozygous and homozygous for a given trait can be described by the Hardy–Weinberg equilibrium. For an autosomal locus where there are only two alleles, A (the dominant allele) and a (the recessive allele), with frequencies p and q, respectively, the frequency of each genotype can be calculated as:

$$(p+q)^2 = p^2 + 2pq + q^2 = 1$$
$$p + q = 1$$

because A and a are the only two alleles at this locus.

This allows the calculation of each phenotype and genotype within a population (Table 2.1).

The Hardy–Weinberg equilibrium is, however, an ideal situation and certain conditions are assumed for it to be true:

- There is **completely random mating** in the population.

Table 2.1 Calculation of each phenotype and genotype within a population using the Hardy–Weinberg equilibrium

Genotype	Phenotype	Frequency
AA	A *(wild-type phenotype)*	p^2
Aa (carrier)	A *(wild-type phenotype)*	$2pq$
Aa	a *(recessive phenotype)*	q^2

The Hardy-Weinberg equilibirum is described above. The relative frequency of the alleles 'A' and 'a' are described by 'p' and 'q' respectively, where p | q = 1

- The population **is infinitely large**.
- There is **no preferential survival** of genotypes.
- **No new alleles will emerge** in the population.

Disturbances of the Hardy–Weinberg equilibrium

There are a few cases where the Hardy–Weinberg equilibrium does hold – notably blood groups. However, in the study of genetic diseases, there are four ways in which the Hardy–Weinberg equilibrium is disturbed within a population:

1 Non-random mating
2 Mutations
3 Genetic drift
4 Selection.

Non-random mating

Humans are likely to choose mates who share characteristics, such as height, intelligence and racial origins. This **assortative mating** can be extended to some genetic traits, e.g. autosomal recessive deafness, which accounts for a large proportion of congenital hearing loss. Such assortative mating will lead to an increase in the allele frequency.

Consanguinity can also alter the Hardy–Weinberg equilibrium. In small communities, individuals are likely to share common relatives, and may inherit recessive alleles from them. This increases the occurrence of individuals who are homozygous for the recessive alleles, which leads to a relative decrease for heterozygotes.

CLINICAL Sickle cell anaemia

Sickle cell anaemia results from a substitution mutation in the gene encoding the β-chain of haemoglobin. In equatorial Africa 10–40% may carry the sickle cell gene, although in Europe this number is much lower (around 0.25% or less). The gene conveys a resistance to malaria in the heterozygote. However, in the homozygote it causes crippling sickle cell disease as a result of the polymerisation of haemoglobin, inducing 'sickle-shaped' red blood cells in a low-oxygen environment. These lead to occlusion of the blood vessels, causing crises. The precise nature of the crisis depends on the site affected, e.g. bone pain can result from bone marrow infarcts. The most severe crises are sequestration crises, where a large number of blood cells become trapped within an organ (commonly the spleen, liver or lungs), causing widespread damage to that organ and also a severe anaemia. Chronic complications result from the repeated occlusion of the vessels in the organ.

Sickle cell anaemia may affect individuals to a varying degree. In its most severe form, it may be an extreme haemolytic anaemia. Jaundice often occurs and an elevated white blood cell or platelet count is not uncommon.

In heterozygotes, the sickle cell trait causes no symptoms, except occasionally in extreme hypoxia.

Mutations

Mutations occur naturally, although the equilibrium does not allow for the entry of new alleles into the population. If a locus has a particularly high mutation rate, there will be an increase in the proportion of mutant alleles in the population. If a mutation is detrimental to survival, it is likely to be quickly eliminated from the population.

Genetic drift

Genetic drift is the effect of fluctuations in the reproduction of individuals in a population. In large populations, the average number of children produced by individuals of a given genotype is normally relatively similar – the frequencies of the genotype are likely to remain constant. In a small population, random fluctuations in the number of offspring inheriting the allele can alter this constancy. If a new allele occurs, even if it is advantageous, it will not survive if none of those individuals who carry it has any children who carry the allele. The effects of these random events on the survival of an allele is called **genetic drift**.

Selection

Selection ensures that the proportion of an allele that conveys a survival advantage is likely to increase within the population. In Africa there is selection for the sickle cell mutation, as heterozygotes have an increased resistance to malaria although homozygotes have a decreased survival. However, there is no such advantage in non-malarial countries and the sickle cell allele occurs at a much lower frequency.

Genetic techniques

Gene mapping

Many polymorphisms are found in non-coding regions of DNA. Such polymorphism can be used to detect different alleles of genes due to linkage, and also allow the prediction of inheritance of genetic diseases in which the gene involved has not been definitively identified. A variety of different polymorphisms can be used:

- **Restriction fragment length polymorphisms** (RFLPs) occur when the variation in the DNA sequence occurs at a **restriction enzyme site**. Two alleles will exist – one that can be cut by the specific restriction enzyme, and one that cannot.
- **Single nucleotide polymorphisms** (SNPs) are single base changes found in the DNA, and as such can be identified directly through DNA sequencing.
- **Micro- and minisatellite DNA** (also known as variable number tandem repeats or VNTRs) are sequences of DNA made up of a repeated pattern, where the number of repeats varies. Such polymorphisms are very heterozygous and can be found spread throughout the genome.

Despite these polymorphisms occurring predominantly in non-coding DNA regions, they can be used to detect different alleles of genes. If two genes are found on a chromosome, they are generally inherited together. If there is **crossing over** of the chromosomes during meiosis, the genes may be passed into different cells.

The closer the two genes are located on the chromosome, the greater the chance of the two genes being inherited from the same parent. If any two loci (such as a gene and an SNP) are placed closely together on a chromosome, they are more likely to be inherited together because there is less chance of crossing over.

The deviation can be determined as a measure of genetic distance, based on the number of recombinants – where crossing over has prevented the inheritance of both loci – within the population.

The measure of genetic distance is a **centimorgan** (cM); 1 cM of distance represents a 1% probability that the two loci would be separated by recombination. A centimorgan does not correlate to a precise physical distance – specific regions of DNA recombine with different frequencies – although **1 cM is typically around 1 megabase.**

Genetic maps

Using genetic markers, a map can be constructed to identify inheritance of specific alleles. In principle, any DNA marker can be used. RFLPs and SNPs are limited in their usefulness, because there are only two alleles – the presence of heterozygotes at a specific location cannot be greater than 50% as determined by the **Hardy–Weinberg equilibrium** and, if an individual is homozygous for a specific marker, then genetic analysis is not informative, because recombination events at that site cannot be detectable.

VNTRs are more advantageous because heterozygosity is frequently greater than 90%. The presence of individuals homozygous at a specific VNTR is very low.

The production of genetic maps allows the detection of the region of DNA where the gene responsible for a condition is likely to reside. It allows prediction of the inheritance of a condition, when the gene responsible has not been identified. However, the accuracy of such analysis is never 100%, because there is a risk of crossing over. In autosomal recessive disorders, a limited number of mutations are likely to be responsible, and associated markers can be used as a direct test.

In dominant conditions the disease is likely to have resulted from a new mutation – each family may possess a different mutation. Linkage analysis may allow identification of markers in this case, if sufficient numbers of family members can be tested.

Molecular techniques: PCR and sequencing

The understanding of the human genome has been helped, by development techniques, to identify specific sequences and the polymorphisms that occur in genes. Four techniques have been crucial to the early development of genetics, and are used nowadays in the identification of inherited disorders:

1 **Gel electrophoresis**
2 **PCR** (polymerase chain reaction)
3 **Sequencing**
4 **Southern blotting**.

Gel electrophoresis

Electrophoresis allows the separation of DNA molecules based on their charge and size. DNA molecules are drawn towards a positive charge as a result of their negatively-charged phosphate groups. The DNA fragments are passed through a porous gel under the electric charge, the migration speed depending on the size of the fragment and the overall charge of the molecule.

PCR

The PCR amplifies a specific DNA sequence. Within a reaction the following are required:

- Sample DNA which acts as a template for the DNA amplification
- *Taq* DNA polymerase which catalyses the replication of DNA and can survive the high temperature of the reaction – necessary to separate the DNA strands
- Nucleotides which are polymerised in the polymerase reaction
- Primers which bind specifically to the DNA template and permit further elongation to create new copies of the DNA sequence in question.

The PCR occurs through the sequential cycling of the reactants through three temperatures:

- 95°C allows the separation of the DNA strands such that they are accessible to the primer sequences
- a lower temperature (often around 55°C) permits the annealing of the primers to the strands (the precise temperature depends on the sequence of the primers themselves, because that determines the temperature at which they bind)
- 72°C allows binding of the polymerase and then elongation of the DNA chains at the primer sites to produce new copies of the DNA sequence.

Repeated cycling through these three temperatures allows the exponential amplification of a specific DNA sequence. The primers allow PCR to be specific, permitting the detection of polymorphisms, or the presence/absence of the gene:

- If the primers are complementary to the target sequence of DNA, there will be amplification of DNA and a band will be detectable by gel electrophoresis.
- If the primers are not complementary (as a result of the target sequence being absent), then amplification will not occur and hence no band will be detectable.

Sequencing reaction

Understanding of the genome sequence has been aided by the development of a method to establish the precise nucleotide sequence. This process uses dideoxynucleotides at low concentrations in a PCR reaction.

Dideoxynucleotides can be added to the growing nucleotide chain, yet lack the necessary hydroxyl group to continue the growth of the chain. When added into a reaction at a concentration of about 1%, it ensures that some of the chains of nucleotides are terminated each time that the specific nucleotide is added.

Four reactions are run for each sequence; in each case a normal PCR reaction is set up and a small (about 1%) concentration of a single dideoxynucleotide added (e.g. ddATP). Only one primer is added so that only one sequence is produced. The completed reactions are then run out by gel electrophores and several bands will be detected. Each band signifies the presence of the chain-terminating dideoxynucleotide at that position in the nucleotide sequence.

The sequencing process has been further sped up by the use of fluorescent molecules in the termination of the DNA chains, which can be read by a computer, allowing automation of the reading process.

Southern blotting

Southern blotting is a method by which specific genes or polymorphisms can be detected – in light of more modern techniques, this is becoming increasingly rare. The genomes of cells can be isolated and broken into fragments by **restriction enzymes**. The resulting DNA fragments are separated by gel electrophoresis. The DNA fragments can then be transferred on to a membrane through blotting of the membrane directly on to the electrophoretic gel.

 DEFINITION Restriction enzymes

Restriction enzymes are endonuclease enzymes that cut DNA at a specific palindromic DNA sequence, where the sequence on the complementary strand is identical (e.g. *EcoR1*, a very commonly used restriction enzyme, cuts DNA with the sequence GAATTC). These enzymes are found in many species of bacteria, where they are thought to be part of the defence against viral infection. The target sequence of the enzymes may be found in the cell's DNA, but they are protected through methylation of the bacterial cell DNA, which does not occur in viral DNA.

In molecular biology, restriction enzymes allow specific cutting of DNA fragments, through the relatively rarity of the target sequence, and this can be used to isolate specific fragments of DNA, or detect polymorphisms.

The fragments can then be 'probed' for a specific sequence. A probe DNA is constructed with a sequence exactly complementary to the region in question, which is then conjugated to a marker – typically a radioactive label. Once the excess probe is washed away an X-ray film can be applied, and the sites where the probe has bound to its complementary sequence will be detectable.

Southern blotting has been used to detect many of polymorphisms that are used in genetic linkage studies and can be used to determine allele of a gene that someone possesses. The northern and western blots are similar techniques that have been developed to investigate RNA and protein, respectively. In the case of a western blot, the presence of a particular protein can be detected by an antibody that is specific to it.

 RELATED CHAPTERS

3

Biochemistry

All processes in the body rely on complex interactions between macromolecules, the precursors of which are obtained through the diet. There are four classes of macromolecules:

1 **Proteins** are made up of amino acids. Some proteins have a structural or transport role, whereas others are enzymes that catalyse metabolic reactions.
2 **Lipids** provide a concentrated store of energy, as well as making up a large component of the cell membrane and – as steroids – have a crucial role in signalling.
3 **Carbohydrates** provide a store of energy and may be involved in signalling through their action as ligands for many cell-surface receptors.
4 **Nucleic acids** encode the genetic information necessary for the synthesis of all other molecules in the cell. Their role is described in more detail in Chapter 2.

Proteins

Proteins are made up of amino acids linked by peptide bonds. The different amino acids in proteins interact to cause a specific folding pattern resulting in a molecule with a complex structure and a specific function.

The **structure of an amino acid** is conserved, with a basic 'skeleton' and a single group (the 'R' group) which differs between molecules. It is a zwitterion, a molecule containing both positively and negatively charged groups. Although around 50 different amino acids are found in nature, only 20 are used by the body. The classification of an amino acid is based on its 'R' group. Amino acids may be classified by charge (Fig. 3.1):

- **Charged polar** – the 'R' group is **ionic** (e.g. glutamic acid)
- **Uncharged polar** – the 'R' group is a **dipole** (e.g. glycine)
- **Non-polar** – the 'R' group carries **no charge** (e.g. alanine).

Proline is an unusual amino acid, because its side chain is bonded back on to the molecule. This creates an unusual shape that can greatly alter protein structure.

The carbon in the skeleton of amino acids is a chiral centre (except in glycine), around which the amino acids exhibit **stereoisomerism**. In the human body, all amino acids are of the L form.

 DEFINITION Stereoisomerism

In organic molecules, a carbon atom is bonded to four different groups. This carbon atom is known as a **chiral centre** and produces **stereoisomerism**. The four groups are arranged tetrahedrally in three dimensions around the chiral centre. It is possible to generate two different arrangements that cannot be superimposed on each other, no matter how the whole molecule is arranged in space. When drawn in two dimensions, the isoforms appear identical; however, they have different structures in three dimensions. This is **stereoisomerism**. Each stereoisomer has two forms: D and L; these refer to their properties in refracting light. The body uses only the L form of amino acids, whereas many microorganisms can utilise the D form (e.g. in the formation of a peptidoglycan).

Biomedical Science Lecture Notes, First Edition. Ian Lyons.
© 2011 by Ian Lyons. Published 2011 by Blackwell Publishing Ltd.

DEFINITION Dipole

A dipole is a molecule that has mild changes in charge; this is usually the result of an electronegative molecule, such as oxygen, attracting electrons to create this mild difference in charge. Although these differences are mild compared with those caused by the gain or loss of electrons, they can create significant effects in interactions between molecules.

Protein structure

There are five forces that contribute to folding of a protein into its three-dimensional structure:

- **Van der Waal's forces** are result from changes of electron density (and thus minute changes in the charge) between neighbouring groups. The sum of all these forces can be significant, although each individual interaction is very weak.
- **Hydrogen bonding** is a non-covalent interaction in polar molecules resulting from the interaction of hydrogen atoms with an electronegative atom, such as nitrogen or oxygen. Hydrogen groups are found in both the backbone of the protein and the side chains, and help to stabilise the structure.
- **Electrostatic interactions** can occur between the different 'R' groups and are found in three types; they are often stronger than the interactions resulting from hydrogen bonding. The different types are a result of combinations of dipoles and charged groups which may interact; from the strongest to the weakest, these are:
  – **charge–charge interactions**
  – **charge–dipole interactions**
  – **dipole–dipole interactions.**
- **Disulphide bonds** are an extremely strong covalent interaction resulting from bonding of sulphide groups on cysteine side chains. These bonds help to stabilise the protein structure.
- **Hydrophobic interactions** rely on the interactions of the 'R' groups and the water in the protein's immediate environment. Hydrophobic regions of a protein interact to pack closely together, and reduce direct contact with water molecules. These interactions result in the formation of hydrophobic pockets within a protein.

Levels of proteins organisation

There are four sequential levels of organisation that are used to explain the structure of a protein.

First, the **primary structure** is the order of the amino acids in the polypeptide chain. It is these amino acids that determine the features of the higher level of structure.

Second, the **secondary structure** results from the complex interactions of amino acids in the protein, as a result of **hydrogen bonding, electrostatic interactions, van der Waal's forces** and **hydrophobic interactions**. These contribute to the production of a structure with the lowest free energy. Three forms of secondary structure can be identified:

1 **α Helices** are the most common form of secondary structure. The amino acids form a right-handed helix with the side chains located on the outside of the helix. α Helices form as a result of hydrogen bonding between the C=O and N–H groups in the amino acid backbone. Some amino acids, such as alanine and methionine, preferentially form α helices. Others, such as serine and tyrosine, tend not to. Proline disrupts the α-helix structure because its cyclic structure prevents the formation of a hydrogen bond.

2 **β Sheets** are made up of many lengths of polypeptide lying next to each other. The side chains of the amino acids appear on alternate sides of the β sheet. Strands in the sheet may be parallel – each strand runs in the same direction in reference to its N and C termini; or they may be antiparallel, when they run in opposite directions.

3 **Loop regions** serve to link other secondary structure regions; typically they contain polar residues, because they are likely to be in contact with water. Loop regions may also have a functional role, forming the binding sites on antibodies and some forms of receptor.

The **tertiary structure** is produced by the organisation of secondary structural regions into functional domains. Such domains are often encoded by individual exons in a gene. Again, there are common structural arrangements the tertiary structure:

- **α-Domain** structures are collections of α helices. The side chains of the α helices interact to cause

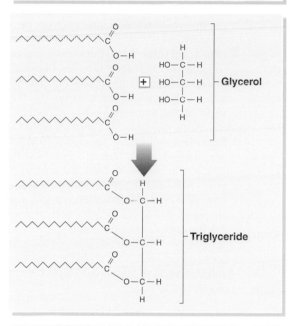

Amino acids

Amino acids share the same conserved structure, varying only in the side chain, marked by the 'R'. It is this chain that contributes to the different properties of the amino acid. Linkage of molecules is through the formation of peptide linkages.

Fats

The triglyceride fat is made up of one molecule of glycerol that is linked to three fatty acids by ester linkages. This produces a highly compact molecule, used for the storage of energy. Phospholipids have a similar structure, although one of the fatty acyl chains is replaced by a polar head group and phosphate molecule.

Carbohydrates

The most common form of carbohydrates in the body is the hexose sugars – of which glucose and fructose are common examples. These hexose sugars are a significant energy source within the body and can be bound together by a glycoside bond to produce sucrose – the form in which sugar is commonly ingested. in addition, there may be five-carbon and three-carbon sugars. They have a similar shape, with a central ring consisting of carbons and a single oxygen molecule.

Figure 3.1 The general structures of amino acids, fats and carbohydrates.

complex folding and mediate the structure of the protein. The side chains may have hydrophobic regions that mediate the tight packing, minimising contact with water molecules.

- **β Domains** are found where there are collections of the β sheets
- **α/β-Domain structures** form from a mixture of α-helix and β-sheet regions and represent a very common structural motif. They often have a structural or a functional role.

Finally a protein may be made up of several distinct polypeptide chains. The way in which these interact is known as the **quaternary structure.**

Lipids

Lipids are non-polar molecules that have a role in the formation of the cell membrane and the storage of energy, as well as in signalling. Three types of lipids with distinct functions can be identified:

- Triglycerides
- Phospholipids
- Sterols.

Triglycerides

Triglycerides are made up of a glycerol molecule joined to one to three fatty acids through ester links (Fig. 3.1). The fatty acid chains contain a long carbon chain that is non-polar and a carboxylic acid group that is charged. The high concentration of carbon in fats makes them a compact energy store. Both saturated and unsaturated fats are used in the human body.

> **DEFINITION Saturated and unsaturated lipids**
>
> Lipids can be defined as saturated and unsaturated, as a result of the presence or absence of double bonds in their acyl chains. Saturated lipids have no double bonds – the carbon chain is fully saturated with covalently bonded hydrogen.

Phospholipids

Phospholipids make up much of the cell membrane. These are made up of glycerol, which binds two fatty acid chains at C-1 and C-2. C-3 is bound to a phosphate and a head group which may be basic, neutral or polar.

Sterols

Sterols contain a well-defined ring structure: three six-carbon rings, a five-carbon ring and a side chain. Sterols can be synthesised in the body, and may be found free or attached to long-chain fatty acids. They form the basis of many hormones and also make up bile salts which help with the absorption of fats.

The role of lipids

Lipids fulfil three major roles in the body:

1 **Energy source**: lipids generate around seven ATP molecules for the oxidation of one carbon, as opposed to five ATP molecules per carbon in carbohydrates
2 **Structural roles**: lipids form barriers to prevent the diffusion of polar molecules. Phospholipids are specialised for the production membranes because their amphipathic nature (having both hydrophobic and hydrophilic components) promotes the formation of a **phospholipid bilayer**.
3 **Signalling molecules**: steroid hormones, which are derived from sterols, cause widespread changes in the body. They are able to diffuse freely into cells and bind cellular receptors that alter gene expression. Signalling is also achieved through other forms of lipids, such as phosphatidylinositol 4,5-bisphosphate (PIP$_2$), which is crucial for calcium signalling. In addition, leukotrienes and prostaglandins, mediators of inflammation, are derived from the lipid arachidonic acid.

Carbohydrates (sugars)

Sugars are made up of a carbon ring, and take the basic form $(CH_2O)_n$:

- **Hexose (six-carbon) sugars** are important as an energy source in the body.
- **Ribose (five-carbon) sugars** are important for the production of nucleic acids.
- **Triose (three-carbon) sugars** may be used in some steps of **glycolysis**.

Types of carbohydrate

Carbohydrates are built up of single sugar blocks – **monosaccharides**. The most important monosaccharide in the body is **glucose** (see Fig. 3.1). This is used in **glycolysis** and can be converted to five-carbon sugars via the pentose phosphate pathway.

Monosaccharides may be linked together to produce **disaccharides**, through the formation of a **glycosidic bond**. Three particularly important disaccharides are:

1 Sucrose – formed from fructose and glucose
2 Maltose – formed from two glucose molecules
3 Lactose – formed from glucose and galactose.

The formation of further glycosidic bonds allows the formation of polysaccharides; in particular **glycogen**, a rapidly mobilised energy source, is produced in the liver and muscles. In the diet starch, a plant polysaccharide, is an important source of carbohydrate.

The role of carbohydrates

Carbohydrates have a role in four main areas:

1 **Energy** through **glycolysis** and further downstream processes. Much of this carbohydrate is obtained by the breakdown of ingested starch.
2 **Structural**, in particular through its contributions to the extracellular matrix.
3 **Modification of other molecules** involved in cell signalling, especially those in the surface.
4 **Nucleotide synthesis.**

Metabolic biochemistry

Principles of metabolism

Metabolism is the process that living systems use to regulate the breakdown and synthesis of the molecules necessary for their continued function and survival. Crucial to this is the conversion of compounds to **adenosine triphosphate** (ATP), the energy currency in the cell. ATP releases energy after the hydrolysis of its phosphate bonds, producing adenosine monophosphate (AMP) or adenosine diphosphate (ADP). The released phosphate groups may be used to phosphorylate a variety of molecules (e.g. proteins) and modulate their function.

 DEFINITION Anabolism and catabolism

Metabolic reactions can be divided into two types:

1 **Catabolic** reactions break down a substrate.
2 **Anabolic** reactions are ones in which a molecule is synthesised from substrate.

Control of metabolism

There are different levels of regulation of metabolism from global control to regulate entire body processes, to controls to meet the needs of individual cells.

Short-term controls

These controls allow tight control of metabolism in the individual cell, in response to the specific conditions experienced:

- **Allosteric regulation** involves the non-covalent interaction of various compounds, triggering conformational changes in the enzyme. Such interactions may enhance or inhibit the function of the enzyme, and allow almost instant changes in response to rapid changes in the immediate environment of the cell.
- **Covalent modification** provides a slightly longer-term form of regulation, which may be in response to the effects of stimuli external to the cell (e.g. hormones). In this case the activity of an enzyme may be modulated by the addition or removal of covalently bound groups (e.g. phosphate) to an enzyme – altering its activity.

Long-term controls

These are the result of chronic changes in the conditions experienced by the cells, or a response to widespread signals such as hormones. This involves modulation of gene expression in a cell, and may take days to come fully into effect.

Cycles between organs

Biochemical cycles can occur between two or more organs. These are controlled by the rate at which a substrate can be delivered to the target organ. This can be illustrated by the **Cori** cycle, in which lactate, produced by anaerobic respiration of glucose, may be converted back to glucose in the liver. Here the rate-limiting step is often the rate of delivery of lactate.

The tricarboxylic acid cycle

The tricarboxylic acid (TCA) cycle is the central step of aerobic respiration. The products of fat, amino acid and glucose metabolism feed into this cycle, which produces reduced co-factors to drive the **electron transport chain**. Intermediates of the cycle are used in a variety of other reactions (Fig. 3.2).

The TCA cycle represents the point at which energy production focuses on the mitochondria.

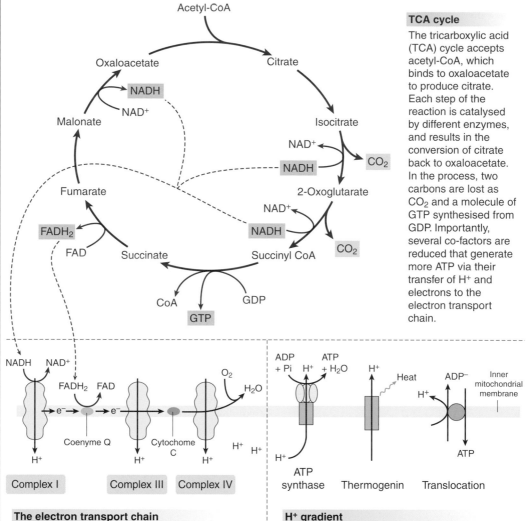

TCA cycle

The tricarboxylic acid (TCA) cycle accepts acetyl-CoA, which binds to oxaloacetate to produce citrate. Each step of the reaction is catalysed by different enzymes, and results in the conversion of citrate back to oxaloacetate. In the process, two carbons are lost as CO_2 and a molecule of GTP synthesised from GDP. Importantly, several co-factors are reduced that generate more ATP via their transfer of H^+ and electrons to the electron transport chain.

The electron transport chain

The electron transport chain is the final acceptor for the reduced co-factors NADH and $FADH_2$ which are produced through many of the metabolic reactions within the cell. NADH contributes its electrons to complex I in the chain, whereas $FADH_2$ is found located within complex II, which is not part of the electron transport chain, although it donates electrons to coenzyme Q. Electrons travel through the chain, being carried between the large complex by coenzyme Q and cytochrome c. The electrons contribute to the reduction of ion centres within the complex, which powers the transport of H^+ ions across the inner mitochondrial membrane. The final acceptor of the electrons is complex IV (cytochrome oxidase) which catalyses its reaction with H^+ and O_2 to generate water.

H^+ gradient

The H^+ gradient generated by the electron transport chain can be discharged through a variety of proteins to power a variety of cellular processes. The vast majority of the gradient is discharged through the enzyme ATP synthase, powering oxidative phosphorylation of ADP to ATP. In addition, the H^+ gradient may be use to generate heat or to mediate the transport of molecules across the inner mitochondrial membrane.

Figure 3.2 The tricarboxylic acid cycle and oxidative phosphorylation.

It occurs in the matrix of the mitochondria and accepts intermediates that are generated in the cytosol or other parts of the cell.

The products of glycolysis and β oxidation of fatty acids enter the TCA cycle as acetyl-coenzyme A (acetyl-CoA). A single acetyl-CoA molecule contributes two ATP molecules and two CO_2 molecules, as well as generating reduced co-factors that contribute to the electron transport chain.

Amino acid metabolism also contributes to the TCA cycle; however, depending on the specific amino acid, the resulting metabolites can enter the cycle at a variety of sites. Similarly, removal of specific TCA cycle intermediates may be used for the synthesis of new amino acids.

Electron transport chain

Throughout the metabolic processes, co-factors are reduced by hydrogen. These reduced co-factors donate H^+ ions and electrons (e^-) to the electron transport chain in the mitochondria (see Fig. 3.2).

The electron transport chain is located on the inner mitochondrial membrane and consists of three major complexes (I, II and IV) linked by mobile electron carriers, which accept e^- and use it to generate an H^+ gradient across the inner mitochondrial membrane.

NADH (reduced nicotinamide adenine dinucleotide) is a co-factor generated during the TCA cycle (and other cellular processes). It donates electrons to complex I, whereas $FADH_2$ (another co-factor, reduced flavin adenine dinucleotide) is part of complex II, and does not contribute to the movement of as many H^+ ions because its electrons join the chain at a later point than those of NADH. The final acceptor is cytochrome oxidase (complex IV), which catalyses the transfer of electrons from cytochrome c to oxygen and H^+ to produce H_2O.

The energy released in the electron transport chain is used to transport H^+ across the inner mitochondrial membrane to create an H^+ gradient; this may be as large as 10 000:1.

Utilisation of the H^+ gradient

The H^+ gradient produced by the electron transport chain has three physiologically important uses:

1 Synthesis of ATP
2 Inner membrane transport
3 Thermogenesis.

Synthesis of ATP

Much of the H^+ gradient is converted into ATP as it flows through **ATP synthase**. This enzyme is made up of F_1 and F_0 subunits; the addition of phosphate to ADP is catalysed in the F_1 subunit, whereas the flow of electrons through the transmembrane F_0 subunit catalyses the release of ATP from the protein's active site. The F_1 particle consists of six subunits which make up three active sites in a rotary arrangement. The reaction is highly efficient: one NADH molecule capable of producing three ATP molecules.

Inner membrane transport

The transport of molecules across the inner mitochondrial membrane is highly regulated; many substances must be transported actively using energy derived from the H^+ gradient. This is an extremely expensive process – around 25% of the H^+ gradient is thought to be expended in the movement of ATP and ADP across the inner mitochondrial membrane.

The proton gradient is used electrogenically – to neutralise an electric charge. In the case of the adenine nucleotide translocator, ATP is translocated out of the mitochondrion for one molecule of ADP^- and one H^+ is expended to neutralise the extra negative charge.

Thermogenesis

The brown adipose tissue, which is particularly prominent in newborn babies because they are incapable of shivering, can utilise the H^+ gradient for heat generation. Thermogenesis is mediated by proton flow through the protein **thermogenin**, which converts the released energy into heat.

Carbohydrate metabolism

Carbohydrates in the diet must be broken down into monosaccharides by a variety of enzymes in the gut. The major carbohydrate metabolised in the body is glucose, although fructose and galactose are also significant additional sources (Fig. 3.3).

In an average individual, a little less than 200 g glucose is essential for the body each day. This may be as glucose, or another sugar (such as **fructose)** that is converted to glucose.

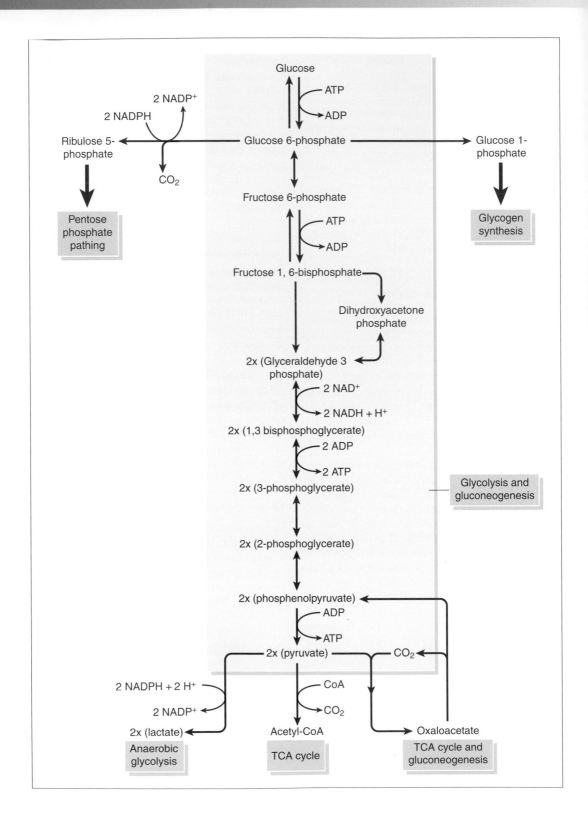

A supply of glucose is essential for the body, because some tissues are capable of using only glucose:

- The **brain** – aerobic respiration, although ketones can be used in starvation
- **Red blood cells** – anaerobic respiration
- **Renal medulla** – anaerobic respiration, due to the low oxygen environment found at the interface of the renal medulla and cortex.

Uptake of glucose

Glucose enters cells by passive diffusion. There are 5 classes of GLUT transporter which are responsible for uptake into many cells of the body:

1 **GLUT1**: found on red blood cells and not regulated by insulin. These transporters constantly take up glucose from the blood.
2 **GLUT2**: expressed in pancreatic β cells and the liver. GLUT2 transporters can transport large amounts of glucose, allowing rapid sensing of changes in the body's glucose levels; GLUT2 is also expressed in the intestines to help absorption of glucose.
3 **GLUT3**: similar to GLUT1 transporters and found in the brain. These transporters also constantly take up glucose in an insulin-independent manner.
4 **GLUT4**: regulated tightly by insulin and responsible for the uptake of surplus glucose to maintain a constant blood glucose level. GLUT4 transporters are expressed in the muscles and adipose tissue; a large number of transporters are stored in vesicles in the cell, such that they can be rapidly expressed on the cell surface.
5 **GLUT5**: transporters are responsible for the uptake of **fructose** from the gut. Glucose is not taken up in the gut by a GLUT transporter, but by a sodium co-transporter (SGLT).

Glycolysis

Glycolysis is the process by which glucose is broken down; Glycolysis directly generates two ATP molecules per glucose molecule, although the products and reduced co-factors formed can contribute to the formation of far more ATP molecules in aerobic respiration. In the glycolytic pathway, there are three critical reactions that regulate the process:

1 Phosphorylation of glucose by **hexokinase** or **glucokinase**
2 Phosphorylation by **phosphofructokinase** (PFK)
3 Phosphorylation by **pyruvate kinase**.

Hexokinase and glucokinase

Both hexokinase and glucokinase phosphorylate glucose; this commits the use of the glucose to that cell, although not necessarily to glycolysis. The presence of two different enzymes with the same task reflects the different needs and roles of the cells in which they are expressed.

Hexokinase is expressed in most cells in the body and capable of phosphorylating many sugars other than glucose. It is inhibited by its own product, **glucose 6-phosphate**, preventing commitment of too much glucose to an individual cell. Hexokinase has a high affinity for glucose, so it is capable of trapping glucose in a cell at low concentrations. The rate at which the enzyme can catalyse its reaction (V_{max}) is very low, preventing it from phosphorylating large amounts of glucose.

Glucokinase has a similar specificity for sugars to hexokinase, and is expressed in the liver and β cells of the pancreatic islets. It is adapted for coping with large amounts of glucose and has a much higher V_{max} than hexokinase; however, it also has a lower affinity for glucose, so that it operates effectively at high glucose levels. Its action is not inhibited by the reaction product.

Phosphofructokinase

The phosphorylation of fructose 6-phosphate to fructose 1,6-bisphospate is the crucial enzymatic step that commits a molecule to **glycolysis**.

Figure 3.3 Glycolysis. Glucose can be used for a variety of reactions. Glycolysis is crucial for the generation of energy and produces a net gain of two molecules of ATP per glucose, although under aerobic conditions it also contributes two NADH molecules and two molecules of acetyl-CoA which may enter the tricarboxylic acid (TCA) cycle. Under anaerobic conditions, the NADH is required to convert pyruvate into lactate. Glucose synthesis is possible in these cells by the conversion of pyruvate or oxaloacetate to phosphenolpyruvate. The three regulatory reactions of glycolysis may be bypassed by the use of alternative enzymes. Glucose can also be sequestered for the production of glycogen or converted to other forms of sugar by the pentose phosphate shunt.

The enzyme is regulated by many substances that reflects the energy needs of the cell:

- **PFK is inhibited by ATP**, signalling a plentiful energy supply in the cell, and hence no need for increased metabolism. It is also inhibited by citrate, an intermediate of the TCA cycle, another indicator of high-energy concentrations.
- **PFK activity is promoted by AMP**, a product of the breakdown of ATP, signalling low energy levels.

In many cells (particularly the liver) the typical concentration of ATP is too high to allow PFK to function. This is overcome by the presence of an activating molecule – fructose 2,6-bisphosphate – which increases the affinity of PFK for fructose 6-phosphate, overcoming the ATP-mediated inhibition of PFK.

Generation and regulation of fructose 2,6-bisphosphate are by the enzyme phosphofructokinase-2; it is broken down by fructose bisphosphatase-2. Both enzymes are found as discrete domains on a single protein molecule. While it is phosphorylated, the phosphatase domain is active; when it is dephosphorylated, the kinase domain is active. This process allows very tight regulation, so that the level of fructose 2,6-bisphosphate, and thus the rate of glycolysis, can be rapidly altered.

Pyruvate kinase

This enzyme controls the release of pyruvate from the glycolytic pathway to the TCA cycle. It is inhibited by ATP, reflecting control in relation to the energy needs of the cell. Pyruvate kinase is also inhibited by alanine, an amino acid that can contribute to the TCA cycle at the same point. In addition, pyruvate kinase is upregulated by fructose 1,6-bisphosphate, anticipating its requirement further down the pathway.

The fate of pyruvate

In **aerobic conditions** the products of glycolysis can be further oxidised by **pyruvate dehydrogenase** to release more energy. This leads to the breakdown of pyruvate, the end-product of glycolysis, into acetyl-CoA in the mitochondrion. Pyruvate dehydrogenase is a large multienzyme complex that contains several copies of the three protein subunits, and the necessary co-factors, including NAD^+ and FAD. The regulation of pyruvate dehydrogenase is inhibited by its products – NADH and acetyl-CoA – through their action to promote activity of the associated pyruvate dehydrogenase kinase. The presence of AMP – a signal of low energy within the cell – promotes the activity of pyruvate dehydrogenase.

In **anaerobic conditions**, pyruvate cannot be converted to acetyl-CoA and is converted to lactate, by **lactate dehydrogenase**. In sites of low oxygen (e.g. the renal medulla) this is common. The conversion of pyruvate to lactate requires the oxidation of NADH. As such, the net gain of ATP per glucose molecule is two ATP molecules released during glycolysis. Lactate formation occurs in muscles under exercise – this is released into the blood, where it can be converted back to glucose in the liver or used as a source of energy.

The utilisation of lactate

Lactate dehydrogenase is a tetrameric isoenzyme made up of two types of subunits. The M subtype is prevalent in muscle, which catalyses the conversion of pyruvate to lactate, as occurs in anaerobic glycolysis. In the liver and heart, the H subtype is prevalent which promotes the conversion of lactate to pyruvate; this generates ATP through the TCA cycle. In the liver lactate is used to generate glucose by gluconeogenesis.

Metabolism of other monosaccharides

Although glucose is the major monosaccharide used by the body, a normal diet contains significant quantities of other monosaccharides, in particular fructose and galactose. These sugars are converted into intermediates that are appropriate for breakdown via the glycolytic pathway.

Fructose makes up 10–20% of a normal western diet; it enters cells in an insulin-independent manner and is phosphorylated by the enzyme, **fructokinase**. Fructose then joins the glycolytic pathway, after its breakdown by aldolase B, to produce glyceraldehyde.

 CLINICAL Hereditary fructose intolerance

Aldolase B is responsible for the breakdown of fructose 1-phosphate. This enzyme is missing in those individuals with hereditary fructose intolerance, leading to accumulation of fructose. This results in hypoglycaemia, vomiting, jaundice and haemorrhage; liver failure may result.

Treatment is by removal of fructose and sugars that contain fructose (such as sucrose) from the diet.

Galactose is derived from dairy products and, similar to other monosaccharides, requires phosphorylation for metabolism. The conversion of galactose to uridine diphosphate (UDP)-galactose allows it to be transformed to UDP-glucose which can be used for glycolysis.

Pentose phosphate pathway

Five-carbon sugars are an essential component in nucleotide bases and produced from glucose.

The first reaction in the pentose phosphate pathway (PPP), catalysed by **glucose-6-phosphate dehydrogenase**, commits the molecule to this pathway. Molecules of glucose 6-phosphate are oxidised to form ribulose 5-phosphate and CO_2. Two molecules of $NADP^+$ are also reduced to NADPH.

The second series of reactions are reversible and produce a series of different length sugars. These reactions are regulated to ensure there is a sufficient supply of different length intermediates which may be required by other metabolic pathways in the cell.

The regulation of the diversion of sugars to the PPP is through the $NADP^+$/NADPH balance. The reduced form (NADPH or reduced nicotinamide adenine dinucleotide phosphate) of the co-factor inhibits the function of glucose-6-phosphate dehydrogenase.

NADPH is a critical co-factor in the body; it is used in the liver in the production of fatty acids and in the adrenal cortex for the production of steroid hormones. It is also involved in the protection against damage by reactive oxygen intermediates.

> **CLINICAL Glucose-6-phosphate dehydrogenase deficiency**
>
> NADPH is a crucial co-factor that can mediate the removal of reactive oxygen intermediates. Glucose-6-phosphate dehydrogenase deficiency is an X-linked recessive disorder in which individuals are less able to detoxify these intermediates due to reduced levels of NADPH. This leads to a chronic anaemia caused by repeated damage to red blood cells, in which the sole means of generating NADPH is via this pathway. Often the deficiency is mild, and does not manifest clinically unless oxidant drugs are used or fava beans are ingested; these require NADPH in their breakdown. In both cases a haemolytic anaemia results.

Storage of glucose as glycogen

The majority of excess glucose is converted to fat, a much more compact storage medium. A small amount of glucose is stored as **glycogen**. This large polymer can be rapidly broken down to glucose to regulate blood glucose levels. The key synthetic reaction is the conversion of glucose 6-phosphate to glucose 1-phosphate, and then its integration into glycogen. The addition of glucose 1-phosphate to glycogen is mediated by **glycogen synthase**.

Glycogen is generated by the progressive addition of glucose to a primer protein, **glycogenin**. This reaction requires UDP-glucose as the glucose donor and is catalysed by the enzyme glycogen synthase. The glycogen molecule is highly branched through the action of a branching enzyme. Branching is beneficial because it:

- makes glycogen highly soluble
- increases the number of terminal residues for breakdown of glycogen into glucose.

Glycogen is broken down from the terminal residues to produce glucose 1-phosphate, which is rapidly converted to glucose 6-phosphate.

Regulation of glycogen synthesis and degradation is achieved through the activation of glycogen synthase by glucose 6-phosphate, ensuring that glycogen is synthesised when there is excess substrate. Similarly, glucose 6-phosphate inhibits glycogen breakdown by inhibiting glycogen phosphorylase, as does ATP.

Gluconeogenesis

Gluconeogenesis, the process by which glucose is generated from non-carbohydrates, occurs in the liver. Those substrates that enter at an intermediate point in the TCA cycle are not completely metabolised before they can be removed from the cycle for gluconeogenesis. Fatty acids enter the TCA cycle as acetyl-CoA and cannot be used to generate glucose; the acetyl-CoA must undergo the complete series of TCA reactions to reach the point where a suitable metabolic intermediate can be removed for gluconeogenesis; in this time two-carbon molecules of acetyl-CoA have been metabolised into CO_2.

The process of gluconeogenesis is very similar to glycolysis; however, the three points of control in glycolysis are bypassed by different reactions (see Fig. 3.3):

1 **Hexokinase** is bypassed by a hydrolysis reaction.
2 **PFK** is bypassed by a hydrolysis reaction.
3 **Pyruvate kinase** is bypassed by two reactions.

The gluconeogenetic pathway occurs in all tissues, but glucose-6-phosphatase is expressed only in the liver. Non-liver tissue lacks this enzyme, so any glucose that is produced by gluconeogenesis must be retained in the cell.

Bypass of pyruvate kinase

Bypass of the reaction mediated by pyruvate kinase is achieved in two stages:

1 **Pyruvate carboxylase** triggers the formation of pyruvate from oxaloacetate.
2 **Oxaloacetate** is removed from the mitochondrion by the **malate shuttle** (where is it reduced to malate for transport and then converted back in the cytoplasm) and is converted to phosphenolpyruvate.

Bypass of PFK and hexokinase

The PFK-mediated phosphorylation of fructose 6-phosphate is reversed by a hydrolysis reaction mediated by fructose-1,6-bisphosphatase.

The phosphorylation by hexokinase is reversed by glucose-6-phosphatase. Most tissues lack glucose-6-phosphatase, so that any glucose produced by the gluconeogenetic pathway is retained in the tissues and not released into the blood. However, the liver expresses glucose-6-phosphatase which allows it to contribute glucose to the blood if needed.

Control of glucose metabolism

Glycolysis and gluconeogenesis must be tightly regulated to prevent the generation of a **futile cycle** in which the products of one are immediately used by the other, resulting in the expenditure of energy for no useful gain. Glycolysis yields two ATP and two NADH molecules per glucose molecule, whereas two pyruvate molecules in gluconeogenesis require two NADH and six triphosphate molecules (four ATP and two GTP) to produce one glucose molecule, representing a net loss of energy.

Control of glucose pathways is through cAMP (adenosine cyclic 3′:5′-monophosphate) signalling in the liver, in response to glucagon. The resulting rise in cAMP and associated signalling stimulates gluconeogenesis and inhibits glycolysis:

- Pyruvate kinase is inhibited by cAMP-dependent protein kinase.
- PFK is activated by fructose 2,6-bisphosphate which is reduced in response to cAMP, preventing glycolysis during glucagon signalling. Conversely, fructose-1,6-bisphosphatase is inhibited by fructose 2,6-bisphosphate and is thus activated during the cAMP-associated events of glucagon signalling.

Fat metabolism

Fats account for around 75% of the total energy stores. They are easily mobilised and there is no loss of body function if such stores become depleted. Each carbon atom in carbohydrates contributes around **five ATP** molecules, whereas each carbon atom in fats contributes around **seven ATP** molecules.

Absorption of fat

Fats are insoluble in water and tend to accumulate in globules on the intestinal lumen. They are emulsified by bile salts to increase their surface area; this improves the activity of pancreatic lipase which breaks triglycerides into two fatty acid chains and a monoacylglycerol molecule for absorption into the epithelial cells.

The fatty acids are packaged in micelles – small spherical particles that are produced as a result of the interactions between water and the hydrophobic elements of fatty acids.

Transport of fatty acids around the body

Fats represent an easily mobilised energy store that can be transported from adipose tissue to sites where energy production is required. The transport of fats is mediated by **lipoproteins**.

After absorption of fats by the intestinal cells, they are packaged into **chylomicrons**, which are secreted into the lymphatic vessels and transported around the body to sites of storage.

DEFINITION Chylomicrons

Chylomicrons are particles made up of a high proportion of lipids packaged around proteins. These particles are produced by the intestinal cells after absorption of dietary fats. They are released into the lymph and taken up by adipose tissue. The latter expresses lipoprotein lipases on the endothelial cells of its capillaries, to release the component fatty acids from chylomicrons for absorption and storage.

Transport of fatty acids into the cell

As fatty acids are lipid soluble, entry into the cell across the cell membrane occurs by diffusion. Fatty acid molecules are rapidly converted to fatty acyl-CoA in the cytosol by **fatty acyl-CoA synthetase**. Fatty acids and acyl-CoA molecules can be transported around the cytoplasm by fatty acid-binding proteins, allowing their transport in the cytoplasm, in which they are otherwise insoluble. The polar nature of the acyl-CoA prevents its transport across the inner membrane, so a specialised **carnitine shuttle** is required to transport the fatty acyl chain into the mitochondrion (Fig. 3.4).

Carnitine acyltransferase I is located in the cytosol and catalyses the transfer of the fatty acyl group from the acyl-CoA to the carnitine molecule, forming *O*-acylcarnitine; a similar enzyme, carnitine acyltransferase II, catalyses the reverse reaction in the mitochondrial matrix. Transport of carnitine (with or without the fatty acid molecule attached) is mediated by a specific carrier protein in the membrane.

Malonyl-CoA, a substrate for the generation of fatty acids, inhibits the action of carnitine acyltransferase I, preventing the simultaneous degradation and synthesis of fatty acids.

β Oxidation of fatty acids

After their transport into the mitochondrial matrix, fatty acids are broken down into two-carbon blocks to release acetyl-CoA, for metabolism by the TCA cycle. As there is less oxygen in fat than in carbohydrates, it is possible to produce more ATP molecules per carbon through aerobic respiration. β Oxidation occurs for fatty acids that are no longer than 16–18 carbon atoms in length. Fatty acids longer than 16–18 carbon atoms in length are first

processed in peroxisomes, although this does not provide any energy for the cell.

Oxidation of other forms of fatty acid chains

The basic β-oxidation pathway is capable of releasing energy from saturated fatty acids with even numbers of carbon atoms. Many fatty acids in the diet are not in this form:

- **Oxidation of fatty acids with odd numbers of carbons** is achieved by β oxidation until a three-carbon molecule remains. This is metabolised to produce succinyl-CoA, an intermediate of the TCA cycle.
- **Branched-chain fatty acids** cannot always be oxidised in the two-carbon blocks seen in β oxidation. The enzyme α-hydroxylase is used to remove single carbon units, allowing β oxidation to proceed. This is particularly important for the metabolism of the plant-derived fatty acid phytanic acid.
- **Longer chain fatty acids** (>16–18 carbon atoms in length) are first oxidised in the peroxisomes, before being transferred to the mitochondria for β oxidation.

Fatty acid synthesis

Excess glucose and amino acids are converted to fatty acids, which are ultimately stored in adipose tissue. The reactions that mediate the production of fatty acids are very similar to those in β oxidation, although there are several important differences:

- **Different enzymes** catalyse the two processes.
- **Different locations:** synthesis occurs in the cytoplasm; β oxidation occurs in the mitochondrial matrix
- **Different carriers:** in β oxidation, the intermediates of the reaction are carried by coenzyme A whereas, in synthesis, the intermediates are carried by the acyl-carrying protein.
- **Different co-factors:** NAD^+ and FAD are co-factors for β oxidation, whereas NADPH is the co-factor for synthesis.

The key regulatory step is the production of malonyl-CoA by acetyl-CoA carboxylase. The remaining synthetic reactions proceed to add two-carbon units on to the fatty acid chain. These reactions are all catalysed by a single enzyme complex, **fatty acid synthase**.

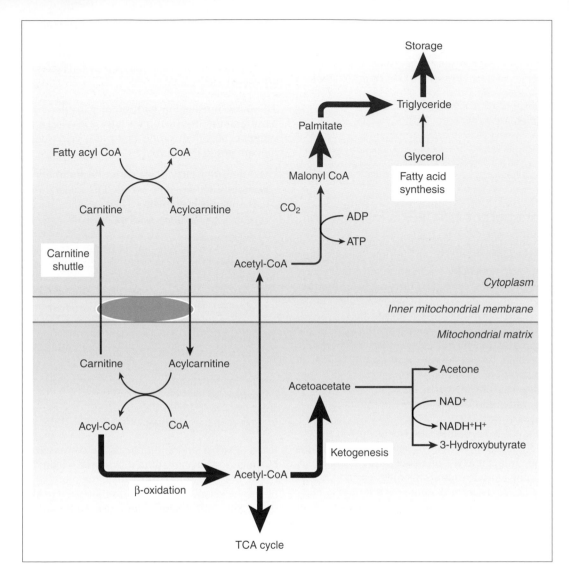

Figure 3.4 The transport and metabolisms of fatty acids. The important steps of transport, and the key metabolic reactions involving fatty acids, occur in the mitochondria and cytoplasm. Transport of fatty acids to the mitochondria is achieved via the carnitine shuttle because fatty acyl-CoA (the form in which it is found within the cell) cannot be transported across the cell membrane. The product of the breakdown of fatty acids by β oxidation is acetyl-CoA, which may be used to generate energy through entering the tricarboxylic acid (TCA) cycle. It may also be used to produce ketone bodies, which are an important source of energy in infants and in adults under starvation. Transport of acetyl-CoA to the cytoplasm allows its conversion into fatty acids by the fatty acid synthase enzyme complex, and its subsequent conversion to triglycerides for storage.

Fatty acid synthase contains several subunits on a single complex; the growing fatty acid chain is retained by an acyl-carrier protein, which is itself part of the complex. This allows rapid production through minimisation of the loss of intermediates.

The final product of fatty acid synthesis is the 16-carbon palmitate. After production, palmitate is bound to glycerol molecules to produce a triacylglyceride, which is how fat is stored in the body.

Ketogenesis

Fatty acids are mobilised and metabolised during fasting through the production of ketones by the liver. These four-carbon derivatives are water soluble and can reach high levels in the blood in prolonged fasting. In addition, they are preferentially metabolised by a wide variety of tissues, maintaining the glucose for tissues incapable of switching to another energy source. Ketone bodies are taken up by cells, where they are converted back to acetyl-CoA.

Regulation of fat metabolism

The regulation of fatty acid synthesis and β oxidation of fats by internal and hormonal signals must be integrated:

- **The presence of malonyl-CoA** in the cytoplasm inhibits the transport of fatty acids into the mitochondria, to prevent β oxidation.
- **Internal signals** may alter the activity of acetyl-CoA carboxylase. Citrate, a sign of surplus in the TCA cycle, activates acetyl-CoA carboxylase to promote the production of fatty acids. Conversely, AMP inhibits the enzyme to signal the lack of energy. Palmitoyl-CoA also inhibits acetyl-CoA carboxylase – this prevents the production of fatty acids in a cell that has already taken up large amounts of fat from the surroundings.
- **Hormonal signals** modulate the process, reflecting the state of readiness of the body as a whole. Adrenaline and glucagon both signal a need for energy and inhibit the action of acetyl-CoA carboxylase. Conversely, the presence of insulin signals the plentiful supply of glucose and promotes its conversion into fatty acids through activation of the enzyme.

Amino acid metabolism

Proteins are broken down into small peptides that are one to three amino acids long, for absorption in the gut. After this, they are converted into free amino acids for release into the circulation; these amino acids are used to synthesise new protein.

Digestion of proteins

Digestion of proteins starts in the stomach, where pepsin cleaves protein to produce peptone, a mixture of oligopeptides, which is released into the small intestine for further digestion.

The digestion of peptides in the intestines is mediated by the enzymes secreted by the pancreas. Endopeptidases, such as trypsin, cleave the peptides at specific sites to produce a series of small peptides, which can be acted on by carboxypeptidases; these remove peptides from the C terminus of a peptide chain.

Di- and tripeptides, the end-products of amino acids, are transported into the cells of the gut by specific transporters, where they are broken down into free amino acids, before release into the portal blood.

Amino acids in the diet

Many amino acids can be synthesised in the body; however, there are a few that are 'essential' – no synthetic pathway exists for them in the body. The essential amino acids include methionine, phenylalanine and tryptophan.

Excess amino acids are not easily stored so instead they are used by the TCA cycle. Depending on the site at which the amino acid joins the TCA cycle, it may contribute to the formation of fatty acids and/or glucose. During this process, the removal of nitrogen from the amino acid is essential. This occurs by producing ammonia and converting it rapidly to urea for excretion from the body.

Transamination and oxidation of amino acids

Only the carbon skeleton of amino acids is used for oxidation, so the amino element must be removed by a transaminase which transfers the amine group of the amino acid to a 2-oxoacid (Fig. 3.5).

The transaminase process typically uses 2-oxoglutarate (α-ketoglutarate) as a recipient for the amine group. 2-Oxoglutarate is itself generated from glutamate, through a reaction catalysed by the enzyme glutamate dehydrogenase. It is the generation of 2-oxoglutarate that regulates much of the transamination (and thus oxidation) of amino acids.

- ATP and GTP are **inhibitors** of glutamate dehydrogenase activity.
- ADP and GDP are **activators** of glutamate dehydrogenase activity.

The transaminases are specific to a limited range of amino acids, although almost all use 2-oxoglutarate as the acceptor.

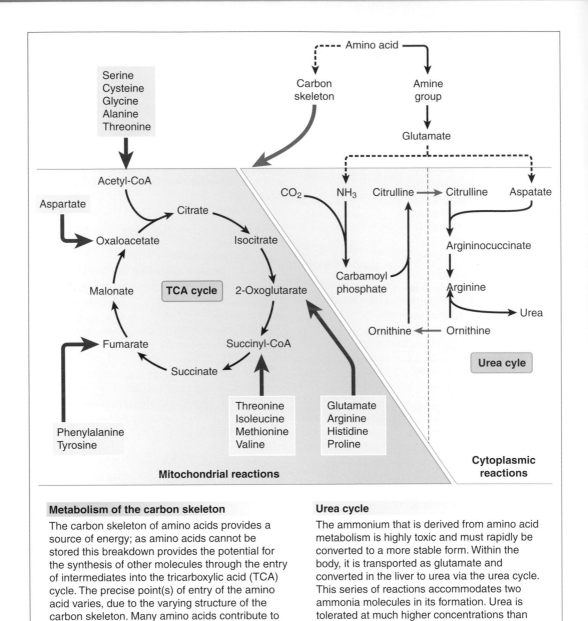

Metabolism of the carbon skeleton

The carbon skeleton of amino acids provides a source of energy; as amino acids cannot be stored this breakdown provides the potential for the synthesis of other molecules through the entry of intermediates into the tricarboxylic acid (TCA) cycle. The precise point(s) of entry of the amino acid varies, due to the varying structure of the carbon skeleton. Many amino acids contribute to the formation of TCA cycle intermediates, which have the potential to produce glucose, or other amino acids. Others contribute to the formation of acetyl-CoA, which can be metabolised or used to generate fat stores.

Urea cycle

The ammonium that is derived from amino acid metabolism is highly toxic and must rapidly be converted to a more stable form. Within the body, it is transported as glutamate and converted in the liver to urea via the urea cycle. This series of reactions accommodates two ammonia molecules in its formation. Urea is tolerated at much higher concentrations than ammonia, and can be transported freely within the bloodstream for excretion by the kidneys.

Figure 3.5 The metabolism of amino acids. The initial step in the metabolism of amino acids is the removal of the amine group – which enters the urea cycle. The remaining portion of the amino acid is processed such that parts of the carbon skeleton are broken down to a form that can enter the tricarboxylic acid (TCA) cycle.

Breakdown of D-amino acids

Although animal cells use L-amino acids in their proteins, plants and microorganisms may use D-amino acids, which humans may ingest. D-Amino acids are deaminated in an oxidative process catalysed by the FAD-dependent enzyme D-amino oxidase. After oxidative deamination, the resulting 2-oxoacids may be reaminated to produce L-isoforms, or broken down for energy.

Generation of ammonia

The excess amine groups produced by the transamination reactions must be removed from the body, either as ammonia or after its subsequent conversion to urea. Free ammonia is very toxic and is transported around the body in glutamate.

The urea cycle

Most of the ammonia produced in the body is converted into urea by the periportal cells of the liver. Urea accounts for around 90% of the nitrogen that is released in the urine. Both the ammonia and aspartate that contribute to urea formation are derived from glutamate:

• Ammonia is released from **glutamate** through **deamination** by glutamate dehydrogenase.
• Aspartate is produced by **transamination** of **oxaloacetate** by aspartate transaminase.

The reactions of the urea cycle are shared between the mitochondria and the cytosol of the cell:

• Glutamate dehydrogenase is found in the mitochondria.
• The first two reactions of the ammonia cycle occur within the mitochondria, because they provide ammonia that can be used to produce **carbamoyl phosphamide**.

The remainder of the urea cycle occurs in the cytoplasm. After synthesis, urea is released into the blood, where it is excreted from the body via the kidneys.

Regulation of the urea cycle is achieved by altering the enzyme activity at the point of entry. There is more chronic control of the cycle: high protein intake results in the upregulation of the urea cycle enzymes, and a fourfold increase may occur in 36 hours.

Location of amino acid metabolism

Metabolism in the liver

Most amino acids are ingested in amounts surplus to the body's needs in terms of protein synthesis, although a few are required in larger amounts than are typically ingested. Consequently, many amino acids are converted to other types or used to provide the body with energy. The breakdown and conversion of amino acids occur in the liver. In particular, around 30% of the amino acids ingested in the diet are glutamate or aspartate, yet these make up a very small proportion of the amino acids released from the liver.

Metabolism in the renal cortex

The kidney can deal with citrulline and glycine using them to form glucose and arginine. The production of arginine is critical to counteract its usage within the liver in several processes:

• Creatinine synthesis
• Urea synthesis
• Protein synthesis.

Functional compartmentalisation of metabolism

The organelles of a eukaryotic cell have adapted to perform specific metabolic tasks. This compartmentalisation allows the localisation of the various enzymes required to mediate a specific process. By isolating a specific pathway to a single location, regulation is helped by mediating the rate of substrate transport. Furthermore, isolation prevents potentially damaging processes in metabolism from affecting the general cell environment, through its limitation to one compartment in the cell (Fig. 3.6). Although the metabolic roles of organelles are discussed below, a more generalised outline of the function of organelles is covered in Chapter 1.

The cell membrane and the cytoplasm

The cell membrane regulates the entry into and exit from the cytoplasm of substances via the presence of transporters and channels. The cytoplasm contains many enzymes that can commit molecules to specific fates and locations.

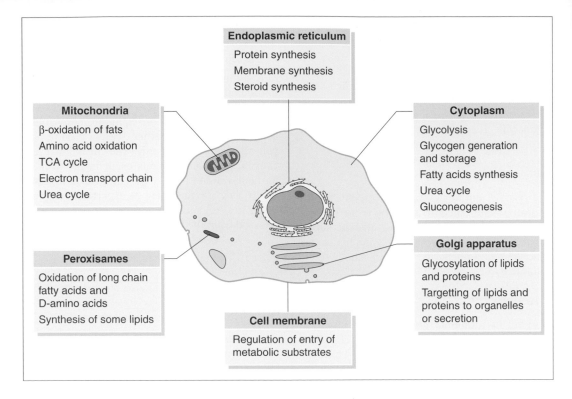

Figure 3.6 Functional compartmentalisation of metabolism. The major metabolic reactions are often compartmentalised within a single organelle. The locations of these reactions are summarised, showing that many organelles may be involved in catabolic and/or anabolic reactions within the body.

Storage of some molecules is possible within the cytoplasm, particularly glycogen which can be mobilised for glucose. In addition, the presence of signalling proteins allows the cytoplasm to integrate metabolism within the cell to ensure that conflicting pathways are not both activated.

The mitochondria

Complementing its role as the major site of energy generation in the cell, the mitochondrion is the site of breakdown of many molecules, leading to release of energy. In particular, β oxidation of fatty acids and the oxidation of amino acids occur in the mitochondrial matrix.

These processes (along with glycolysis, which occurs in the cytoplasm) feed into the TCA cycle, which also occurs in the mitochondrial matrix. The final pathway in the generation of ATP is the electron transport chain, located on the inner mitochondrial membrane.

In the liver, the mitochondrial membrane is the site of the early reactions of the urea cycle,

separating the ammonia from the rest of the cell, to reduce the damage that it may cause.

The endoplasmic reticulum and the Golgi apparatus

The endoplasmic reticulum (ER) and the Golgi apparatus are involved in synthetic processes. First, they are responsible for the production of the proteins needed for the metabolic processes occurring in the rest of the cell. More directly, the ER and Golgi apparatus are responsible for the following:

- Synthesis of **phospholipids**
- Synthesis of **membrane proteins**
- **Detoxification**
- **Assembly of sugars on glycoproteins and lipids**.

The lysosomes

Lysosomes are responsible for the breakdown of molecules into their constituent parts. These can then be transferred to other regions of the cell for reuse in synthetic reactions. Lysosomal enzymes require an acidic environment to function properly, which prevents them from acting on other regions of the cell and damaging the cell's integrity.

Peroxisomes

Peroxisomes contribute to both the oxidation of substrates and the synthesis of lipids and carbohydrates.

- **Oxidation of long-chain fatty acids** can occur in peroxisomes. This does not produce ATP; instead it produces H_2O_2 which is removed by catalase in the peroxisome, to restrict any damage that may occur if the H_2O_2 were to enter other compartments of the cell.
- **Breakdown of D-amino acids** is aided by peroxisomes, where they are converted into 2-oxoacids.
- **Synthesis of lipids can occur within peroxisomes;** in particular **bile salts** are produced in peroxisomes through modifications to cholesterol.

 CLINICAL Zellweger syndrome

Zellweger syndrome results from the lack of functional peroxisomes. The features of the condition vary, but include motor abnormalities, high forehead, epicanthus and other facial abnormalities, epileptic seizures, cataract and hepatomegaly. Given the severe nature of the condition, few individuals live longer than 6 months.

Structural biochemistry

Many of the molecules in the body are concerned with metabolism and generation of energy, and others with the reactions that maintain the state of the cell. However, other molecules contribute to the architecture and organisation of the cell, providing a framework to allow transport and compartmentalisation of the cell. The cell itself can contribute molecules to influence the architecture of the tissue in which it resides.

Intracellular architecture

In the cell, structural components contribute to three main areas:

1 The organisation of DNA
2 The cytoskeleton
3 The organisation of cellular compartments.

These areas are closely linked, but each is associated with a particular group of structures allowing a (somewhat artificial) distinction to be made.

Histones

DNA in the cell nucleus is an enormously long molecule, yet it is efficiently organised and packaged into the nucleus. Much of this packaging is achieved by histone proteins, which associate with the DNA to aid packaging and also act to regulate gene expression. The role of histones is discussed in detail in Chapter 2.

Cytoskeleton

The cytoplasm of the cell is not merely made up of fluid and ions; it contains a complex protein architecture that organises the various cellular compartments through a scaffold of fibres, allowing transport between them. Three major classes of fibres can be identified:

1 **Microtubules** (around 20 nm in diameter) contain the protein tubulin and are particularly important in intracellular transport.
2 **Intermediate filaments** (around 10 nm in diameter) are found throughout the cell, reinforcing cells and organising them within tissues, by supporting the cell membrane.
3 **Actin filaments** (around 7 nm in diameter) rapidly polymerise to produce microfilaments. These can regulate the formation of protrusions in cells, such as lamellopodia – projections of cell membranes that aid cellular migration – and changes in cell morphology, as occurs in phagocytosis.

Organisation of cellular compartments

Cellular compartments are held in place through being tethered to the cytoskeleton. This also aids vesicular transport of materials between cellular compartments. Special families of proteins allow the transport and trafficking of compartments, by exploiting the cytoskeleton's filamentous network.

Kinesin is a protein that binds to vesicles through the kinesin receptor. The other end of kinesin contains two globular heads that bind to microtubules. Hydrolysis of ATP is required to power the repeated binding and unbinding that allows a 'stepping' process; this moves the kinesin proteins along the microtubule. Microtubule fibres are defined as having a $(+)$ end, which is the end at which the microtubule is polymerised, and a $(-)$ end where the microtubule is broken down. Kinesin is a motor protein capable of moving towards the $(+)$ end.

There are processes that require movement of vesicles in the opposite direction, towards the $(-)$ end of the microtubule. This retrograde process is achieved by **dyneins** which work in a similar way to kinesin.

Extracellular architecture

Cells are organised into tissues that may be connected directly with each other and/or bathed in a surrounding material, the extracellular matrix. There are many key components in the extracellular matrix that are crucial for the organisation and integrity of the tissue. Two key components that make up a large proportion of the extracellular matrix can be observed:

- Collagen
- Proteoglycans.

Collagen

Collagen accounts for up to a third of the protein in the body. A collagen fibril is made up of a repeating unit of glycine–X–Y (where, frequently, X is proline and Y is hydroxyproline). This repeating unit of three amino acids produces a polypeptide helix with a left-hand twist. Three identical chains make up a collagen fibre, which is held together by hydrogen bonding between the different chains – there is no hydrogen bonding between residues on the same chain. The resulting fibre is a triple helix with a right-hand twist.

The collagen fibres align themselves in strong fibrous sheets, which form a large portion of the connective tissues in the body. There are different chains of collagen that can contribute to fibres. The composition of chains within a fibre allows them to associate in a variety of ways to generate covalently linked collagen fibrils or sheets with various properties. There are at least 13 types of collagen in the body, which may be found as fibrils, as sheets or in a variety of other arrangements; this is governed by the types of chain making up the fibres and the orientation of the fibres in relation to each other.

Collagen synthesis occurs from the production of procollagen chains, with large additional amino acid sequences at both their N and C termini. These regions allow chain alignment and promote the proper folding of the chains into a collagen fibre. In the extracellular space, the N and C termini are removed and collagen is linked into another collagen fibril by covalent association.

Hyaluronan and proteoglycans

Proteoglycans – large molecules made up of protein and carbohydrates – are found in all extracellular matrices. A key component is **hyaluronan**.

Hyaluronan

Hyaluronan is made up of repeating subunits of the disaccharide gluronic acid-β–N-acetylglucosamine-β. An individual molecule may have over 50 000 repeats within it, and the whole molecule folds into a coiled structure about 500 nm in diameter. The constituent subunits of hyaluronan are negatively charged, which allows the repulsive forces between the subunits to produce regions that are rigid, within the coiled structure.

Hyaluronan can provide stiffness to the extracellular matrix and yet act as a lubricant in other areas, such as joints. This is aided by the hydrophilic nature of the molecules, which allows them to bind large amounts of water to produce a hydrated gel. Hyaluronan can be bound by the cell surface receptor CD44, aiding the migration of cells in the extracellular matrix.

Proteoglycans

Proteoglycans consist of a central protein core to which large numbers of glycosaminoglycans are attached. Similar to hyaluronan, they may contribute to the nature of the extracellular matrix. Of particular importance is the molecule **aggrecan**, which is found in cartilage. This proteoglycan associates with hyaluronan to generate an enormous macromolecule that is responsible for the weight-bearing and gel-like nature of cartilage.

Some forms of proteoglycans – particularly those found in the basement membranes of epithelia – may be attached to cells, anchoring them into place in the matrix. Proteoglycans can also bind many signalling molecules (e.g. cytokines and growth factors), which retain them in the area where they were secrete, maintaining and prolonging their effect.

 DEFINITION Glycosaminoglycans

Glycosaminoglycans are long unbranched polysaccharides that are made up of repeating disaccharide units. Typically one sugar is either D-glucosamine or D-galactosamine, where the amino group has been acetylated, eliminating the positive charge of the molecule.

The negative charge in the molecule ensures that it efficiently recruits large amounts of water as well as ensuring that neighbouring glycosaminoglycan molecules are repulsive, to allow them to move past each other with ease.

RELATED CHAPTERS

4

Physiology

The function of the human body depends on ions, most importantly sodium (Na^+), potassium (K^+) and calcium (Ca^{2+}). In particular, the asymmetrical distribution of Na^+ and K^+ is responsible for the electrical excitability of cells, which allows transmission of nervous signals. Ca^{2+} is a crucial intracellular messenger that regulates many processes including release of chemical mediators at synapses and muscular contraction.

Membrane potential

The membrane potential is the voltage (electrical potential) difference across the cell membrane. In most cells, the interior of the cell is negative with respect to its exterior. Cells have different membrane potentials; the typical resting membrane potential of a neuron is −70 mV.

Ion distribution across a membrane

Three ions, Na^+, K^+ and Cl^-, are the main species that generate the membrane potential. Ca^{2+} has no role in the formation of the membrane potential, although it is a crucial **second messenger**, controlling many cellular processes. In each case, the function of the ion is aided by an **electrochemical gradient** that exists across the cell membrane.

Generation and maintenance of the resting potential

These processes are closely related and the relative contributions of different mechanisms are discussed below:

- The **resting potential** may be gradually discharged due to the small flow of ions across the membrane. To prevent this, the gradient must be **maintained** by the further active transport of ions.
- Following an **action potential**, the distribution of ions across the membrane differs considerably from their resting potential; the electrochemical gradients of Na^+ and K^+ must be re-established through active transport.

Table 4.1 Concentrations of the ions across a typical cell membrane

Ion	Extracellular concentration (mmol/L)	Intracellular concentration (mmol/L)
Sodium (Na^+)	140	15
Potassium (K^+)	4	140
Chloride (Cl^-)	110	4
Calcium (Ca^{2+})	1.0	10^{-4}

Biomedical Science Lecture Notes, First Edition. Ian Lyons.
© 2011 by Ian Lyons. Published 2011 by Blackwell Publishing Ltd.

DEFINITION **Active transport**

Active transport can move molecules against their natural diffusion gradient, so it **requires energy**. It is mediated by transport proteins in the cell membrane:

- **Primary active transport** is powered by energy derived directly from the hydrolysis of ATP.
- **Secondary active transport** is **not** powered directly by ATP and so is not really active. It uses energy stored in the **electrochemical gradient** of another molecule created by primary active transport.

 DEFINITION **Electrochemical gradient**

The **electrochemical gradient** for any ion describes the combined energy stored as a result of the difference in both ionic concentrations and electrical potentials. The electrochemical gradient is released to power important cellular functions.

The electrical and ionic concentration gradients can be in either the same or opposing directions. If the electrical and concentration gradients are opposite and balance each other, there will be no net movement of ions across the cell membrane (i.e. the movement of ions in one direction balances the movement of ions in the opposite direction). The ion is said to be in **electrochemical equilibrium**.

Ionic basis of the membrane potential

Three mechanisms contribute to the resting membrane potential:

1 Passive ionic diffusion
2 Active ionic transport
3 The Gibbs–Donnan equilibrium.

Passive ionic diffusion

Passive ion movements contribute most of the effect of the membrane potential. Charged ions can cross the membrane passively via protein channels embedded in the lipid bilayer. The passive diffusion of an ion (e.g. Na^+) across the membrane via a protein channel is determined by two factors:

1 The **electrochemical gradient**
2 The **permeability** of the membrane to the ion, resulting from the number of channels that allow the ion to flow through.

The principles of ion movement can be applied to demonstrate how passive ionic diffusion can generate a membrane potential. Consider an idealised cell that contains a high concentration of non-diffusible negatively charged proteins and that is permeable only to K^+ ions, so that there is a high concentration of K^+ inside the cell (140 mmol/L) and a low concentration of K^+ outside (4 mmol/L). The concentration gradient of K^+ from the inside to the outside of the cell will tend to drive K^+ ions out of the cell before they can completely neutralise the negative charges on the proteins. This creates a negative membrane potential – the inside of the cell is negatively charged whereas the outside is positively charged. The K^+ ions will eventually reach electrochemical equilibrium as described above. The **equilibrium potential** can be modelled by the **Nernst equation** (see below).

Only a few ions need to cross the cell membrane to maintain an electrical potential, e.g. to change the membrane potential of a cell by 100 mV, about 0.001% of the total number of K^+ ions inside the cell will cross the membrane.

Active ionic transport

Na^+/K^+ ATPase pumps three Na^+ ions out of a cell for every two K^+ ions that it transports. This results in the net movement of a **single positive charge**, which directly contributes to the generation of the resting membrane potential. Na^+/K^+ ATPase is **electrogenic** because it directly moves charge through its action. However, in the short term, this direct contribution is small – if the activity of Na^+/K^+ ATPase is stopped, the membrane potential drops by around 10 mV. Na^+/K^+ ATPase also contributes indirectly by **establishing** and **maintaining** ion gradients across the cell membrane.

The Gibbs–Donnan equilibrium

The Gibbs–Donnan equilibrium describes the contribution of impermeant (those that cannot cross the membrane) cellular anions, such as proteins, to the resting membrane potential. The cytoplasm of most cells contains many impermeant anions that contribute around $-10\,\text{mV}$ to the resting membrane potential.

The Nernst equation

The **Nernst equation** can be used to calculate the **equilibrium potential**:

$$E_X = \frac{RT}{zF} \ln \frac{[X]_i}{[X]_o}$$

where E_x is the **equilibrium potential** for the ion 'x', R and F are **constants** (gas and Faraday's constants, respectively), T is the **absolute temperature** in kelvins (K), z is the **charge of the ion** (e.g. $+1$ for Na^+, $+2$ for Ca^{2+} and -1 for Cl^-), ln is logarithm to the base e – the natural logarithm, $[X]_i$ is the intracellular concentration of the ion, and $[X]_o$ is the extracellular concentration of the ion.

If the logarithm to the base e is converted to logarithm to the base 10, and it is assumed that **the temperature is 37.5°C** and the ion has **a single positive charge** (e.g. Na^+), the Nernst equation can be simplified to:

$$E_x = -61.5\,mV \log_{10} \frac{[X]_i}{[X]_o}$$

If the intracellular and extracellular concentrations of K^+ are 140 mmol/L and 4 mmol/L respectively, as was the case in the idealised cell described above, permeable only to K^+ ions, the equilibrium potential is:

$$E_x = -61.5\,\text{mV} \log_{10} \frac{[140]_i}{[4]_o}.$$

$$= -95\,\text{mV}$$

If the intracellular and extracellular concentrations are varied, the equilibrium potential will be different.

Na^+, K^+ and Cl^- all contribute to the membrane potential in real cells, generating a membrane potential determined by not only the equilibrium potential of each ion, but also the relative permeability of the ions. The more permeable the membrane to an ion, the greater its flow across the membrane, and the greater its contribution to the membrane potential. When considering multiple ions, the membrane potential (E_m) can be determined by:

$$E_m = \frac{P_{K^+}}{P_{tot}} E_{K^+} + \frac{P_{Na^+}}{P_{tot}} E_{Na^+} + \frac{P_{Cl^-}}{P_{tot}} E_{Cl^-}$$

where E_x is the equilibrium potential of that ion, P_x the relative permeability of that ion and P_{tot} the total permeability, which is the sum of the relative permeabilities.

The permeability of a cell membrane to an ion is determined mainly by the availability of ion channels through which a particular ion can pass: membranes tend to be **most permeable to K^+ ions** because cell membranes contain many protein channels known as K^+ **leak channels**. As a result, the typical membrane potential of $-70\,\text{mV}$ lies close to the **equilibrium potential of K^+**.

Action potentials

An action potential is a rapid depolarisation of the cell **membrane potential** which travels along the length of the cell without decrease in magnitude. It occurs in excitable cells, where rapid transmission of a signal is essential; it is caused by the opening of voltage-gated channels which change membrane conductance and therefore alter the membrane potential (Fig. 4.1a). Action potentials are an **all-or-nothing response,** triggered once a threshold level of depolarisation has been reached.

> **DEFINITION Membrane conductance**
>
> Membrane conductance is a measure of how easily ions are able to cross the cell membrane and is altered by the opening of membrane channels.

Mechanism of the action potential

Action potentials can be divided into four phases (Fig. 4.1):

1 **Initiation**: a stimulus that changes membrane permeability causing a depolarisation which reaches threshold.
2 **Upstroke**: a rapid increase in membrane potential to a peak of about $+40\,\text{mV}$.

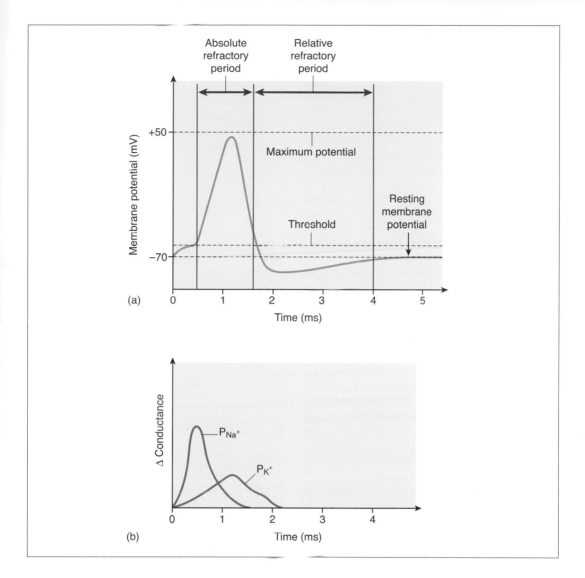

Figure 4.1 (a) **Membrane potential changes during the action potential of a typical neuron**. The cell is depolarised to threshold and then fires an action potential. A maximum potential of around $+50\,mV$ is reached before the neuron repolarises. The absolute and relative refractory periods are shown. During the absolute refractory period the neuron is unable to fire another action potential as voltage-gated channels are inactivated, although, during the relative refractory period, a larger than usual stimulus is required to generate an action potential. (b) **Changes in membrane conductance associated with the action potential of a typical neuron**. There is a rapid increase in Na^+ conductance associated with opening of voltage-gated Na^+ channels, which corresponds to depolarisation. This is followed by a slower and smaller increase in K^+ conductance caused by opening of voltage-gated K^+ channels and a decrease in Na^+ conductance as Na^+ channels inactivate. These changes correspond with the repolarisation of the neuron.

3 **Repolarisation**: a decay in the membrane potential. **After hyperpolarisation** – a transient undershoot occurs, in which the membrane potential falls below the resting membrane potential before returning to it.

4 **Refractory period**: the period following repolarisation of the cell membrane, in which triggering of a further action potential is impossible or requires a significantly stronger stimulus.

DEFINITION Depolarising and hyperpolarising currents

A **depolarising** current causes the membrane potential to become more positive, e.g. from $-55\,\text{mV}$ to $-40\,\text{mV}$.

A **hyperpolarising** current causes the membrane potential to become more negative, e.g. from $-55\,\text{mV}$ to $-60\,\text{mV}$.

Initiation of the action potential

Action potentials are initiated by a localised depolarisation of the cell membrane as a result of the opening of cation channels, leading to an increased flow of cations into the cell. In a neuron, this change usually results from the binding of a transmitter to a ligand-gated ion channel although other stimuli, such as heat and pressure, can also alter membrane permeability.

An action potential will occur if the membrane is depolarised to a **threshold value**. Those currents that do not reach the threshold value will not cause an action potential and are defined as **local circuit** currents; they rapidly decrease as they spread along the length of the cell.

 DEFINITION Threshold value

The **threshold value** is the value to which the membrane potential of a cell must be depolarised to cause an action potential through opening of voltage-gated channels.

Upstroke of the action potential

When the membrane is depolarised to its threshold potential it triggers the opening of **voltage-gated Na^+ channels**, greatly elevating the conductance of the membrane to Na^+. As more and more Na^+ channels open, Na^+ ions move into the cell down their electrochemical gradient and the membrane potential rapidly heads towards the equilibrium potential of Na^+, which is about $+65\,\text{mV}$. The peak of the upstroke of the action potential is usually around $+40\,\text{mV}$.

Voltage-gated ion channels

These channels are sensitive to membrane potential and can exist in one of three states:

1 **Closed**: there is no movement of ions but the channel will open if stimulated.
2 **Open**: ions can freely pass into or out of the cell.
3 **Inactivated**: after channel opening, voltage-gated channels become inactivated. In this state the channel does not allow the flow of ions, and cannot be opened again until the cell membrane repolarises, allowing the channel to return to its closed state.

 CLINICAL Local anaesthetics

Local anaesthetics (e.g. lidocaine) bind to the open voltage-gated Na^+ channels and, while allowing them to become **inactivated**, prevent them returning to a 'closed' state. As a result, local anaesthetics prevent voltage-gated Na^+ channels from reopening and stimulating subsequent action potentials.

Repolarisation

During repolarisation the membrane potential returns towards its resting value through two processes:

1 The **inactivation** of voltage-gated Na^+ channels
2 The **opening** of voltage-gated K^+ channels.

As the membrane potential becomes more positive, voltage-gated Na^+ channels become **inactivated** and conductance of Na^+ ions decreases. Membrane depolarisation to the threshold also affects voltage-gated K^+ channels, increasing the probability that these channels will be open. The activation of these K^+ channels is much slower than that for voltage-gated Na^+ channels, occurring at around the same time as the Na^+ channels become inactivated (see Fig. 4.1b). For this reason, they are known as **delayed-rectifier channels**; they cause an outward flow of K^+ ions which, together with inactivation of the voltage-gated Na^+ channels, quickly drives the membrane potential towards the equilibrium potential for K^+. This is usually slightly more negative than the membrane resting potential, resulting in the phase know as after hyperpolarisation.

After hyperpolarisation

There is usually a hyperpolarising after-potential, in which the membrane potential is lower than the usual resting membrane potential due to the elevated permeability to K^+ ions. As the delayed rectifier channels close, the membrane potential returns to its resting value.

Refractory period

During the refractory period the resting ionic gradients are re-established, restoring the excitability of the cell. This can be divided into two important periods:

1 **The absolute refractory period**: no further action potential can be elicited because the channels are **inactivated**.
2 **The relative refractory period**: a stronger than usual stimulus is required to elicit an action potential because many channels are still in an inactivated state. A greater proportion of the closed channels must therefore be stimulated to cause sufficient depolarisation.

Conduction of the action potential

There are two forms in which a depolarisation can be propagated along an axon:

1 **Local circuit currents** are the result of a membrane of a depolarised region drawing the charge from neighbouring regions. As this process does not require channel opening, local circuit currents move extremely rapidly along the cell membrane; however, as there is no movement of ions across the cell membrane, these currents rapidly diminish.
2 **Action potentials** are propagated along the axons of neurons through opening of voltage-gated channels, which reinforces the depolarisation of the cell membrane. As the channels must open, the speed of conduction is less rapid than for local circuit currents, but action potentials are capable of travelling along the length of an axon.

The speed of conduction increases as the **cross-sectional area of the axon** increases due to a decreased internal resistance; however, to achieve the conduction velocities required by this means alone, nerves cells would have to be exceedingly large.

In humans, most neurons are **myelinated** which increases the speed of conduction. The myelination of neurons is achieved by different cells in the peripheral and central nervous systems (CNS):

- **Schwann cells** myelinate peripheral nervous system neurons. These wrap tightly around a single axon.
- **Oligodendrocytes** myelinate CNS neurons. These cells myelinate several different axons because they project processes that wrap around the neuron to generate a myelin sheath.

> **DEFINITION Myelin**
>
> Myelin is a phospholipid layer produced within Schwann cells and oligodendrocytes; it plays an important role in insulating neurons because the cells wrap their cell membrane (containing myelin) around the neurons.

Myelin insulates the neuron and increases membrane resistance. This causes conduction along myelinated areas of the membrane by (faster) local currents. At regular intervals in a myelinated neuron, there are gaps in the myelin sheath known as **nodes of Ranvier**. Only action potentials that express a high density of voltage-gated Na^+ channels can occur at the nodes of Ranvier. **Local circuit currents** are set up between adjacent nodes of Ranvier so action potentials 'jump' rapidly between nodes, missing out whole sections of the axon. This is called **saltatory conduction**. In this way, a long nerve fibre can conduct an action potential very rapidly.

> **CLINICAL Multiple sclerosis**
>
> Multiple sclerosis (MS) is a CNS disease in which there is gradual loss of the myelin sheath surrounding neurons, affecting nerve conduction. This causes the characteristic symptoms of **blurred vision**, **limb numbness** and **vertigo**. MS is thought to be caused by an autoimmune response to myelin proteins.

Synapses

A synapse is the **junction between a neuron and its target cell**, over which a signal can be transmitted. Synapses typically occur between two or more neurons, or between a neuron and a muscle cell. However, there can be synapses between other cell types. There are two important types of synapse:

1 **Electrical synapses**: the action potential passes directly between the two cells via **gap junctions**.
2 **Chemical synapses**: the signal is transmitted between cells by a **neurotransmitter**.

Electrical synapses

The transmission at electrical synapses is **rapid** and can be **bidirectional.** Electrical synapses can be seen in the heart where **gap junctions** are found between neighbouring **cardiac muscles** and for which the rapid spread of current is important in coordinating contractions. Electrical synapses do not allow for integration of signals in the same way as chemical synapses. They are predominantly found in smooth and cardiac muscles to aid coordinated contraction of the tissues.

 DEFINITION Gap junctions

Gap junctions provide a direct physical connection between two cells, permitting passage of small molecules, such as ions and water. A gap junction is made up of two **connexons**, one from each connecting cell. Each connexon is formed from six protein subunits known as **connexins**. A complete gap junction made up of two connexons contains 12 connexins.

Chemical synapses

Chemical synapses allow communication between cells by the release of neurotransmitters across the synapse. The arrival of an electrical signal at the nerve terminal causes release of a neurotransmitter from transmitting cells, which diffuses across the synapse to the receiving cells; there it binds to receptors, altering the membrane permeability, and thus the membrane potential. The nerve terminals of neurons are typically unmyelinated and contain neurotransmitters within **vesicles** at the nerve terminal (Fig. 4.2).

 DEFINITION Neurotransmitter

A neurotransmitter is a chemical released in response to the depolarisation of a nerve terminal, which diffuses across a synapse. The neurotransmitter binds to receptors on the postsynaptic cell membrane, triggering an inhibitory or excitatory response.

In contrast to electrical synapses, chemical transmission is less rapid and **unidirectional** – at a synapse most synaptic membranes will only be able either to release neurotransmitters or to express the receptors that allow a response, not both (though the pre-synaptic membrane, which releases the neurotransmitter, may express some receptors related to the regulation of further neurotransmitter release). However, chemical synapses allow the **integration of many inputs** into a single target neuron, which is crucial for processing of signals. Chemical synapses can also be modulated presynaptically, altering its behaviour in future action potentials.

Neuromuscular junction

The neuromuscular junction (NMJ) is a specialised **chemical synapse** between a **motor neuron** and a **skeletal muscle fibre**. It is one of the best-understood synapses.

Anatomy of the NMJ

Although each skeletal muscle fibre is innervated by only **one neuron**, each neuron may branch and innervate **many skeletal muscle fibres** (the motor unit). The fine **demyelinated-terminal branches** that innervate individual skeletal muscle fibres release acetylcholine at the NMJ. The space between the motor neuron and the skeletal muscle cell is known as the **junctional cleft**. The membrane of the postsynaptic skeletal muscle cell is highly folded into **junctional folds**.

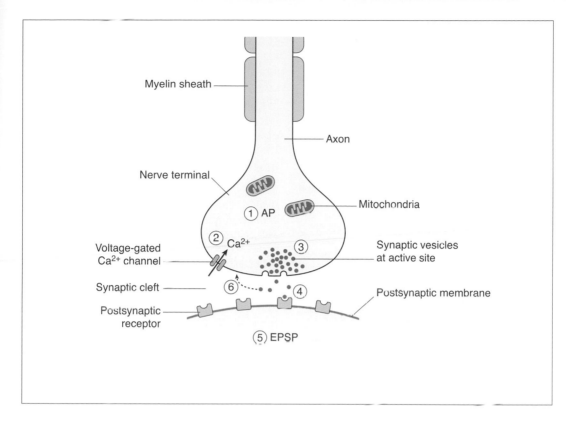

Figure 4.2 Transmission at a chemical synapse. (1) An action potential arrives at the nerve terminal of the presynaptic neuron. (2) Depolarisation causes the opening of voltage-gated Ca^{2+} channels, allowing calcium to move into the neuron, down its electrochemical gradient. (3) The rise in intracellular calcium triggers the exocytosis of the neurotransmitter into the **synaptic cleft**. (4) The neurotransmitter binds to receptors on the target cell. (5) These receptors are either **ligand gated** or **G-protein coupled** and alter membrane conductance. This results in either an **excitatory postsynaptic potential** (EPSP) or an **inhibitory postsynaptic potential** (IPSP). An EPSP is when the change in membrane conductance causes the cell to **depolarise**, whereas an IPSP is when the change in membrane conductance causes the cell to hyperpolarise. The action of the neurotransmitter is terminated by **reuptake** into the presynaptic axon, **diffusion** away from the synaptic cleft or **enzymatic breakdown** by a specific enzyme.

Physiology of the NMJ

The neurotransmitter at the NMJ is **acetylcholine**. There are several important steps involved in transmission at the NMJ (Fig. 4.3, overleaf):

- **Synthesis of acetylcholine**
- **Release of acetylcholine** from the nerve ending
- **Receptor activation and depolarisation** of the muscle fibre after binding of the neurotransmitter
- **Deactivation of acetylcholine.**

Synthesis of acetylcholine

Acetylcholine (Ach) is synthesised and stored in the nerve ending. The enzyme **choline-O-acetyltransferase** catalyses its formation from **choline** and **acetyl-coenzyme A** (acetyl-CoA):

- **Acetyl-CoA** is synthesised within the nerve ending.
- **Choline** cannot be synthesised by the neuron and is actively transported into the neuron.

Release of acetylcholine

The arrival of an action potential at a nerve ending triggers the opening of **L-type voltage-gated Ca^{2+} channels**, resulting in an inflow of Ca^{2+} ions. Increased intracellular Ca^{2+} triggers the release of ACh into the synapse by exocytosis, where it diffuses into the muscle cell.

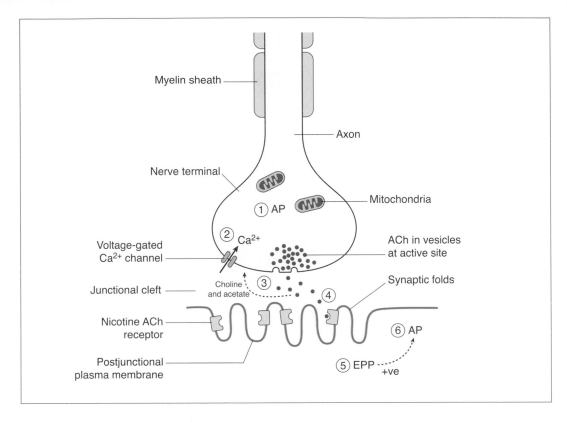

Figure 4.3 **Transmission at the neuromuscular junction**. (1) An action potential arrives in the nerve terminal of the presynaptic neuron. (2) Depolarisation causes the opening of voltage-gated Ca^{2+} channels, allowing Ca^{2+} to move into the neuron, down its electrochemical gradient. (3) Acetylcholine (ACh) is released into the junctional cleft by exocytosis in response to a rise in Ca^{2+}. (4) ACh diffuses across the junctional and binds to nicotinic ACh receptors found on the postsynaptic membrane of the skeletal muscle fibre. These are known as ligand-gated ion channels, because the binding of the ligand will cause the channel to open. The binding of ACh directly causes the opening of an ion channel. (5) The skeletal muscle fibre is **depolarised**. The depolarisation spreads to the surround cell membrane, which expresses voltage-gated Na^+ channels, triggering an action potential (6) that travels along the skeletal muscle fibre. ACh is broken down to form choline and acetate by acetylcholinesterase and the products recycled.

 CLINICAL Botulinum toxin

Botulinum toxin is a poisonous bacterial exotoxin that prevents the release of ACh from the nerve ending and causes severe motor and parasympathetic paralysis.

Receptor activation and depolarisation

Acetylcholine binds to **nicotinic acetylcholine receptors** on the muscle fibres. These are ligand-gated cation channels which open in response to binding of ACh. The membrane conductance to both Na^+ and K^+ is increased and the skeletal muscle fibre is **depolarised**; this is known as an **end-plate potential** (EPP). An action potential cannot occur at the NMJ itself, because it does not express voltage-gated Na^+ channels. Instead, the positive charge spreads by local circuit currents to the membrane surrounding the NMJ, where voltage-gated Na^+ channels are expressed, allowing initiation of an action potential. The action of ACh is terminated by the enzyme **acetylcholinesterase** which hydrolyses ACh to form choline and acetate. The components of the breakdown are reabsorbed by the synapse cells, and recycled to produce more neurotransmitter.

Pharmacology of the NMJ

There are two ways of blocking the NMJ:

1 A **depolarising blocking** agent (e.g. suxamethonium) activates the nicotinic ACh receptor to cause sustained depolarisation of the end-plate region. After an initial action potential, the membrane is unable to repolarise, preventing triggering of subsequent action potentials; the voltage-gated channels in the muscle cell remain inactivated. Depolarising blocking agents may be metabolised by acetylcholinesterase present at the NMJ.

2 A **non-depolarising** blocking agent (e.g. atracurium) is a competitive antagonist at the NMJ and so prevents the binding of ACh to its receptors.

There are two important differences between using a non-depolarising and a depolarising blocking agent:

1 Depolarising blocking agents cause **transient fasciculations** (muscle twitches) when used, which is not seen with non-depolarising agents.

2 Inhibitors of acetylcholinesterase, such as **eserine,** are effective at reversing non-depolarising blocking agents, whereas depolarising agents are unaffected by these drugs.

> **CLINICAL** **Myasthenia gravis**
>
> Myasthenia gravis (MG) is an autoimmune disease characterised by generalised muscle weakness. It is caused by antibodies that destroy the ACh receptors at the NMJ. Treatment is by anticholinesterases, which prevent the breakdown of ACh, so increasing the effective ACh concentration which helps transmission, counteracting the decreased number of receptors at the NMJ.

Skeletal muscle

Three important types of muscle – **skeletal, smooth** and **cardiac** – can be distinguished according to their properties and organisation, although the basic contractile mechanism is similar in each type of muscle. Both skeletal and cardiac muscles are classified as **striated muscle**, whereas smooth muscle is classified as **non-striated**.

> **DEFINITION** **Striated and non-striated muscle**
>
> Striated muscle (skeletal and cardiac muscle) contains filaments that have an alternating light and dark appearance when viewed under a microscope, and are said to have a characteristic 'striated pattern'. This is due to the orderly organisation of the contractile elements within the cells. In contrast, there is no regular arrangement of the contractile elements in smooth muscle and these striations are not visible.

Skeletal muscle is generally attached to the bones of the skeleton, where it maintains posture and initiates movement. It is also found in the oesophagus, where it is involved in the voluntary phase of swallowing, and in the anal and urethral sphincters.

Structure of skeletal muscle

Skeletal muscle is made up of muscle fibres, responsible for contraction and the protective covering. There are also various sensory structures to provide feedback on the state of the muscle; these are discussed in Chapter 17.

The connective tissue that protects the muscle's contractile elements comprises:

- The **epimysium**: a layer of connective tissue that surrounds skeletal muscle
- The **perimysium**: another layer of connective tissue that surrounds bundles (fascicles) of skeletal muscle fibres or **myofibres**
- The **endomysium**: a layer of connective tissue that surrounds individual myofibres bundled within the fascicles.

Ultrastructure of myofibres

Myofibres are **multinucleate cells** formed during embryonic development from the fusion of many early cells known as **myoblasts.** In myofibres, the cell cytoplasm is called the **myoplasm** and the cell membrane is called the **sarcolemma.** Deep invaginations in the sarcolemma, called **T-tubules**, are closely associated to sac-like structures known as the **sarcoplasmic reticulum** (an adapted form of endoplasmic reticulum), which contain a store of calcium ions that are released to initiate muscular contraction.

Each myofibre contains many **myofibrils**, which are bundles of protein filaments or myofilaments arranged in parallel along the length of the cell, giving the cell a striated appearance. The filaments bundled within the myofibrils are known as **myofilaments** and these are the contractile elements of the cell.

Myofilaments

There are two types of myofilament in the sarcomeres – **thick** and **thin filaments**:

1 The **thin filaments** are composed primarily of **actin**, but also contain **troponin** and **tropomyosin**. Troponin is a regulatory molecule that binds actin, tropomyosin and Ca^{2+} ions. Tropomyosin regulates the binding of actin and myosin.
2 The **thick filaments** are made of **myosin molecules**. Each myosin molecule consists of two head regions and a tail region. In a chain of myosin molecules, the tail regions are bundled together, leaving the head regions free to bind actin.

The myofilaments are divided into functional units known as **sarcomeres** (Fig. 4.4) which are distinct contractile units organised in a specific way:

- The **Z-line** is the site where the thin filaments attach to the edge of the sarcomere.
- The **I band** is the region to which the thin filaments do not extend, appearing light under a microscope.
- The **M-line** is found in the centre of the sarcomere and is the site of attachment of the myosin-containing thick filaments, which do not extend to the very edge of the sarcomere.

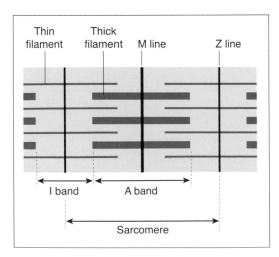

Figure 4.4 The structure of a sarcomere.

- The **A band** is where the thin and thick filaments overlap, appearing as a dense region under a microscope.

When there is a muscular contraction, the I band shortens as the thin filaments are drawn together by the contractile myosin in the thick filaments. As a result, the overlapping A band will become thicker.

Mechanism of contraction

The molecular mechanism of contraction is similar in all three types of muscle. In order to contract, muscles require ATP, as a source of energy, and Ca^{2+}, as a link between excitation and contraction.

Excitation–contraction coupling

Excitation–contraction coupling links the action potential with muscular contraction through the release of Ca^{2+}. The chain of events is as follows:

1 The action potential travels down the motor neuron to the NMJ.
2 ACh is secreted into the neuromuscular cleft and binds to nicotinic receptors on the postsynaptic membrane, causing an **end-plate potential** in the myofibre through influx of Na^+.
3 Local depolarisation spreads down the myofibre and triggers an action potential, which is propagated along the length of the myofibre.
4 The action potential spreads down the **T-tubules**, spreading the action potential to the interior parts of the cells.
5 Depolarisation of the T-tubules allows Ca^{2+} to be released from the closely associated **sarcoplasmic reticulum** (SR) through **ryanodine receptors** (RyRs) which are Ca^{2+} channels anatomically coupled to the T-tubular system. The activation of Ca^{2+} channels in the membrane triggers the release of further Ca^{2+} ions from intracellular SR.
6 Ca^{2+} flows into the myoplasm down the electrochemical gradient. **Troponin C**, a domain of troponin, then binds four ions of Ca^{2+}; this causes conformational changes in several components in **tropomyosin**, exposing binding sites are and allowing **myosin** and **actin** to interact to form cross-bridges (links between myosin and actin) and allow **cross-bridge cycling**.
7 The muscle relaxes when Ca^{2+} is pumped back into the SR by Ca^{2+} ATPase. Intracellular calcium levels are **lowered**, so that actin and myosin can no longer interact.

Troponin is a protein made up of three subunits: troponin C, I and T. Troponin C is capable of binding four Ca^{2+} ions, troponin I binds to actin and troponin T binds to tropomyosin. The latter two are both involved in the regulation of skeletal muscle contraction.

Cross-bridge cycling

The **sliding-filament** theory describes the molecular basis of contraction. During contraction, actin (thin filaments) slides across the myosin (thick filaments), which remains stationary, shortening the overall length of the myofibre. The movement of actin across myosin is generated by **cross-bridge cycling**. Myosin and actin can interact only with each other when intracellular Ca^{2+} is raised. The chain of events during cross-bridge cycling is represented in Fig. 4.5.

Rigor mortis is muscle rigidity after death; it is caused by the failure of myosin to dissociate from actin because there is no ATP. The filaments are joined for up to 72 hours after death, after which the proteins begin to degrade.

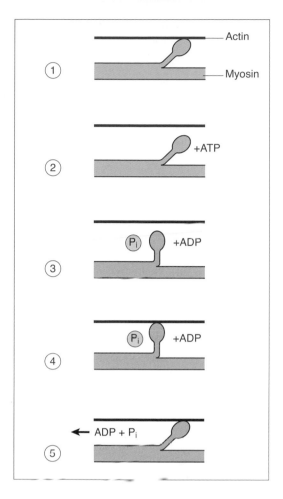

Figure 4.5 Cross-bridge cycling. (1) The myosin head is attached to actin. (2) ATP binds to myosin which causes the myosin head to dissociate from the actin filament. (3) Myosin hydrolyses ATP to ADP and inorganic phosphate (P_i). This causes a conformation change in the angle of the myosin head so that it is ready to bind to actin. (4) The head of myosin binds to actin. (5) P_i and ADP are released and this causes a conformational change in the myosin head, which completes a power stroke through $45°$, sliding the actin filament along, and myosin is ready to rebind ATP so starting another cycle.

Force of contraction

It is important that the amount of force generated by a muscle can be varied. The force of contraction can be varied both physiologically and mechanically. It can be altered **physiologically** in **two** ways:

1 The **number of motor units** recruited can be varied: the more motor units recruited, the greater the force generated.
2 The **frequency of stimulation** can be changed. A single stimulus causes a **twitch tension**. A train of stimuli allows **summation** of tension, increasing the contractile force – there is a progressive increase in cytoplasmic Ca^{2+} because there is insufficient time to remove all the Ca^{2+} released in response to the previous stimulus. If the train of stimuli is at a high enough frequency, they may cause a **fused tetanus**, which is a prolonged contraction. There is no decline in calcium levels during a fused tetanus, allowing cross-bridge cycling to generate a maximal force.

There are **three mechanical factors** that influence the force generated by a muscle.

1 There is an optimal **resting muscle length** at which the maximum number of cross-bridges can be formed, so that the most force is

generated by cross-bridge cycling. If a muscle is stretched, there will be less overlap between actin and myosin filaments; consequently fewer cross-bridges will form during contraction, reducing the force generated.

2 The **shortening velocity** will affect the force generated: the faster the velocity, the greater the force. The shortening velocity is dependent on:
  (a) the type of muscle fibre
  (b) the load against which it is acting: the heavier the load, the smaller the shortening velocity. A muscle may contract but not shorten at all – this is **isometric contraction** which is different to **isotonic contraction**, in which there is shortening against a constant load.

3 A myofibre with a larger **cross-sectional area** will contain many myofibrils, so there will be a larger number of myofilaments contributing to contraction. Training increases the cross-sectional area of myofibres rather than the number.

Cardiac muscle

Cardiac muscle generates contractile force in the heart. It shares many features of both smooth and skeletal muscle but there are also important differences: cardiac muscle is **myogenic** – contraction arises in the muscle itself and not from a motor neuron, unlike skeletal muscle.

The link between excitation and contraction in cardiac muscle again relies on Ca^{2+}. However, in cardiac muscle the source of Ca^{2+} is different. During the cardiac action potential, Ca^{2+} enters the cell via specialised calcium channels. This triggers the release of more Ca^{2+} from intracellular stores, a process known as **calcium-induced calcium release**. In a similar way to skeletal muscle, intracellular Ca^{2+} changes are able to regulate cellular contraction although the cardiac troponin molecule has only three Ca^{2+} ions.

 CLINICAL **Calcium channel blockers in the treatment of hypertension**

Antagonists of voltage-gated calcium channels, such as **amlodipine**, can be used in the treatment of hypertension because they reduce tone in the smooth muscle present in blood vessel walls.

Smooth muscle

Smooth muscle is **non-striated** and found in the walls of **blood vessels** and the lining of **hollow organs**; it is adapted to contract tonically for sustained periods of time. The degree of contraction that smooth muscle achieves is greater than both cardiac and skeletal muscle. Smooth muscle does not always require an action potential to contract and can be generally classified as two types:

1 **Neurogenic** smooth muscle which shows no spontaneous electrical or mechanical activity. It is innervated and contracts only after stimulation.
2 **Myogenic** smooth muscle shows **spontaneous mechanical activity**, although its activity can be modulated by the innervation that it receives.

Structure of smooth muscle

Smooth muscle tissue consists of sheets of smooth muscle cells that are adapted for tonic contraction. They can contract to a much shorter length but the speed of contraction is much less important. Smooth muscle cells have characteristic features:

• They are small, spindle-shaped cells 4–8 µm in diameter and 80–200 µm long, with a single nucleus. Smooth muscle cells do not possess any T-tubules and have a much smaller SR.
• There are **no cross-striations** because the thick and thin filaments are not arranged in an orderly way. Thin filaments insert into **dense bodies** rather than a Z-line. There is a much higher ratio of actin:myosin filaments which allows a greater degree of contraction.
• **Gap junctions** allow coordinated contraction of muscle cells by linking depolarisation.
• **Dense bands** allow **mechanical coupling** between the cells.

Coupling in smooth muscle

There are two forms of coupling in smooth muscle:

• **Excitation–contraction coupling** where contraction of smooth muscle follows membrane depolarisation. Depolarisation of the cell activates voltage-gated Ca^{2+} channels. Increased Ca^{2+} subsequently activates **myosin light chain kinase** (MLCK).
• **Pharmomechanical coupling** where contraction is linked to the binding of a molecule to a cellular receptor; this can either be through the direct activation of ligand-gated Ca^{2+} channels or via a second messenger system that triggers Ca^{2+} release, such as the G_q protein.

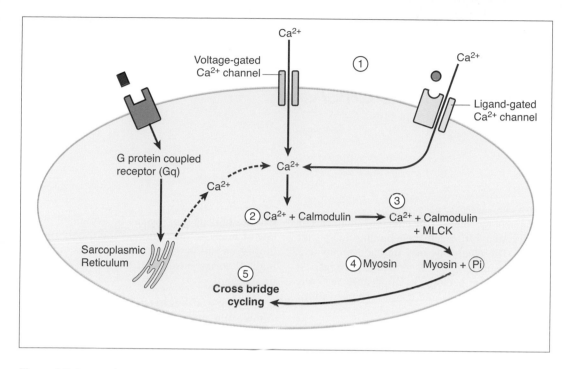

Figure 4.6 Contraction in smooth muscle. (1) There is a rise in intracellular Ca^+ caused either by influx from the extracellular fluid or release from internal stores. (2) Ca^{2+} binds to a cytoplasmic protein known as calmodulin, which can then activate an enzyme myosin light chain kinase (MLCK). (3) MLCK phosphorylates myosin. (4) Interaction between myosin and actin leads to contraction through cross-bridge cycling. (5) Contraction is terminated by the dephosphorylation of myosin by the enzyme myosin light chain phosphatase.

Mechanism of contraction

The basic molecular mechanism of contraction in smooth muscle is similar to that in skeletal muscle, although the sequence of events that triggers the cross-bridge cycle differs markedly. The following steps lead to contraction (Fig. 4.6):

1 There is a rise in intracellular Ca^+ caused by either influx from the extracellular fluid (ECF) or release from internal stores.
2 Ca^{2+} binds to a protein known as **calmodulin** which can then activate MLCK.
3 **MLCK** phosphorylates myosin light chains allowing interaction between myosin and actin; this leads to contraction through cross-bridge cycling.
4 Contraction is terminated by dephosphorylation of myosin by **myosin light chain phosphatase**. However, smooth muscle does not necessarily relax because cells can maintain contraction without cross-bridge cycling.

> **✓ DEFINITION Myosin light chain kinase**
>
> MLCK phosphorylates myosin light chain allowing cross-bridge cycling to take place; it is regulated by Ca^{2+}. In this way, it controls the contraction of smooth muscle and can be compared with the regulatory role played by troponin in skeletal muscle.

> **→ RELATED CHAPTERS**

5

Pharmacology

Pharmacology refers to the effects of chemicals on living systems, through their binding to specific targets. The chemicals may be endogenous (e.g. neurotransmitters) or exogenous (e.g. drugs). As a result pharmacology is applicable to every pathway in the body and can be exploited in the treatment of a condition.

Exogenous and endogenous molecules may act on a variety of targets, usually proteins, to modify their function. Targets include specific receptors, enzymes, ion channels and carrier proteins. The precise interactions that occur may vary: in the case of endogenous molecules, many are substrates for enzymes or carrier proteins, whereas others are signalling molecules that bind and activate receptors. Exogenous drug molecules can mimic or inhibit the behaviour of endogenous molecules, or may act as 'false substrates' to subvert specific pathways.

Crucial to a drug's action is the absorption, distribution, metabolism and excretion of a molecule, which can alter the amount of active molecule that reaches its target.

More recently the field of pharmacogenetics has emerged, whereby the drug and therapies used exploit genetic variation of an individual to improve the effectiveness of a treatment.

The principles of drug action: pharmacodynamics

The binding of a drug

For a drug or endogenous substance to act, it must bind to its target site on the molecule. The kinetics of drug binding can be explained by the **law of mass action**, whereas the theory behind how drugs bind is not well understood. Two main theories have been used to explain this interaction:

1 The **lock-and-key hypothesis** suggests that the molecule and its target are complementary and fit together, much like a lock and key. This explains how a drug and its receptor are specific, but does not serve to explain the basis of efficacy.

2 The **induced fit hypothesis** suggests that a molecule bears an almost complementary structure to its target. The interaction between the two molecules induces conformational changes that can promote or inhibit the activation of the target molecule; this gives rise to the effect that the pharmacological agent has on its target.

The kinetics of drug binding and the law of mass action

The law of mass action explains the kinetics of a drug binding to its target. It can be stated as:

> The rate of a chemical reaction is directly proportional to the effective concentrations of the reacting molecules.

In this way, the binding between the free drug molecule and its binding sites can be modelled using this law, where the binding between the drug and its receptor is reversible:

$$\text{For the binding reaction by drug A :}$$
$$A + \text{Receptor} \Longleftrightarrow A - \text{Receptor}$$

Biomedical Science Lecture Notes, First Edition. Ian Lyons.
© 2011 by Ian Lyons. Published 2011 by Blackwell Publishing Ltd.

The rate of the forward reaction, $k(\mathrm{f})$
    is directly proportional to : $X_A \times (N - N_A)$
The rate of the reverse reaction, $k(\mathrm{r})$
    is directly proportional to : N_A
At equilibrium $k(\mathrm{f}) = k(\mathrm{r})$
N is the number of drug-binding sites; X_A
    the concentration of the drug; and N_A
    the number of sites binding the drug.

In almost all cases, the number of drug molecules is far greater than the number of receptors, such that the concentration of free drug is not greatly changed by those drug molecules that bind.

> ✓ **DEFINITION Drug potency, affinity and efficacy**
>
> The potency of a drug is its ability to trigger an effect at a specific receptor. More potent drugs require much smaller doses to elicit a given effect. Potency is determined by a variety of different factors:
>
> - **Affinity**: the ability of a molecule to bind to its receptor. In most cases this binding is non-covalent and transient. The affinity provides an indication of the proportion of receptors that will be bound at any one time.
> - **Efficacy**: after binding, a drug must activate its receptor. The ability of a drug to achieve this is its efficacy; although some drugs can induce a maximal response, having bound only a small proportion of receptors, others are unable to induce a maximal response even when all the available receptors are bound because they have a lower efficacy.
> - **Potency**: the effect of a drug. This is determined by a combination of its affinity and efficacy, as well as the number of receptors present on the tissue and the access of the drug to its target.

Drug–receptor actions

For a drug to be effective it must, after binding, induce a conformational effect that activates the receptor molecule. The property is distinct from the ability to bind to the target.

The effects of drugs can be described using a log dose–response curve, where the dosage is plotted (on a log scale) against the response. The effects of drugs on the activation or inhibition of receptors can be used to describe them (Fig. 5.1):

- **Antagonists** bind receptors without activating them. Antagonists typically have an efficacy of 0 – having bound a receptor they are unable to activate it.
- **Agonists** are drugs that activate the receptors to which they bind.

Antagonists

Most drugs are antagonists – preventing the activity of their target molecule. There are different forms of antagonists, based on the site to which they bind and the nature of the binding:

- **Competitive inhibitors** bind reversibly to the same site as the substrate, without activating the receptor. The molecules **compete** with the agonists for receptor-binding sites, preventing binding of the natural ligand. This is reflected in the shift to the right of the log dose–response curve, such that a higher concentration of agonist is required to generate an equivalent effect.
- **Non-competitive inhibitors** act at a different site on the target molecule to that of the agonist, and prevent the action of the agonist, triggering a conformational change in the active site. The use of a non-competitive antagonist causes a different effect on the log dose–response curve. The maximal response is reduced, although the ability of the agonist to bind the receptor is not affected. Non-competitive antagonists reduce the number of receptors available, so a greater proportion of the remaining receptors must be bound to induce a maximal response.
- **Irreversible inhibitors** bind covalently to their target, effectively removing the molecule permanently as a target.

Competitive

The addition of a competitive inhibitor results in a rightward shift of the response curve, which is proportional to the concentration of the competitive inhibitor. As the name suggests competitive inhibitors compete for the same sites as the drug, such that a higher concentration of the agent is required to ensure that necessary number of sites are occupied to induce a response of particular magnitude.

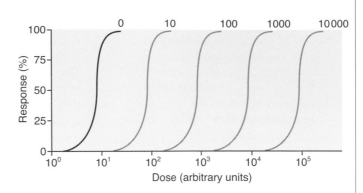

Non-competitive

A non-competitive inhibitor acts on a different site of the target molecule to that of the normal ligand. As a result it effectively removes a proportion of the receptors from binding their natural ligand. The progressive increase in the dose can be such that a large enough proportion of the receptors can be effectively removed, so that the natural ligand will not be able to elicit a maximal response, at any concentration.

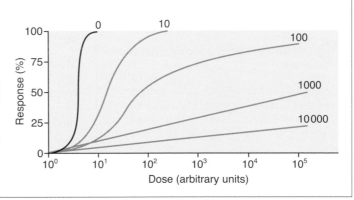

Figure 5.1 Drug dose-response under competitive and non-competivite inhibitors. When the response of a pharmacological agonist is plotted against the log of the dose administered, a characteristic sigmoidal curve is generated. The dose refers to the amount of agent reaching the receptor, and in a physiological situation this may be modulated by the agent's metabolism and the access that it has to its target receptor. The administration of antagonists alters the properties of the log dose–response curve. Here for varying doses of drugs competitive and non-competitive inhibitors have very distinct effects on the response at a given dose. Here, the dose of the inhibitor (arbitrary units) is given next to the appropriate dose-response curve.

 DEFINITION Pharmacological agents

Two groups of pharmacological molecules can be determined:

1 **Endogenous agents** are produced by the body itself to elicit a change, such as hormones and neurotransmitters.
2 **Exogenous agents** originate outside the body but can exert an influence on an endogenous system, by promoting or inhibiting its activation. Some exogenous agents may act indirectly, through modulation of the release or metabolism of an endogenous agent.

 CLINICAL Physiological antagonists

Some conditions can be treated by physiological antagonists, which oppose the symptoms of a problem, but do not act through the same receptor pathway, e.g. in asthma, a bronchodilator is administered to counteract the bronchoconstriction resulting from the various inflammatory mediators.

Agonists

Most endogenous signalling molecules are agonists:

- **Full agonists** elicit a maximum response from target cells if given in an appropriate concentration. This is through a combination of a high **affinity** for the target and a high **efficacy** to activate the receptors once bound.
- **Partial agonists** are unable to generate a maximal response even if every available receptor is bound; although they may have a high **affinity**, they usually have a low **efficacy**. Partial agonists can be used as **competitive inhibitors**, by preventing the binding of the natural agonist to sufficient target receptors to elicit a maximal response.

Targets of drug action

Any molecule in the body is a potential drug target. Four classes of molecules, which cover the majority of drug targets, can be identified:

1 Receptors
2 Ion channels
3 Enzymes
4 Carrier proteins.

Receptors

In the body, signals must be passed between different tissues and organs by the transmission of chemical or electrical signals around the body. Chemical transmission requires the binding of a transmitter to its target receptor.

Receptors can vary enormously in the response that they elicit and its time course. Similarly, the magnitude of the response may range from a brief depolarisation of a cell to a massive change in the entire gene expression profile of the cell. Based on the structure and nature of the downstream effects, four types of receptor can be distinguished (Fig. 5.2):

1 Ligand-gated ion channels
2 G-protein coupled receptors
3 Enzyme-linked receptors
4 Nuclear receptors.

Ligand-gated ion channels

Ligand-gated ion channels are the fastest-acting form of receptor. The binding of a ligand triggers a rapid conformational change in the structure of the protein, allowing a channel to open through which ions flow. A key role of such channels is in the neuromuscular junctions, where depolarisation of the cell is triggered by the functions of the nicotinic acetylcholine receptor, which is a cation channel. Ligand-gated ion channels exhibit a series of features:

- **Rapid response** (milliseconds)
- **Short-term effect**, usually complete within seconds, although channels can induce other elements leading to longer-term effects
- The **effects are specific,** typically limited to individual cells.

G-protein-coupled receptors

G-protein-coupled receptors (GPCRs) create a slower, although larger, response than the ligand-gated ion channels. GPCRs are associated with trimeric **GTP-binding proteins** in the cytoplasm. The binding of a ligand to its receptor causes activation and release of the associated G-protein, which modulates specific **second messenger pathways** in the cell.

G-protein structure

G-proteins are made up of three subunits – α, β and γ. When associated with a GPCR, they are typically in an inactivated state, in which the protein is associated with a molecule of GDP. Activation of the G-protein results from the displacement of the GDP molecule by a molecule of GTP.

The binding of GTP to the G-protein causes it to dissociate; $G\alpha$ is released from $G\beta\gamma$. $G\alpha$ travels across the membrane and binds to specific enzymes, modulating a second messenger cascade.

The G-protein contains a GTPase that can hydrolyse GTP to deactivate the G-protein. GDP-$G\alpha$ cannot activate second messenger enzymes and reassociates with a $G\beta\gamma$ subunit.

Types of G-protein

Various different G-proteins exist, which associate with specific receptors, to modulate specific second messenger cascades.

- G_s **activates adenylyl cyclase** to increase the levels of cAMP in the cell.
- G_i **inhibits adenylyl cyclase** to reduce the levels of cAMP in the cell
- G_q **activates the protein kinase C** (PKC), resulting in an increase in the cytoplasmic concentration of Ca^{2+}.

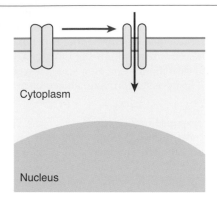

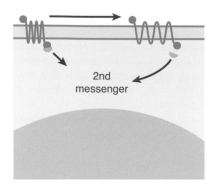

Ligand gated

Ligand-gated ion channels are the most rapidly acting class of receptor. The binding of the ligand to its binding site triggers a conformation shift in the receptor, opening a channel to allow the passage of ions into, or out of, the cell down their electrochemical gradient. The specificity of the ions is determined by the structure of the channel.

GPCR

Protein receptors bind a ligand on the extracellular side, which triggers the activation of G proteins, which are found on the cytoplasmic side. The activation triggers the separation of the α subunit from the $\beta\gamma$ subunits and allows the α subunit to activate a variety of second messenger cascades or directly act on other proteins within the cell to modulate their function.

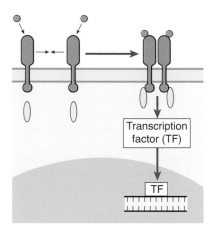

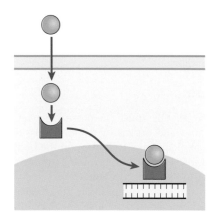

Tyrosine kinase

The binding of the ligand to the extracellular part of the enzyme-linked receptor, and its subsequent dimerisation with another receptor, allows activation of the downstream pathways. Typically this results in the phosphorylation of tyrosine kinases, which leads to a signalling cascade that alters the activation and transcription of genes within the nucleus. Other downstream mechanisms may also be recruited. Instead of tyrosine kinases, some enzyme-linked receptors activate the second messenger molecule cGMP.

Steroid

Steroid hormones are lipid soluble and pass through the cell membrane to bind directly to their receptors in the cytoplasm. The binding of the ligand to its receptor triggers its translocation to the nucleus, where it can bind to specific DNA sequences and modulate the expression of genes. In this way steroid receptors can trigger huge changes in gene expression within a cell, although the induction of a response is relatively slow because new proteins must be synthesised subsequent to the modulation of transcription.

Figure 5.2 **Classes of receptor**. There are four main classes of receptor found in the body; they vary both in their mechanisms of action and in the site and longevity of their effects. TF, transcription factor.

Alternative methods of activation of GPCRs

Although most GPCRs are activated by the binding of an endogenous ligand, there are two major exceptions in which other mechanisms trigger the activation of proteins in this family:

1 **Rhodopsin** in the retina is activated by light, causing a change in the conformation of the pre-bound retinal molecule.
2 The **thrombin receptor** is activated by thrombin, cleaving a proportion of the N-terminus of the receptor. This cleavage exposes a series of residues that can bind to and activate the receptor itself, as a 'tethered agonist'.

Targets of G-proteins

G-proteins, depending on their subtype, can act to promote or inhibit many different proteins. There are three main paths through which they act:

1 Cyclic nucleoside monophosphates
2 Calcium signalling
3 Modulating ion channels.

Enzyme-linked receptors

Enzyme-linked receptors develop enzymatic activity in their intracellular domain on binding an appropriate ligand to the receptor's extracellular domain. The signal transduction of enzyme-linked receptors typically requires the receptors to dimerise, after the phosphorylation of specific domains. The net result of this phosphorylation is the activation and translocation of transcription factors to the nucleus. Many of these factors are associated with regulating cell growth and the cell cycle. The following are two particularly common examples of this system:

1 **Tyrosine kinases** (e.g. the insulin receptor): activation of a tyrosine kinase receptor results in the enzyme catalysing the phosphorylation of specific tyrosine residues on target proteins. In turn, this modulates further enzymes downstream of the receptor to induce widespread cellular effects.
2 **Guanylyl cyclase**: the second messenger cGMP can be produced after the activation of guanylyl cyclase in the cytosolic domain of some receptors. The elevated cGMP activates cGMP-dependent protein kinases to mediate a variety of different effects through the phosphorylation of target proteins. The gaseous messenger **nitric oxide** acts by triggering guanylyl cyclase production in the target cell.

Intracellular receptors

Intracellular receptors are typically nuclear factors that cause long-term changes induced over the course of hours and days. Due to their intracellular location these receptors often bind thyroid and steroid hormones which, being fat soluble, are capable of diffusing directly into a cell.

Intracellular receptors all share a similar structure and, in most cases, are found in the cytosol until they bind their ligand, upon which they travel to the nucleus. Typically, nuclear receptors dimerise before they become active – the dimers form with either the same receptor or different factors. Occasionally, receptors are bound to DNA in an inactive state, maintained by the presence of an inhibitory complex. The binding of the ligand triggers the inhibitory complex to dissociate.

Binding of the ligand recruits activating proteins, to initiate gene transcription. This initial activation targets a few genes and occurs in the course of minutes, resulting in the primary response. The protein products of the primary response will, in turn, act on other genes to produce a larger, secondary response. The precise nature of the response caused depends on both:

- Which intracellular receptor has been activated
- The molecules and transcription factors already expressed in the cell, which can be determined by both the cell type and other signals that it receives.

Ion channels

Ions cannot pass across the cell membrane because of their charged nature. Any transport into, or out of, the cell is achieved through the ion channels or carrier proteins. There is a variety of channels which can be categorised based on:

- their selectivity for an ion species
- the mechanism of gating
- their molecular architecture.

Selectivity

Channels may vary in their selectivity. The nature of the selectivity is determined by the size and charge of the pore in the channel. Some channels are broadly selective for ions (e.g. the nicotinic acetylcholine receptor is selective for cations), whereas others may be far more restricted to a single species of ion (e.g. the L-type Ca^{2+} channel):

Gating

The three main forms of ion channels classed by gating are:

1 Voltage-gated ion channels
2 Ligand-gated ion channels
3 Mechanically gated ion channels.

Voltage-gated channels

Voltage-gated ion channels open in response to changes in the cell membrane potential (usually depolarisation), permitting the flow of ions down their concentration gradient. This is typically seen in the propagation of an action potential in a cell. Voltage-gated channels may also have an **inactivated** state, to ensure membrane repolarisation before they can reopen.

Ligand-gated ion channels

The binding of a specific ligand to its target channel triggers a conformational shift in the structure of the channel to promote opening. The ligand that triggers the opening of the channel typically binds to a site in the extracellular domain of the receptor, and the rapid opening that occurs is advantageous in **synaptic transmission**.

There are some channels where the ligand-binding site is found in its cytoplasmic portion, allowing the channel to open in response to changes in the cell's internal condition (e.g. the ATP-sensitive K^+ channels in β cells).

Although ligand-gated ion channels are typically found on the cell membrane, they can be found at other locations in the cell. In particular, the endosomal compartment may be used as a store for the release of Ca^{2+} into the cytoplasm. Inositol 1,4,5-trisphosphate (IP_3) or ryanodine receptors on the sarcoplasmic reticulum (a specialised form of endoplasmic reticulum) can bind IP_3 or cytoplasmic calcium, respectively, triggering the opening of channels and release of Ca^{2+} from the stores; in the muscle this is used to regulate contractions.

Mechanically-gated ion channels

Some channels open in response to mechanical deformation of the tissue.

Modulation of receptor gating

Many drugs and pharmacological compounds modulate the behaviour of ion channels. These compounds do not directly trigger or inhibit the opening of channels; rather they change the response of the channel to its natural ligand:

- **Binding of ligand to modulatory sites**: distinct from the ligand-binding site. These increase or decrease the likelihood of a channel opening in response to the ligand binding.
- **Indirect modulation of channel opening**: many compounds act through the modulation of different pathways (particularly through the opening or closure of G-protein-coupled channels) resulting in covalent modification of the protein, especially through phosphorylation, to alter the channel's behaviour.
- **Intracellular signals**: many channels possess modulatory sites in their intracellular domains, permitting internal signals such as Ca^{2+} or ATP to modulate the behaviour of the channel.

Intracellular pathways

In most cases, the binding of a ligand to its appropriate receptor modulates a second messenger pathway. Second messenger systems have two main benefits:

1 **Amplification of responses** – the binding of a single molecule to its receptor can contribute to the activation of many second messenger molecules.
2 **Integration of responses** – a variety of different receptors may target a single second messenger pathway, allowing many different stimuli to be integrated through a common second messenger pathway.

Many different second messenger pathways exist, although there are three particularly prominent examples (Fig. 5.3):

1 Cyclic adenosine monophosphate (cAMP)
2 Cyclic guanosine monophosphate (cGMP)
3 Ca^{2+}.

Cyclic adenosine monophosphate (cAMP)

Production

cAMP is produced from ATP by the enzyme adenylyl cyclase.

Actions

cAMP activates a variety of proteins, in particular protein kinase A (PKA). PKA is made up of four subunits – two regulatory and two catalytic. The binding of cAMP to each regulatory subunit results in their dissociation from the catalytic subunits, allowing PKA activity. The cAMP is rapidly inactivated through the action of cyclic nucleotide phosphodiesterase, which converts cAMP into a 5′-AMP molecule. The action of PKA ceases with the re-association of the regulatory subunits with the catalytic subunits.

Effects

Increased cAMP levels result in the phosphorylation of many cellular proteins through the action of cAMP-dependent protein kinases, causing many effects, including:

- **Activating phosphorylase kinase**, which acts on many metabolic enzymes to promote the breakdown of glycogen
- **Promoting the breakdown of lipids** through the activation of hormone-sensitive lipase
- **Activating L-type Ca^{2+} channels** in the cardiac myocytes to promote cardiac contraction.

Pharmacological modulation of cAMP

The predominant mechanism by which cAMP levels are modulated is through the activation or inhibition of the GPRCs which act through G_i or G_s. In addition, increased cAMP levels can be achieved through inhibition of the phosphodiesterase enzymes that degrade cyclic nucleotide monophosphates.

Methylxanthines act in this manner. They are occasionally used in the treatment of asthma. This class of drug also includes active compounds found in tea and coffee.

Cyclic guanosine monophosphate (cGMP)

Production

cGMP is produced by the enzyme guanylyl cyclase and is not usually regulated by G-proteins; rather, it is directly coupled to a receptor. cGMP is a more specialised messenger than cAMP. In addition, the gaseous messenger nitric oxide (NO) can diffuse into cells and activate cGMP production. This is a crucial mechanism in endothelium-mediated vasodilatation.

Actions

cGMP mediates its effects through the activation of a variety of different cGMP-dependent protein kinases and is selectively degraded by the enzyme phosphodiesterase type V.

Pharmacological modulation

There are relatively few drugs that target cGMP. There are two main sites of action in the cGMP pathway:

1 **NO donors** (e.g. glyceryl trinitrate) release NO, which activates cGMP synthase. They are potent vasodilators, often used to treat angina.
2 **Phosphodiesterase inhibitors** (e.g. sildenafil citrate), which inhibit degradation of cGMP, are used to aid erection by causing vasodilatation in the blood vessels of the corpus cavernosum.

Calcium

The concentration of free calcium is much higher outside the cell than inside it (2.4 µmol/L vs 0.1 µmol/L). Ca^{2+} is a crucial second messenger in cells and can be either released from intracellular stores or obtained extracellularly. Ca^{2+} in cells is commonly regulated through the phospholipase C/inositol phosphate pathway. This pathway is regulated through the signalling of G-proteins, namely G_q, which regulate the breakdown of the membrane lipid phosphatidylinositol 4,5-bisphosphate (PIP$_2$) and activation of phospholipase C (PLC), through G-protein subunits (G_q). PLC catalyses the breakdown of PIP$_2$ into two subunits that promote an increase in Ca^{2+}:

- **Inositol 1,4,5-trisphosphate** acts on the IP$_3$ receptor, a ligand-gated ion channel, increasing the concentration of free Ca^{2+} within the cytoplasm.

- **Diacylglycerol** (DAG) activates protein kinase C (PKC), which phosphorylates many intracellular proteins. Most PKC isoforms require an increased level of Ca^{2+} to become activated, which is induced through G-protein signalling.
- Ca^{2+} itself is capable of binding to many enzymes in addition to PKC, to modulate their activity.

Other targets of drug molecules

There are a few other mechanisms by which drugs may act that are usually specific to individual classes of drugs. In particular:

- **Sequestration of cellular proteins**, e.g. colchicine inhibits the structural protein tubulin
- **Modulation of the osmolality of a fluid compartment**, e.g. osmotic diuretics.

Cell-to-cell communications

Cell-to-cell junctions permit the passage of small soluble molecules and ions between cells. This is important in the communication between some epithelial cells, and also within cardiac and smooth muscles to coordinate contractions. These junctions are made up of many connexin proteins on each cell, which are linked to form a connexin channel. Many different connexin proteins exist, which can give channels different permeabilities to different molecules.

Modulation and regulation of pharmacological responses

The repeated administration of a drug may result in changes in the response elicited. In particular, desensitisation and modulation occur widely in the body.

Desensitisation

The repeated administration of a drug can result in a decrease in the effect that a given dose has. This desensitisation can be divided into two types, although the distinction is not well defined:

1 **Tachyphylaxis** is a rapid desensitisation to a drug, which may occur over the course of minutes.
2 **Tolerance** is a more gradual and long-term decrease in the response to an agent.

A variety of mechanisms may be responsible for desensitisation:

- Change in the receptors
- Loss of receptors
- Exhaustion of mediators
- Increased metabolic degradation
- Physiological adaptation.

Change in receptors

A change in the conformation of a receptor, or its modification (e.g. phosphorylation), can alter the behaviour of the receptor. In ligand-gated ion channels, such a change can be rapid – often a conformational change in the receptor, such that it binds to its ligand without resulting in channel opening. This is seen in voltage-gated Na^+ channels in the action potential; it results in a refractory period to allow re-establishment of the ion gradients so that another action potential can be propagated.

In GPCRs, three steps of modification can occur to modulate receptors. At each step, the desensitisation is more pronounced and recovery takes longer:

1 The **phosphorylation of serine residues** in the receptor's cytoplasmic tail can result in desensitisation, such that the receptor is less able to activate its G-protein, despite binding of the appropriate ligand.
2 The protein **arrestin may bind to phosphorylated serine**, which further limits receptor activity and may mark it receptor for internalisation.
3 The **receptors may be internalised** by **endocytosis**.

Loss of receptors

Prolonged exposure to an agonist can promote the gradual removal of receptors through endocytosis. As a result, a progressively larger dose of an agent is required to mediate a similar effect, because there are fewer targets on which the agent may act.

Exhaustion of mediators

Desensitisation can result from a decrease in the availability of an endogenous ligand. This can be through either release of the agent faster than it can be produced or depletion of an intermediate.

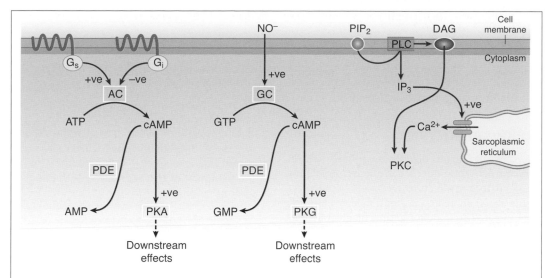

cAMP

Cyclic AMP is a very common second messenger pathway. It is commonly altered by the G proteins Gs and Gi, which promote and inhibit the activity of adenylyl cyclase respectively. Adenylyl cyclase (AC) is the enzyme responsible for converting ATP in the cell into cAMP.

The cAMP primarily acts by binding to, and thus activating, the enzyme protein kinase A (PKA), which goes on to phosphorylate many other enzymes downstream, to trigger many other intracellular pathways. It is degraded via the action of phosphodiesterase (PDE), which converts cAMP into its active form AMP.

cGMP

Cyclic GMP functions in a similar way to cAMP, and is produced from GTP, by the enzyme guanylyl cyclase (GC). GC is activated by a variety of methods, most notably by the gaseous molecule nitric oxide (NO). The resulting cGMP activates the enzyme protein kinase G (PKG), which triggers further pathways downstream. The cGMP is degraded to GMP through the actions of type V PDE.

Ca²⁺

The Ca^{2+} is a crucial signalling pathway, responsible for many biological processes, including exocytosis, and muscular contraction. The major trigger of Ca^{2+} is activation of the enzyme phospholipase C (PLC). This can be triggered by many methods, in particular, the G protein Gq. PLC triggers the breakdown of the phospholipid phosphatidylinositol-4,5-bisphosphate (PIP_2) into diacyglycerol (DAG) and inositol-1,4,5-trisphosphate (IP_3).

IP_3 acts on its specific receptor within the cell which triggers release of Ca^{2+} from the endoplasmic reticulum to increase the cytoplasmic concentration. At the same time the DAG, together with Ca^{2+}, can activate the enzyme protein kinase C (PKC). Many different forms of PKC can be found, with different downstream targets. The activation of PKC triggers a downstream effect. In addition, the increased Ca^{2+} within the cytoplasm can bind to and activate a variety of other enzymes, such as the activation of calmodulin to trigger muscular contraction.

Figure 5.3 Second messenger pathways. Second messenger pathways integrate the signals caused by the binding of receptors at the cell surface with internal signals, altering many intracellular systems. In each case the pathways focus on the activation of enzymes, which are typically associated with phosphorylation. AC, adenylyl cyclase; DAG, diacylglycerol; GC, guanylyl cyclase; IP_3, inositol 1,4,5-trisphosphate; NO, nitric oxide; PDE, phosphodiesterase; PIP_2, phosphatidylinositol 4,5-bisphosphate; PKA, PKC, PKG, protein kinase A, C and G; PLC, phospholipase C.

Physiological adaptation

Many agents perturb homoeostatic systems. As a result the body adapts to counteract the response, e.g. the effects of thiazide diuretics gradually decrease as the renin–angiotensin system becomes progressively activated.

Action on enzymes

Enzymes are involved in the synthesis and/or breakdown of compounds in the body; modulating their activity can affect a wide variety of pathways within the body which is a particularly common drug target. Three main pharmacological actions can target enzymes:

1 Enzyme inhibitors
2 False substrates
3 Prodrugs.

Enzyme inhibitors

Enzyme inhibitors are the most common form of agent. Common examples of such drugs are the cyclooxygenase COX-2 inhibitors used to treat acute inflammation.

 CLINICAL COX-2 inhibitors

COX-2 is an important inflammatory enzyme and the target of many non-steroidal anti-inflammatory drugs. These can be broken down into two groups:

1 **Aspirin** irreversibly inhibits COX-2. This property allows aspirin to be used as an anticoagulant, because it can effectively remove platelet COX-2. As platelets are not nucleated, they are unable to synthesise new COX-2
2 **Ibuprofen** and other COX-2 inhibitors are competitive inhibitors. Although they are able to reduce inflammation, they do not have the antiplatelet activity of aspirin.

COX-2 inhibitors also inhibit the housekeeping gene, *COX-1*. This can lead to damage to the gastric mucosa, because COX-1 mediated production of prostaglandins normally inhibits acid secretion. As a result, gastric ulceration, nausea, bleeding and vomiting are all well-recognised side effects of treating with COX-2 inhibitors.

False substrates

False substrates are metabolised by their target enzyme to produce a molecule that is not usually found within the body. False-substrates exert actions in two ways:

1 Through competing with the natural substrate for the enzyme
2 Through generating an abnormal product that is improperly used by the downstream pathways. Nucleoside analogues (e.g. lamivudine) used in the treatment of HIV are examples of this type of drug.

Prodrugs

Prodrugs are given to the recipient in an inactive form and are activated by enzymatic conversion in the body, e.g. L-**dopa** is given to treat **parkinsonism** and must be converted to dopamine at the blood–brain barrier; this then acts in the substantia nigra.

Action on carrier proteins

Many molecules used by cells are not lipid soluble, and must enter cells through a variety of carrier protein mechanisms. Through modulation of the activity of a carrier protein, the availability of the molecules that it transports can be altered, affecting the rate of reaction of all pathways dependent on that compound. Three major classes of agents can target carrier proteins:

1 Inhibitors
2 False substrates
3 Normal compounds.

Inhibitors

Inhibitors prevent the transport of the physiological target of the transport protein. Such compounds are often used at synapses to modulate stores of neurotransmitters. A common class of compounds used to treat depression is the **tricyclic antidepressants** which inhibit the reuptake of noradrenaline at synapses.

False substrates

False substrates are compounds that, although transported by the carrier, cannot be appropriately used by the systems in the cell. They act by out-competing the natural ligand for the carrier protein or specific elements of the downstream pathway, because they cannot be fully metabolised into an active product.

Normal compounds

In some cases, where disease results from the deficiency of a specific molecule, treatment can be efficiently managed through replacement of this molecule. This is often used to treat hormonal disorders such as **Addison's disease**, whereby cortisol is supplied by regular injection because the adrenal gland is unable to produce sufficient amounts.

Pharmacokinetics

The effect of a drug depends not only on its precise actions with a target receptor, but also through the administration, distribution, metabolism and excretion of the agent in the body. This can alter its availability at the site of the target receptor. Pharmacokinetics refers to the processes that affect the availability of a drug to its target and can be divided into four main areas:

1 Administration
2 Distribution
3 Metabolism
4 Excretion.

Administration of a drug

The rate at which a drug is absorbed into the body is dependent on three major factors:

1 Route of administration
2 Chemical nature of the compound
3 Formulation.

 DEFINITION Bioavailability

Bioavailability is the fraction of a drug dose that reaches the systemic circulation via a specific route, in comparison with intravenous administration (which, by definition, has a bioavailability of 1, whereas all other routes will be between 0 and 1).

The precise route of administration depends on the target site of the drug, and the rate at which absorption is required, as well as the convenience of the individual taking the drug. Four broad routes of administration can be identified:

- Through the mucosa
- By inhalation
- By injection
- By topical application.

Mucosal absorption

Absorption of a drug through the mucosa is the route of choice for most drugs. The large surface area of the mucosa allows the drugs to be absorbed into the bloodstream, and, although slower and more difficult to regulate than intravenous routes, there is no need for injection.

Sublingual administration

Absorption by this route is directly into the bloodstream, permitting a rapid effect and also avoiding potential breakdown if the compound is unstable at the low pH of the gut. In addition, the drugs avoid entering the portal system enter the bloodstream without the potential for metabolism within the liver. Glycerol trinitrate is typically administered in this fashion.

Oral administration

Many drugs are administered orally, because it is a convenient way for patients to take them. Absorption of the agent occurs typically in the gastrointestinal tract, although little usually occurs until the small intestine. Weak acids can be absorbed in the stomach, although the vastly larger (about 1000 times) surface area of the intestines results in it being the favoured site of absorption for almost all drugs. Absorption in the gut relies on diffusion and the factors regulating absorption are the same in the gut as for any other barrier:

- Membrane solubility
- Diffusivity
- Concentration gradient.

There are some drugs (e.g. proteins) that cannot be given orally. Passage through stomach acid and the gastrointestinal enzymes is likely to break down the agent so that it is not effectively absorbed.

Partitioning through pH and the Henderson–Hasselbalch equation

In general, lipid-soluble substances are better absorbed; strong acids and bases are poorly absorbed because they remain fully ionised in the gut. Most drugs that are administered through orally are weak acids or bases, which exist within the body in both ionised and non-ionised forms.

The weaker the acid or base, the more readily absorbed it will be because less of the drug is in the ionised form. Even if there is only a small proportion in the non-ionised form, the large surface area of the gut ensures that a significant proportion can be absorbed.

The kinetics of dissociation are determined by the Henderson–Hasselbalch equation. For a weak base, in the body it exists in equilibrium:

$$\text{For a } weak \text{ base}: XH^+ \Longleftrightarrow X + H^+$$
$$\text{For a } weak \text{ acid}: YY^- + H^+.$$

The dissociation constant for the reaction is given as the pK_a, which would be the pH if the protonated and unprotonated forms of the drug were to exist at the same concentration:

$$pK_a = pH + \log_{10}[\text{Protonated compound}]/$$
$$[\text{Unprotonated compound}].$$

In most cases the Henderson–Hasselbalch equation provides a good calculation of the pK_a, although it has two assumptions that may affect the values at particularly high or low concentrations:

- The dissociation of H_2O to H^+ and OH^- has no effect.
- Once the concentrations of the protonated and unprotonated forms of the compound have been established, they do not change.

Factors affecting absorption of a drug

In general, around 75% of an orally administered drug is absorbed in 1–3 hours. Three major factors can alter this:

1 Gastrointestinal motility
2 Blood flow
3 Particle size and formulation.

Gastrointestinal motility

The motility of the gastrointestinal (GI) tract has a potentially huge effect on absorption. Conditions such as migraines and diabetic neuropathy can reduce the GI motility, increasing absorption from the gut. In addition, excessive GI motility may result in impaired absorption if the drug has insufficient time for absorption.

Drugs themselves may alter GI motility and thus affect their own absorption, or the absorption of other agents that have been co-administered, e.g. metoclopramide increases GI motility and is often given with analgesics in those who have migraines to counteract the GI stasis that occurs in this condition.

Blood flow

A reduced blood flow decreases absorption as the rate of diffusion from the gut is reduced. This can be crucial in hypovolaemia where the absorption of any drugs given orally will be reduced.

Particle size and formulation

The formulation of drugs can be altered to produce the desired absorption characteristics. In some cases, capsules can be designed to break down slowly to delay release (and subsequent absorption) of a drug. A mixture of fast- and slow-release particles can be produced to generate sustained absorption over a longer period.

This may reduce the adverse effects that can be seen at the peak high plasma concentrations of a drug. However, such mechanisms may lead to a higher concentration of drug in the gut, leading to side effects at this site.

Rectal absorption

Rectal administration can be used for drugs required to produce a local effect, or as a route of administration for systemic drugs. Rectal administration is often used to give diazepam to patients who have **status epilepticus** because it is difficult to obtain intravenous access.

Topical administration of drugs

Most drugs are not very lipid soluble and absorbed poorly through the skin. This can be used to advantage to restrict local effects while avoiding systemic side effects. Other drugs (e.g. steroids) are absorbed significantly through the skin, which can be exploited through transdermal administration (e.g. nicotine patches) to generate systemic effects. Such patches are applied to areas of thin skin; they release the drug over a long period of time. Furthermore, the patch can easily be removed from the skin if the drug generates unwanted effects.

Administration to the eye

Drugs can be applied as eye drops, which are absorbed through the epithelium of the conjunctival sac. The absorption of drugs through this route requires significant lipid solubility. Systemic side effects are generally limited.

Administration by inhalation

Three groups of drugs are typically administered by inhalation for distinct reasons:

1 **Volatile gases and anaesthetics** exploit the large surface area of the lungs to allow rapid adjustments to the plasma concentration of the drug, providing tight control of the drug level. Here, the lungs are the site of both administration and excretion of the drug
2 Drugs that **target the lungs** allow the development of a high concentration in the target tissue, while minimising the potential for systemic effects. Drugs given by this route are often modified to reduce the potential for absorption into the system.
3 **Drugs that would be susceptible to breakdown in the GI tract** can be given nasally. This allows rapid entry of the drug to the systemic circulation without the need for injections. This route of administration is typically used for peptide drugs (e.g. gonadotrophin-releasing hormone [GnRH] and desmopressin, a synthetic form of antidiuretic hormone [ADH]) which work at relatively low concentrations, although they would be broken down in the GI tract.

Administration by injection

Injection provides the most rapid and certain route of administration of a drug to the desired body compartment. Three main routes of injection are typically used in medicine:

1 **Intravenous injection**
2 **Subcutaneous or intramuscular injection**
3 **Intrathecal injection** into the subarachnoid space allows administration of drugs that would not normally pass the blood–brain barrier.

Intravenous administration

Intravenous injection is commonly used to administer drugs because it is reliable and rapid. However, the rapid delivery can present problems with the dosage of drug. A single bolus injection can result in a very high concentration of the drug, before it becomes distributed evenly across the body compartment. The peak concentration depends on the rate of the injection – the more rapid the injection, the greater the concentration. To maintain a steady concentration of drug in the plasma, a steady infusion must be given.

Subcutaneous and intramuscular injections

Subcutaneous and intramuscular injections are a significantly slower route than intravenous administration. The rate of absorption varies with the tissue used, and in particular with the rate of blood flow through the tissue. These routes of injection are often favoured for 'slow-release' preparations. Subcutaneous and intramuscular administration can also be used to generate local effects.

Intrathecal injection

Intrathecal injection is via a lumbar puncture needle. This is usually performed for drugs that target sites in the central nervous system (CNS) but do not cross the blood–brain barrier; this precludes intravenous administration. Intrathecal injection of local anaesthetics can be used to develop a spinal or regional anaesthesia (e.g. epidural).

 CLINICAL Epidural anaesthesia

In childbirth an epidural anaesthetic is often used. For this the needle is inserted into the epidural space, a potential space outside the dura that is created by injection of the anaesthetic. The anaesthetic diffuses from this space and acts on the nerve roots as they exit the spine. An epidural needle can be attached to a catheter which allows repeated infusion of the anaesthetic, whereas a spinal anaesthetic needle, which enters the spinal canal, must be removed immediately after injection.

Distribution of drugs in the body

The distribution of drugs in the body refers to factors that affect the concentration of a drug at its site of action. The distribution of a drug between the body compartments is affected by:

- The compartment into which a drug is administered
- Movement between body compartments
- Fat solubility of the drug
- The binding of the drug to cellular and plasma proteins.

The body can be modelled as four compartments, which can be further subdivided (Fig. 5.4). Typically, total body water accounts for around 70% of body weight; in a 70-kg individual the size of the relevant body compartments can be estimated as:

Extracellular fluids	14 L
Blood plasma	3 L
Interstitial fluid	10 L
Transcellular fluid	1 L
Intracellular fluid	28 L

Intracellular fluid is the fluid contained within all the cells in the body.

Transcellular fluid includes the cerebrospinal fluid (CSF), intraocular, peritoneal, pleural and synovial fluids.

 DEFINITION Volume of distribution (V_d)

V_d is the volume of plasma that would contain the total body content of the drug at a content equal to that in the plasma. This measure provides an indication of the distribution of a drug:

Drugs that are mainly protein bound stay mainly in the plasma compartment, resulting in a small V_d.

Drugs that accumulate outside the plasma may have a large V_d, often greater than the total body volume. This is often seen in lipid-soluble drugs, which can accumulate in fats.

There are two main methods of drug transport within the body:

1 **Bulk flow transfer** (i.e. in the bloodstream) is the mass movement of particles through a compartment, and is not influenced by the chemical nature of the drug.
2 **Diffusion** occurs over very small distances. The differences in the pharmacokinetics of

drugs are the result of their diffusional characteristics.

The body can be modelled as a series of compartments. The crucial effects of distribution are mediated through the movement of drugs across the diffusion barriers between the different compartments.

Movement of drugs across diffusion barriers

The barriers between different compartments are made up of cell membranes:

- A **single cell membrane** separates intracellular and extracellular compartments.
- **Epithelial barriers** between two extracellular compartments are made up of two cell membrane layers – the drugs must pass through both the apical and the basolateral membranes. There is limited scope for paracellular absorption between the cells, due to the tight junctions in place.

The nature of the endothelial barriers between the bloodstream and the interstitial fluid is more complex:

- In most tissues **capillaries are fenestrated**, such that small molecules do not need to pass across a diffusion barrier. Larger molecules (>30 kDa) cannot pass through fenestrations (i.e. most proteins).
- In some sites **continuous endothelium** can be found – especially in the central nervous system (CNS) and the placenta. These sites require transport or diffusion of all molecules across the diffusion barrier, which can severely affect the distribution of a drug.

Molecules can pass across cell membranes in one (or more) of four ways:

1 **Diffusion** across the lipid bilayer
2 Transport across a bilayer by a **carrier protein**
3 By **pinocytosis**
4 **Diffusion through aqueous pores** in the lipid bilayer.

Diffusion across lipid

As many drugs are weak acids or bases, the ratio of ionised to unionised forms of a drug depends on the pH.

The different pH in different body compartments can modify the distribution between compartments. In each compartment, the ratio of

Administration

The majority of routes into the body focus on administering drugs directly or indirectly into the bloodstream. In particular, this may be achieved by intravenous injection, when drugs directly enter the bloodstream; or through inhalation, when the large diffusible area of the lungs assures rapid entry of drugs into the blood.

CSF

The brain is separated from the blood by the blood–brain barrier, and is bathed in cerebrospinal fluid (CSF). The blood–brain barrier prevents the movement of many drugs from the blood and, instead, access is often sought by intrathecal injection.

Oral

One of the most common forms of administration is orally, when drugs enter the portal circulation via the gastrointestinal tract. This route of administration is reliable and does not require individuals taking the drugs to be able to inject themselves. However, oral administration may not be effective if the drugs are readily metabolised by the liver ('first-pass metabolism').

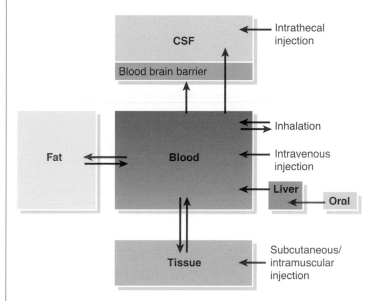

Fat

Although most drugs are polar, and do not enter body fat, there are a few rare cases where the drugs do, and they can act as a reservoir in equilibrium with the blood. This may prolong presence of the drug in the body far longer than would otherwise be expected (fat: water coefficient).

Tissue

In most cases, specific cells in the tissues are the target of a specific drug – equilibrium is set up between the concentration of the drug in the blood and that in the fluid surrounding the tissue. In addition, drugs may be administered directly into the tissue, to slow the release into the blood or to generate specific localised effects.

Blood

The blood forms the central storage of most drugs within the body – it is in equilibrium with the fluid surrounding the tissues; it carries the drug from its route of administration to its site of action and also to the locations where it may be metabolised and/or excreted.

Figure 5.4 Distribution of drugs in different body compartments. Drugs are often administered to compartments of the body different from the site at which they act. Between each compartment of the body, there is equilibrium which alters partitioning of the drug. Furthermore, barriers between compartments may selectively prevent movement of the drug, or, in some cases, result in its metabolism and inactivation. CSF, cerebrospinal fluid.

ionised:unionised drug is determined by the pK_a of the drug and the pH of the compartment. The resulting distribution of a drug can be predicted using the assumption that unionised species can freely cross the membranes, whereas ionised species cannot cross the membrane. However, large distributions between compartments are unlikely to be as large as predicted, because small 'leaks' contribute to a significant decrease in the gradients that can be generated:

- **Charged species are not totally impermeable**. A small degree of permeability can considerably reduce the concentration gradient between compartments.
- **Equilibrium between the different body compartments is almost never achieved**. The fluid in the gastrointestinal (GI) tract and renal tubule is constantly in motion, leading to a flux of drug molecules.

Despite these obstacles, pH partitioning explains many factors of drug distribution, particularly in relation to the blood–brain barrier and renal excretion. However, it is not a major factor in absorption of drugs from the GI tract. The huge surface area of the intestines abrogates any pH effect.

 CLINICAL Exploitation of pH partitioning

The partitioning of the pH can be exploited clinically to concentrate drugs in a body compartment, to increase their action or the rate of excretion:

- Urinary acidification increases the excretion of weak bases and inhibits that of weak acids.
- Increasing plasma pH causes the extraction of weak acids from the CNS.
- Reducing pH can concentrate acidic drugs within the CNS.

Carrier-mediated transport of drugs

Cells regulate the transport of physiologically important molecules (many of which cannot diffuse across a lipid bilayer unaided) by carrier proteins. Drugs may use these carrier systems, because they are often structurally related to endogenous molecules. The transport of a drug may be active or passive, and show similar kinetics to the transport of endogenous molecules. Furthermore, the presence of the drug can act as a competitive inhibitor for the transport of endogenous molecules, and vice versa, because they compete for the same binding sites.

Partitioning of drugs into body fat

Fat typically makes up around 15% of the body weight and is essentially non-polar. Two major factors influence the distribution of drugs between the body fat and the plasma:

1 The fat:water coefficient
2 Blood supply to the fatty tissue.

Fat:water coefficient

The fat:water partition coefficient determines the distribution of a drug, at equilibrium, between the fat and body water. Body fat can act as a large store that communicates with the plasma, slowly releasing a drug as it is cleared from the plasma.

Most drugs have a very low fat:water coefficient; as such this has little impact on the use of the drug. Partitioning in body fat is a crucial consideration in drugs with a high fat:water coefficient (e.g. thiopental).

Blood supply

Fatty tissue receives a very low proportion of the blood supply (<5%), resulting in slow delivery to the fatty tissues, requiring a long time to reach equilibrium.

Accumulation of drugs in other tissues

There are rare instances of drugs that accumulate in other locations within the body, and there are three of particular importance:

1 **Drugs with an affinity for nucleic acids** (e.g. mepacrine, an antimalarial drug): these drugs are typically taken up by the nuclei of hepatocytes.
2 **Chloroquine has an affinity for melanin.** It is also taken up in the retina, and can cause retinitis in overdose.
3 **Tetracyclines accumulate in the bones and teeth** because they have a high affinity for calcium; this can result in bone and dental deformities seen in children.

Binding of drugs to plasma proteins

Many drugs bind plasma proteins, effectively reducing the concentration of free drug, which is able to diffuse into another body compartment. The bound drug acts as a reservoir, similar to the effect seen in fat partitioning. The most important molecule with regard to drug binding is albumin, which binds a large proportion of acidic drugs, as well as some basic drugs. The amount of drug bound depends on three factors:

1 **Concentration of free drug**
2 **Affinity** of the drug for binding sites
3 **Concentration of binding protein**, which determines the number of available binding sites.

Binding of drugs to protein is a reaction similar to drug–receptor binding, although more complex because albumin has at least two binding sites:

- The normal concentration of plasma albumin is about 0.6 mmol/L, although the existence of two binding sites allows it to bind drugs at 1.2 mmol/L.
- In many drugs **the therapeutic concentration of the drug approaches saturation of binding sites**. Consequently, addition of more drug results in a disproportionate increase in the free plasma concentration. This is particularly important when a patient is taking several drugs.

The binding of a drug to plasma protein reduces its potential for renal clearance because proteins, and the molecules bound to them, are not filtered.

Metabolism of drugs

Drugs can be enzymatically modified or broken down within the body to abolish their activity, typically in the liver. Metabolism of drugs is less crucial in polar drugs, which are typically excreted in the urine in an unchanged state.

Drug metabolism is a relatively non-selective system that is used to detoxify the body of both exogenously and endogenously derived molecules. The enzymes involved in detoxification are commonly found on the smooth endoplasmic reticulum (ER) of cells. The reactions can be broken down into two phases, both of which take place predominantly in the liver, which means that the drugs have to cross the hepatocyte cell membranes to be metabolised:

1 **Phase I reactions** often make the drug molecules more reactive. This helps their subsequent conjugation to other molecules for excretion and also reduces the lipid solubility of the molecule, retaining it in the plasma.
2 **Phase II reactions** utilise the reactive groups added in phase I reactions to conjugate larger groups to drug molecules. The resulting polar groups aid excretion of the molecule and prevent its diffusion to another body compartment.

Phase I reactions

Phase I reactions often result in the production of a more reactive molecule, which may be more toxic than the parent drug. Three major reactions that occur in phase I can be identified:

- Oxidation
- Reduction
- Hydrolysis

Oxidation

Oxidative reactions include the hydroxylation of nitrogen and carbon as well as oxidative deamination. These reactions are usually catalysed by the **cytochrome P450 system** on the smooth ER.

 DEFINITION Cytochrome P450 system

The cytochrome P450 pathway is made up of a series of closely related enzymes with broad specificities. It is commonly used in the metabolism of many drugs, and its inhibition can result in many drug-related side effects. In particular, grapefruit juice and St John's wort contain chemicals that inhibit the activity of P450, which accounts for their potentially serious interactions with other drugs. The net result is the addition of a hydroxyl group using O_2 as the oxidant and NADPH to provide a source of H^+ for H_2O.

Reduction

Reduction is a less common method of drug metabolism. Warfarin is one agent, the metabolism of which involves reduction – a ketone group is converted to a hydroxyl group. Reduction can also be used to activate drugs: glucocorticoids may be given as ketones but must be reduced to become active.

Hydrolysis

Hydrolysis typically occurs in the plasma and tissue, and does not involve the hepatic smooth ER enzymes. Ester and amide bonds in drugs are commonly hydrolysed.

Phase II reactions

The reactive groups added in phase I reactions are used to allow the conjugation of larger groups to the molecules. Phase II reactions commonly occur in the liver but can also occur in other tissues.

Sugar conjugation

Conjugation usually results in the addition of glucuronide, catalysed by **UDP-glucuronsyl transferases** (UDP is uridine diphosphate). The resulting conjugate can be excreted from the body in the bile (e.g. chloramphenicol).

Sulphation

The addition of sulphur groups is catalysed by **sulphotransferase enzymes** in the liver and blood cells. Soluble conjugates resulting from this process can be excreted in the urine or bile. An example of a product metabolised by sulphation is salbutamol.

Glutathione

Glutathione (GSH) is a tripeptide added to molecules in a reaction catalysed by glutathione-*S*-transferase, found in the cytosol, particularly of the lungs. The resulting conjugate is metabolised to mercapturic acid and excreted in the urine (e.g. **paracetamol**). There is variability in the activity of the transferase enzymes involved in this process, particularly as a result of **glucose-6-phosphate dehydrogenase deficiency**.

Acetylation

Acetyl coenxyme A (acetyl-CoA) may be transferred as a conjugate using the enzyme *N*-acetyltransferase. Acetylation is important for the clearance of sulphonamides, with the resulting conjugate being excreted in the urine.

Induction of metabolic enzymes

Many drugs can induce the activity of the phase I and II enzymes if given repeatedly due to increased synthesis of the metabolic enzymes. Although such increases are usually restricted to the few enzymes involved in metabolism of the drug, some compounds (e.g. phenobarbital) cause a more non-selective increase, resulting in a general acceleration of the drug's action.

The induction of metabolic enzymes can increase the effects of a drug. Paracetamol toxicity is predominantly the result of the phase I metabolite of paracetamol. The induction of additional enzymes results in more rapid production of metabolites, increasing the likelihood of toxicity.

 DEFINITION First-pass metabolism

Drugs that given orally enter the body's circulation via the portal system and must pass through the liver. They can be metabolised and inactivated before reaching the systemic circulation – this is known as **first-pass metabolism**. First-pass metabolism can require a larger dose of a drug given orally, compared with other routes. Also, marked variation in the extent of first-pass metabolism can lead to unpredictability in the plasma level of the drug.

Metabolism of a drug may alter its effects: aspirin (salicylic acid) is an anti-inflammatory drug that also has anti-platelet activity. However, after hydrolysis to salicylate, the platelet activity is abolished, due to changes in the nature of its binding to its target molecule.

Excretion of drugs

Drugs or their metabolites can be removed from the body by several routes:

- Renal excretion – the major route by which drugs are removed from the body
- Biliary and faecal excretion
- Milk – important in breastfeeding women
- Sweat – generally not significant.

Renal excretion of drugs and metabolites

In drugs that do not undergo significant metabolism, excretion is the major factor determining the duration of action. This may have implications in patients with impaired renal function. Renal handling of drugs varies: penicillin can be cleared almost entirely in a single pass through the kidneys, whereas diazepam is cleared extremely slowly. In most cases the products of phase I and II metabolism are cleared more quickly than the parent drug molecule. Three broad processes in the kidneys can affect drug excretion:

1 Glomerular filtration
2 Tubular secretion and reabsorption
3 Passive diffusion across the tubular epithelium.

Glomerular filtration

The fenestrations in the glomerular capillaries allow the filtration of most free drug molecules (a molecular weight or M_r of less than about

20 000). Some drugs bind significantly to plasma proteins, which are not filtered; as a result the concentration of drug entering the nephron is correspondingly reduced.

Tubular secretion and reabsorption

Around 20% of fluid is filtered from the plasma into the nephron, the remaining 80% passing on to the peritubular capillaries; here two systems may transport drug molecules further into the nephron. Both systems can transport a variety of molecules against their concentration gradients, potentially reducing the plasma concentration to close to 0. This mechanism allows the clearance of drugs that are mostly bound to plasma protein, over the length of the peritubular capillaries.

Most drugs that are secreted share the same transport system, so competition between drugs for the transport system is possible, e.g. probenecid has been used clinically to reduce excretion of penicillin because both molecules compete for the same transporter.

Diffusion across the renal tubule

Water is progressively removed along the length of the nephron. If the tubule is permeable to drug molecules the concentration of the drug will remain similar to that of plasma, such that large proportions of the drug will be reabsorbed with the water.

Diffusion trapping

Polar drugs are poorly lipid permeable, and can be concentrated in the urine as water is removed. Weak acids and bases change their ionisation with pH, and this can be exploited to affect excretion. Low pH will favour the ionisation of a basic drug, increasing its trapping within the tubule.

Urinary alkalisation can be used to increase the excretion of acidic drugs (e.g. aspirin in cases of overdose)

Acidification of urine can accelerate excretion of basic drugs, although this has few clinical applications.

 CLINICAL Pharmacogenetics

Pharmacogenetics is the study of the genetic variation in an individual, to anticipate his or her potential responsiveness to a drug. This may allow doctors to predict which drugs are likely to be effective and which will cause side effects.

Biliary excretion and circulation

Some drugs are excreted from the liver into the biliary system. This can be achieved by one of three systems:

- Acidic handling system – similar to that in the renal tubule
- Basic handling system – similar to that in the renal tubule
- Concentration of hydrophilic drug conjugates in bile.

Drugs are frequently conjugated to glucuronide. During release, glucuronide conjugates can become hydrolysed in the intestine, allowing the reabsorption of the free drug. This recirculation can create a reservoir of a drug, prolonging its action. Morphine is recycled in this manner.

Variation of drug effect between individuals

A similar dose of drug can affect different individuals to different extents. Even if controlling for differences in size and weight, in one individual a drug may function well, whereas in another it can cause serious side effects. Four major causes of such differences in drug effect:

- Genetic differences
- Age
- Underlying diseases
- Drug–drug interactions.

Genetic differences

Differences in every individual's genetic code can affect the ability to process different drugs. These differences are typically the result of genetic variation in the drug target molecule, or enzymes involved in processing of the drug. **Pharmacogenetics** aims to profile such differences in individuals, allowing prediction of an individual's susceptibility to a specific therapy.

Some genetic differences are already well known to account for the side effects of drugs (e.g. glucose-6-phosphate dehydrogenase deficiency affects glutathione-mediated drug metabolism).

Age

Age-related differences in drug tolerance are due to the reduced kidney function of young children and elderly people.

In newborn children, particularly those born preterm, the kidneys function poorly. This function rapidly increases in the first few months.

As people age, the glomerular filtration rate decreases. It is around 50% of its starting value at the age of 70. Correspondingly, excretion of a drug requires a significantly longer period.

There is a similar factor of age in relation to the metabolism of drugs and partitioning:

- Many liver enzymes involved in detoxification are not fully expressed until 8 weeks after birth.
- In elderly people, the level of detoxifying enzymes tends to be reduced. Furthermore, the increased level of lipids in the body can increase the partitioning of lipid-soluble drugs.

 CLINICAL Pregnancy and sensitivity to drugs

Pregnancy is an important consideration with the administration of drugs for three main reasons:

1 The **fetus may be affected** by drugs at much lower doses than the mother, often causing serious developmental abnormalities.
2 During pregnancy, there is **increased renal excretion**, as a result of the mother's increased cardiac output increasing systemic blood flow.
3 **Plasma protein concentration is reduced** during pregnancy, altering drug binding in the compartment.

The fetus effectively forms a separate compartment and this can be exploited. Drugs that do not cross the placenta can be used to treat the mother, while not affecting the fetus.

Effects of disease on drug sensitivity

Diseases can affect every step of drug sensitivity, through altering both the pharmacokinetics and the pharmacodynamics. All four processes that alter the pharmacokinetics of a drug may be affected by disease:

1 **Absorption** of a drug from the gut can be altered if blood flow to the gut has been affected or if there is an abnormality in gut movement.
2 **Distribution** of a drug may be impaired by breakdown of the barriers between compartments (e.g. breakdown of the blood–brain barrier in many infectious diseases).
3 **Metabolism** in the liver is affected by chronic liver disease, because this reduces function.
4 **Excretion** is reduced by renal failure.

Disease can affect the pharmacodynamics of drug interaction:

- In **myasthenia gravis**, the nicotinic acetylcholine (ACh) receptor at the neuromuscular junction is reduced due to the presence of autoantibodies. As such, drugs acting on this receptor may require higher concentrations to elicit a similar result to that seen in a healthy individual.
- Some individuals have **diabetes insipidus** due to a mutation in their ADH receptor. Such individuals cannot be treated by synthetic ADH molecules because their diabetes insipidus results from production of non-functional ADH.

Drug–drug interactions

Many patients, particularly those with chronic conditions, are often treated by many drugs. Should they also develop an infection or other acute condition, additional treatment may be required. The use of multiple drugs (**polypharmacy**) can result in interaction between the different drugs, which can alter their effects.

Pharmacodynamic interaction of drugs

There are many forms of pharmacodynamic interaction, many of which are very specific. Although some such interactions can be extremely beneficial, most are detrimental, due to either excessive side effects or the drugs cancelling each other out:

- Antagonist and agonist drugs that **act on the same receptor** will cancel each other's effects (e.g. β blockers and β-adrenoceptor agonists).
- Drugs that target the same pathway may act synergistically to cause an excessive response, e.g. sildenafil acts by inhibiting type V

phosphodiesterase, which breaks down cGMP. If used together with a nitric oxide donor, which increases the activity of guanylyl cyclase, they can cause extreme hypotension.

Many interactions are more complex than these examples, as a result of the interaction between different pathways in the body.

Pharmacokinetic interactions

Absorption

Drugs that alter the activity of the GI tract are likely to affect the absorption of drugs through this route. Absorption from intramuscular locations can be modulated by adrenaline, which vasoconstricts arterioles and reduces movement of drug into the blood. This effect can be exploited by local anaesthetics, where confining drugs can prolong their effect.

Distribution

In general, drugs rarely alter the distribution of a drug sufficiently to be clinically significant. The addition of a second drug to the plasma compartment may displace the drug from its binding to plasma proteins; however, the free drug will be rapidly cleared to restore equilibrium. In the meantime, the elevated concentration may be sufficient to cause side effects.

Metabolism

As drugs can cause induction of enzymes or inhibit enzymes, drugs that modify metabolism may be hazardous or have potential benefits:

- **Enzyme induction** can decrease the activity of a drug, commonly through upregulation of enzymes in the cytochrome P450 (CYP) system (see earlier). The upregulation may also cause potentially harmful side effects through an increase in the production of metabolites (e.g. paracetamol toxicity)
- **Enzyme inhibition** can reduce the metabolism of drugs and increase their action. In addition, some dietary elements – particularly grapefruit juice – inhibit the CYP pathway, and can cause reduce drug metabolism.

Excretion

There are three major mechanisms by which one drug can affect the excretion of another:

- **Altering filtration** is generally due to modulation of the binding of a drug to plasma protein. Increasing the concentration of free drug will increase the amount filtered.
- **Altering pH partitioning** may aid or restrict diffusion trapping. This can be used either to reduce excretion of a drug or to increase removal of a drug in an overdose (e.g. aspirin overdose).
- **Altering secretion into the nephron** can be achieved if both drugs are secreted by similar transport systems. This will increase the clearance time, particularly if one drug is preferentially secreted.

→ RELATED CHAPTERS

6

Cardiovascular system

The cardiovascular system transports nutrients to tissues, removes waste to be processed, and carries hormones and other signals throughout the body. It is made up of three components: the heart, the vasculature and the blood.

Contraction of the heart forces blood from its chambers into the pulmonary arteries and the aorta, to be carried around the systemic circulation. Blood flows from the heart through the arteries to the capillaries, the narrow vessels where diffusion is possible to allow movement of molecules between the blood and tissues. After this, blood drains back to larger veins before it enters the other side of the heart to be pumped around the pulmonary circulation. The distribution of the blood varies with the need of the tissues themselves, and is achieved through a series of regulatory mechanisms.

Given the important function that the cardiovascular system performs, it is not surprising that many pathologies affect it. In particular, there is a potential for fatty deposits to build up, leading to the development of atherosclerotic lesions; these cause narrowing of the vessels and restricted blood flow.

Functional anatomy of the heart

External anatomy of the heart

The external anatomy of the heart and its relations are covered in Chapter 14. However, a few structures of particular functional importance are covered below. The heart is located in the mediastinum, enclosed within a fibrous sac – the pericardium. It is connected to the **systemic circulation** by the aorta and the vena cava, and to the **pulmonary circulation** by the pulmonary vessels.

> **DEFINITION** Systemic and pulmonary circulations
>
> There are two circulatory systems in the body, arranged in series so that blood from one circulation flows into the other:
>
> - **The systemic circulation** carries the blood to the tissues of the body to supply it with oxygen and nutrients for respiration.
> - **The pulmonary circulation** carries blood to and from the lungs where waste CO_2 can be removed and the blood reoxygenated.

Pericardium

The pericardium is made up of two layers of tissue surrounding a potential space:

- The **visceral layer** is attached directly to the heart tissues.
- The **fibrous layer** is attached to other mediastinal structures.

The **pericardial** space between the two layers is lined by a single layer of **mesothelial** cells, which secrete fluid to allow movement of layers of the pericardium without friction.

Biomedical Science Lecture Notes, First Edition. Ian Lyons.
© 2011 by Ian Lyons. Published 2011 by Blackwell Publishing Ltd.

The **fibrous pericardium** is attached to other mediastinal structures:

- The central tendon of the diaphragm
- The sternum, by the sternopericardial ligaments
- The posterior structures of the mediastinum
- The great vessels which must pierce the pericardium to enter the heart.

The **visceral layer of the pericardium** is reflected to become a parietal layer and forms two sinuses at these folds:

1 The **transverse pericardial sinus** is located where the aortic and pulmonary trunks leave the heart.
2 The **oblique pericardial sinus** is found where the vena cavae and pulmonary veins enter the heart.

The pericardium is innervated by the **phrenic nerve** (C3–5). As a result, damage to the pericardium can result in **referred pain** to the shoulder on the same side.

 CLINICAL Cardiac tamponade

The pericardial space may become filled with fluid (i.e. blood) during trauma, which prevents adequate filling of the heart if the pressure in the pericardium exceeds that in the atria. This is **cardiac tamponade**. Typically, mean atrial pressure is 0–3 mmHg, so little fluid is needed to limit the filling of the heart.

Great vessels entering and exiting the heart

The heart is divided into right and left sides. The large vessels entering and leaving the various chambers of the heart receive blood from one entire circulatory system and distribute it to the other (Fig. 6.1):

- The **aorta** receives blood from the **left ventricle**. The coronary arteries leave the aorta at the aortic sinuses, located immediately distal to the aortic valve.
- The systemic circulation drains into the **right atrium**. The **superior vena cava** enters the right atrium superiorly at the level of the third costal cartilage and the **inferior vena cava** at the level of the fifth costal cartilage. The **coronary sinus**, which drains the heart tissue itself, enters the

heart between the right atrioventricular (AV) orifice and the opening of the inferior vena cava.
- The pulmonary circulation drains into the **left atrium**. Two **pulmonary veins** are derived from each lung: one vein from each lung enters superiorly and one inferiorly.
- The **right ventricle** pumps blood to the pulmonary circulation, through the **pulmonary trunk** which divides into the left and right pulmonary arteries.

Interior anatomy of the heart

The heart contains four chambers, each with a specific function. The atria receive venous blood and transfer to the corresponding ventricle, to be pumped around either the systemic or the pulmonary circulation.

- The **right atrium** possesses an auricle, a muscular pouch that increases the volume of the chamber. The atrial septum, which separates the left and right atria, contains an oval-shaped depression, the **fossa ovalis,** which is the remains of the foramen ovale in the fetus.
- The **right ventricle** receives blood from the right atrium through the right AV orifice, which is sealed by the tricuspid valve. The right ventricle expels blood through the **pulmonary valve** into the **pulmonary trunk**.
- The **left atrium** receives blood from four pulmonary veins. The atrial wall is smooth except within the auricle, which has a different embryological derivation. The left atrium has a slightly thicker wall than the right atrium and discharges blood through the left AV orifice into the left ventricle.
- The **left ventricle** receives blood from the left atrium via the left AV orifice, which is sealed by the mitral valve. Contraction of the left ventricle expels blood into the aorta.

Heart valves

There are two distinct types of heart valve with different structures and functions:

1 The **AV valves** consist of fibrous leaflets covered in endothelium tethered by the chorda tendinae. These mitral (two-cusp) and tricuspid (three-cusp) valves permit the flow of blood from the atrium to the left and right ventricles respectively, while preventing flow in the opposite direction.

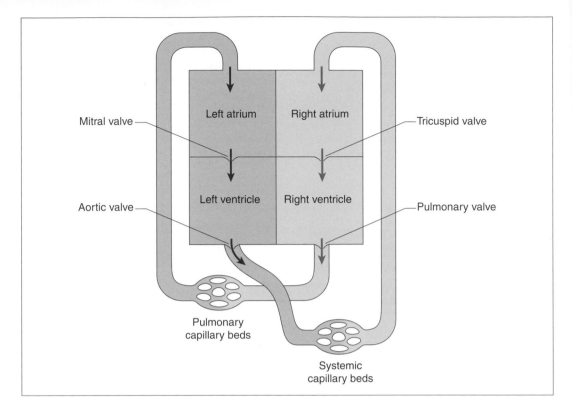

Figure 6.1 **The heart and circulation**. The heart is made up of four chambers; the vessels, valves and flow of blood between the chambers are indicated.

2 The **semilunar valves** are found between the ventricles and their outflow vessels. They are made of three semilunar cusps, which fill and close as blood attempts to regurgitate into the heart chambers. The **aortic valves** are situated in swellings in the aorta, known as the **aortic sinuses**. The **pulmonary valves** are found at the start of the pulmonary trunk.

 DEFINITION Chordae tendinae and papillary muscles

During ventricular contraction, the pressure within the chamber rises drastically. To prevent their opening, the cusps of the mitral and tricuspid valves are tethered by the **chorda tendinae**. These tendons are linked to the **papillary muscles** found on the ventricle walls; the muscles contract to oppose the opening of the valve leaflets. The papillary muscles are more developed in the left ventricle, to oppose the greater force generated.

 CLINICAL Valve sounds

The competency of the valves can be assessed by listening at specific points on the chest surface. These points reflect the transmission of the valve sound, based on the flow of blood through the valves, and may be some distance from the site of the valve:

- The **mitral valve** is heard close to the apex beat.
- The **tricuspid valve** is heard close to the sternum at the fifth intercostal space.
- The **aortic and pulmonary valves** are best heard at the second intercostal space on the right and left sides, respectively.

Blood supply to the heart tissue

The heart requires a blood supply to its tissue, provided through the **coronary circulation**. The left and right coronary arteries arise at the **aortic sinuses** and branch around the heart to supply the

CLINICAL Valve abnormalities

Valve defects are detectable by changes in the valve sounds. Two main classes of abnormalities produce distinctive murmurs:

1 **Stenosis**. This is the narrowing of the valve so that a higher pressure is required to force the blood out of the chamber.
2 **Incompetence**. This occurs where the valve does not shut efficiently. The regurgitation of blood is detectable as a murmur during systole of that chamber.

entire tissue. Blood flow is intermittent, entering the coronary arteries as a result of turbulence in the aortic sinuses during **diastole**. Although there are side branches connecting the major coronary arteries, these branches are rarely sufficient to provide adequate blood flow if a blockage develops in the major supply vessel. The organisation of the circulation discussed below is the most common arrangement, although there is considerable variation between individuals.

Right coronary artery

The right coronary artery (RCA) arises from the **right aortic sinus** and is usually the dominant artery (in around 90% of individuals), in that it provides the **posterior interventricular artery**. This branch travels towards the apex of the heart and supplies much of the diaphragmatic surface of the heart and the posterior part of the interventricular septum.

The RCA runs in the AV groove of the heart and usually provides a branch to the sinoatrial (SA) node of the heart. As the artery descends down the AV groove it provides a **right marginal branch**, which supplies the right border of the heart.

Left coronary artery

The left coronary artery (LCA) arises from the **left aortic sinus**, passing through the coronary groove before dividing into two branches:

1 The **circumflex artery** travels along the left border of the heart to the posterior aspect. In around 40% of people, the **SA nodal branch** arises from the circumflex artery; this gives rise to the **left marginal artery** which follows the left margin of the heart and supplies the left ventricle.

The artery terminates on the posterior surface of the heart, often anastomosing with the **posterior interventricular branch**.
2 The **anterior interventricular branch** is the larger branch of the left coronary artery, and passes along the interventricular groove towards the apex of the heart. Its **anterior interventricular-branch** supplies the anterior two-thirds of the interventricular septum.

 CLINICAL Myocardial infarction

The myocardial tissue is highly dependent on receiving a rich blood flow to meet its metabolic needs. On occasion, a blockage of one of the coronary vessels may occur due to a blood clot, or other embolus. The tissue downstream of the blockage initially becomes ischaemic, causing pain – **angina**. If the blockage continues it leads to death of a region of the heart.

Initial treatment of a myocardial infarction (MI) is, where possible, by stenting open the blocked vessel to restore blood flow. At-risk patients may be given long-term anticoagulant therapy to limit the risk of thrombus formation. Myocardial tissue cannot regrow, so damaged tissue is replaced by fibrous tissue and, even if the individual survives the heart attack, the functionality of the heart is likely to be compromised.

Venous drainage of the heart

These veins draining the heart tissue eventually drain into the **coronary sinus** which runs in the AV groove of the heart and opens into the right atrium. It receives venous blood from three main veins within the heart:

• The **great cardiac vein** drains the regions supplied by the LCA.
• The **middle and small cardiac veins** drain the regions supplied predominantly by the RCA and its branches.

Some parts of the heart do not drain into the coronary sinus. Instead they are drained by other vessels into the right atrium:

• The **anterior cardiac veins** arise on the anterior surface of the right ventricle, and mostly drain directly into the right atrium, although some enter the small cardiac vein.
• The **smallest cardiac veins,** which are direct communications with the capillary beds of the heart muscle, may drain blood directly into the heart chambers.

Histology of cardiac tissue

Cardiac myocytes are long, branched, cylindrical cells that form a network throughout the tissue. These cells typically contain one or two nuclei, found in the middle of the cell, and are contained in a collagenous extracellular matrix with large numbers of capillaries.

Cardiac cells are connected to each other by intercalated discs, which serve as points of insertion for the contractile fibres; they also contain gap junctions allowing transmission of the cardiac action potential between cells. There is marked heterogeneity in the cardiomyocytes; most are adapted for contraction, although others have more nerve-like characteristics, reflecting their role in coordinating contraction.

The cardiac impulse

Although most cells in the heart function to contract and expel blood, this contraction is coordinated by specialised bundles of tissue running through the heart via the propagation of a cardiac action potential. These cells do not contribute directly to the contractile force of the heart.

The conduction system in the heart

In a normal sinus rhythm it takes around 200 ms for depolarisation of the sinoatrial (SA) node to result in contraction of the ventricles. The conduction system is relatively complex to ensure that the correct sequence of contractile events in the heart. The conducting system in the heart has five components:

1 The SA node
2 The atrial conducting pathways
3 The AV node
4 The bundle of His
5 The Purkinje system.

The sinoatrial node

This small region of tissue is located in the right atrium close to the entry point of the superior vena cava. The SA node has the highest rate of depolarisation of cardiac cells with intrinsic activity, such that it acts as a pacemaker to the rest of the heart, triggering impulses before depolarisation occurs in other regions. Autonomic nerve fibres directly synapsing at the SA node can modulate the heart rate.

The atrial conducting pathways

Conducting pathways carry impulses generated by the SA node across the rest of the atrial tissue at a relatively slow pace (around 0.3 m/s). Impulses carried by the **internodal bundles** of the conducting system trigger synchronous contraction of the atrial cardiomyocytes to pump blood into the ventricles; they also transmit the cardiac impulse to the atrioventricular node.

The atrioventricular (AV) node

The cardiac impulse is carried to the AV node by the internodal bundles in the atrium. The AV node is found in the right atrium, close to the septum and inferior to the coronary sinus. It has a very slow conduction velocity, ensuring that ventricular contraction occurs subsequent to the atrial contraction. The AV node is the only site that allows an impulse to pass from the atria to the ventricles; the ventricles and atria are separated by the layer of non-conductive tissue at all other points.

The cells around the AV node form the AV junction. In the event that the SA node loses its pacemaker activity, it is these junction cells that have the next highest intrinsic rate of firing, and take over the pacemaker responsibility.

 CLINICAL Wolff–Parkinson–White syndrome

The Wolff–Parkinson–White syndrome results from the presence of a second set of conductive fibres linking the atria and ventricles. This can result in the formation of a **re-entry loop** through which the action potential stimulates the ventricles by travelling down one of the tracts; the impulse is then retransmitted to the atria via the other tract. The rapid rhythm may provide insufficient time for relaxation of the ventricles. As a result, they do not fill adequately to sustain efficient function. Treatment of the Wolff–Parkinson–White syndrome is by **cardiac ablation** to remove the additional conducting tissue.

The bundle of His

The bundle of His is the sole group of fibres that carries the cardiac action potential to the ventricular myocytes. Depolarisation of the bundle of His is regulated by the **AV node**, with which it is directly connected. At its lower portions the bundle of His is divided into three conducting bundles which propagate the cardiac action potential to the ventricles:

- The **right ventricle** is supplied by a single group – the **right connecting bundle**.
- The **left ventricle** is supplied by the remaining two bundles: the **left anterior bundle** supplies the anterior and superior parts, while the **left posterior bundle** supplies the posterior and inferior aspects.

The Purkinje system

The large fibres in the Purkinje system rapidly conduct impulses across the ventricular tissue to ensure even and rapid ventricular contraction. The Purkinje fibres trigger depolarisation of neighbouring cardiomyocytes, allowing contraction of the whole ventricular mass.

Measuring electrical activity of the heart: the ECG

The electrical activity of the heart can be detected as very small potential changes in the skin which can be monitored by an **electrocardiogram** (ECG) and can help in the diagnosis of a variety of heart conditions. ECG recordings may be made from three leads, by comparing the potential differences of the leads. However, for more accurate diagnosis a 12-lead ECG is required, where 6 leads are placed on the chest to measure the conduction changes across the front of the heart and 6 monitor the changes across the other planes.

A series of distinct waves can be identified within the ECG (Fig. 6.2):

- The **P wave** is triggered by depolarisation of the atria.
- The **QRS complex** is triggered by depolarisation of the ventricles.
- The **T wave** is the result of repolarisation of the ventricles.

The **atrial repolarisation** is not detectable on the ECG, because it is masked by the greater electrical activity of depolarisation of the ventricles, which occurs at the same time.

Cardiac arrhythmias

Arrhythmias are pathological disturbances in cardiac contraction as a result of abnormal generation or transmission of an impulse. Such arrhythmias are detected clinically by ECG. Treatment is by either drug therapy or **cardiac ablation**.

 CLINICAL Cardiac ablation

When an arrhythmia results from the presence of abnormal conducting tissue in the heart, one method of treatment is to remove the affected conducting tissue. This is achieved through inserting a catheter into the heart, typically through the femoral vein, and then destroying the conducting tract responsible for the pathology. Typically, cardiac ablation is used to treat the **Wolff–Parkinson–White syndrome** or **supraventricular tachycardia**; both conditions result from abnormal impulse conduction to the ventricles.

Abnormal impulse initiation

Arrhythmias may result from abnormal initiation in the SA node, altering the frequency of impulse generation. Typically, these are either sinus tachycardia (fast heart rate) or sinus bradycardia (slow heart rate), whereby the elements of the ECG look normal but the interval between impulses is altered.

AV conduction block

A block in the transmission of impulses from the atria to the ventricles can generate severe disturbances in cardiac contraction. A block at the AV node may vary in severity and lead to uncoupling of the atrial and ventricular contractions. Three classes of AV block, differing in severity, are distinguished:

1 **First-degree AV block** is characterised by a lengthened P–R interval because impulse transmission is delayed
2 **Second-degree AV block** leads to some atrial contractions not being followed by ventricular contraction. On the ECG, all QRS complexes

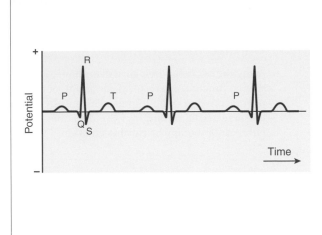

ECG

The electrical heart on the ECG can be divided into three main sections: (1) the P wave is the result of atrial depolarisation. (2) The large wave of electrical activity, the QRS complex, is produced by depolarisation of the ventricles and masks repolarisation of the atria. (3) The later T wave is triggered by the repolarisation of the ventricles, followed by a refractory period where there is little electrical activity.

Specific conduction problems are associated with typical ECG patterns.

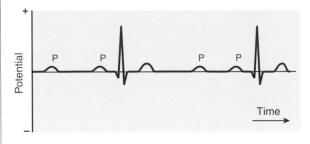

AV block

In an atrioventricular (AV) block, transmission of the action potential between the atria and the ventricles is impeded, which can result in only a proportion of P waves being followed by a QRS complex. In complete AV block, atrial depolarisation is completely unable to trigger ventricular depolarisation – as such the ventricles begin to depolarise intrinsically at a slow rate, which is not coupled to atrial depolarisation.

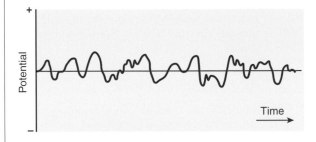

Fibrillation

In fibrillation the heart is contracting in an uncoordinated fashion. In atrial fibrillation, there is sporadic triggering of ventricular contractions, which can be detected on the background of a 'wavy' ECG. Ventricular fibrillation is observable because there is no discernable pattern of features to the electrical currents detectable.

Figure 6.2 **The electrocardiogram**. The ECG detects the electrical activity of the heart, which is achieved by comparing the potentials between two of the three leads attached to an individual. The representations are ideal ones, because actual ECGs are often significantly different in shape as a result of variations between individuals in measurement, although the major electrical complexes should always be visible.

will be triggered by a P wave, although not all P waves will lead to a QRS complex.

3 **Third-degree AV block** occurs when atrial impulses are completely inhibited from being propagated to the ventricles. The resulting slow ventricular rhythm is not coupled to the atrial contraction and requires treatment by a pacemaker.

CLINICAL Cardiac pacemaker

In some conditions, the ventricles may contract ineffectively. To overcome this problem, a pacemaker may be fitted. This device triggers regular depolarisation of the ventricular tissue, through electrodes that are implanted into the heart muscle at appropriate positions. The precise nature of the pacemaker and the location of the electrodes depend on the condition that is being treated.

Abnormal depolarisation

The cardiac tissue has intrinsic electrical activity. Although the SA node usually depolarises first to regulate cardiac contraction, premature depolarisations in other regions of the heart may occur. This happens occasionally in healthy individuals, although it is more common in some pathologies. Depolarisations may be initiated at any point in the heart tissue, and is followed by a prolonged refractory pause, because the SA nodal rhythm is not disturbed but the other tissues in the heart have yet to recover from the previous premature impulse.

Paroxysmal tachycardia

Paroxysmal, or ectopic, tachycardias start and end abruptly and can arise from a variety of different mechanisms:

- The **rapid spontaneous firing of impulses** from a region of the heart which results in it becoming an 'ectopic' pacemaker
- Repetitive cycles of a **re-entry loop**
- An **after-potential that reaches threshold values**, immediately triggering further impulses.

 DEFINITION Re-entry loop

Cardiac cells are capable of transmitting impulses in all directions, although, due to their typical pattern of depolarisation, inactivation impulses travel in a single direction from the atria to the ventricles. In some conditions, areas of the heart conduct the impulse more slowly, such that they are capable of triggering other parts of the heart (which have already repolarised) to carry the impulse in the reverse direction, resulting in a circuit impulse being created. This 're-entry loop' can prevent adequate regulated contraction of the heart and may proceed for a significant time before a correct rhythm is re-established.

Fibrillation

Fibrillations occur when the muscle undergoes irregular contractions in either the atria or the ventricles; this results in no effective pumping of blood through the affected chambers:

- **Atrial fibrillations** can be detected on the ECG as an irregular rippling potential interspersed by **ventricular depolarisations**. The ventricular depolarisations occur at irregular intervals as the AV node is activated intermittently. Although not directly life-threatening, atrial fibrillation increases the risk of blood clots forming and can lead to emboli in the pulmonary or systemic capillary beds.
- **Ventricular fibrillation** is a serious, immediately life-threatening condition. The fibrillations prevent effective pumping of blood; the rhythm must be rapidly corrected or death will result through lack of circulation. Treatment is achieved by **defibrillation** whereby a large electrical current is used to depolarise the entire myocardium, so that the SA node reasserts its control over the cardiac rhythm.

Antiarrhythmic drugs

The drugs used to correct arrhythmias are classified into four groups (**Vaughan–Williams classification**) based on their mechanisms of action, and hence the types of arrhythmias that they can treat:

1 **Class I antiarrhythmics** (e.g. lidocaine) reduce the excitability of cells by blocking the voltage-gated Na^+ channels in a use-dependent fashion, inhibiting the generation of ectopic rhythms. The drugs inhibit high-frequency rhythms but do not affect the heart beating at normal frequencies.
2 **Class II drugs** are β **blockers** (e.g. propranolol); they suppress the arrhythmic effects of adrenaline and sympathetic activity.
3 **Class III drugs** (e.g. amiodarone) increase the length of the cardiac action potential by inhibiting K^+ **channels** in the myocytes, slowing repolarisation of the cell and increasing the refractory period during which the cell cannot be restimulated.
4 **Class IV drugs** (e.g. verapamil) block the **voltage-gated calcium channels**, shortening the cardiac action potential and reducing the force of contraction via the subsequently decreased calcium-induced calcium release.

Treatment of bradycardia

Some pathologies result in an abnormally slow heart beat and require treatment by agents to increase heart rate and, potentially, cardiac output. Typically **atropine**, an antagonist of muscarinic acetylcholine receptors, is used. This **blocks parasympathetic stimuli** to the heart, restricting suppression of the heart rate and contraction by the autonomic nervous system.

Cardiac contraction

Cardiac contraction is coupled to the cardiac action potential, which spreads through the conducting tissue of the heart. The nature of the cardiac action potential varies in different regions of the heart, related to whether it is involved in the regulation of cardiac rate or in triggering and coordinating the contraction of the cardiac myocytes.

The cardiac action potential

Two distinct action potentials, related to their function in conduction or contraction, can be identified (Fig. 6.3):

- Pacemaker action potential
- Ventricular action potential.

Pacemaker action potential

Cells throughout the heart will spontaneously depolarise, although those of the SA node do so at the highest rate. In the SA node depolarisation of the membrane potential to a threshold potential occurs through four main factors, the balance of which regulates heart rate (Fig. 6.3):

1 An activating depolarising influx of Ca^{2+} ions – I_{Ca}
2 An efflux of K^+ that restricts depolarisation – I_K
3 An influx of Na^+ ions in response to hyperpolarisation of the cell known as the 'funny current' – I_f
4 A background influx of Na^+ ions – I_{Na}.

Once the threshold potential has been released, an action potential is triggered through the opening of voltage-gated channels, and spreads between adjacent cells through the gap junctions. Although I_{Ca}, I_K and I_{Na} are also present in the ventricular action potential, the I_f is found in only pacemaker regions, and is the result of expression of a specific Na^+ channel that opens in response to hyperpolarisation of the cell.

Ventricular action potential

Most cells in the heart are specialised for contraction and this adaptation is reflected in the nature of their action potential (see Fig. 6.3). There are four stages to the ventricular action potential:

1 Depolarisation
2 Plateau
3 Repolarisation
4 Refractory.

The general mechanisms of an action potential are discussed in Chapter 4.

Depolarisation

Initial depolarisation of the myocyte is the result of depolarisation of the neighbouring cell membrane, which triggers the activation of the voltage-gated Na^+ channels. The sodium current (I_{Na}) is the largest current in the muscle, responsible for the sharp upstroke in the membrane potential. Once depolarised, the Na^+ channels are rapidly **inactivated** until there is repolarisation of the membrane; this initial depolarisation triggers the brief opening of **transient outward** K^+ channels, resulting in a slight repolarisation.

Plateau

The outward flow of K^+ is matched by an inward flow of Ca^{2+} (I_{Ca}) through L-type Ca^{2+} channels, resulting in a 'plateau' where the flow of charge is balanced, maintaining a constant potential for 100–300 ms. The entry of Ca^{2+} couples depolarisation of the cell to its contraction. This plateau is also maintained by the **Na^+/Ca^{2+} exchanger** which transports one Ca^{2+} ion for three Na^+ ions; this in turn maintains charge by transporting Ca^{2+} out of the cell, and Na^+ into it, to balance the Ca^{2+} entering the cell across the cell membrane.

Repolarisation

The final repolarisation of the cell results from increased inflow of K^+ ions (I_K) and reduced

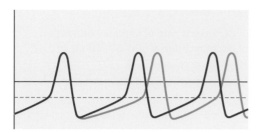

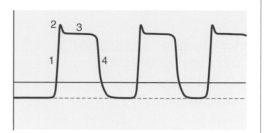

SA potential

The depolarisation of the SA node occurs gradually, driven in particular by the outward flow of K^+ ions and the inward Ca^{2+} current, and the 'funny' Na^+ current, which is triggered by hyperpolarisation. On reaching a threshold potential, rapid depolarisation of the cell occurs (a) triggering an action potential that is propagated around the rest of the heart. After inactivation of the voltage-gated channels, repolarisation occurs and leads to the gradual depolarisation once again.

Altering the slope of the initial depolarisation by altering the rate of flow of ions across the cell membrane. This can lead to an increased or decreased slope, resulting in shorter (red) or longer (blue) intervals between action potentials, respectively.

Ventricular action potential

The resting potential within a ventricular myocyte is maintained at a constant voltage, and the propagation of an action potential from the conducting fibres of the heart triggers the rapid depolarisation by opening of the voltage-gated Na^+ cells (1).

Closure and inactivation of the Na^+ channels is followed by a slight repolarisation as K^+ outflow is also reduced (2). The long plateau phase of the action potential (3) is the result of the influx of Ca^{2+} ions through L-type Ca^{2+} channels being balanced by the outward flow of K^+. It is this influx of Ca^{2+} that is responsible for calcium-induced calcium release.

Eventually, the plateau phase ceases, as the Ca^{2+} flow is decreased, and this results in repolarisation (4) of the cell followed by a refractory period where the cell cannot be restimulated because the voltage-gated channels have yet to recover from inactivation.

Figure 6.3 The cardiac action potential.

Ca^{2+} flow due to inactivation of the **L-type calcium channels**. The Ca^{2+} ions in the cell are rapidly expelled or returned to the sarcoplasmic reticulum to end the contraction. There is additional removal of Ca^{2+} across the cell membrane through the Ca^{2+} ATPase, and the Na^+/Ca^{2+} exchanger.

Refractory phase

After the inactivation of the channels, there is a **refractory phase**, in which there are insufficient closed (not inactivated) channels to permit depolarisation and trigger another impulse. The resulting refractory period of the myocytes is relatively long, preventing the generation of tetany in the heart muscle.

Excitation–contraction coupling in the heart

Contraction of the myocytes is triggered by an increase in free Ca^{2+} in the cytoplasm. The action potential results in a small influx of Ca^{2+} across the plasma membrane, although this is insufficient to allow the contraction of the myocyte. T tubules penetrate into the cell to ensure that that action potential is carried to the interior of the cell, particularly to the sarcoplasmic reticulum (SR). The Ca^{2+} that enters across the cell membrane triggers the release of large amounts of Ca^{2+} from the SR, an internal store of calcium, through activation of ryanodine receptors. This process is termed **calcium-induced calcium release**. The mechanisms relating increased Ca^{2+} levels to contraction are very similar in skeletal and cardiac muscle and are covered in detail in Chapter 4.

Physiological modulation of cardiac contraction

The heart is regulated by the autonomic nervous system and hormones.

The sympathetic response

The sympathetic innervation is derived from the cervical and superior thoracic ganglia. There are various effects caused by sympathetic stimulation of the heart:

- **Increased heart rate** through effects on the SA node
- **Increased contractile force** through actions on the cardiac myocardium
- **Dilatation of the coronary arteries** to increase blood supply to the heart muscle.

Sympathetic stimulation of the SA node

Noradrenaline release by sympathetic nerve fibres acts on the β_1-adrenoceptors on the membranes of SA nodal cells. These G-protein-coupled receptors activate adenylyl cyclase production and, in turn, increase the Ca^{2+} current into the cell to potentiate its depolarisation. Adrenaline released from the adrenal gland may also act to increase the heart rate by increasing both I_{Ca} and I_f.

Sympathetic stimulation of the contractile tissue

The release of noradrenaline from the sympathetic nerves supplying the heart, as well as from circulating adrenaline, can modulate contraction. These hormones act on the β_2-adrenoceptors, increasing Ca^{2+} influx across the cell membrane and a corresponding increase in release of Ca^{2+} from the SR. In addition, the Ca^{2+} ATPase proteins on the SR are upregulated, triggering greater uptake of calcium from the cytoplasm, and allowing greater release in subsequent heart beats.

The parasympathetic response

The parasympathetic innervation of the heart is derived from vagus nerve fibres, which act on the SA and AV nodes and on the coronary circulation. Parasympathetic stimulation of the heart causes:

- a **decreased rate** of cardiac contraction
- a **decreased force** of contraction.

Parasympathetic effects on the SA node

The activation of muscarinic M_2-receptors on the SA nodal cells by the release of acetylcholine (ACh) causes a decrease in the pacemaker current; this happens via decreasing Ca^{2+} influx because of the inhibition of cAMP production by **adenylyl cyclase**. There is a direct action on a ligand-gated K^+ channel which causes cell **hyperpolarisation**.

Parasympathetic effects on the contractile tissue

The released ACh binds to M_2-receptors and reduces the influx of Ca^{2+}, thus reducing calcium-induced calcium release, and hence the length and force of the cardiac contraction.

Sensory innervation of the heart

Sensory innervation of the heart is provided by nerve fibres originating in the upper four thoracic nerves. Damage to the heart leads to referred pain to the left arm, neck and chest – the sites in the skin innervated by the same nerve roots.

Cardiac mechanics

Coupling of the cardiac action potential to contraction triggers a build-up of pressure in the chambers of the heart, so that it expels blood into the arteries. This process forms a cycle of filling and relaxation that must be regulated to ensure that the demands of the tissue are met and that both sides of the heart adequately match their output.

The cardiac contractile cycle

The mechanical events in cardiac contraction are made up of four stages:

1 Atrial contraction
2 Ventricular contraction
3 Ventricular filling
4 Diastasis.

Atrial contraction

Atrial contraction aids the movement of blood into the ventricles. At rest, flow into the ventricles occurs passively with little contribution from atrial contraction. However, as heart rate increases, the period for ventricular filling decreases and atrial contraction becomes essential to ensure adequate filling. Atrial contraction produces pressure waves that can be detected in the **jugular venous pulse**, and may also be detectable as a **fourth heart sound**.

Ventricular contraction

During ventricular contraction, pressure in the ventricles increases until it opens the outlet valves and ejects blood into the circulation. This process occurs in three phases:

1 **Isovolumetric contraction**. There is an increase in the pressure in the ventricular chamber without a change in its volume
2 **Ejection of blood** from the ventricle into the corresponding great vessel
3 **Isovolumetric relaxation**. There is a decrease in the pressure in the ventricular chamber without a change in its volume.

Isovolumetric contraction

The initial phase of ventricular contraction results in the increasing pressure of blood forcing the AV valves closed. The closure of the AV valves causes the **first heart sound** and the **'c' pressure wave within the jugular venous pulse**. After closure of the valves, the ventricles continue to contract, increasing the pressure in the chamber without any change in the volume. The isovolumetric phase ceases when the pressure in the ventricle exceeds that of the aorta, or pulmonary arteries, at which point the corresponding valves are forced open.

Ventricular ejection

Initially, blood is expelled faster than can be accepted by the arteries and, as a consequence, the vessels become distended. At rest, the ventricular ejection phase lasts around 300 ms, most (75%) of the blood volume being expelled in the first 150 ms, allowing efficient expulsion at higher heart rates when the interval decreases. Ventricular ejection ends when the pressure of the ventricles falls to below that of the corresponding artery. At this point, the backflow of blood closes the semilunar valves, which is detectable as the **second heart sound**.

Ventricular isovolumetric relaxation

Once the aortic and semilunar valves have closed, the ventricles relax and the pressure falls without a change in volume, until the pressure is exceeded by that within the atria.

Ventricular filling

The AV valves have a large diameter to allow rapid filling from the atria and veins. Most of the blood flow occurs early in the phase to allow shortening of the filling interval during exercise.

Ventricular filling reduces the volume of blood stored within the reservoirs of the great veins, and the resulting decrease in pressure can be detected as the **'y' wave** in the jugular venous pulse.

Diastole

This phase is where the heart is relatively inactive. The atria and the large veins fill with peripheral blood, although there is little electrical activity in the heart. Diastole accounts for the reserve time, which can be reduced as the heart rate increases without compromising the heart's function. Diastole ends with the P wave of the ECG, when atrial contraction occurs.

Regulation of stroke volume of the heart

The stroke volume of the heart is regulated by two factors:

1 The metabolic needs of the body
2 The stroke volume of the other ventricle.

The stroke volume of one ventricle in relation to its counterpart is regulated by the Frank–Starling mechanism.

The Frank-Starling mechanism in the heart

It is essential that the cardiac output of both sides of the heart be matched, otherwise there will be a build-up of fluid immediately in one side of the heart – as seen in **heart failure**. If the filling of a ventricle is increased, it results in greater contraction to clear the additional fluid. This process appears to contradict **La Place's law**, because the enlarged ventricle would be expected to be less efficient and thus expel a smaller volume of blood.

This process results from the force generated during contraction and is proportional to the initial length of the sarcomere before contraction. The ideal length of a sarcomere for optimal contraction is around 2.2 μm; either side of this length, the force generated in contraction is decreased. This relationship applies for both cardiac and skeletal muscles, although in the heart there is rarely stretching of the sarcomeres beyond this point.

The **Frank–Starling mechanism** is apparent in cases when premature ventricular ejection occurs – as a result of early contraction, a smaller than normal volume of blood is expelled. Consequently a larger volume of blood fills the left ventricle – the Frank–Starling mechanism results in the following contraction being larger, returning the end-systolic volume of the ventricle to normal.

Functional values of cardiovascular performance

A series of normal values can be used to assess the function of the heart. In particular, the amount of fluid expelled by the (left side of the) heart in a given time – the cardiac output – provides a measure of the function of the heart and the strain that it may be under.

The cardiac output

Cardiac output (CO) is defined as:

Left ventricular stroke volume (mL)
   × heart rate (beats/min) = Cardiac output (mL/min).

At rest, the cardiac output is around **5 L/min**. During exercise the increased metabolic demands of the skeletal muscle result in an increase in both the stroke volume and the heart rate, and can allow the cardiac output to reach up to around **20 L/min**.

Stroke volume

The stroke volume is the total amount of blood expelled from the ventricles in a single contraction and is determined by two opposing factors:

1 The contractile force generated by the myocardial cells
2 The arterial pressure against which the blood is expelled.

Not all the blood is expelled from the ventricles in a single stroke; the end-systolic volume is retained and can be used as a reserve to expel further blood when increased cardiac output is required.

Assessment of the central venous pressure

If a patient sits back and relaxes their neck, it is possible to view the point at which the external jugular vein collapses; the vertical height between this point and the atria (estimated as 5 cm below the manubrium of the sternum) gives an indication of the central venous pressure (CVP).

In heart failure, the accumulation of fluid behind the affected ventricle can result in an increase in the CVP. In right heart failure the accumulation of fluid will be reflected in the systemic circulation. Afflicted individuals are likely to have a CVP that can be viewed when they are upright. In normal individuals, the point of collapse of the jugular veins is usually occluded by the clavicle.

The jugular pulse

The pressure waves generated by the contraction of the atria and closure of the AV valves are reflected as pressure waves in the large veins. The emptying of the veins to fill the atria and ventricles also results in pressure changes in the veins. Assessment of the jugular pulse can provide an indication of pathologies of the heart (Fig. 6.4).

Heart sounds

Four heart sounds may be detected; these reflect the closing of valves and the movement of blood. In normal individuals only the first and second heart sounds may be detected. The detection of the third and fourth heart sounds, as well as changes in quality of all the heart sounds, may be indicative of pathology:

1 The **first heart** sound is the result of closure of the mitral and tricuspid valves.
2 The **second heart** sound results from closure of the aortic and pulmonary valves. It is often a 'split' sound due to earlier closure of the aortic than the pulmonary valve.
3 The **third heart** sound is caused by the movement of blood from the atria to the ventricles during relaxation. It is commonly heard in young people, although it is of low frequency and relatively difficult to detect. In older people it is pathological and may reflect a degree of heart failure.
4 The **fourth heart** sound just precedes the first heart sound and results from contraction of the atria. The fourth heart sound is always pathological.

'a' wave	'c' wave	'x' wave	'v' wave	'y' wave
The peak pressure in the 'a' wave results from the contraction of the right atrium to expel blood into the right ventricle.	The contraction of the right ventricle forces the closed atrioventricular (AV) valve back, generating a brief increase in pressure.	The x wave is the lowest pressure in the jugular venous pulse, and occurs during ventricular contraction. Here the change in the heart draws blood into the atrium, with the AV valve remaining closed.	The pressure gradually rises in the veins as the atrium begins to fill. The 'v' wave represents the maximum pressure in the atrium, before the AV valve opens. This is accompanied by a transient drop in venous pressure as blood rushes into the ventricle.	The filling of the ventricle after the opening of the AV valve leads to a decrease in pressure. The pressure subsequently increases because the rate of atrial filling exceeds the rate at which blood leaves the atrium to enter the ventricle.

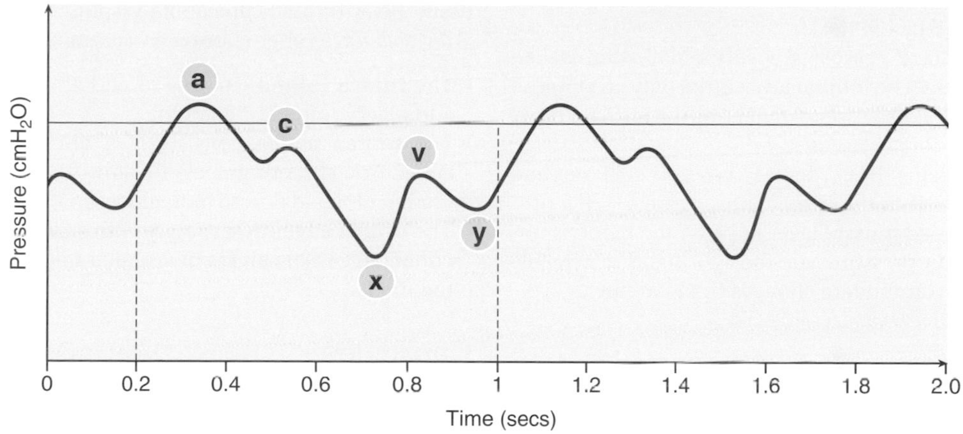

Figure 6.4 **The jugular venous pulse**. The closure of the various valves and contraction of the chambers of the heart are reflected backwards in the venous blood. These changes are seen as a series of peaks in the venous pressure and can be related to the function of the right side of the heart.

Functional anatomy of circulation

The circulatory systems carry blood from the heart to the tissues and lungs, where gas exchange occurs. The vasculature shares a common design, although this varies depending on the role of the vessels. Arteries must be strong and muscular to support the high pressure of the blood, whereas capillaries are thin to allow efficient diffusion.

Veins are distensible to accommodate varying volumes.

There is insufficient blood volume, or cardiac output, to maximally perfuse every capillary bed. Instead, the flow of blood is regulated to best serve the needs of the body at the time. During exercise, the skeletal muscle beds are highly perfused to supply the respiring tissue with the oxygen and nutrients that it needs, whereas at rest the flow to the muscle beds is low and that to the gastrointestinal tract and kidneys much higher.

Structure of blood vessels

The blood vessels share a similar common structure of three functional layers:

1 **Tunica intima**. A single layer of endothelial cells on a basement membrane
2 **Tunic media**. The middle layer characterised by layers of smooth muscle
3 **Tunica adventitia**. The outermost layer, which is continuous with surrounding connective tissue.

There are three distinct types of blood vessels, each with a different function:

1 **Arteries** are thick muscular vessels that carry blood from the heart and regulate the distribution of blood to the capillaries. They have developed media to tolerate the high pressures generated by the heart.
2 **Capillary vessels** are very small, thin-walled vessels. The intimal layer is the only layer found in capillary vessels – reflecting the need for rapid diffusion.
3 The **veins** receive blood from the capillaries and return it to the heart. These vessels lack a pronounced muscle layer because the blood is under low pressure, and they are highly distensible to accommodate changes in blood flow.

Arteries

Arteries serve the dual function of tolerating the high pressure of blood within the vessels and regulating the distribution of blood to the different capillary beds through muscular contraction. Two forms of vessel can be distinguished which vary in the constitution of the vessel walls; this is related to the stress tow which the vessel must be subjected and the function that it performs:

- Elastic arteries
- Muscular arteries.

Elastic arteries

Elastic arteries are the largest arteries in the body, carrying blood at high pressure and flow rates:

- There is a prominent layer of connective tissue rich in elastin between the intimal and medial layers of the vessel walls, allowing accommodation of large pressure changes.
- The elastic arteries are extremely large and possess their own blood vessels to supply their tissue – the vasa vasorum.

Muscular arteries

Muscular arteries are the vessels of larger distribution. The vessel walls are well innervated and have a highly developed muscular layer to modulate blood flow, so that the blood can be appropriately distributed as demand requires:

- The smooth muscle in the tunica media is arranged in a series of concentric layers for significant contraction and restriction of blood flow.
- The tunica adventitia is made up of predominantly collagen and elastin, allowing contraction to limit the flow.

Arterioles

Arterioles are the major resistance vessels in the vasculature; they control blood flow into individual tissue beds through precapillary sphincters. The arterioles have other features in common:

- The **tunica intima** consists of endothelial cells and a very thin elastic lamina.
- The **tunica media** consists of a few rings of concentric smooth muscle to allow further regulation of blood flow to individual capillary beds.
- The **tunica adventitia** merges with surrounding connective tissue and is of a similar thickness to the media.

Capillaries

The capillaries are the major site of exchange of substances across the endothelium and are made up of three layers:

1 The endothelium
2 The basement membrane
3 The pericytes are that surround the intima and can regulate both blood flow and vessel growth. They are also stem cells for endothelial cells.

Veins

Veins accept blood from the capillaries, carrying it back to the heart:

- **Small venules** drain the capillary beds. These vessels possess a limited tunica media and carry the blood through progressively larger vessels as it goes back to the heart. The venules around the lymph node are distinct; these **high endothelial venules** are the site of migration of lymphocytes from the blood into the lymph nodes.
- **Veins** accept blood from the venules and possess a thicker muscular wall to accommodate the

larger volume of blood. The veins have a poorly developed elastic lamina and the tunica adventitia is continuous with the surrounding connective tissue.

Special circulations

Some sites in the body require other circulatory arrangements:

- **Arteriovenous shunts** are direct connections between the arterial and venous systems, allowing the bypass of an intervening capillary bed. By opening a shunt vessel, blood bypasses the capillary bed. Such shunts are common in the skin, where they are important for **thermoregulation**.
- **Portal systems** involve a series of vessels that connect two capillary beds together. The hepatic portal system is particularly prominent; here blood from the capillary beds in the intestinal tract drains into the tributaries of the hepatic portal vein, which transport the nutrient-rich blood to the liver for processing. Portal blood is transported to the sinusoids of the liver and from there enters the hepatic veins, via which it returns to the main circulation.

Endothelium: regulation of the vasculature

Endothelial cells line the lumen of every blood vessel. There are four broad functions to which the endothelium contributes:

1 It acts as a barrier regulating exchange across the vessel wall
2 It regulates haemostasis
3 It regulates vascular tone
4 It regulates angiogenesis.

Endothelium as a barrier regulating exchange

Three classes of endothelial arrangement found in capillaries have been defined, related to the 'leakiness' of the vessels (Table 6.1):

- **Continuous endothelium**
- **Fenestrated endothelium**
- **Discontinuous endothelium (sinusoids)**.

Transport across the endothelium

Transport across endothelium can occur by a variety of routes:

- **Passive diffusion** of small non-polar molecules occurs across the endothelium down their concentration gradient.
- **Carrier-mediated transport** may be through facilitated diffusion or by active transport.
- **Pinocytosis** is used to transport larger molecules such as proteins.
- White blood cells are able to travel between the endothelial cells (**diapedesis**) to leave capillary vessels.
- **Paracellular transport** can occur between the endothelial cells, down a concentration gradient.

Table 6.1 The endothelial arrangements found in capillaries

Type of endothelium	Location	Features
Continuous	Where tight regulation of transport is required (e.g. blood–brain barrier)	Tight cell junctions: transport is entirely transcellular and large numbers of mitochondria are present to provide energy for active transport
Fenestrated	Most capillaries	Fenestrations in the endothelium – small bilayers of cell membrane with no intervening cytoplasm. Allows the free flow of small molecules by diffusion. Basement membrane is continuous with the fenestrations. Transport across the endothelium is less regulated, although it does not have the high energy costs
Sinusoids	Where blood interacts directly with underlying cells (e.g. liver)	Endothelial cells are discontinuous and lack a basement membrane

The relative contribution of the paracellular route is governed by the 'leakiness' of the tight junctions that join the endothelial cells.

The endothelium in haemostasis

The endothelial cells are perfectly placed to detect changes in blood flow and damage to the vessel. They can secrete and express molecules that may be anti- or procoagulant, especially in response to tissue damage.

Endothelium as a regulator of vascular tone

Vascular tone is regulated by molecules and neural signals. The endothelium is responsible for the production of various substances that modulate contraction, including:

- **Nitric oxide** (NO) is a gas produced by nitric oxide synthase (NOS) in the endothelium in response to parasympathetic nervous stimulation. NO diffuses to smooth muscle cells where it causes relaxation through its activation of the cGMP signalling cascade.
- **Endothelin** triggers long-term vasoconstriction and is released by the endothelial cells.
- **Angiotensin II**, a potent vasoconstrictor, is converted from angiotensin I by the angiotensin-converting enzyme (ACE) expressed on the endothelial surface. In addition, ACE inactivates several vasodilators, in particular bradykinin.

Blood

Blood is made up of four components, each with a distinct role:

1 **Red blood cells**
2 **White blood cells**
3 **Platelets**
4 **Plasma**.

All blood cells are derived from haematopoietic stem cells, which are found in different locations at different ages:

- In the **fetus,** haematopoiesis occurs initially in the yolk sac in the first 8 weeks, and then progresses to the liver and spleen.
- By **birth and during infancy**, the major site of haematopoiesis is the bone marrow (which is found in almost every long bone).

- In **adults,** the sites at which bone marrow is found are more restricted, primarily the ribs, sternum, pelvis and more proximal parts of the femur.

A single haematopoietic stem cell gives rise to the cellular components of blood; however, two major progenitor cells – both derived from the stem cells – can be identified:

- The lymphoid progenitor cell generates lymphocytes – discussed in Chapter 15.
- The myeloid progenitor cell gives rise to all the other cellular components of the blood.

Red blood cells

Red blood cells are enucleated cells responsible for carrying oxygen from the lungs to the respiring tissues. They contain large amounts of the oxygen-carrying protein haemoglobin,

---

 CLINICAL Anaemia

Anaemia is a defect in the oxygen-carrying capacity of the blood, as a result of low haemoglobin. The chief symptoms of anaemia are persistent tiredness and pallor. In more severe cases, shortness of breath on exertion may be noticeable, as well as palpitations and sweating caused by the extra strain put on the heart to maintain adequate oxygenation of tissues. There can be many different causes of anaemia, each of which may require a different treatment:

- **Inadequate production of haemoglobin**, typically due to a lack of iron, is the most common form of anaemia. This causes a microcytic anaemia, where the red blood cells are smaller than usual.
- Anaemia can result **through overall loss of haemoglobin**, without changes in the red blood cells (normocytic anaemia); this is often due to severe chronic blood loss or excessive destruction of red blood cells.
- In some cases, there may be **defects in the production of haemoglobin or of the red blood cells themselves**. This is particularly apparent in pernicious anaemia, where there is a deficiency in vitamin B_{12}, which is essential for DNA synthesis, and therefore impaired production of the numerous precursor cells of mature red blood cells.

and make up around 45% of the blood volume. These cells are **biconcave flattened discs**, shaped to generate a large surface area to allow rapid diffusion, while maintaining high volume.

Red blood cells have a typical lifespan of 120 days and are found in the blood at a concentration of approximately 7×10^7 cells/mL. Maintenance of enough red blood cells is essential to maintain effective oxygen transport around the body. Shortage of haemoglobin, is referred to as **anaemia**, and may have many different underlying causes.

Generation of red blood cells (erythropoiesis)

Red blood cells (erythrocytes) form by **erythropoiesis**. Burst-forming units derived from the myeloid progenitor cells differentiate through three stages to develop into mature red blood cells.

1 **Normoblasts** are the nucleated precursors of red blood cells in the bone. The presence of **normoblasts** in the blood is abnormal.
2 **Reticulocytes** are the direct precursors of mature red blood cells. These cells lack a nucleus although they possess large amounts of RNA, to allow translation as the cells mature. These cells are released into the blood, where they account for around 1% of the circulating red blood cells.
3 **Erythrocytes** are the mature red blood cells. They possess no nucleus or RNA, and have a short lifespan as a result. With no mitochondria, energy required for biological processes is achieved solely by **glycolysis**, making the cells dependent on glucose for ATP generation.

Regulation of erythropoiesis

The major regulator of erythropoiesis is the hormone **erythropoietin** (EPO), which is released by the kidneys in response to low oxygen tension in the blood. EPO triggers increased division of progenitor cells, resulting in the production of more erythrocytes. Dysregulation of EPO secretion can result in overproduction of red blood cells (polycythaemia).

 CLINICAL Polycythaemia

Polycythaemia is a clinical condition in which there is overproduction of red blood cells. Although sometimes symptomless, polycythaemia may present with a generalised itching and classically, although rarely, with burning pains in the limbs accompanied by discoloration of the skin (erythromelagia).

The underlying cause of polycythaemia may vary:

- Primary causes are usually due to abnormal processes in the bone marrow.
- Secondary causes are usually due to chronic low oxygen or an EPO-secreting tumour.

Individuals with polycythaemia are at risk of increased thrombosis:

- Treatment of **primary polycythaemia** focuses on reducing the risk of clotting, such as through the administration of aspirin or through removing the excess blood cells via blood letting.
- **Secondary polycythaemia** is usually corrected by treating the underlying pathology.

White blood cells

White blood cells make up the cellular part of the immune system; their role and generation are discussed in Chapter 15.

Platelets

Platelets are cell fragments around 2–3 μm in size. They express many surface proteins and receptors and regulating the clotting process. Platelets are formed from the **megakaryocyte** fragments. There are usually around 2.5×10^8 platelets/mL and they typically have a lifespan of 7–10 days. Platelets carry numerous granules containing a variety of factors associated with their function:

- **Alpha granules** contain many mediators of blood clotting (e.g. fibrinogen and thrombospondin), and are released on platelet activation.
- **Dense bodies** are electron dense when viewed by an electron microscope, and are fewer in number than the alpha granules. They contain ATP, ADP and serotonin, all of which are important mediators released by platelets during activation.
- **Lyosomes**.

Generation of platelets

The megakaryocytes differentiate from the myeloid progenitor cells and go through nuclear replication, although with no cytoplasmic cleavage. During this process the volume of the cytoplasm increases markedly. The resulting cell may have gone through several rounds of nuclear division, having up to 32 times the normal copies of the genome ($64n$). As the megakaryocyte matures, its cytoplasm becomes more granular, and then fragments to release many platelets into the blood. A single cell may give rise to around 4000 platelets.

 CLINICAL Thrombocytopenia

A reduced number of platelets can result in clotting defects, and is associated with rapid bleeding and bruising. The method of treatment varies with the underlying cause of the condition, although in severe cases transfusion of platelets may be used to boost the circulating numbers.

Plasma

Plasma is the fluid and medium that carries the other components of the blood. It contains many components involved in regulating and powering cellular processes. Many ions also regulate pH buffering of the blood. The protein components are predominantly produced by the liver and perform many functions:

- **Proteins**, such as albumin, regulate the oncotic pressure of the blood, regulating the fluid volume of the body's compartments.
- **Carrier proteins** allow transport of ions or hormones around the body in a more stable form, so that they do not come out of solution or get excreted inappropriately.
- **Protein cascade precursors** (e.g. complement and blood clotting) are often contained in the plasma.
- **Antibodies** are found in the blood to protect against pathogens.
- **Hormones** allow the regulation of the function of widespread, dispersed tissues.

Haemodynamics

Haemodynamics refers to the movement of blood through the vessels. The body must regulate the distribution and flow rate of the blood to ensure that the needs of different tissues are met. Furthermore, the nature of the flow can be determined by the vessels and the properties of the blood, and by the forces exerted.

Distribution of blood within the systemic circulation

Typically the veins in the body act as a reservoir for blood volume; they can undergo a large change in volume relatively easily. The standard distribution between the vessels is:

- about 20% in the arteries
- 5% in the capillaries
- 75% in the veins.

There is typically around 5 litres of blood in an individual, although this varies with body size. The total blood volume is insufficient to maximally perfuse all the capillary beds at the same time; instead the arterioles supplying the capillary bed are maintained at varying degrees of vasoconstriction to provide an adequate balance of the perfusion of the capillary beds so that the needs of the respiring tissue are met but do not exceed the limited blood volume.

The process of vasoconstriction relies on the contributions of the smooth muscles and elastic connective tissue in the arteriole walls. The factors that regulate peripheral blood flow through causing alterations in vessel tone are in three groups:

1 **Local factors** produced in response to the metabolic needs of the tissue itself
2 **Extrinsic factors** resulting from the regulation of blood flow to the different organ beds, ensuring that demand does not exceed cardiac output
3 **Global homoeostatic regulation** of other systems, such as temperature, may require alterations in the blood flow that conflict with other factors. This regulation may override the needs of individual capillaries.

Local factors

Despite changes in the amount of blood passing through it, constriction of the arterioles in the vascular bed maintains a constant perfusion pressure over a wide range of systemic blood pressure. This process is called **autoregulation** and is most prominent in the vascular beds where the tone is not vastly altered by neural signals (e.g. the brain).

There are various local factors that regulate peripheral blood flow. These are mainly vasodilatory agents which are produced in response to inadequate capillary perfusion:

- **Myogenic effects** result from changes in the transmural pressure (the pressure difference across the wall of the blood vessel). To prevent the vessel walls expanding, the vessels oppose any increase in transmural pressure by further constriction.
- **Local metabolites** (e.g. adenosine) promote vascular relaxation to increase perfusion which washes them from the tissue.
- **Endothelial factors** are produced in response to changes in the tissue (e.g. acute inflammation) or to circulating hormones.

Extrinsic regulation of peripheral blood flow

Extrinsic mechanisms acting via the autonomic nervous system promote control of blood flow, and function through three sets of autonomic fibres:

- Sympathetic vasodilator fibres
- Sympathetic vasoconstrictor fibres
- Parasympathetic vasodilator fibres.

Neural control dominates in capillary beds, which tolerate ischaemia and have vastly variable metabolic requirements, depending on tissue activity, e.g. skeletal muscle. Tissue beds that do not tolerate ischaemia, e.g. the heart and brain, are predominantly regulated by intrinsic mechanisms to ensure adequate perfusion at all times.

Hormones may modulate vascular resistance. Within skeletal muscle, adrenaline acts via the β_1 adrenoceptors to trigger vasodilatation, in readiness for anticipated physical activity. At high concentrations, adrenaline may also act on α_1-adrenoceptors in vascular beds that supply tissues not required for physical activity. The action of adrenaline on α_1-adrenoceptors triggers vasoconstriction.

Regional circulation

If all tissues were to receive sufficient blood to operate at maximal capacity, the oxygenated blood required would be vastly greater than the maximum pumping capacity of the heart. Control systems are in place to ensure that the needs of different tissues are met as far as possible.

Starling's forces

Fluid travels from the capillaries into the interstitial tissue as a result of bulk flow. The rate of flow into the tissues is far higher than can happen by diffusion alone, and results from differences in the osmotic and hydrostatic pressures between the capillaries and tissue. The net transfer of fluid between the body compartments is governed by **Starling's forces**.

Four factors contribute to Starling's forces:

- Oncotic pressure of the blood
- Oncotic pressure of the tissue
- Hydrostatic pressure of the blood
- Hydrostatic pressure of the tissue.

The blood pressure within the capillaries forces large volumes of fluid out of them. In contrast, the hydrostatic pressure in the interstitial spaces is very low and is counteracted by the oncotic pressure of the blood, which is maintained by the presence of proteins within the fluid. In the blood, the oncotic pressure is high, because plasma proteins are too large to be forced out of the fenestrations in the endothelial cells. This high concentration of proteins contributes a pressure equivalent to around 25 mmHg.

The balance of forces results in a small net volume of fluid entering the tissues. This tissue fluid enters the lymphatic system and is eventually returned to the blood.

 DEFINITION Oncotic pressure

Oncotic pressure is generated by proteins in the fluid. Although small ions will be easily filtered out of blood vessels, proteins are retained in the blood. The proteins increase the osmolality of the compartment, drawing fluid into it to equalise the osmotic gradient.

 CLINICAL Oedema

When the balance of Starling's forces is affected, the rate at which fluid enters the tissue may increase; this can cause loss of function within the tissue. This **oedema** can be caused by a variety of different factors:

- Increase in the hydrostatic pressure of blood
- Decreased concentration of plasma proteins, leading to a lower blood oncotic pressure
- Increased permeability of capillaries
- Increased extracellular fluid volumes
- Blockage of lymphatic vessels, preventing drainage of tissue fluid.

Blood pressure

Blood pressure is given as two values: the **systolic** blood pressure is the highest arterial pressure, and is reached during ejection of blood from the heart. The **diastolic** blood pressure is the lowest arterial blood pressure, and is reached immediately before the next ejection phase starts in the heart. The effects and regulation of blood pressure are discussed in Chapter 11.

The difference between the systolic and diastolic blood pressures is referred to as the **pulse pressure**; the pressure wave associated with the changes in blood pressure during the heart beat can be felt at points on the body's surface that lie close to major arteries. The characteristics of the pulse wave can reflect the characteristics of distension of the aorta and the profile of ejection of blood from the heart.

Mean arterial pressure

Much of the time the blood pressure is far closer to the diastolic value than to the systolic value. A true average can be determined by dividing the area under the pulse pressure wave profile by the number of heart beats, although in practice the diastolic pressure + a third of the pulse pressure provides a good estimate. Using ideal values, the mean arterial pressure can be calculated as around 93 mmHg.

Total peripheral resistance

As blood must be pushed through a series of branching tubes, there is significant resistance to the flow of blood. Over the entire systemic circulation this resistance is referred to as total peripheral resistance (TPR):

$$TPR = (Mean\ aortic\ pressure - Mean\ right\ atrial$$
$$pressure)/Cardiac\ output.$$

However, for most purposes this right atrial pressure is negligible, so this can be simplified to:

$$TPR = Blood\ pressure/Cardiac\ output.$$

The main sites of such resistance are the arterioles which regulate the flow of blood into specific capillary beds. For a given cardiac output to be sustained, the greater the TPR, the higher the blood pressure that must be reached.

Haemostasis and vascular pathologies

Haemostasis is the series of physiological changes that prevent blood loss as a result of injury to blood vessels. Blood loss is limited by formation of a clot, although this clot must eventually be removed to allow tissue repair. There are four mechanisms that contribute to haemostasis:

1 Vasospasm
2 Endothelial changes
3 Platelet activation
4 Coagulation of blood.

Vasospasm

Vasospasm is the contraction of arterial vessels due to the actions of the vascular smooth muscle. Initially, injury to the vessel and tissue triggers constriction, which is subsequently maintained by the factors produced by the platelets to reduce blood loss.

Endothelial changes

Damage to a blood vessel will result in loss of or damage to the endothelial lining, which triggers several regulatory changes:

• Loss of endothelium exposes the basement membrane of the vessel to blood. This exposed surface can recruit platelets and promote blood clotting, because it is negatively charged, stimulating the intrinsic pathway.
• Activation of endothelium can cause the upregulation and expression of various proinflammatory molecules on the surface. The von Willebrand factor (vWF) can bind platelets, whereas **tissue factor** activates the **extrinsic pathway** of blood coagulation.

 CLINICAL The Von Willebrand factor

This factor is a glycoprotein produced by the endothelial cells, and stored in Weibel–Palade bodies until activation. It is also found in platelets and the subendothelial space. The vWF binds factor VIII to stabilise it, bind the glycoprotein Ib, recruit platelets and promote their aggregation. It can also bind collagen to promote clotting at sites where the endothelium has been disrupted, exposing the underlying basement membrane.

CLINICAL Von Willebrand disease

Von Willebrand disease is one of the most common genetic clotting diseases. It results from a defect in vWF. The severity of the disease is related to the specific mutation or production of autoantibodies. In mild cases of the disease individuals bruise easily, and may suffer from heavy blood loss during menstruation. In more severe forms of the disease there is no detectable vWF, resulting in severe internal bleeding, particularly at the joints.

In severe cases of von Willebrand disease, factor VIII is administered as a long-term treatment.

Platelet activation

Platelets contribute to haemostasis through many different mechanisms:

- Adherence to damaged endothelial cells and sub-cndothelial tissues by binding to collagen and vWF
- Activation of platelets triggers release of granules; both fibrinogen and ADP are released and cyclooxygenase-2 is activated to synthesise thromboxane A_2 (TxA$_2$)
- Aggregation of platelets to form a 'plug': this in teraction is the result of glycoprotein IIb and IIIa, expressed on the surface of platelets, binding to fibrinogen to stabilise the aggregation of platelets.

Blood clotting

The end-stage of clotting is the formation of a mesh of fibrin by the cleavage and binding of many fibrinogen monomers (Fig. 6.5). Commonly blood factors are referred to by a number (e.g. factor VII) and if activated are denoted by an '**a**' (e.g. factor VIIa). The coagulation cascade can be divided into three parts:

- The **extrinsic pathway** is the main trigger of blood clotting. It is initiated by the release of **tissue factor**, which cleaves **factor VII** to VIIa. Widespread activation of the extrinsic pathway is prevented by the presence of the extrinsic pathway inhibitor, which restricts the activation of factor X.
- The **intrinsicpathway** is activated by negatively charged surfaces, which can cause coagulation on surfaces such as artificial heart valves, hence the need for anticoagulant drugs. The crucial stage in the intrinsic pathway is the activation of factor VIIIa, which may also be activated by enzymatic cleavage by thrombin, serving to amplify coagulation responses that have been triggered by the extrinsic pathway.

- The **common pathway** in blood clotting is responsible for the production of **thrombin** (factor IIa) from **prothrombin** (factor II). Prothrombin is activated by factor Xa, which is itself activated from factor X by factor Va in a Ca^{2+}-dependent fashion.

Deficiencies in factors VIII or IX, which are part of the intrinsic pathway, are the normal causes of **haemophilia**.

 CLINICAL Haemophilia

Haemophilias are inherited deficiencies in one of the blood clotting factors. In most cases (around 90%) this is factor VIII. The disease is inherited in an X-linked recessive fashion. Afflicted individuals have very poorly clotting blood so that the smallest bruise becomes a serious injury. Thankfully treatment is now possible by giving patients the deficient human blood factor.

 DEFINITION Fibrinogen

Fibrinogen is a large plasma protein. On cleavage by thrombin there is a conformational change in the molecule; it becomes insoluble and rapidly aggregates. This aggregation is aided by cross-linking catalysed by factor XIIIa to form a large meshwork.

Production of clotting factors

Clotting factors are produced by the liver, and their activation catalyses further cleavage of the pathway, to amplify the response. The production of many clotting factors (II, VII, IX and X) relies on vitamin K. The anticoagulant **warfarin** acts through inhibition of vitamin K's role in the synthesis of these factors.

 CLINICAL Warfarin

Warfarin is a commonly used anticoagulant. It inhibits the enzyme vitamin K reductase, to prevent the reduction of vitamin K – essential for the production of many clotting factors. Warfarin takes a significant time to establish its effect. Heparin, which works by a different mechanism and acts immediately, is often given until the anticoagulant effect of Warfarin has been established.

Intrinsic pathway

The intrinsic pathway is so named because all components of it are found within the blood. It is triggered by factor XII, which is activated when it comes into contact with a negatively charged surface. The intrinsic pathway is not crucial for blood coagulation *in vivo* because it serves to reinforce coagulation through the extrinsic pathway.

Common pathway

The common pathway is activated by either the intrinsic or the extrinsic pathway. The two pathways converge through their cleavage of factor X to Xa, which in turn activates thrombin (factor IIa). This is the crucial step, because thrombin can activate fibrinogen, and also contributes to the action of many other factors in the cascade, promoting their activity.

Extrinsic pathway

The extrinsic pathway is triggered by tissue damage, through the release of a tissue factor. The tissue factor, together with Ca^{2+}, binds and catalyses the cleavage of factor VII into its active form VIIa.

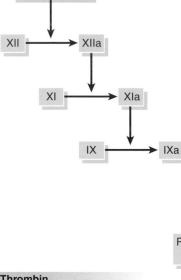

Thrombin

Prothrombin (factor II) becomes activated to thrombin (factor IIa) and acts to cleave fibrinogen into fibrin, which polymerises to form clots. Thrombin also acts on factor XIII which, when activated, stabilises the fibrin clots. Thrombin also has other roles. It can bind to specific receptors on platelets and smooth muscle, activating platelets and promoting vasospasm. It also promotes the activation of many other clotting factors in the cascade. Thrombin may also have anticoagulant roles, through binding to thrombomodulin, which allows it to activate promoters of fibrinolysis.

Fibrin

The final stage of the coagulation cascade is the production of fibrin from its precursor, fibrinogen. The fibrin molecules polymerise to form a tight meshwork of fibres. These are stabilised through the action of factor XIIIa to generate a stable clot, preventing the loss of blood.

Regulation of clotting

The endothelium is typically anticoagulant to restrict the development of thrombi in healthy vessels:

- Endothelial cells secrete **antithrombin III** which inactivates thrombin.
- Endothelial cells express **thrombomodulin**, which binds thrombin, modifying its activity to activate protein C, which is fibrinolytic.
- Endothelial cells are coated in **heparan sulphate**, which has a similar structure and function to heparin.

 DEFINITION Heparin

Heparin refers to a family of glycosaminoglycan molecules that have potent anticoagulant properties. Heparin binds antithrombin III which promotes its action. Heparin and antithrombin III can bind thrombin, or factor Xa, inhibiting their action and reducing coagulation.
Clinically, low-molecular-weight heparin is administered as an anticoagulant.

Fibrinolysis

Once bleeding has stopped, it is necessary to remove the clot, because it no longer serves a purpose, and is likely to impede both repair and function of the tissue. Clot breakdown (fibrinolysis) is achieved using plasmin, which is generated by cleavage of plasminogen.

It is also essential to ensure that clotting does not continue in healthy vessels. This can be achieved through the interaction of **antithrombin III** and heparin. Heparin and 'heparin-like' molecules can bind antithrombin III, which in turn recruits and inactivates thrombin.

Thrombosis

In some situations haemostatic mechanisms may be activated inappropriately, which can lead to severe clinical consequences:

- **Arterial thrombosis** results from the activation of platelets, often due to disruption of the endothelium in **atherosclerosis**.
- **Venous thrombosis** results from blood clotting.

The factors that promote venous thrombosis can be described in **Virchow's triad**:

- **Changes in the surface of the blood vessels** can lead to activation of the endothelium. Systemic inflammation is itself a major risk factor for thromboses through endothelial activation.
- **Changes in the pattern of blood flow**, in terms of both speed and turbulence, may increase the propensity for thrombus formation. Stasis of blood within the veins promotes blood clotting, as is seen in **deep vein thrombosis** (DVT). Turbulent flow of blood across the endothelium can activate the endothelium to express procoagulatory factors.
- **Changes in the constituents of blood** are likely to vastly alter the risk of thrombosis. Increased viscosity of the blood, as in dehydration, will affect the pattern of flow and hence alter the risk of the thromboses.

Virchow's triad applies to both arterial and venous thromboses, although the precise changes vary in different conditions.

 CLINICAL Deep vein thrombosis

The deep veins of the leg require the action of surrounding muscles to return blood to the heart. During periods of physical inactivity, blood may pool and become susceptible to clotting. Dehydration increases the blood viscosity, further promoting clotting. On moving with a DVT, there is a significant risk that the thrombus may detach and lodge at another site as an **embolus**.

Embolism

An embolus is a mass that is transported by the bloodstream. It may lodge in vessels and prevent blood flow to capillary beds. Emboli may form from many different materials:

- Detached thrombus
- Air
- Fat
- Atherosclerotic plaque rupture.

Figure 6.5 Blood clotting factors. The coagulation cascade is made up of a series of proteolytic enzymes, which each become activated (denoted by an 'a') and cleave one or more further enzymes in the cascade. The coagulation cascade can be broken down into three pathways – the intrinsic and the extrinsic, both of which converge through the common pathway.

As over 95% of all emboli result from detached thrombi, the major risk factors of embolism are very similar to those associated with thrombus formation.

Pulmonary embolism

An embolus may pass through the right side of the heart and occlude the pulmonary vessels, restricting adequate blood flow to the lungs for oxygenation. If the embolus is sufficiently large, death will result. The most common cause of pulmonary embolism is a deep vein thrombosis (DVT).

Systemic embolism

Typically originating as an arterial thrombus, often in the left side of the heart, systemic emboli may block systemic capillary beds. Thrombus formation may commonly be triggered by **atrial fibrillation** or **myocardial infarction**, both of which will result in abnormally turbulent blood flow. The precise effect of the thrombus depends on the capillary bed that is blocked.

Treatment of thrombi

Treatment of thrombi focuses on three different mechanisms, the use of which varies depending on the type of thrombus (e.g. whether it is arterial or venous):

1 **Angioplasty** to open blocked vessels
2 **Thrombolytic agents** to break down the thrombus
3 **Antiplatelet agents** (e.g. aspirin) to prevent platelet activation and aggregation; they are effective in inhibiting arterial thrombosis
   • **Anticoagulants** to prevent coagulation and promote fibrinolysis: **heparin** is often given, although it is associated with uncontrolled bleeding due to the inactivation of the clotting cascade; **warfarin** is given as a long-term treatment for venous thrombosis.

Atherosclerosis

Atherosclerotic lesions are fatty deposits that accumulate in vessels, leading to their gradual occlusion. These legions may rupture and trigger formation of an arterial thrombus. Such thrombi may further occlude the vessel, or break off and block a downstream vessel. The precise symptoms of an atherosclerotic lesion depend on the vessels that it affects.

Mechanisms of atherosclerotic formation

Atherosclerosis can be viewed as an unusual form of **chronic inflammation** initiated by the entry of cholesterol-rich, low-density lipoproteins (LDLs) into the subendothelial space between the tunica intima and media (Fig. 6.6). There are three crucial phases in the development of an atherosclerotic lesion:

1 **Initiation**
2 **Progression**
3 **Complication**.

Initiation

Initiation of the formation of a lesion is caused by the entry of LDL into the subendothelial space. Oxidative damage to the LDL can trigger inflammation and activate endothelial cells. As a result, the endothelium recruits monocytes that migrate into the tissue and differentiate into macrophages.

Macrophages express scavenger receptors and take up modified LDLs. They become progressively laden with oxidised LDLs and develop into 'foam cells', forming a **fatty streak** – a preatherosclerotic lesion – because they are unable to leave the subendothelial space in the fatty state.

Progression

The **progression** of a fatty streak into an atherosclerotic lesion is the result of continued recruitment of foam cells. This recruitment progressively forms a necrotic core of tissue. Furthermore, smooth muscle cells migrate into the tissue and form a fibrous cap which stabilises the lesion. The long-term accumulation of cells generates raised plaques which narrow the vessel. These plaques may indirectly cause thromboses downstream, due to the turbulent blood flow that they create.

Complications

Atherosclerotic plaques are associated with two main complications:

1 **Rupture of the plaque** can trigger platelet activation on an exposed core, promoting an arterial thrombus. Rarely, material from the ruptured plaque may enter the bloodstream as an embolus.
2 **Aneurysms or arterial rupture** can result from weakening in the vessel wall caused by the presence of the plaque.

Initiation

LDL carried in the blood may enter the subendothelial space, and become oxidised to Ox-LDL. These molecules become taken up by macrophages in the vascular tissue. The macrophages ingest the Ox-LDL molecules and become overloaded as they are unable to process the LDL, resulting in their conversion to 'foam cells'. The gradual accumulation of foam cells in point in the arteries leads to fatty streaks.

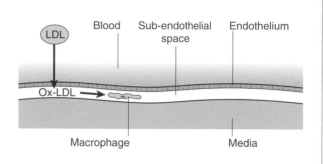

Progression

Fatty streaks further develop as more macrophages ingest Ox-LDL, resulting in the accumulation of foam cells . This process recruits more macrophages and also smooth muscles cells from the media. The smooth muscle cells secrete various connective tissue components, such as collagen, and act to stabilise the lesion. Due to the increasing number of cells, the lesion bulges out into the vessel, which can occlude blood flow downstream. The additional shear stresses occurring in an atherosclerotic lesion result in activation of the overlying endothelium, further increasing recruitment of macrophages and other cells.

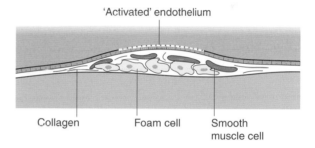

Complication

Atherosclerotic lesion may progress such that foam cells begin to die and produce a necrotic core. This may destabilise the lesion such that it ruptures, exposing the necrotic core directly to the blood. The ruptured lesion rapidly attracts platelets to form a thrombus , and the contents of the lesion may also escape into the blood supply as a fatty embolus .

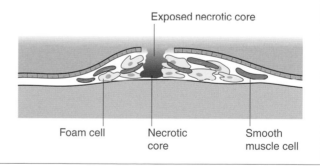

Figure 6.6 Atherosclerosis is a process that occurs in most people. However, progressive build-up of these fatty lesions can result in many health problems. Cardiovascular disease is the biggest killer in the western world. LDL, low-density lipoprotein.

Risk factors for atherosclerosis

Atherosclerotic processes occur within everyone, although there are risk factors that increase their occurrence. Key modifiable risk factors that have been identified are:

- **High plasma LDLs**
- **Low plasma HDLs** (high-density lipoproteins), a type of lipoprotein that can acquire cholesterol, so reducing its deposition in the tissues
- **Physical inactivity**
- **Smoking** which increases the oxidation of LDLs, promoting the inflammatory processes initiating atherosclerosis
- **High blood pressure**: this is likely to increase the shear stress to which the endothelium is exposed, increasing its propensity to be activated
- **Diabetes**.

Other non-modifiable risk factors have been identified:

- Being male
- **A family history** of atherosclerosis
- **Age**: atherosclerosis is a process that takes many years to manifest, so older people are more likely to develop such conditions
- **Genetic disorders**, such as **familial hypercholesterolaemia** (FH), in which there is altered regulation of lipoproteins, vastly increase the risk of atherosclerosis.

Prevention of atherosclerosis

Much of the treatment of atherosclerosis is through lifestyle and dietary changes to reduce the risk factors associated with an increased risk of the condition. Drugs may be used to reduce the levels of cholesterol (and, hence, LDLs) within the body:

- **Diet** is a crucial factor to manage the development of atherosclerosis. The typically western diet contains far more fat and cholesterol than the body has evolved to tolerate. As a result cutting down cholesterol can slow the progression of developing atherosclerotic lesions.
- **Exercise**.
- **Statins** inhibit **hydroxymethylglutaryl (HMG)-CoA reductase**, which is crucial for the endogenous synthesis of cholesterol. Increases in the expression of LDL receptor on the liver have been observed which are likely to further reduce plasma levels. Statins have proved to be extremely effective drugs with few side effects.

 CLINICAL Familial hypercholesterolaemia (FH)

FH is a genetic disorder resulting from mutations in the proteins regulating the transport and uptake of LDLs. High levels of LDLs result, which are taken up by scavenger receptors on macrophages, so promoting atherosclerosis. There are a number of common features for people with FH:

- Family history of atherosclerosis and heart disease
- Early onset cardiovascular disease
- Cholesterol deposition in the tissues, in particular:
  – tendon xanthomas – yellow cholesterol deposits in the tendons
  – deposition of cholesterol in the eyelids, discolouring them
  – discoloration of the iris.

Mutations resulting in FH occur either in the LDL receptor, making it non-functional, or in the transport protein ApoB100. Individuals who are hetero- and homozygous for FH mutations have been reported; these require different treatments:

- Heterozygous FH individuals still express the LDL receptor, allowing statins to be used as treatment.
- Homozygous FH individuals are extremely rare, and have significantly more severe symptoms. Apheresis may be used instead, in which LDLs are removed directly from the patient's blood, or a liver transplantation may be undertaken, replacing the patient's liver with one that expresses functional LDL receptors.

Treatment of atherosclerosis

Surgical intervention is required if an atherosclerotic lesion prevents sufficient blood from reaching the tissues. Three major procedures are commonly used:

1 **Balloon angioplasty**. a balloon is inserted through an incision in the femoral artery up to the stenosis. The balloon is then inflated to open the lumen of the affected vessel. There is a significant risk, with a balloon angioplasty, that the vessel will collapse again because there is nothing to hold the vessel open.

2 **Stenting**. A vessel is opened by a balloon angioplasty and a metal tube placed at the site of stenosis to hold the vessel open. Although this guarantees that the vessel will remain open, the body is likely to react against the stent, despite being coated in drugs to prevent this. Smooth muscle cells may migrate to the site and contribute to further stenosis, which must be corrected by more drastic intervention.

3 **Coronary artery bypass graft (CABG)**. A blocked vessel can be bypassed by the attachment of a grafted vessel either side of the blockage.

Typically, an artery from the thoracic wall is used because it can cope with the high-pressure arterial blood flow and does not severely compromise blood flow to the thoracic wall tissues.

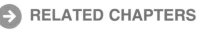 **RELATED CHAPTERS**

7

Respiratory system

The respiratory system's principal role is ensuring the oxygenation of the blood and the removal of carbon dioxide from the body through gaseous exchange which occurs in the alveoli of the lungs.

The gaseous exchange that occurs in the lungs relies on diffusion, and is reflected in the large surface area that the lungs provide, through the many millions of small alveoli which are the sites of gas exchange.

Although carbon dioxide is readily soluble in the blood, the transport of oxygen is through a specialised transport protein – haemoglobin. In the lungs the ventilation of the alveoli is matched to the blood flow, to allow sufficient time for the diffusion of oxygen. This large blood flow and surface area also allow the regulation of many other processes: in particular, the short-term regulation of pH, as a result of the effect of CO_2 in bicarbonate buffering of the blood, and as a site of enzymatic activity allowing the modulation of protein hormones carried in the blood.

Anatomy of the respiratory system

The gross anatomy of the lungs and their relation to other thoracic structures is discussed in the anatomy chapter, whilst the detailed anatomy of the airways and lungs are discussed below.

The pleura

The pleurae cover the lungs to allow their movement against the chest wall during breathing, without causing irritation. They are made of two layers surrounding a potential space:

- The **visceral pleura** surrounds the lungs, and protrudes into the fissures, so that all the lobes are covered. They receive their blood supply from the **bronchial arteries**.
- The **parietal pleura** lies outside the visceral pleura. It is in contact with structures directly adjacent to the lungs – the mediastinum, thoracic wall and diaphragm. The parietal pleura is vascularised by the thoracic wall blood.
- The **pleural sac** is the potential space between the two layers of pleurae. It contains a layer of **pleural fluid** which acts as a lubricant. The surface tension of the pleural fluid is sufficient to ensure that the pleural layers (and, hence, the lungs and thoracic wall) remain in contact so that the lungs expand as the chest does.

The airways

The airways transport air to the sites of gas exchange while limiting entry of pathogens and harmful particles into the fragile lung tissue, as well as moistening the air to aid diffusion. The airways can be divided into three sets of structures:

1 The **upper airways and sinuses** are found in the head and neck, and share many conduits with the gastrointestinal tract.

Biomedical Science Lecture Notes, First Edition. Ian Lyons.
© 2011 by Ian Lyons. Published 2011 by Blackwell Publishing Ltd.

2 The **larynx** connects the upper airways to the **respiratory tree** and is separate from the gastrointestinal tract.

3 The **respiratory tree** is the branching structure of airways that carries air from the trachea to the **alveoli** – the site of gas exchange.

 CLINICAL Pneumothorax

Pneumothorax is an accumulation of air in the pleural cavity, reducing the vital capacity; this causes a 'collapsed lung'. Occasionally, a one-way valve forms that causes air to be drawn into the pleural space, although it prevents it from leaving. This **tension pneumothorax** is a medical emergency and causes rapid inflation of the pleural space and an accompanying shift of the mediastinum, detectable by deviation of the trachea at the neck.

Treatment of a pneumothorax depends on its size:

- A **small pneumothorax** will resolve spontaneously.
- **Larger pneumothoraces** require the insertion of a **chest drain** – a tube containing a one-way valve to remove air from the pleura.
- **Tension pneumothorax** is treated rapidly by the insertion of a needle into the chest (at the second intercostal space in the midclavicular line) to allow removal of air from the chest. A chest drain is then inserted to clear the pneumothorax.

The upper airways and sinuses

The nose and sinuses are the site of entry of air, and are responsible for warming inhaled air. In addition, they are involved in removing particles by the hairs and mucus present in the nose.

The trachea

The trachea is the large single tube through which inhaled air flows. The trachea starts directly below the larynx at the level of C6, and ends at the **carina**, where it bifurcates into the two bronchi; this occurs at the level of the T4–5 intervertebral disc. The trachea is held open by incomplete rings of cartilage, which contain gaps posteriorly (where the oesophagus lies) to allow expansion of the oesophagus for passage of food to the stomach.

The respiratory tree

The respiratory tree is a series of branching tubes, which form in the lungs by **branching morphogenesis**. The 23 generations of branches carry air from the trachea to the millions of alveoli; gas exchange occurs in only the last six generations. The first few branches of the respiratory tree reflect the gross anatomical organisation of the lungs:

- The **trachea** is the first airway in the respiratory tree.
- One **bronchus** carries air to each lung, entering at the **hilum** of the lungs. The bronchi are supported by rings of cartilage in their walls.
- **Lobar bronchi** are branches of the main bronchi. There are two lobar bronchi on the left and three on the right.
- The **segmental bronchi** are the branches of the lobar bronchi. Each segmental bronchus supplies a distinct **bronchopulmonary segment**.
- The **bronchioles** branch into progressively smaller branches in each bronchopulmonary segment, carrying air to the alveoli.

The lungs

For gas exchange to occur, inspired air must be brought close to the blood in the pulmonary capillaries, so that diffusion can occur. The branching structure of the airways terminates in small air sacs – the **alveoli** – which are surrounded by blood vessels. The numerous alveoli generate an enormous surface area to facilitate diffusion.

Gross anatomy of the lungs

The lungs are found on either side of the **mediastinum** and are broadly pyramidal in shape. Three sides can be identified (Fig. 7.1):

- The **costal surface** is the large curved surface that lies adjacent to, and follows the course of, the sternum, ribs and costal cartilages.
- The **mediastinal surface** is adjacent to the mediastinum. The left lung has a 'cardiac notch' in its mediastinal surface, which accommodates the **pericardium**.
- The **diaphragmatic surface** forms the bottom of the lung which lies on the superior surface of the diaphragm.

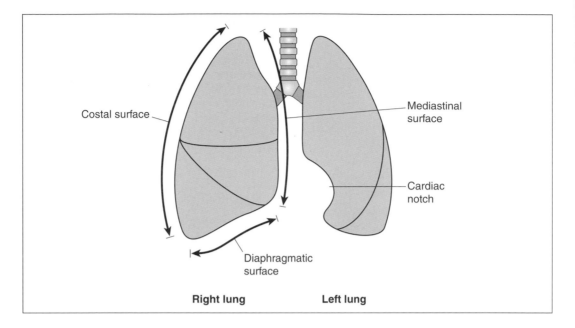

Figure 7.1 **Gross anatomy of the lungs**. Each lung has a similar gross structure, possessing costal, diaphragmatic and medial sides. The apex of the lungs ascends into the neck. Although the right lung has both horizontal and oblique fissures, the left lung has only an oblique fissure because it is divided into just two lobes. The oblique fissure runs from the level of T2 on the posterior aspect to the level of the sixth costal cartilage anteriorly. The horizontal fissure runs along the level of the fourth rib. The left lung possesses a pronounced cardiac notch on the medial side. The pleurae (red) surround the lungs. Should a wound occur allowing air to enter the pleura, a **pneumothorax** occurs. The presence of air between the pleurae prevents the proper expansion of lungs, limiting ventilation.

A variety of structural features of the lungs can be identified:

- The lungs are divided into lobes. The **left lung has two lobes** separated by the horizontal fissure, whereas the **right has three lobes**, separated by horizontal and oblique fissures.
- The **hilum of the lungs**, located on the medial surface, is the site of entry of the bronchi, vasculature and nerves.
- The **apex** is the blunt superior end of the lungs which ascends above the level of the first rib and into the lower part of the neck.

Bronchopulmonary segments

Both lungs are organised into 10 **bronchopulmonary segments** separated by connective tissue; each receives its own blood supply and airway:

- A **segmental bronchiole** carries air to each bronchopulmonary segment.
- A **segmental pulmonary artery** supplies each segment.

- **Pulmonary veins** run in the connective tissue between the segments, and receive blood from both segments.

The respiratory zone

The respiratory zone contains the last 6 generations (17–23) of the respiratory tree. These airways are lined with alveoli, which account for around 10% of the gas exchange surface. The final generation of airways terminates in many alveoli, which accounts for the remainder of the gaseous exchange surface.

Alveoli

The alveoli are the basic functional unit of the lungs. Each lung contains around 300 million, the development of which is not completed until the age of around 8 years. The alveoli are made up of a single cellular layer, which is closely apposed to capillary vessels, containing blood in the pulmonary circulation.

Vasculature and innervation of the lungs

Arterial supply

The lungs receive two arterial supplies:

1 The **pulmonary arteries** carry blood from the heart for oxygenation.
2 The **bronchial arteries** carry oxygenated blood to supply the tissue of the lungs.

The pulmonary arteries

The right and left pulmonary arteries originate from the pulmonary trunk and enter the lungs at the hilum. They descend posterolaterally to the main bronchus and divide progressively following the bronchial tree, with the arterial branch running anterior to its corresponding bronchiole.

The bronchial arteries

The **bronchial arteries** are part of the systemic circulation, oxygenating the lung tissues:

- The **left bronchial artery** arises from the thoracic aorta.
- The **right bronchial artery** arises from either the superior branch of the left bronchial artery or an intercostal artery.

The bronchial arteries supply the bronchial tissue as far as the respiratory bronchioles.

Venous drainage

There are two different venous systems in the lungs:

- Two **pulmonary veins** leave each lung and carry oxygenated blood to the left atrium.
- The **bronchial veins** drain part of the blood supplied by the bronchial arteries whereas the remainder is drained by the pulmonary veins. The right bronchial vein drains into the **azygos** vein whereas the left drains into the **hemiazygos** vein.

Lymphatic drainage

The lymphatic drainage of the lungs contains two main groups of lymphatics in the connective tissue, one superficial and one deeper. Both drain to the hilar lymph nodes. Lymph from the parietal pleura drains to the lymph nodes of the thoracic wall. In the cervical region, there is some drainage to the axillary lymph nodes.

Innervation

The lungs receive sensory innervation from both arms of the autonomic nervous system:

- **Sensory fibres** are derived from the vagus nerve. These sense stretching of the vessels and bronchi, and can detect irritation that may initiate a cough reflex.
- **Sympathetic fibres** cause relaxation of the bronchial smooth muscle and decrease secretion. Sympathetic stimulation also triggers pulmonary vasoconstriction.
- **Parasympathetic fibres** from the vagus nerve trigger bronchoconstriction as well as dilatation of the pulmonary vessels. They also stimulate secretion in the bronchioles and alveoli.

The **parietal pleura** receives a rich sensory innervation resulting in pain on irritation:

- The **phrenic nerves** supply the mediastinal side of the lungs and the central part of the diaphragmatic surface. Those areas innervated by the phrenic nerve develop referred pain over the C3–5 dermatomes – the base of the neck and shoulder.
- The **intercostal nerves** supply the costal surface of the lungs and the peripheral regions of the diaphragmatic surface. Regions innervated by the costal nerves have referred pain from the area of skin innervated by the same intercostal nerves.

The **visceral pleura** receives no sensory innervation.

Tissue types in the lungs

There is pronounced specialisation of the respiratory tract. Three distinct groups of tissues with different functions can be identified:

1 The **respiratory epithelium** allows carriage of air to the alveoli while removing any debris present.
2 The **alveolar cells** are adapted to ensure that the alveoli are open and capable of gaseous exchange.
3 The **connective tissue** of the lungs supports the rest of the structures involved in ventilation.

Respiratory epithelial cells

The predominant cells in the airways are the **ciliated epithelial cells**; however, these are interspersed with secretory cells which release mucus and other secretions to protect the airways:

- The **ciliated epithelial cells** provide a physical barrier to the movement of mucus, and anything caught within it, out of the respiratory tract. The cells are classified as **pseudostratified columnar epithelial cells**.
- **Goblet cells** contain mucus droplets, which they secrete into the lumen of the airways. The mucus catches debris in the air and facilitates its removal through the **mucociliary escalator**.
- **Clara cells** produce surfactant and express detoxifying enzymes to protect the airways. They are also the stem cells that replicate and differentiate to replace other cell types that may be lost through damage.
- **Brush cells** have microvilli on their apical surface and are innervated, suggesting that they have a sensory role.
- **Neuroendocrine cells** may have a sensory role in the lungs, as well as secreting regulatory factors.

 DEFINITION Mucociliary escalator

Inhaled particles in the lungs are trapped by mucus secreted by the goblet cells. This is then moved out of the respiratory tract by beating of the cilia on the epithelium. This movement draws the mucus to the epiglottis where it is swallowed.

 CLINICAL Emphysema

Emphysema is the destruction of the alveolar walls, decreasing the available surface for gas exchange. Many inhaled pollutants from smoking and air pollution damage the alveoli and cause emphysema, which decreases surface area for gas exchange to the point where it is inadequate to meet the body's needs. Emphysema is a major cause of death in the industrialised world.

Alveolar tissue

The alveolar surface is extremely thin (less than $1\,\mu$m thick), and can be divided into three layers:

1 Surface epithelium
2 Basement membrane and supporting matrix
3 Capillary cell wall.

The alveolar walls contribute to the high surface area and contain pores that allow the passage of alveolar macrophages between the different alveoli.

The surface epithelium

Two cell types are found in the diffusion surface of the alveoli:

- **Type I pneumocytes** make up around 95% of the surface area of the alveoli.
- **Type II pneumocytes** are the most numerous cells in the alveoli, yet account for <5% of the alveolar surface area. The two main roles of the type II cells are secretion of **surfactants** and being precursors of type I pneumocytes.

The basement membrane

The basement membrane of the pneumocytes and the capillaries contains **collagen** and **elastin** fibres, to provide recoil for expulsion of air from the alveoli during expiration. As with other alveolar layers, the basement membrane is thin, to help diffusion.

Alveolar capillaries

The pulmonary capillaries form a plexus of thin vessels around the alveoli to minimise the diffusion distance. The alveolar capillaries are continuous and do not contain fenestrations, to prevent fluid leaving the capillaries as a result of Starling's forces.

Alveolar macrophages

Alveolar macrophages do not contribute to the diffusion surface of the alveoli. Instead, they provide innate immune protection and are responsible for the clearance of particulate matter that reaches the alveoli. These cells are derived from circulating **macrophages** and can travel between alveoli, through pores in the alveolar wall.

Supporting tissue of the lungs

The airways contain connective tissue that supports and maintains the airways as conduits to the alveoli:

- **Cartilage** reinforces the large branches of the respiratory tree. These branches maintain the vessels during expiration, when the increased force can cause collapse, preventing further expulsion of air. Initially cartilage is found as rings, although, as the bronchioles become narrower, they are found in small plates before disappearing entirely.

- **Smooth muscle cells** are found throughout the respiratory tree. These receive autonomic innervation, allowing regulation of the size of the airways, and of the vessel resistance.
- The **elastic connective tissue** provides the lungs with the recoil to contract and expel air during expiration. This elasticity also allows the expansion necessary for inspiration.

Ventilation

Ventilation is the physical process by which air is drawn into the lungs so that gas exchange can occur in the alveoli. It is achieved by contraction of the diaphragm and ribcage, increasing the volume of the thoracic cavity. This, in turn, causes expansion of the lungs, which reduces the pressure, allowing the inflow of air down the pressure gradient.

 DEFINITION Ventilation

Ventilation (V) is defined as the **volume of gas breathed out in 1 min**, which is determined by the formula:

$$V(mL/min) = \text{Volume of one breath (mL)}$$
$$\times \text{Breaths/min.}$$

A better measure of the air entering the lungs is the volume available for gaseous exchange – **alveolar ventilation (V_A)** – which takes into account the volume of dead space (V_D) in the lungs:

$$V_A(mL/min) = (\text{Volume of one breath} - V_D)$$
$$\times \text{Breaths/min.}$$

Mechanics of ventilation

There are two stages to ventilation: **inspiration**, when air is drawn into the lungs, and **expiration**, when air is expelled. Inspiration is always an active process, requiring contraction of muscles, whereas expiration is initially a passive process, relying on the elastic properties of the lung tissue. At higher rates of breathing, forced expiration occurs.

Inspiration

The following are two main groups of muscles involved in inspiration:

1 The **diaphragm** contracts and flattens to increase the size of the thorax.
2 The **external intercostal muscles** pull the ribs upwards and outwards, to increase the volume of the thoracic cavity.

On inspiration, the **sternocleidomastoids** and other neck muscles aid breathing, particularly if the individual's arms are braced against a surface, allowing the pectoral muscles to contribute to inspiration.

Expiration

Expiration is mainly a passive action, relying on the elastic nature of the tissues to expel the air, although the **internal intercostal** muscles can contract, pulling the ribs downwards and inwards. During exercise, forced expiration increases the rate of expiration. Contraction of the **abdominal muscles** aids the expulsion of air from the lungs by forcing the roof of the diaphragm up into the thorax.

Static mechanics of ventilation

The static values measured in respiration refer to those determined by the static properties of the lungs, and are not a direct measurement of the rate of air flow through the airways and the related effects. A variety of different lung volumes can be measured by **spirometry** or **helium dilution**. These static volumes reflect the total volume available in the lung as well as that proportion usually used in ventilation (Fig. 7.2):

- The **total lung capacity** (TLC) is the total volume of air that the lungs can accommodate; however, not all the air can be removed, even during maximal ventilation.
- The **residual volume** (RV) of the lungs is the volume that remains at maximal expiration.
- The **functional residual capacity** (FRC) is the volume of gas that is in the lungs at the end of a normal breath. This cannot be calculated without knowledge of the RV of the lungs.
- The **vital capacity** (VC) is the maximum volume of air that can be inhaled and expelled by the lungs.

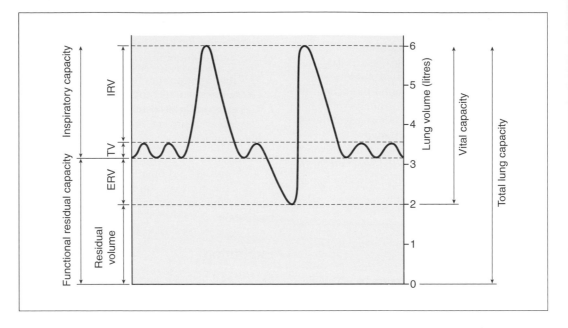

Figure 7.2 The spirometer allows measurement of many of the static respiratory values which allows assessment of the functionality of the lungs.

- The **tidal volume** is the volume of air that is ventilated during normal breathing.

> **DEFINITION Spirometry**
>
> A **spirometer** is used to measure breath functions. There are two sets of values that a spirometer may measure: volume and flow rate. Spirometers require the patient to breathe into a tube attached to the machine, and the volume of air in relation to time taken is measured. From these data many different values can be calculated.

> **DEFINITION Helium dilution**
>
> It is not possible to measure the total lung volume (and the residual volume) using spirometry. Instead, helium dilution is used. The patient breathes from a spirometer containing a known volume of helium. As helium is effectively insoluble, repeated re-breathing allows the helium to become evenly diluted between the lungs and the spirometer. The magnitude of the dilution of the helium, together with the initial concentration and volume of the spirometer, can be used to calculate the total lung volume.

Dead space

Gas exchange occurs only in the **respiratory zone** which is made up of the last six generations of the respiratory tree (branches 17–23). Before this point, the airways of lungs are **anatomical dead space** in which no diffusion occurs:

- The **anatomical dead space** has a volume of around 150 mL.
- The **respiratory zone** has a volume of around 3000 mL.

Physiological dead space

Physiological dead space is a better measure of the volume in the lungs that does not permit gas exchange. It consists of two components:

1 The **airways in the anatomical dead space**, which do not contribute to diffusion
2 The **alveolar dead space,** which is the area in the respiratory zone where there is little perfusion or ventilation, preventing adequate gaseous exchange. In situations where there is damage to the alveolar tissue, there may be a significant contribution from the **alveolar dead space**, as in emphysema.

Partial pressures

The partial pressures of O_2 and CO_2 vary between the arteries and the veins. Gas exchange is a passive process, and occurs through diffusion down a concentration gradient. In most cases, there is sufficient time to allow equilibrium between the arteries and the alveoli. The values of arterial O_2 and CO_2 pressures are virtually identical to those of the alveoli (Table 7.1).

 DEFINITION Partial pressure

This describes the concentration of a gas in the air, or dissolved in a fluid. The partial pressure of a gas is defined as the pressure that it would exert if all other gases were removed, yet the volume in which it is contained were kept constant.

The partial pressure of a gas can be calculated by multiplying its relative concentration by the total pressure of the gas in which it is found. However, the pressure resulting from water must also be accounted for. The lungs saturate the air with water vapour, resulting in a partial pressure of water of 47 mmHg, which must be 'removed' from the initial gas pressure. Thus the partial pressure of a gas is:

(Atmospheric pressure (mmHg) – 47) × Relative concentration of gas = Partial pressure.

To get the partial pressure in the correct units of kilopascals, 1 mmHg = 133 Pa.

The contribution of water vapour becomes more significant at high altitudes, because it effectively removes a proportion of the air that can carry O_2.

Table 7.1 The values of O_2 and CO_2 partial pressures

Gas and location	Partial pressure (mmHg/kPa)
Inspired O_2 (PiO_2)	150 (20)
Arterial O_2 (PaO_2)	100 (13.3)
Venous O_2 (PvO_2)	40 (5.3)
Inspired CO_2 ($PiCO_2$)	0
Arterial CO_2 ($PaCO_2$)	40 (5.3)
Venous CO_2 ($PvCO_2$)	45 (6)

Regional ventilation

Ventilation of the lungs is altered by:

- **Gravity**: the weight of the lung tissue alters the interpleural pressure, resulting in a more negative pressure at higher regions. The lower regions are more compressed, have a greater potential to expand and can draw in a greater volume of air, proportionally increasing the ventilation that they receive.
- **Speed of inspiration**: fast breathing promotes better ventilation of the higher regions of the lungs at FRC. Under slow breathing, the lower regions of the lungs are better ventilated.

Dynamic respiratory mechanisms

The dynamic effects on ventilation are the result of the airflow through the airways, and the changing resistance, which depends on the pattern and rate of flow.

At **low velocities** air flows through a tube in a smooth stream – **laminar flow**. At higher flow rates the air becomes **turbulent**, resulting in a disrupted stream, and large changes in the resistance of the airflow. Although the airflow is **laminar**, the resistance of the flow through the tube can be determined by Poiseuille's equation:

$$R = (8\eta l)/(\pi r^4)$$

where η is the coefficient of viscosity, P the pressure difference, l the length and r the radius.

The tube size has a huge effect on the resistance during laminar flow – halving the radius of the tube increases the resistance 16-fold.

The nature of the airflow tends to vary throughout the lungs. Pure laminar flow occurs when the air is moving in parallel stream lines, with the air at the centre moving far faster than the air at the edges. In contrast, turbulent flow is more disorganised and lacks the high-velocity flow seen at the centre of tubes with laminar flow:

- **Airflow is turbulent** in the trachea.
- Most of the respiratory tree carries **air in transition** (neither truly laminar nor truly turbulent).
- **True laminar flow** is seen only in the smallest bronchioles.

Airway resistance

Airway resistance is governed by the total cross-sectional area. The point at which the maximal resistance is encountered is in the first seven generations of branching. After this point, the large number of airways generates a larger total cross-sectional area, although each individual airway is of a very small diameter. The cross-sectional area of the lung airways may vary during breathing, altering resistance:

- The **lung volume** alters the support that the connective tissue fibres provide to the lung, drawing open the airways.
- The **tone of the airway smooth muscle** can be altered by a variety of stimuli – from both the environment and the body.

Measurement of airway resistance

Measurement of airway resistance allows detection and diagnosis of pathologies in the lungs. Airway resistance can be determined by the difference between mouth pressure and alveolar pressure. Two key values are used to assess the airway resistance:

1 The **forced expiratory volume in 1 second (FEV$_1$)** is the maximum volume of air that an individual can expel in 1 second. Changes in this ratio allow the distinction between restrictive and obstructive pulmonary diseases.
2 **Peak expiratory flow** (**PEF**) provides a measurement of airway resistance. It is relatively constant regardless of the force with which one tries to expire. As the pressure on the lungs increases, the airways are constricted, increasing the potential resistance for a given airflow velocity.

DEFINITION Restrictive and obstructive pulmonary diseases

In **restrictive diseases** (e.g. fibrosis) the ability of the lung to expand has been impeded. As such, people with the condition are likely to have a markedly reduced FVC, although their FEV$_1$ is probably quite normal, because the airways themselves are not obstructed.

Obstructive diseases lead to the obstruction of airflow through the lungs. As a result the FEV$_1$ of infected individuals is likely to be rather lower than average, although the vital capacity is unlikely to be as affected as in restrictive disorders.

CLINICAL Asthma

Asthma is an obstructive pulmonary disorder caused by a chronic inflammatory response within the lungs. The closure of the airways in people with asthma can be managed by steroids to reduce inflammation and also acutely by the administration of **salbutamol**, a β$_2$-adrenoceptor agonist, which causes dilatation of the bronchial smooth muscle.

Compliance and airway closure

In normal breathing, the lungs are very compliant. At higher volumes, the lungs become less compliant – there is an increased amount of effort required to allow further tissue expansion.

DEFINITION Compliance

Compliance of the lungs is measured as the change in volume of the lungs for a change in pressure. This provides a measure of how easily the lungs can be inflated. The compliance of the lungs and the chest wall differ slightly, because they are separated by the pleura.

Changes in compliance can be associated with pathology and tissue damage. Common causes of reduced compliance are:

- **Pulmonary fibrosis** due to the increased fibrous tissue hindering expansion
- **Pulmonary oedema** which causes increased compliance through prevention of the inflation of some of the alveoli, as they become filled within fluid
- **Emphysema** which leads to increased compliance as a result of loss of connective tissue in the alveoli, including the elastic fibres
- **During asthma attacks** there is an increase in compliance although the mechanisms are not fully understood
- **Normal ageing of the lungs** which leads to increased compliance, due to changes in the alveolar connective tissues.

The relationship between the interpleural pressure and the lung volume at a given pressure differs on inspiration and expiration (Fig. 7.3). This is known as **hysteresis** and results from airway closure.

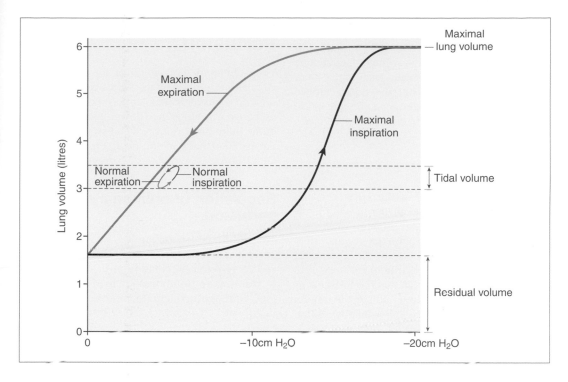

Figure 7.3 **Intrapleural pressure during ventilation**. The intrapleural pressure of the lungs differs on inspiration and expiration and at different lung volumes, as a result of the effect of surfactant and the collapse of the smaller vessel before complete expulsion of air from the lungs. There is a difference in the effort (as reflected in the changes in intrapleural pressure) required to inflate and deflate the lungs. This hysteresis becomes progressively more pronounced for bigger breaths.

In less well-ventilated regions (i.e. base of the lung), it is not possible for all the air to be expelled from the lungs, because the smaller airways tend to collapse before the alveoli. In elderly people, this effect may be significant during normal breathing, due to changes in the elastic connective tissue. Regions where airway closure occurs are poorly ventilated and, as a result, have poor gas exchange. Surfactant in the alveoli also contributes to hysteresis because it alters the alveolar surface tension.

Movement of air in the respiratory zone

The later branches of the respiratory tree are termed the respiratory zone, because they are the site of gaseous exchange. At this point the cross-sectional area of the airways is so large that the movement of air by diffusion is greater than that occurring as a result of ventilation. The result is that gas partial pressures of in this region remain relatively constant and do not change with each breath.

Alveolar ventilation

In the respiratory zone, the partial pressures of CO_2 and O_2 remain relatively constant, and can be calculated by the **alveolar gas equation**:

$$P_AO_2 = P_IO_2 - PaCO_2[F_IO_2 + (1 - F_IO_2)/R]$$

where P_IO_2 is the partial pressure of inspired O_2, P_ACO_2 the partial pressure of alveolar CO_2, F_IO_2 the fraction of air, i.e. O_2 and R the respiratory quotient.

 DEFINITION Respiratory quotient

The **respiratory quotient** (RQ) provides a ratio of CO_2 production and oxygen consumption:

RQ = CO_2 production/O_2 consumption.

At rest, the average man consumes around 250 mL O_2/min and has a respiratory quotient of 0.8. In exercise his RQ may increase to 2, and his intake of O_2 increases to around 3000 mL, and thus CO_2 production increases to 6000 mL.

Surfactant and surface tension

The alveoli are all lined with fluid, resulting in a surface tension due to the stronger interactions of the liquid molecules with each other than with the gases. As a result the liquid surface area tries to contract, generating a pressure in the gas in the alveoli. This is determined by La Place's Law:

$$\text{Pressure} = 2 \times \text{Surface tension}/\text{Radius}.$$

As the alveoli are not all the same size, the tension should trigger the smaller alveoli to collapse because the increased pressure causes the gases within to be expelled into the neighbouring, larger alveoli. This is overcome by the presence of surfactant within the alveolar fluid.

Surfactants are unusual in that the surface tension changes with the volume. It is made up of a phospholipid – dipalmitoylphosphatidylcholine (DPPC). The molecules of DPPC repel each other. As a result the more tightly the molecules are packed, the more strongly they repel each other, opposing the effects of surface tension. Surfactant contributes to lung function by:

- **increasing compliance** of the lungs such that the work required to inflate the lungs is reduced
- **promoting alveolar stability** by opposing the La Place equation
- **preventing the transduction of fluids** into the alveoli. Surface tension promotes the accumulation of liquids in a discrete location. By disrupting surface tension, surfactant hinders this accumulation of fluids within the alveoli.

 CLINICAL Respiratory distress syndrome

Preterm babies frequently lack surfactant production, which causes collapse of the alveoli within the lungs so the work required for inspiration is correspondingly increased. As the neonate is unable to breathe well, he or she becomes underventilated and retains CO_2, which can contribute to damage to the respiratory epithelium and pulmonary capillaries; it forms a fibrous tissue that gives the disease its other common name, **hyaline membrane disease**.

Perfusion

The pulmonary circulation is the low-pressure circulation pumped by the right side of the heart. It carries deoxygenated blood to the lungs for gas exchange. The blood then flows into the tributaries of the pulmonary veins, which carry the reoxygenated blood back to the heart for the systemic circulation.

Regulation of pulmonary perfusion

The pulmonary circulation transports blood a short distance but must carry the same volume as the systemic circulation with each beat. As a result, the pulmonary blood pressure is low, although it fluctuates markedly with each heartbeat.

- **Pulmonary systolic blood pressure** is typically 25 mmHg.
- **Pulmonary diastolic blood pressure** is typically 8 mmHg.

The low pressure of the pulmonary circulation is essential because the pulmonary vessels have much thinner walls than their corresponding systemic vessels, reflecting two major differences in the roles of the circulation:

1 **There is little need to distribute the blood asymmetrically**: in the systemic circulation the blood is allocated depending on the metabolic needs of different tissues. In the pulmonary circulation, all the blood requires oxygenation, so there is little need to direct it. As a result the blood vessels do not possess a significant muscular layer. **The pulmonary circulation remains in the chest**.

2 **The transmural pressure of the alveolar capillaries must be kept low**: the alveolar vessels are effectively surrounded by gas – there is little interstitial fluid as there is around the endothelium of systemic capillaries. As a result there is little hydrostatic force in the interstitium to prevent flow of the plasma into the alveoli through **Starling's forces**. There is a small net pressure in the lungs forcing fluid from the capillaries. This is reflected in the small lymph flow drained by the lymphatic system. Increased pulmonary blood pressure can increase the

movement of fluid out of the capillaries and lead to **pulmonary oedema** in severe cases.

 CLINICAL Pulmonary oedema

An increase in the pressure inside the pulmonary capillaries can result in increased fluid leaving the capillaries. This increased fluid is **pulmonary oedema**. The oedema may directly damage the fragile alveolar tissue, as well as filling the alveoli with fluid, thereby reducing the available surface for gas exchange.

Pulmonary oedema is treated by reducing the pulmonary blood pressure, which is typically achieved by improving cardiac function. Although the pulmonary function is being corrected, oxygen is typically given to ensure adequate oxygenation of the blood.

Distribution of blood flow in the pulmonary circulation

The level of perfusion of the lungs varies across the height of the lung as a result of the hydrostatic pressure differences, the weight of lung tissue and fluid on the vessels. As a result, in the upper regions of the lungs, the pressure within the alveoli tends to exceed that in the pulmonary vessels, constricting blood flow. Further down, towards the bottom of the lungs, the pulmonary arterial pressure is greater, exceeding the alveolar pressure, which allows for increased perfusion. The difference in pressure between the top and bottom of the lungs may be around 25 mmHg.

Regulation of pulmonary vascular resistance

The pressure in the pulmonary circulation must be kept low. However, there is a vasoconstrictive response in hypoxia. Regions of low alveolar O_2 trigger vasoconstriction of the arterioles in this region. It is thought that this mechanism may ensure that pulmonary blood flows to well-ventilated areas of the lungs, allowing gas exchange and diverting it from regions of the lungs where the airways are compressed or blocked.

The hypoxic vasoconstriction response can present a clinical problem at high altitude, where the low oxygen levels may trigger a widespread vasoconstriction, which leads to increased pulmonary pressure.

Matching of ventilation and perfusion

To ensure that there is efficient gaseous exchange, both the ventilation of the lungs and the perfusion of the pulmonary capillary beds must be regulated so that sufficient O_2 reaches the alveoli and the blood flow allows effective loading of O_2 on to haemoglobin:

- **Ventilation** ensures that sufficient O_2 reaches the diffusion surfaces within the alveoli. If the amount of gas reaching the alveoli is reduced, less diffusion will occur.
- **Perfusion** of the alveoli will affect loading. If the blood flow is too low, there is sufficient time for equilibration of the blood gases, although total oxygen transport to the tissues must still be sufficient to meet its requirements. At high perfusion levels, more blood flows through the alveoli although there may be insufficient time for equilibration of the gases between the alveoli and the blood. In general, perfusion is the limiting factor.

The matching of ventilation ($\dot{V}$) and perfusion ($\dot{Q}$) is stated by the ratio $\dot{V}/\dot{Q}$. The necessity for a regulated $\dot{V}/\dot{Q}$ can be illustrated by the three-compartment model, modelling a normal alveolus and the two extremes (Fig. 7.4):

- Pulmonary shunt
- Alveolar dead space
- Matched ventilation and perfusion.

Pulmonary shunt

The situation in which there is no ventilation is seen to a small extent within the body and contributes to a small reduction in the final arterial PO_2. The main physiological causes result from systemic venous blood draining into the pulmonary venous circulation:

- A small amount of bronchial arterial blood is drained by the pulmonary veins.
- Some coronary venous blood drains directly into the left ventricle. There are pathological reasons that may result in alveoli with adequate perfusion but inadequate ventilation:
- Blockage of airflow to a region of the lungs prevents ventilation. Asthma can also contribute to a similar mismatch, although not a complete blockage of ventilation. The natural response of the body is to divert airflow to better-ventilated

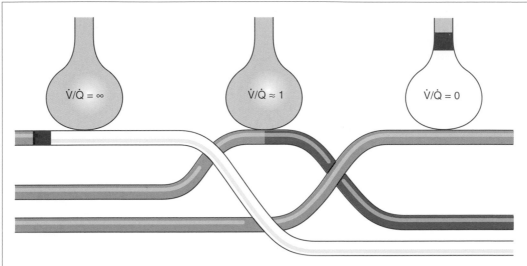

No perfusion	Matched V/Q	Shunt
Should a blockage occur within the pulmonary vessels, alveoli may be well ventilated although, due to the lack of perfusion, unable to contribute to gaseous exchange. Such a situation may arise pathologically through an embolus.	The majority of alveoli receive adequate ventilation and a good supply of blood, and allow gaseous exchange to occur supplying the tissues with oxygen. The precise ventilation-perfusion (V/Q) ratio varies throughout the lungs between around 0.5 and 3.0. Within this range the lungs are well adapted for efficient gas exchange.	In some cases blood may not reach ventilated alveoli, so gaseous exchange cannot occur and such blood results in a depression in the overall PO_2 in arterial blood.

Figure 7.4 The three-compartment model. The importance of matched ventilation and perfusion is best shown by comparing the three situations (the two extremes and a balanced system). At the extremes blood will not be adequately oxygenated as a result of failure of perfusion or ventilation.

regions, which can contribute to hypoxic pulmonary vasoconstriction.

No perfusion

Regions of the lungs with adequate ventilation but no perfusion can occur, often as a result of pulmonary emboli; they cause the blockage of blood flow to portions of the alveoli. Ventilation of this **alveolar dead space** causes two downstream effects:

1 An alkalosis develops in the surrounding tissue, due to the loss of CO_2, which causes bronchiolar constriction. The constriction contributes to returning the $\dot{V}/\dot{Q}$ ratio to a suitable value.
2 Alveolar cells become starved due to the lack of blood reaching them. A prolonged decrease in

perfusion can result in a loss of **surfactant production**, which can reduce compliance and ventilation in an attempt to rematch $\dot{V}/\dot{Q}$.

Matched ventilation and perfusion

The vast majority of alveoli in the lungs have a $\dot{V}/\dot{Q}$ within acceptable values. The ventilation and perfusion of the alveoli vary from the top to the bottom of the lungs:

- The top of the lungs is well ventilated and relatively poorly perfused, generating a high $\dot{V}/\dot{Q}$ – typically around 3.
- The lower regions of the lungs are less ventilated, although better perfused, resulting in a much lower $\dot{V}/\dot{Q}$ – often 0.5.

If the overall $\dot{V}/\dot{Q}$ across the lungs is mismatched, it prevents adequate transport of O_2 into the blood, and may also restrict removal of CO_2. As a result both **hypoxia** and **respiratory acidosis** may occur.

Gaseous transport

Gaseous exchange in the alveoli

Once gases have reached the respiratory regions of the airways, their movements into the alveoli and then into the blood depend primarily on diffusion. The rate of diffusion is determined by a variety of factors:

- The gradient of the concentrations of the substance
- The solubility of the substance
- The surface area of the diffusion surface and the diffusion distance.

Conditions altering the available diffusion surface can severely impede the body obtaining sufficient O_2 to function properly. This is seen in both **emphysema** and **pulmonary oedema**.

Oxygen transport

Oxygen reaching the alveoli must diffuse into the blood for transport to tissues where respiration can occur. O_2 is very poorly soluble in water, so adequate amounts of oxygen cannot merely dissolve. O_2 is transported by haemoglobin, which is contained within erythrocytes, to overcome this and allow adequate transport.

Dissolved oxygen

A small amount of O_2 dissolves in the fluid proportional to the partial pressure. At a PO_2 of 100 mmHg (13.3 kPa), there is typically 0.3 mL O_2/100 mL blood, which is insufficient for the needs of the body.

Erythrocytes

Erythrocytes (red blood cells) are biconcave disc-shaped cells that are specialised for the transport of O_2 from the respiratory regions of the lungs to the respiring tissues. The formation and other features of these cells are discussed in Chapter 6. The structure of erythrocytes helps their function:

- Erythrocytes contain large amounts of the oxygen-carrying protein **haemoglobin**.

- Erythrocytes lack a nucleus which would increase the volume available for haemoglobin.
- The **biconcave shape of erythrocytes** provides a large surface area to help diffusion while maintaining a large volume in the cell.

Haemoglobin

Haemoglobin is a globular protein made up of four polypeptide chains – typically two α chains and two β chains. Each chain is attached to a **haem** group, which is the site of oxygen binding; here O_2 binds reversibly to the Fe^{2+} irons carried by the haem group to form oxyhaemoglobin. In the genome there are typically four copies of genes encoding the α chain, and two copies of the genes encoding the β chain.

Different types of haemoglobin result from the presence of different chains within the haemoglobin molecule; three are particularly significant:

1 α chains are found in adult haemoglobin.
2 β chains are found in adult haemoglobin.
3 γ chains replace the β chain in fetal haemoglobin.

 CLINICAL Fetal haemoglobin

In adults, adult haemoglobin (HbA) makes up around 98% of the haemoglobin found in the body. In the fetus the predominant type is fetal haemoglobin (HbF), which is made up of two α chains and two γ chains. HbF is not regulated by 2,3-diphosphoglycerate which allows it to bind O_2 with a higher affinity than HbA.

Haemoglobin disorders

Disorders in haemoglobin cause defects in oxygen transport. There are two genetic disorders that are particularly common:

1 **Sickle cell anaemia** is an autosomal recessive disorder that is the result of a point mutation in the β chain of haemoglobin. This causes polymerisation of haemoglobin at low oxygen tensions. The clinical implications and basis of the condition are discussed in Chapter 2.
2 **Thalassaemia** is caused by the underproduction of either of the chains that make up haemoglobin.

CLINICAL Thalassaemia

Thalassaemia results from a disrupted production of one of the chains in the haemoglobin molecule. Thalassaemias can be classified based on the genes affects:

- **α-Thalassaemia**: results from disrupted production of the α chain. This leads to production of a haemoglobin molecule containing four β chains. The phenotype may vary in the number of copies of the α chain gene that are affected. Although disruption of a single copy of the gene results in a silent carrier phenotype, disruption of all four copies is not compatible with life.
- **β-Thalassaemia**: is categorised into β-thalassaemia minor and β-thalassaemia major. The former is the heterozygotic phenotype and is usually asymptomatic, although it can cause a mild microcytic anaemia. Where there are mutations in both alleles, β-thalassaemia major results, which causes a severe hypochromic/microcytic anaemia; this requires treatment by blood transfusion.

The oxygen dissociation curve

The four polypeptide chains of haemoglobin act cooperatively, so that binding of oxygen to one chain increases the affinity of the other chains for O_2. A sigmoidal relationship results between the partial pressure of oxygen and its haemoglobin saturation – the percentage of available oxygen-binding sites that have been filled.

At normal arterial PO_2 there is almost complete O_2 saturation. In highly metabolising tissues, the PO_2 is lower and this promotes even more rapid O_2 unloading. In addition, other factors associated with active metabolism can promote oxygen dissociation, by shifting the oxygen dissociation curve (Fig. 7.5):

- **Temperature**: increases in temperature, as generated in actively respiring tissues, promote oxygen dissociation. Active cells undergo more respiration, thus requiring more oxygen. During hypothermia, the body's metabolism slows, the need for O_2 is less and more remains in the blood.
- **H^+ ions**: increases in respiration can result in the occurrence of anaerobic respiration, of which lactic acid is a by-product. In addition, CO_2 readily forms carbonic acid. Both signals lead to an increase in the H^+ concentration, which acts directly on haemoglobin to promote oxygen dissociation.
- **2,3-Diphosphoglycerate**: (2,3-DPG) is produced by an isomerase enzyme from 1,3-diphosphoglycerate, an intermediate in glycolysis. Increased levels of 2,3-DPG act directly on haemoglobin to reduce its oxygen affinity. Many hormones associated with increased metabolism promote the production of 2,3-DPG, e.g. thyroxine, adrenaline and human growth hormone. Fetal haemoglobin has a higher affinity for O_2 than maternal haemoglobin; as a result of its ability to bind 2,3-DPG less well, O_2 is readily transferred from mother to child.

Transport of carbon dioxide

Although it is around 20 times more soluble than O_2, only a relatively small proportion of CO_2 transport is mediated directly by dissolving into solution. Three main mechanisms contribute to CO_2 transport by the blood:

1 **Bicarbonate-mediated transport of CO_2**
2 **Transport by carbamino compounds**
3 **Dissolution of CO_2**.

Bicarbonate-mediated transport

Bicarbonate (HCO_3^-) is responsible for transport of around 60% of the body's CO_2 through an equilibrium in the plasma of CO_2, carbonic acid (H_2CO_3) and bicarbonate; this equilibrium is important in the regulation of pH. The formation of H_2CO_3 from CO_2 is catalysed by the enzyme **carbonic anhydrase** and carbonic acid rapidly dissociates into bicarbonate and H^+:

$$H_2O + CO_2 \Longleftrightarrow H_2CO_3 \Longleftrightarrow H^+ + HCO_3^-$$

HCO_3^- is capable of diffusing out of the cell; however, the cell membrane is impermeable to H^+, so transport of Cl^- into the cell is required to maintain neutrality of the overall electric charge across the cell membrane. As H_2CO_3 is constantly being removed from the cell, it allows its continuous production from H_2O and CO_2.

Transport of CO_2 by carbamino groups

The N-terminus of proteins (such as haemoglobin) contains a free NH_2 group, which can combine with CO_2 to produce a carbamino group on the

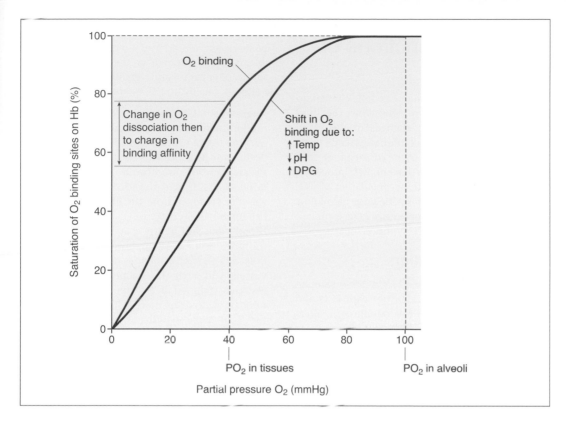

Figure 7.5 **The binding of oxygen to haemoglobin.** This is not a linear relationship. At low saturations, the proportion of oxygen binding increases rapidly for small increases of partial pressure. The shape of the oxygen dissociation curve permits rapid loading in the lungs and rapid unloading in the respiring tissues. Furthermore, there is a shift in O_2 binding in response to increases in temperature and 2,3-diphosphoglycerate or decreases in pH, all of which are typical in heavily respiring tissues. This enhances the unloading of oxygen in the sites that need it most.

N-terminus of the protein molecule. This effect is thought to contribute to around 30% of total CO_2 transport.

Dissolution of CO_2

Although CO_2 is soluble, allowing significant transport, in normal conditions this transport mechanism accounts for only around 10% of the total CO_2 transport in the blood.

The CO_2 dissociation curve

CO_2 carriage in the blood related to its partial pressure forms a much more linear arrangement than seen with O_2. However, there is also a shift in the dissociation curve related to O_2 saturation of haemoglobin. Haemoglobin reduced through unloading O_2 more readily accepts H^+ ions produced by splitting of H_2CO_3. The reduced haemoglobin is a much better acceptor of H^+ ions than oxyhaemoglobin, promoting the formation of HCO_3^- in

low oxygen conditions. Conversely, in oxygenated blood the ability of haemoglobin to bind H^+ is reduced, and so in the lungs this promotes the unloading of CO_2 from the blood. The effect of haemoglobin on CO_2 loading is known as the **Haldane effect**.

Gaseous exchange between the blood and respiring tissues

The transport of O_2 and CO_2 between the blood and respiring tissues also relies on diffusion. The respiring tissues are not as highly vascularised as the lungs; the diffusion distance to some cells may be around $40\,\mu m$, whereas in the alveoli the figure is $<1\,\mu m$. As the demands of the respiring tissues increase, extra capillary beds open to increase blood flow and therefore O_2 supply. The additional capillaries also increase the surface area available for diffusion and reduce the diffusion distance.

Regulatory functions of the lungs

The lungs are unusual in that the whole circulation goes through a single organ. This allows the lungs to regulate and mediate changes to the blood rapidly. In particular, regulation of gaseous compounds can be achieved by rapid exchange with the atmosphere. Although most of these processes are concerned with breathing, regulation of CO_2 contributes to pH regulation. The large blood flow and surface area of the lungs can also be exploited in the metabolism of blood components.

Acid–base regulation

The major pH buffer in the blood is bicarbonate (HCO_3^-) which is in equilibrium with H_2O and CO_2 in the blood. Due to this equilibrium, alteration in the CO_2 level can be used to temporarily correct blood pH. Alterations in the dissolved CO_2 can shift the equilibrium to modulate H^+ levels. The systemic regulation of this mechanism is discussed in Chapter 11, although the mechanism employed by the lungs is described briefly below.

Ventilation of CO_2 removes it from the body, preventing the reaction with H_2O and subsequent generation of H^+. However, any change in this mechanism is relatively limited. In the longer term, alterations to the H^+ balance require changes in the excretion of H^+ ions from the kidneys; respiratory mechanisms to regulate pH may also be employed to compensate for metabolic disturbances of pH.

Respiratory alkalosis

In cases where there is excess removal of CO_2 from the blood (e.g. prolonged periods at high altitude), the shift in the equilibrium reduces the H^+ concentration, causing a respiratory alkalosis. The lungs also act to compensate for changes in H^+ resulting from other systems, because an increase in ventilation will be seen to compensate for a **metabolic acidosis**.

Respiratory acidosis

If there is restricted ventilation, the PCO_2 of the blood will increase, causing a respiratory acidosis. The body may restrict ventilation as compensation secondary to a **metabolic alkalosis**.

Metabolic function

The large surface area of the lungs can modify substances and variables in the blood. As a result a variety of enzymes and signalling molecules may be altered, inactivated or cleared in the blood:

- **Angiotensin I is converted to angiotensin II** predominantly by the angiotensin-converting enzyme (ACE) expressed on the pulmonary endothelium. **Bradykinin** is also inactivated by ACE.
- **Prostaglandins**, **serotonin** (5-hydroxytryptamine or 5-HT) and **noradrenaline** are inactivated or removed from **the blood by uptake in the lungs**.
- **Blood clots and debris** may become lodged in the lungs, removing them from circulation where they may occlude capillaries in the brain or other vessels. Although the pulmonary vessels may become occluded as a result, the blockage can often be cleared and there is sufficient functional tissue to avoid significant long-term damage. Rarely, large clots may occur which result in **pulmonary embolism**.

Control of ventilation

Ventilation is unusual in that it is under automatic control which can be heavily overridden by higher functions. It is possible to hold one's breath for a significant length of time, or to voluntarily hyperventilate. Most of the time, an individual is not consciously aware of breathing, and it is regulated automatically.

Sensors involved in the regulation of breathing

Automatic control of ventilation ensures that sufficient O_2 enters the lungs and CO_2 is adequately removed. There are four types of sensors that provide information in the regulation of ventilation:

1 Central chemoreceptors
2 Peripheral chemoreceptors
3 Stretch receptors
4 Irritant receptors.

Central chemoreceptors

The central chemoreceptors are located on the surface of the medulla, near the exit of cranial nerves IX and X. The chemoreceptors detect changes in the pH of the cerebrospinal fluid (CSF). As CO_2 freely diffuses across the blood–brain barrier, where it combines with H_2O to generate HCO_3^- and H^+. A corresponding change due to increased CO_2 results in a larger pH change in the CSF than in the blood, as a result of less buffering by proteins. Central chemoreceptors are thought to drive over 80% of the breathing response caused by a change in PCO_2.

Peripheral chemoreceptors

The peripheral chemoreceptors are located in the aortic arch and carotid bodies, at the site of the bifurcation of the common carotid artery. In humans, the **carotid bodies** have a more significant contribution to breathing than their aortic counterparts.

The peripheral chemoreceptors respond to O_2, pH and changes in PCO_2 and respond rapidly enough to detect changes during each breath. They are responsible for the increased drive that is seen in **hypoxaemia**. The carotid bodies are able to respond to a fall in arterial pH, whereas the aortic bodies are not.

 CLINICAL Response to hypoxaemia

The body's drive in response to hypoxaemia is relatively weak. As CO_2 is the main regulator of ventilation, PaO_2 must fall to <60 mmHg (8 kPa) for it to trigger significant increases in ventilation so that loss in O_2 is detectable through the significant unloading of oxygen from haemoglobin; this is reflected in the oxygen dissociation curve. Hypoxaemia is detected by type I cells in the peripheral chemoreceptors.

Stretch receptors

Pulmonary stretch receptors in the smooth muscle of the airways sense distension of the tissues, signalling via the vagus nerve afferent fibres. The stretch receptors trigger the **Hering–Breuer reflex**, which regulates the volume of the lungs to prevent overinflation. If the lungs are inflated more than usual, there is a slowing of breathing such that the next breath is not as big. Similarly, if the lungs are deflated excessively, the Hering–Breuer reflex anticipates the next breath to promote inflation of the lungs. The Hering–Breuer reflex contributes significantly to breathing shortly after birth, but contributes little in adults.

Irritant receptors

The airways are in contact with the outside world, which presents a risk of irritants and harmful particles entering the lungs. Irritant receptors located in the walls of the airways sense noxious stimuli such as cigarette smoke, dust particles and cold air. The nervous impulses from irritant receptors are transmitted up the vagus nerve and trigger bronchoconstriction to reduce the risk of the irritant travelling deeper into the airways; the increased breathing aids the expulsion of the irritant from the lungs. Irritant receptors show rapid adaptation to stimuli and may also respond to mechanical stimuli, such as the presence of a foreign body within the airways.

J receptors are a group of chemoreceptors that respond to the presence of chemicals within the blood. Stimulation of the J receptors by the presence of chemical stimuli within the pulmonary circulation triggers rapid shallow breathing. J receptors appear to be activated by an increase in fluid volume in the alveoli, and may contribute to the shallow breathing seen in left heart failure and interstitial lung disease.

C FIBRES

C fibres are found in the connective tissue of the lungs. These fibres detect mechanical distortion of the tissue which may be caused by inflammation or oedema, or an irritant. The activation of the fibres triggers a rapid hyperventilation as well as increased mucus secretion and bronchoconstriction in an attempt to remove the irritant from the lungs.

Respiratory centres in the brain

In the **medulla** a natural breathing rhythm is generated; the **medullary respiratory centre** is located in the reticular formation of the medulla. There are two main groups of cells: those located in the dorsal region of the medulla are associated with inspiration, and those in the ventral area are involved in expiration.

The **cortex** can influence and override the actions of the respiratory centres to allow voluntary control of breathing. Hyperventilation is possible such that PCO_2 can be reduced to half its normal values, causing **respiratory alkalosis**. It is possible to consciously hypoventilate, although to a lesser extent than seen with hyperventilation. Other regions, associated with emotion (e.g. the limbic system), can also modulate breathing, as shown in fear and anger. Two modulatory centres have been identified in the pons. Although neither is essential for breathing, ablation of either results in abnormal ventilation:

- The **apneustic area** appears to promote inspiration by exciting the inspiratory area of the medulla.
- The **pneumotaxic centre** acts to inhibit inspiration in response to inspired volume.

Disorders of breathing during sleep

Breathing disorders during unconsciousness result from the cessation of breathing – an **apnoea**. Apnoeas may be due to a central error in the regulation of breathing or obstruction of the airways. Some apnoeas may be mixed.

Obstructive sleep apnoeas

Obstructive sleep apnoeas result from the decrease in muscle activity that occurs during sleep. The relaxation of the palate may completely obstruct the airflow, despite the activity of the inspiratory muscles. This state may continue for many seconds and the PO_2 will drop whereas the PCO_2 rises. The apnoea ends in arousal as a result of chemical and mechanical stimuli associated with lack of ventilation and the increased breathing cycle. Apnoea usually causes transition to a lighter stage of sleep which increases the activity of the airway muscles. Apnoeas may occur many times an hour, leading to a poor quality of sleep, and can cause tiredness during the day.

Central sleep apnoeas

Central sleep apnoeas occur when breathing stops but the airway remains open – there is no attempt to breathe and no activation of the inspiratory muscles. Types of central sleep apnoea can be described in three groups:

- A defect in the respiratory control system
- Transient fluctuations in the respiratory drive
- Reflex inhibition of the central respiratory drive.

Periodic breathing

This is a form of central apnoea in which ventilation increases and decreases in a periodic fashion due to changes in the respiratory drive.

Cheyne–stokes breathing

This is a type of periodic breathing characterised by a periodic apnoea in which there is decreased ventilation, or a series of apnoeas interspersed with hyperventilation. As a result of this varied pattern of breathing, the levels of CO_2 and O_2 within the blood and alveoli may vary. During consciousness there is an internal threshold for the level of CO_2 within the blood, and during sleep this value is reset to a different level. Cheyne–Stokes breathing may occur during the transition to sleep as the new threshold is set.

 CLINICAL Ondine's curse

There are rare cases where there is congenital or acquired disruption of the automatic control of breathing. This failure, Ondine's curse, may become apparent only while the individual is unconscious, because, while awake, a patient is consciously able to control breathing. Such individuals may need to be ventilated while asleep, because the brain-stem centres are unable to regulate breathing.

 CLINICAL 'Locked-in syndrome'

Locked-in syndrome is caused by a lesion that severs the brain stem from the spinal cord. All four limbs are paralysed. The patient is also unable to voluntarily regulate their breathing; the patient cannot speak as they cannot regulate their breathing voluntarily. Although the patient experiences emotion and has thoughts, their only way of expressing it is through their eyes (the oculomotor nucleus that controls eye movements is intact).

 RELATED CHAPTERS

8

Gastrointestinal system

The gut breaks food down and absorbs the products of digestion in the gastrointestinal (GI) tract, while the waste is compacted and eliminated from the body. The GI tract is a single tube, around 15 metres long that is responsible for all these processes. Supporting organs produce a variety of secretions to aid digestion and process the absorbed nutrients. The GI tract also provides a route for removal of substances not readily cleared by the kidneys.

Features of the abdominal cavity

The GI tract and its supporting organs are located mainly in the abdominal cavity, contained within a thin membranous structure, the **peritoneum**. The abdomen also contains organs not associated with the function of the GI tract. These are discussed in Chapter 14.

Anatomy of the GI tract

The GI tract is a single, convoluted tube that conveys and processes food. It is aided by the pancreas and salivary glands which produce enzymes to help break down ingested material, and the gallbladder aids the digestion and absorption of fats through the storage of bile, which acts to emulsify fats. Regions of the GI tract are specialised to perform specific functions that are discussed later in the chapter.

The gut wall

The wall of the GI tract has a common structure throughout its length, although individual areas are specialised for particular functions. It is a muscular tube lined by a mucous membrane and can be divided into four distinct portions (Fig. 8.1):

1 The mucosa
2 The submucosa
3 The muscularis propria
4 The adventitia.

The mucosa

The mucosa is the tissue in contact with the **lumen** of the gut. It is responsible for the absorption of digested nutrients through its walls, and is richly innervated and vascularised to perform this function. Three distinct layers can be identified in the mucosa:

1 The **epithelium** forms the interface between the tissue and the lumen and is lined by different cell types, depending on function of the GI tract at that point.
2 The **lamina propria** is the layer of loose connective tissue beneath the epithelium. It is highly cellular, containing many lymphocytes and plasma cells. The lamina propria is highly vascularised and possesses many capillaries and lymphatic vessels, which transport absorbed nutrients from the mucosa.
3 The **muscularis mucosa** is made up of smooth muscle. The superficial layers are made up of circular muscle layers whereas the deeper layers run parallel to the lumen. The activity of the smooth muscle keeps the glands and tissue constantly moving, preventing the clogging of crypts in the tissue and helping the luminal contents to be in contact with the epithelium for absorption.

Biomedical Science Lecture Notes, First Edition. Ian Lyons.
© 2011 by Ian Lyons. Published 2011 by Blackwell Publishing Ltd.

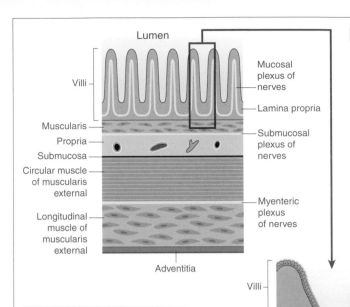

Villi

The epithelial cells on the surface of the villi possess a thick brush border of microvilli which further increases the surface area available for transport. The epithelial cells express a wide variety of proteins on the surface for the transport of nutrients, as well as enzymes involved in processing some of the substrates.

Transitional region

The cells that form the epithelia on the villi are derived from the division of stem cells within the crypts and must replace the villi epithelium as it is removed by mechanical trauma from the ingested material passing over it. Those cells that develop into absorptive cells migrate out of the crypts, and as they do so develop the characteristic features of the villous cells – expressing the relevant proteins, and developing a brush border. The life of a villus epithelial cell is typically around 2–4 days.

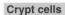

Intestine

The wall of the gastrointestinal (GI) tract is made up of many different layers. The most internal layer is that of the GI epithelium, which is arranged in a series of folds, to increase the surface area in contact with the lumen. Immediately below the epithelium is the connective tissue in the lamina propria, which contains many of the vessels supplying and draining the epithelium, and the mucosal plexus of nerve. Muscularis propria is responsible for contracting the epithelium to generate the villi.

Below the mucosa is the submucosa, a layer of connective tissue carrying the vessels and nerves supporting mucosal layer. The major smooth muscle of the GI tract is made up of two layers: the inner is circularly arranged, while the outer is longitudinally arranged. The outermost layer of the GI tract is the adventitia, a connective tissue covering.

There are three nerve plexus found within the GI tract – the most prominent are the myenteric plexus, found between the circular and longitudinal layers of muscle, and the submucosal plexus, located in the inner layers of the submucosa. Finally, there is a plexus of nerves in the lamina propria that involved regulating the behaviour of the epithelial cells, and the secretion and transport of substances.

Crypt cells

Cells can be grouped into those with one of two major functions. First, stem cells located at the base of crypts are those proliferating cells with progeny that develop into the other cell types found in the intestinal epithelial layer. The other cell types found in the crypts are primarily involved in secretion:

- Paneth cells form part of the innate immune response, through the secretion of defensins.
- Enteroendocrine cells are involved in the release of GI hormones.
- Goblet cells are responsible for the production of mucus to lubricate the passage of material through the gut.

The basic structure of the mucosa throughout the gut is conserved, although in each region the precise structure of the villi and crypts, and the cell types, vary. Nevertheless, the tissue layers below the mucosa remain, to an extent, very much conserved. Within the mucosa the villi vary in terms of the nature of the cells, while in the small intestine they possess large numbers of microvilli to allow absorption; in the large intestine the microvilli are far less prominent, because mass absorption of nutrients is no longer needed.

The submucosa

The submucosa is made up of supporting tissue, namely elastin and collagen, which links the mucosa to the muscular wall of the GI tract. It contains many of the large blood vessels and lymphatics that supply the lamina propria as well as the nerve plexus of the mucosa. The many small parasympathetic ganglia found in the submucosa form the submucosal plexus.

The muscularis propria

The muscular layer of the gut consists of two layers of smooth muscle: an inner circular layer and an outer longitudinal layer. Between the layers is the **myenteric plexus** of nerves.

The muscularis propria undergoes synchronised contraction to produce peristaltic waves that move food through the gut. Although peristaltic activity is intrinsic to the smooth muscle, it is regulated by the **enteric nervous system** and **hormones**, as well as by other environmental factors.

The role of the gut mucosa

The role of the GI tract gradually changes down its length and allows classification of its mucosa into four types, based on function:

1 **Protective epithelium**, found in the oral cavity, pharynx and anal canal, is squamous in nature and has no role in absorption or digestion. It acts merely as a conduit or storage region.
2 **Secretory epithelium** is found only in the stomach and is typified by many glandular structures for secreting acid and other factors.
3 **Absorptive epithelium** is found throughout the entire small intestine. The mucosa is arranged in a series of pronounced folds, 'villi', which increase the surface area of the mucosa to increase absorption.
4 **Absorptive/protective epithelium** in the large intestine is more closely packed and there are fewer glands. The cells are specialised primarily for water reabsorption. Clara cells, which secrete mucus, are also present to lubricate the gut.

Regional specialisation of the GI tract

The GI tract contains distinct regions specialised for distinct functions. Four main regions with different functions can be identified:

1 The **oral cavity** is the site of food ingestion. Physical breakdown occurs through the action of the teeth, while enzymatic breakdown and lubrication result from secretions of the salivary glands.
2 The **stomach** contributes to physical breakdown of food and the digestion of proteins. Due to its low pH, the stomach plays a protective role by killing pathogens that may contaminate ingested food.
3 The **small intestine** digests food into its constitutive components. It also absorbs the products of digestion into the blood and lymph for processing and use by the body.
4 The **large intestine** packages the waste from digestion and regulate of ions through both secretion and absorption. It predominantly absorbs water to produce faeces for excretion.

The oral cavity

Food is ingested through the mouth; and detailed anatomy of the mouth is discussed in Chapter 14. The mouth performs several functions related to the breakdown of food:

- **Mechanical breakdown** of food is achieved by the action of the teeth.
- **Secretion of saliva** aids the shaping of food into a bolus and lubricates it for travel to the stomach via the oesophagus.
- **Salivary amylase** initiates the digestion of carbohydrates.

Figure 8.1 **The basic structure of the mucosa**. The basic structure throughout the gut is conserved, although in each region the precise structure of the villi and crypts, and the cell types of which they are composed, vary. Nevertheless, the tissue layers below the mucosa remain very much conserved. Within the mucosa the villi vary in terms of the nature of cells; although the small intestine possesses large numbers of microvilli to allow absorption, in the large intestine they are far less prominent, because mass absorption of nutrients is no longer needed.

The oesophagus

The oesophagus is a long muscular tube that connects the mouth with the rest of the GI tract. It runs in the neck posterior to the trachea and slightly to the left of the midline. After this it runs within the posterior mediastinum, through the thorax, before penetrating the diaphragm and joining with the stomach.

The oesophagus is made up of an inner circular layer of muscle and an outer longitudinal layer and is lined with squamous epithelium. The type of muscle making up the oesophagus walls changes down its length:

- The upper third is made up of striated (skeletal) muscle.
- The lower third is made up of smooth muscle.

Stomach

The stomach is a dilated region of the gut, with a distinct role and structure. It secretes many compounds, in both an endocrine and an exocrine manner, performing a variety of functions:

- It continues digestion of carbohydrates initiated within the oral cavity.
- It adds acid to the food to kill pathogens and promote protein digestion.
- It helps digestion of lipids by the production of gastric lipase.
- It secretes **intrinsic factor** to enable absorption of vitamin B_{12}.
- It breaks down food into a thick soup – chyme – to increase the effective surface area available to the enzymes that continue digestion.

The stomach, when empty, is not much bigger in diameter than the large intestine, although it is capable of expanding significantly so that it may hold 2–3 litres of food in an average individual. Grossly, the stomach is a dilated region of the intestines, in the shape of the letter J.

Mucosa

In places the surface epithelium of the stomach protrudes into the lamina propria to form gastric pits, into which many glands enter. Different regions of the stomach contain different cell types with different functions. Six main cell types related to digestion are found within the stomach:

1 **Simple epithelium** lines the gastric mucosa. The cells secrete mucus which forms a thick layer to protect the stomach walls from the stomach acid.
2 **Parietal (oxyntic) cells** are found in the upper parts of the gastric glands. These pyramidal cells have a single central nucleus, many mitochondria and a deep central invagination. Their major role is the secretion of acid, produced from the dissociation of H_2CO_3 mediated by the enzyme carbonic anhydrase. The secretion is regulated by a variety of mechanisms discussed elsewhere. Intrinsic factor, which is crucial for the absorption of vitamin B_{12}, is also produced by the parietal cells.
3 **Mucous cells** are located in the neck of gastric pits, between the parietal cells. They possess many granules at their apical surface and have their nuclei located near to the base. Their precise function is not clear.
4 **Chief (zymogenic) cells** are found in the lower regions of the gastric glands. The cells have large amounts of rough endoplasmic reticulum (ER) and contain granules of the protein pepsinogen. When released into the acidic stomach, the pepsinogen becomes activated by cleavage to form the enzyme pepsin.
5 **Enteroendocrine cells** in the base of gastric glands secrete a variety of hormones.
6 **Stem cells** are mainly found in the neck region of the gastric glands. These cells divide rapidly to replace epithelial cells in the gastric pits and on the surface of the stomach.

The pylorus of the stomach possesses gastric pits with many glands that secrete lysozyme as well as the products discussed earlier, and there are many gastrin-secreting cells (G-cells), which are involved in stimulating acid secretion. Other enteroendocrine cells are also present, secreting many different hormones.

Small intestine

The small intestine is the final site of food digestion. It absorbs the products of digestion and secretes hormones regulating appetite and other processes. This part of the GI tract is 6–7 metres long and consists of three main sections, which share many common adaptations:

1 The duodenum
2 The jejunum
3 The ileum.

The duodenum

The duodenum is the first and shortest part of the small intestine, immediately distal to the stomach. It forms a C-shaped region located near the head of the pancreas.

The duodenum provides the point of entry of the common bile duct into the intestines at the ampulla of Vater; it marks the boundary between the derivation of the intestines from embryological foregut and the midgut.

The jejunum and ileum

The jejunum and ileum together contribute a huge length to the intestines – around 6–7 metres in an average individual. The jejunum starts at the duodenojejunal flexure and the ileum ends at the ileocaecal junction, which marks the transition from small to large intestines. Although there is no defined boundary that demarcates the transition, there are a variety of clinically important distinctions between the jejunum and ileum:

- The jejunum is **slightly wider** than the ileum.
- The jejunum is **more vascularised**.
- The vascular arcades, the loops of arterial vessels that supply the intestinal tissue, differ. In the jejunum, the arcades consist of a few large arterial loops, whereas in the ileum there are many much shorter loops.
- The mesentery of the jejunum is **less fatty** than in the ileum.
- **Peyer's patches** are more commonly found in the ileum

Organisation of the mucosa in the small intestine

The small intestine is adapted for the absorption of nutrients into the body. The surface area is increased in the small intestine though the formation of villi and crypt structures:

- The **small intestine is also pulled into large folds,** each of which further increases the potential area of contact between the digestive mixture and the tissue.
- **Villi** are finger-like projections of the mucosa, which are produced through contraction of the muscular tissue within the mucosa.
- The apical surfaces of the villous epithelial cells possess many **microvilli**. These minute projections further increase the surface area in contact with the intestinal lumen.

The progressive damage caused by food results in the progressive loss of cells from the villi, which must be replaced by new cells derived from stem cells in the intestinal crypts.

The crypts of Lieberkühn

Deep crypts between the villi contain many cells types that differ from those found on the villi. They have a variety of different functions, including:

- Production of **secretions** to help digestion and lubricate the mucosal surface
- **Replacement of cells** lost from the villi or crypts. These are produced by differentiation of stem cells at the base of the crypts.

The cell types in the small intestines

The cell types found in the villi are mainly involved in the absorption of digested substances. Within the crypts of Lieberkühn there are other cells that are differentiated for secretion:

- **Absorptive cells** make up almost all the cells on a villus. The cells possess a 'brush border' on the apical surface, which is made up of a layer of densely packed microvilli. Moreover, there are enzymes and transporters bound to the apical surface to facilitate the last stages of digestion ready for mediation of absorption.
- **Goblet cells** are found between the absorptive cells and increase in frequency along the length of the small intestine. The goblet cells secrete mucus that lubricates the lining of the gut.
- **Paneth cells** are located deep in the crypts of Lieberkühn. They secrete lysozyme and other antimicrobial substances (e.g. defensins) to control the growth between the intestinal flora and prevent the colonisation of pathogens.
- **M (microfold) cells** are specialised cells found over **Peyer's patches**. The M cells do not have a basement membrane to help transport antigens to Peyer's patches.
- **Stem cells** located at the base of the crypts proliferate at a constant rate. The rate of proliferation is relatively slow, because the daughter

cells also possess significant proliferative activity. Daughter cells progressively differentiate as they travel up the walls of the crypt to replace the absorptive cells that have been removed through mechanical damage. They also replace all the cell types found in the crypts.

Lamina propria and serosa of the small intestine

The **lamina propria** of the small intestine projects into the villi carrying blood vessels, lymphatics, nerve fibres and smooth muscle cells. Many leukocytes, found below the lamina, provide an immunological barrier to protect against infection.

The **muscularis mucosa** is relatively consistent throughout the small intestine. However, in the duodenum the submucosa contains many coiled tubular glands, known as Brunner's glands. These glands secrete an alkaline fluid, which contributes to the neutralisation of the stomach acid and creates an environment for the optimum activity of pancreatic enzymes.

The **lamina propria** and **submucosa** of the small intestine possess regions of lymphoid tissue involved in the immune response – Peyer's patches. These are important in the adaptive immune response in the gut and are found on the side of the tissue opposite the mesentery. There are usually around 30 Peyer's patches in the small intestine, mostly in the ileum.

Large intestine

The large intestine does not contain the folds or villi seen in the small intestine. Glands in the large intestine are characterised by many goblet and absorptive cells, and a few enteroendocrine cells. The cells of the large intestine have three main functions:

1 The large numbers of the goblets cells **produce mucus to lubricate** the intestinal surface.
2 The absorptive cells **reabsorb water** from the gut lumen for the active transport of Na$^+$ out of the lumen.
3 The large intestine is the site of **formation of faecal mass** for subsequent elimination.

The large intestine contains many lymph cells that extend into the submucosa, and are likely to be required to control the large bacterial population present.

Features of the large intestine

The large intestine is made up of the caecum, appendix, and the ascending, transverse, descending and sigmoid colon. There are four major features that allow the distinction of large intestine from small intestine:

1 **Taeniae coli**: these are three thickened bands of muscle that make up most of the longitudinal muscle in the large intestine. As the taeniae are shorter in length than the large intestine, they cause the large intestine to adopt a sacculated shape.
2 **Haustra**: these are large folds (sacculations) that are found within the large intestine as a result of the short nature of the taeniae coli.
3 **Omental appendices**: small fatty projections are found in the omentum around the large intestine.
4 **Calibre**: the large intestine has a far greater diameter than the small intestine.

> **CLINICAL Appendicitis**
>
> Acute inflammation of the appendix is a common cause of acute abdominal pain. Appendicitis may be caused in young people by hyperplasia of the lymphoid nodes located around the appendix. Within older individuals appendicitis probably results from accumulation of faecal matter. The blockage causes swelling of the appendix, resulting in irritation of the visceral peritoneum.
>
> Initially, appendicitis causes referred pain to the periumbilical region of the abdomen – the appendix and the periumbilical skin are both innervated by nerve roots entering the spinal cord at T10. More acute pain develops later due to direct irritation of the peritoneum. This localises to a point two-thirds of the way from the umbilicus to the midinguinal point – referred to as McBurney's point.
>
> Acute infection may sometimes result from thrombosis of the appendicular artery. This can lead to ischaemia or gangrene and perforation of the inflamed appendix, which can contribute to infection of the peritoneum – peritonitis.
>
> Acute appendicitis is often treated surgically through an appendicectomy.

The vasculature of the gut

The vascular supply of the gut develops in accordance with the embryological derivation of the gut tissue. Three major vessels supply the gut, each arising directly from the abdominal aorta:

1 The **coeliac artery** supplies foregut derivatives and originates from the abdominal aorta immediately after it passes through the diaphragm.
2 The **superior mesenteric artery** supplies the midgut and arises at the level of L1.
3 The **inferior mesenteric artery** supplies the hindgut derivatives, and arises at the level of L3.

The course and details of their supply are covered in Chapter 14.

The hepatic portal circulation

Blood draining from the intestines is rich in absorbed nutrients, many of which require processing before being released into the systemic circulation. As a result, a specialised circulation has evolved whereby the blood from the GI tract drains into the hepatic portal vein, which transports it to the liver. In the liver, the portal blood passes through a second capillary bed, allowing the absorption of the products of digestion into the hepatocytes, and the subsequent release of suitable products of processed nutrients into the systemic circulation. The liver is drained by the hepatic veins, which drain directly into the inferior vena cava.

The portosystemic anastomoses

The portal and systemic venous circulation must meet at various points. These anastomoses can form varicosities – swellings – in the case of portal hypertension. There are three major sites of anastomosis:

1 **Oesophageal veins** may drain into either the left gastric vein (part of the portal circulation) or the azygos vein (part of the systemic circulation).
2 The **veins draining the rectum** contribute to both circulations. The superior and middle rectal veins drain into the portal vein, whereas the inferior rectal vein contributes to the systemic circulation.
3 The **paraumbilical veins** in the anterior abdominal wall may anastomose with the superior epigastric veins of the portal circulation.

Enteric nervous system

The gut possesses its own complex system of neurons, which make up the enteric nervous system. The enteric nervous system is thought to contain

 CLINICAL Portal hypertension

The flow of blood through the portal vein may become blocked – most frequently due to fibrosis and scarring within the liver itself (e.g. cirrhosis). As pressure in the portal vein rises, the flow of blood through anastomotic sites within the systemic circulation will increase. The increased pressure causes the walls of the anastomoses to swell and potentially rupture. In particular, rupture of the oesophageal varices causes severe, often fatal, bleeding.

The enlargement of the paraumbilical veins can lead to the formation of caput medusae – which look like snakes radiating from the umbilicus.

over 100 million neurons, arranged in a complex fashion. These receive inputs from both the sympathetic and the parasympathetic nervous systems, as well as receiving sensory afferents and sending out effector neurons.

The enteric nervous system is localised in two plexus:

1 The **myenteric (Auerbach's) plexus** is found between the longitudinal and circular layers of muscle in the muscularis propria. It is involved in regulating motility within the gut.
2 The **submucosal (Meissner's) plexus** is found between the circular muscle layer in the muscularis propria and the longitudinal muscle layer in the muscularis mucosae. It is associated with the regulation of transport of fluid and ions across the luminal boundary.

Though it receives a whole host of inputs, an isolated enteric nervous system can respond to internal stimuli to control peristalsis, secretion and absorption effectively. The ENS also triggers release of secretions from supporting organs, such as the gallbladder.

Supporting organs in the gut

The gut requires the support of many organs, to provide enzymes that mediate digestion and secretions to modulate the conditions within the GI tract so that they are optimal. Moreover, the absorbed products of digestion must be processed to allow them to be used by the rest of the body. Four main organs can be identified that help the function of the gut:

- The **liver** is responsible for receiving and processing most of the products of digestion. It also produces bile, which is essential for the absorption of lipids
- The **gallbladder** stores and concentrates bile.
- The **pancreas** is the main secretory gland of the GI tract, producing many of the enzymes essential for the breakdown of ingested food.
- The **salivary glands** release many digestive enzymes into their secretions. Unlike the other structures, the salivary glands are not located within the abdomen.

Liver

The liver is a large solid organ located in the upper right quadrant of the abdomen. It receives the blood supply draining from the intestines, and hence most nutrients that have been absorbed from the gut. The liver also contributes secretions to the intestinal tract.

Features of the liver

The liver is the largest solid organ in the human body and is made up of **left** and **right lobes** which are delineated by the falciform ligament that attaches it to the peritoneum. The **right lobe** is further subdivided into quadrate and caudate lobes by the gallbladder and the fissure for the ligatmentum teres.

The hepatic blood supply

The liver receives two blood supplies, each with different functions:

- The **hepatic artery** is a branch of the coeliac trunk that contributes around 30% of the total blood flow to the liver. The hepatic artery supplies the tissue with oxygen for respiration, being derived directly from the aorta.
- The **hepatic portal vein** delivers around 70% of the total blood to the liver. It is formed from the veins draining the gut, spleen and pancreas, and carries the nutrients absorbed from the gut to the liver, as well as hormones secreted by the endocrine pancreas.

Histology of the liver

The liver is covered by thin connective tissue, the stroma, which encloses the hepatocytes, the basic cell type. The capillary vessels in the liver, sinusoids, have a particularly irregular vessel wall, so that the blood cells may escape the vessels and bathe the liver cells themselves. Specialised macrophages – the Kupffer cells – are found in the sinusoids (Fig. 8.2).

The hepatocyte

The hepatocyte is the predominant cell type within the liver. Hepatocytes group together into liver lobules, which usually have portal spaces at their corners, where the **portal triad** can run. The hepatocytes are responsible for performing most of the functions of the liver. Functionally, the liver may be split into units known as acini, which represent regions that deliver blood to the same draining vein.

The hepatocyte itself is a cell with six or more sides and is around 25 μm in diameter. It possesses many mitochondria and large amounts of smooth ER, although there are differences depending on the distance of the cells from the portal triad. Each hepatocyte is in direct contact with blood through gaps in the endothelium of the sinusoids.

At sites where hepatocytes meet they generate a space between them – a **bile canaliculus**. This is the first stage of the bile duct system and is sealed by tight junctions. Gap junctions between hepatocytes are common, allowing communication between the cells.

The portal triad

About three to six portal triads supply an individual liver lobule. Each triad consists of three vessels – a venule, an arteriole and a lymphatic vessel – and a duct:

- The **venule** is derived from the hepatic portal vein and normally represents the largest vessel in the triad.
- The **arteriole** is a branch of the hepatic artery.
- The **duct** carries bile to the hepatic duct from where it may enter the gallbladder or gut.

Sinusoids

The sinusoids are made up of irregular blood vessels that contain plates of endothelial cells, so that blood can leak out of the vessel and surround the hepatic cells. Blood can enter the subendothelial space of Disse where it is in direct contact with the hepatocytes, allowing rapid exchange of solutes as

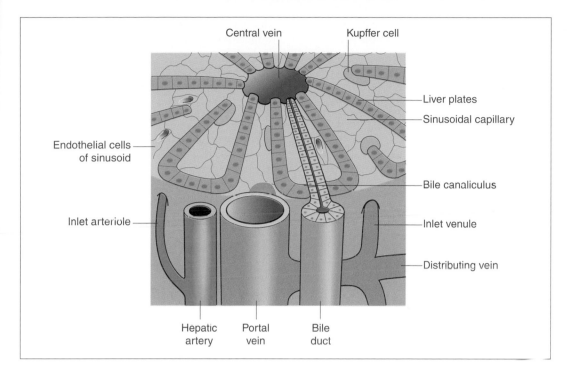

Figure 8.2 **The hepatocytes and the portal triad**. The hepatocytes are organised around a portal triad. These vessels provide hepatocytes with a mixture of nutrient-rich portal venous blood and oxygen-rich arterial blood, which bathes them. Hepatocytes process the nutrients and release the products into the blood, which is drained into a central vein and carried to the hepatic vein. The portal vein also contains a bile duct that drains bile to the gastrointestinal tract and gallbladder.

well as uptake and secretion of many macromolecules. The sinusoids also contain many macrophage-like **Kupffer cells** which are involved in the removal of senescent red blood cells and the digestion of haemoglobin, as well as having immune functions.

The biliary ductal system

The bile ductal system carries liver secretions to the intestine. The cells lining the bile duct are remarkably similar throughout. These epithelial cells are joined by tight junctions that limit the flow of water or solutes between the bile and the plasma. They are adapted for secretion and absorption, allowing them to regulate the composition of the bile. The biliary tree is organised as follows:

- The **initial ducts** that contribute to this system are the small bile canaliculi on the opposing surfaces between two hepatocytes.

- The **canaliculi** contribute to progressively larger vessels which anastomose to drain into the interlobular bile ducts, which are carried in the portal triads.
- The **common hepatic duct** emerges from the liver and merges with the **cystic duct** to form the **common bile duct**.

The common bile duct and the pancreatic duct both emerge in the small intestine through the sphincter of Oddi at the ampulla of Vater.

Gallbladder

The gallbladder is a small organ located between the left and right lobes of the liver. It stores and concentrates bile. The body and neck of the gallbladder are surrounded by peritoneum that binds it to the liver. The liver and the gallbladder are also connected by fibrous tissue layers.

The gallbladder is supplied by the cystic artery, a branch of the right hepatic artery, and is drained by the cystic vein into the portal circulation. It receives innervation from the parasympathetic and sympathetic nervous systems, as well as sensory innervation through the right phrenic nerve.

 CLINICAL Gallstones

If bile is too concentrated it may accumulate into deposits of gallstones. Although small gallstones easily pass into the gut, larger stones may block one of the ducts or damage the wall of the gallbladder itself. Surgical removal of the gallbladder may be required to prevent repeated inflammation. Gallstones are particularly common in women aged over 40 and in obese individuals, as a result of excess cholesterol.

Pancreas

The pancreas is the main secretory gland in the GI tract. It can be divided into two components:

1 An **endocrine** pancreas is involved in the regulation of blood sugar and other metabolic processes – discussed in Chapter 10.
2 An **exocrine** pancreas which secretes digestive enzymes.

Structure and location

The pancreas is a retroperitoneal organ that lies behind the stomach across the abdomen, so that its head is located between the spleen and the duodenum, with the transverse colon attached to its anterior margin.

The histology of the exocrine pancreas

The exocrine tissue of the pancreas, similar to the salivary glands, is made up of acini. These are consist of several serous cells that empty into a central duct. Between the acini of the pancreas are centroacinar cells, which are the terminal cells lining the ducts. The acinar cells are highly polarised and possess many zymogen-containing granules.

The supporting tissue of the pancreas is made up largely of collagen and contains many capillaries to supply the acinar cells. The pancreas itself is surrounded by a capsule of connective tissue which penetrates the pancreas, dividing it into lobules. The acini are separated from each other by a richly vascularised basal lamina.

Salivary glands

Salivary glands are exocrine glands that secrete into the mouth. The saliva produced has a role in lubricating the passage of food and initiating digestion as well as some immunological functions. Many small salivary glands are found throughout the mouth. In addition, there are three large pairs of glands:

- The submandibular
- The sublingual
- The parotid.

The secretory cells of the salivary glands

There are two main groups of cells that can be identified within the gland structure, these contribute different components to the saliva:

- Serous cells
- Mucous cells.

Serous cells

Serous cells are pyramidal – they have a narrow apical membrane that has small microvilli. Serous cells contain many mitochondria, reflecting the energy requirements for transport of ions. Typically the cells are formed in a spherical mass – an acinus – which has a lumen at the centre leading to the duct.

Mucous cells

Mucous cells are cuboidal or columnar and responsible for the secretion of mucus-like components into the salivary gland secretions. In the submandibular gland, the tubules are organised in a characteristic pattern – mucous cells are found in tubules that are capped at the ends with serous cells.

Myoepithelial cells

These are often known as **basket cells** and surround the acini of serous cells. Myoepithelial cells possess muscular elements that allow contraction to expel the glandular secretions.

The ductal system of the salivary glands

The secretory portions of the glands empty into intercalated ducts, which are lined by cuboidal epithelium. The intercalated ducts join to form interlobular structures, which further converge to form striated ducts and then excretory ducts. The main ducts of the salivary glands empty into the mouth.

The large salivary glands are encased in fibrous connective tissue, which also divides them into lobes.

Vasculature and innervation of the salivary glands

The vessels and nerves enter the glands and form a branching structure to supply the lobules. The ductal system of the glands is also highly innervated and vascularised. Parasympathetic innervation directly stimulates secretion of the glands. There is no direct sympathetic innervation to the secretory tissue of the duct; sympathetic stimulation of the vasculature alters blood flow to the gland, although this has less effect than parasympathetic stimulation.

Gut motility: transport and mechanical breakdown of food

The gut must efficiently transport food along its length, so that the different functions that contribute to the digestion and absorption of nutrients from food and the formation of faeces from waste can occur. The muscular action of the gut also contributes to the breakdown of food, particularly within the stomach where the muscular actions contribute to converting ingested food into chyme.

Chewing and swallowing

The ingestion of food occurs in the mouth which is the site of the initiation of digestion – both chemical and mechanical. The resulting bolus of food is shaped by the tongue and passed into the rest of the gut through the act of swallowing.

Mechanical breakdown of food begins with the action of the teeth, three types of which are found:

Incisors are located at the front of the mouth and possess a single thin cutting edge, allowing the cutting of food such as fruit and vegetables.

Canines are located further back in the mouth and possess a single point or cone, adapted for the tearing of meat.

Premolar and **molars** are wider teeth located in the back of the mouth. Their flatter and wider surface area allows the grinding and crushing of food.

Children typically have 20 primary (milk teeth) which are lost as they grow and replaced by permanent secondary teeth. On either side of each jaw children possess (from front to back):

- Two incisors – one medial and one lateral
- One canine
- Two premolars.

Adults possess 32 teeth. On each side of the jaw, the permanent teeth on the upper and lower jaw are:

- Two incisors
- One canine
- Two premolars
- Three molars: these include the 'wisdom teeth' which may not erupt until the later teens and frequently have to be removed because there may not be sufficient space for them to sit in the mouth.

The structure of a tooth

Each tooth has a common structure of three distinct parts:

1 The **root** is located beneath the gingiva (gums) and attaches the teeth into the jaw.
2 The **crown** is the part of the tooth that is exposed within the mouth and is responsible for the chewing action of the tooth.
3 The **neck** connects the crown to the root.

Most of the tooth is made up of dentine, a calcified tissue that contains hydroxyapatite in higher concentrations than found in bone. The exterior of the tooth is covered in a layer of enamel, which is the hardest substance in the human body, consisting of over 90% calcium salts. At the centre of the tooth is the pulp, a connective tissue containing the supporting cells in the tooth. The pulp is highly innervated and vascularised.

Vasculature and innervation

The superior and inferior alveolar arteries supply the upper and lower teeth, and are supplied by the maxillary and mandibular arteries, respectively. The teeth are innervated by the maxillary and mandibular branches of the trigeminal nerve.

Swallowing

After ingestion of food and its mechanical breakdown in the mouth, it must be swallowed and transported to the stomach via the oesophagus. There are a series of steps that transport food from the mouth to the stomach:

- The tongue pushes the food up against the roof of the mouth to form a bolus.
- The first stage of swallowing is voluntary and causes the muscles of the larynx and tongue to guide the food into the oesophagus, as a result of constriction of the constrictor muscles in the pharynx. The epiglottis prevents food from entering the trachea.
- The bolus of food is pushed down the oesophagus by a wave of constriction behind the food.

Stomach motility

The food enters the stomach through the oesophagus. The stomach is responsible for mixing the food and adding many secretions to help digestion, particularly of protein. Mixing occurs mainly in the pylorus of the stomach. Small amounts of food can be forced into the small intestine through the pyloric sphincter for continued digestion and absorption of nutrients.

The fat and acid contents of the stomach can be sensed, as can the state of breakdown of the bulk of the food. Local hormone secretion can alter the rate of gastric activity while chemoreceptors signal to the central nervous system (CNS); this can modulate activity, particularly via activity of the autonomic nervous system.

Storage of food in the stomach

The release of food from the stomach into the small intestine occurs slowly. The stomach retains food to release it into the bowels at a slow rate, even after ingestion of large quantities of food. If too much food has been ingested, a **dumping syndrome** may result, when the stomach empties too early leading to dramatically altered osmolality in the gut.

Peristalsis

Peristalsis is the process by which food is propelled through the gut. The process is tightly regulated and also involves non-propulsive contractions of the gut, which help both the breakdown and the absorption of the food.

GI motility in the small intestine

The small intestinal smooth muscle can generate both propulsive and non-propulsive movements.

Non-propulsive movements

Such movements are associated with mixing of the food:

- **Segmentation** occurs as a result of contraction of the circular smooth muscle in the muscularis mucosa. The gut divides into compartments around 5–10 cm long; this allows mixing of food in the gut and modulation of the properties of individual compartments.
- **Pendular motion** can be induced in individual compartments, whereby the compartment and its contents are moved back and forth vigorously to mix the contents.

Propulsive movements

Food is passed along the intestines as a result of contraction of the circular muscle behind the bolus. The longitudinal muscles in the gut also help the process by moving the walls of the intestine over the food. In the small intestine peristaltic movements that move the food from the duodenum to the jejunum result from myenteric reflexes and not from CNS involvement.

Movement of food from the small intestine to the large intestine occurs through the ileocaecal valve. Several reflexes and stimuli aid this process:

- **Sensors** within the gut may detect stretch (mechanoreceptors), chemical stimuli (such as lipids or aromatic amino acids) or irritants.
- **Intrinsic smooth muscle activity** results from large migrating motor complexes. These are waves of electrical activity (accompanied by muscular contraction) that migrate down the small intestine during fasting.
- **Hormonal signals** can modulate the motor activity in the gut.

Defecation

The rectum stores faeces until a suitable time for voiding. The peristaltic actions that aid the expulsion of faeces are coordinated in part by the enteric nervous system.

Retention of faeces and voiding

Faeces are stored in the rectum at low pressure, although pressure can be rapidly increased by the myenteric reflexes. There are both voluntary and autonomic components to voiding: reflex pathways can increase the abdominal pressure and allow relaxation of the sphincters, although the pelvic floor is under somatic control.

The anal sphincter is made up of two layers.

1 The **inner layer** is made up of both circular and longitudinal layers of smooth muscle, under involuntary control.
2 The **outer layer** is made up of striated muscle controlled by both involuntary and voluntary pathways.

Both layers are maintained by a variety of inhibitory nerves, which release acetylcholine or nitric oxide. During voiding, adrenergic nerves release noradenaline which acts on α_1-adrenoceptors found on the muscle cells in both layers to trigger contraction.

During voiding, peristaltic activity in the colon triggers the movement of the contents of the colon into the rectum. The sensory nerve fibres in the gut wall provide the CNS and enteric nervous systems with information about the state of the rectum which, when appropriate, signal the need for voiding. This triggers the **rectosphincteric reflex** which both stimulates the inhibition of the anal sphincters and triggers reflex peristalsis in the rectum to expel the contents. To prevent voiding, the external anal sphincter can be voluntarily stimulated to contract, i.e. prevent unwanted voiding of faeces, until a suitable time.

Pharmacological modulators of gut motility

Conditions may arise that result in either decreased or increased gut motility.

Laxatives

Laxatives are used to help gut immotility resulting from inadequate hydration or decreased bowel movement. Initial treatment attempts to counter the precipitating factors, through alteration of the hydration and fibre within the diet. In addition, some drugs may cause constipation, as can immobility. There are four major classes of laxative with different mechanisms of action:

1 Lubricants
2 Bulk formers
3 Osmotic laxatives
4 Motility stimulants.

Lubricants

The typical lubricant laxative is **liquid paraffin**. Lubricants help the motility of faeces through the gut, although they do nothing to rectify the underlying cause of the constipation.

Bulk formers

Bulk formers stimulate activity in the gut, decreasing the transit time of food through the gut. This helps the retention of water within the colon, which in turn helps lubricate the gut. Fibre in the diet is a bulk former, and where possible such natural bulk formers (e.g. oats and bran) are used. **Sterculia**, a large polysaccharide that is not digested, is often used clinically.

Osmotic laxatives

Osmotic laxatives act by promoting the retention of water in the colon, increasing both the faecal bulk and the lubrication. They are rarely used as a front-line treatment for constipation because it is difficult to control the dose so that diarrhoea does not result. Osmotic laxatives do not address the underlying cause of the constipation.

Motility stimulants

Motility stimulants act to vigorously promote peristaltic activity through either direct actions on the gastrointestinal smooth muscle or stimulation of the enteric nervous system. Motility stimulants can promote extremely strong contractions and, as a result, are frequently contraindicated after gut surgery. **Bisacodyl** is an example of a motility stimulant.

Treatment of diarrhoea

Diarrhoea can result from a variety of different causes which may warrant different treatments. Frequently, treatment focuses on the correction of water loss or ion imbalance by oral administration of isotonic solutions. Often this is accompanied with glucose or starch, which helps absorption.

If diarrhoea is a result of infection, treatments that reduce gut motility are contraindicated because there is a risk that they may prolong infection. In diarrhoea caused by diet, **kaolin,** an adsorbent agent, may be used.

Antiemetics

Drugs that prevent vomiting act by antagonising receptors which may contribute to triggering vomiting. H_1- and H_3-receptor histamine antagonists and muscarinic antagonists all have antiemetic effects.

Antiemetics are often used to combat the side effects of other therapeutic agents:

- **Domperidone**, the dopamine antagonist can be used with chemotherapy drugs, which frequently trigger vomiting.
- **Prochlorperazine**, another dopamine receptor antagonist maybe administered to prevent the vomiting and nausea that results from administration of morphine for pain relief.

Secretion and digestion in the gut

Most digestive enzymes enter the gut through the ducts at the ampulla of Vater that link the gut to the gallbladder, pancreas and liver. These organs provide most of the secretions responsible for catalysing the breakdown of food into its constituents. The secretory organs supporting the GI tract recycle the fluid and secretions, so that the total volume of fluid that is secreted into (and reabsorbed from) the gut each day far exceeds the volume of fluid ingested.

Salivary enzymes

The total secretion of the salivary glands is around 1 litre of fluid a day – most of which (80–90%) is produced by the major salivary glands: the parotid, submandibular and sublingual. Saliva contains a mixture of ions, mucins and enzymes with both protective and digestive qualities, and has a variety of functions:

- **Moistening** of the mucosa
- **Salivary amylase** is responsible for initiating digestion of carbohydrates

- **Lubrication** – for eating and for speech
- **Protection** from potential pathogens.

Formation of saliva

Initially, the secretion from serous cells of the salivary glands is isotonic. Anions (Cl^-, HCO_3^-) are secreted by a symporter (although not the classic cystic fibrosis Cl^- transporter), as is K^+. The movement of Na^+ is passive, following the movement of anions. Human saliva is typically alkaline as a result of the presence of HCO_3^- in the secretions. The ionic composition of saliva varies with the flow rate, due to the progressive reclamation of ions:

- At **low flow rates** Na^+ and Cl^- are reabsorbed while K^+ is secreted. This generates a hypotonic solution.
- At **higher flow rates** the salivary secretions are more similar to plasma in their composition, because there is less time for the transporter to remove secreted ions. Nevertheless human saliva is typically hypotonic and contains higher levels of K^+ than plasma.

Proteins in saliva

Protein components are secreted into saliva, which can be divided into three main groups:

1 **Enzymes** are secreted to initiate the first steps of digestion. In particular α-amylase breaks down starch, whereas salivary lipase initiates fat digestion.
2 **Mucins** are antimicrobial and lubricate the food, to allow easy passage in the pharynx and oesophagus.
3 **Proline-rich proteins** are antimicrobial and lubricants. In addition they have been implicated in binding Ca^{2+} and strengthening tooth enamel.

Regulation of secretion

Secretion is regulated in a complex manner, requiring the integration of both central and sensory inputs. The CNS nuclei regulating salivation are located at the junction of the pons and medulla. They receive inputs from taste buds and tactile senses, as well as from higher centres. The salivary nuclei stimulate the parasympathetic system to trigger secretion. Sympathetic stimulation can affect blood flow to the gland to reduce activity.

The stomach and gastric acid

The secretions of the stomach into the GI tract can be broken down into four groups:

- **Stomach acid** is secreted to kill pathogens and help the activity of other secretions.
- **Mucus** is secreted to protect the mucosa from acid.
- **Pepsin and other enzymes** are secreted to digest food.
- **Intrinsic factor** is secreted to protect vitamin B_{12} from degradation by acid.

The mechanism of gastric acid secretion

The secretion of gastric acid is due to the activity of the H^+/K^+ ATPase, which actively transports K^+ into the parietal cells in return for secretion of H^+. The K^+ is able to leave the parietal cells through K^+ channels allowing it to re-enter the stomach (Fig. 8.3).

Regulation of H^+ secretion

The pH of the stomach is around 2.5, creating a potentially dangerous environment. As a result the level of H^+ secretion is tightly regulated at a variety of different levels:

- **Paracrine regulation** is achieved by the entero-chromaffin-like (ECL) cells, which secrete histamine; this triggers H^+ release through its action on H_2-receptors.
- **Parasympathetic nerves** derived from the vagus can release acetylcholine, which acts directly on M_3-receptors on parietal cells to stimulate H^+ release. In addition, acetylcholine can act on the ECL cells to stimulate histamine release.
- **Gastrin**, a GI hormone, is released by cells within the GI tract, and can act through the cholecystokinin B (CCK-B) receptor found on both parietal cells and ECL cells.

In most cases, increased acid secretion results from a second messenger cascade within the parietal cells, which in turn results in the insertion of additional H^+/K^+ ATPase proteins into the cell membrane.

Enzyme secretion in the stomach

The **chief cells** of the stomach release **pepsins** into the gut. These are stored within the cells as granules of inactive zymogens (known as **pepsinogen**). The low pH of the gut triggers cleavage of the inactive pepsinogens into their active pepsin form, which is irreversibly inactivated in the small intestines by the neutral pH. The action of pepsins in the gut accounts for around 20% of protein digestion.

 CLINICAL Peptic ulcers and *Helicobacter pylori*

An ulcer is an area of damage within an epithelium. In the stomach this may occur as a result of acid eroding away the mucosa if the mucus layer is insufficient. A peptic ulcer may lead to a haemorrhage, which is a relatively common complication. The continual damage and repair of the mucosa can promote neoplastic changes in the epithelial cells, which may result in the formation of a gastric carcinoma.

The typical causes of gastric ulcers are:

- Diet: smoking, alcohol and hypoglycaemia have all been linked to an increased risk of developing a stomach ulcer
- Excess acid: this may be due to hypoglycaemia or, very rarely, a gastrin-secreting tumour in Zollinger–Ellison syndrome
- Loss of mucosal protection due to defective mucus secretion
- The presence of *H. pylori* infection has been shown to be a common factor in gastric ulcer. Elements of the bacterium are thought to mimic molecules expressed by the gastric epithelium, promoting an autoimmune attack.

Treatment of gastric ulcers aims to remove the predisposing factors. Typically antibiotics are given to treat *H. pylori* infection. Dietary factors such as alcohol and smoking must also be removed. Finally, stress is a significant predisposing factor that can be targeted.

 CLINICAL Zollinger–Ellison syndrome

Zollinger–Ellison syndrome is an extremely rare condition that results from the presence of a gastrin-secreting tumour, often within the pancreas. The tumour triggers the unregulated secretion of stomach acid, which precipitates damage to the lining of the stomach and the small intestine.

Secretion of mucus

Mucus is made up of large numbers of mucin glycoproteins that are secreted by the neck cells of the gastric glands. It lines the stomach in a thick coat to protect it from the highly acidic environment that it has developed. To help

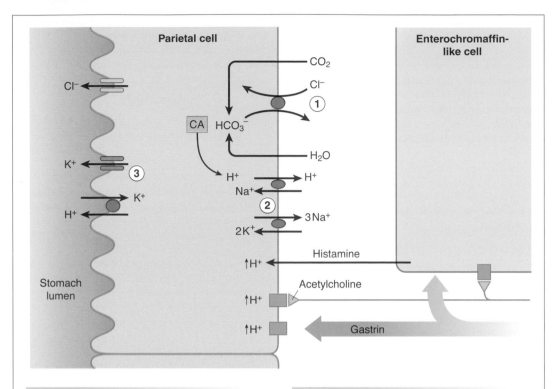

H+ regulation

The ion transport processes resulting in production of HCl by the parietal cells have three major steps associated:

1. CO_2 and H_2O are able to freely enter the cell by diffusion where carbonic acid catalyses the production of H^+ and H_2CO_3. The H_2CO_3 leaves the cell by exchange with Cl^-, which enters the stomach lumen through an apical channel. H^+ is pumped out of the basolateral membrane by exchange with Na^+, allowing the regeneration of H_2O and CO_2 from the H^+ and HCO_3^-.

2. The Na^+ that enters the cell through the Na^+/H^+ exchanger has done so down an electrochemical gradient generated by the Na^+/K^+ ATPase, which has transported K^+ into the parietal cell.

3. K^+ leaves the cell through channels in the apical membrane and is then returned to the cytosol by the K^+/H^+ exchanger, allowing the pumping of H^+ into the stomach to lower the pH.

Hormone regulation

The secretion of H^+ to acidify the stomach lumen is tightly regulated. This regulation involves inputs from both the nervous and the endocrine systems, which may work directly on the parietal cells, or indirectly via the enterochromaffin-like (ECL) cells.

Direct stimulation of the parietal cells is achieved by the actions of the hormone gastrin, or through the release of acetylcholine from nerves that synapse with the parietal cells. These stimuli trigger an increase in acid secretion.

Indirect stimulation occurs through the release of histamine from ECL cells, which triggers increased H^+ secretion by parietal cells. The release of histamine is triggered either by gastrin or through acetylcholine released from nerves that synapse with the ECL cells.

Figure 8.3 Stomach acid. This is produced by the parietal cells, which transport H^+ and Cl^- into the cell lumen through a complex series of ion transports. The process of H^+ transport is tightly regulated directly by nervous and hormonal signals or through paracrine interactions with enterochromaffin-like cells.

protection, the secretion of mucus and stomach acid is regulated by similar stimuli.

The surface epithelium of the stomach also secretes a watery fluid that is high in K^+ and HCO_3^- which makes the mucus alkaline, further protecting the stomach lining from the acid. The mucins retain the HCO_3^- close to the lining of the stomach, preventing it from neutralising the stomach acid entirely. This arrangement allows the surface of the stomach to be maintained at a neutral pH, despite the cavity of the stomach having a highly acidic pH.

The pepsins active in the stomach are capable of cleaving some of the bonds in the mucins; as a result the mucus lining of the stomach must be constantly replenished.

Intrinsic factor

Although the highly acidic environment helps to kill potentially harmful bacteria, and the digestion of proteins, it is also capable of mediating the breakdown of vitamin B_{12} which is essential for correct synthesis of DNA and fatty acids.

The body has developed a method of overcoming this degradation, through the production of **intrinsic factor**. This glycoprotein is produce by the Parietal cells and binds Vitamin B_{12} within the stomach, protecting it from the action of stomach acid and degradative enzymes.

Production of intrinsic factor is the only essential function of the stomach, because it safeguards vitamin B_{12}, without which **pernicious anaemia** results.

 CLINICAL Pernicious anaemia

Vitamin B_{12} is essential for cell division. Owing to their large turnover, red blood cells are the first cells affected by a lack of vitamin B_{12}. Pernicious anaemia results from a deficiency in intrinsic factor, usually caused by the body's production of auto-antibodies against it. As a result, vitamin B_{12} is degraded in the stomach. Treatment is typically regular injections of vitamin B_{12}, thus bypassing the need for intrinsic factor.

Digestion of protein

There are groups of enzymes responsible for the digestion of proteins:

1 **Stomach**: digestion of protein is mediated by the acid-dependent enzymes secreted into the gut, e.g. pepsin.

2 **Pancreatic** and **intestinal** secretions mediate most protein digestion, cleaving large polypeptide chains into many small peptides.
3 The **membrane-bound enzymes** include many aminopeptidases and dipeptidases, which cleave small peptides into single amino acids for transport out of the lumen.

Pancreatic enzymes

The pancreatic secretions contain many enzymes, secreted in their inactive form as proenzymes. The major proenzymes secreted are trypsinogen, chymotrypsinogen and procarboxypeptidase which are activated in a series of cleavage reactions initiated by enterokinase in the intestinal mucosa. Enterokinase acts on trypsinogen to convert it to active trypsin. Trypsin is, in turn, capable of cleaving trypsinogen, chymotrypsinogen and procarboxypeptidase into their active forms.

Trypsin, chymotrypsin and other pancreatic enzymes cleave proteins into small fragments, accounting for about 50% of protein digestion. Trypsin, chymotrypsin and proelastase are all **endopeptidase**s, which cut the polypeptides at internal sites to produce oligopeptides. In contrast, **procarboxypeptidases** cleave amino acids directly from the carboxyl terminal of the peptide to release single amino acids for absorption.

The role of brush border peptidases in the digestion of peptides

The action of the various gastric and pancreatic proteases results in the formation of single amino acids and many small peptides. The brush border peptidases cleave the small peptides into single amino acids for transport out of the lumen.

The digestion of carbohydrates

Carbohydrates supply around 50% of body energy requirements. They are ingested in varying lengths, from single sugar monosaccharides up to long polysaccharides, which are made up of many monosaccharides joined by glycosidic links. As the intestines can absorb only single sugar monosaccharides, polysaccharides are broken down into their constituent monosaccharides. There are some large polysaccharides that the body is unable to break down; these form **fibre**.

Much of the carbohydrate in the diet is supplied as starch, which is broken down by three series of enzymes:

1 **Salivary amylase** initiates the breakdown of starch into oligosaccharides. Salivary amylase is not crucial to the breakdown of polysaccharides, and is inactivated by stomach acid.
2 **Pancreatic α-amylase** hydrolyses internal links in the starch to release many oligosaccharides. Pancreatic amylase secretion is triggered by the gut hormone CCK.
3 **Membrane-bound enzymes** act in combination to convert a variety of oligosaccharides into their constituent monosaccharides which are readily absorbed into enterocytes.

Membrane digestion of oligosaccharides

The brush border of the small intestine expresses a variety of enzymes that can break down oligosaccharides into their constituent monosaccharides:

- **Sucrase** splits sucrose into glucose and fructose,
- **Maltase** breaks down the α-1,4 linkages found in straight chains of oligosaccharides,
- **Lactase** breaks down lactose into glucose and galactose.
- **Isomaltase** is found bound to the enzyme sucrase and can catalyse the breakdown of α-1,6 linkages found in polysaccharides.

 CLINICAL Lactase deficiency

Lactase deficiency is relatively common, and occurs after weaning. In people with the condition, ingestion of lactase results in cramps and diarrhoea. Many factors may alter the effect of lactase deficiency, including colonisation of the gut by lactose-metabolising bacteria. Treatment of the condition is to reduce intake of dairy products or to use products treated with lactase.

Bile and the digestion of fats

Bile is a product of the liver that serves three functions:

1 To **emulsify fat** in ingested food to aid its absorption from the gut
2 To **neutralise stomach acid**, producing a mild alkaline environment in which pancreatic enzymes function optimally

3 As a mechanism to **excrete the products of the breakdown of haemoglobin** and other substances not removed by the kidneys.

Bile is made up of a variety of different components:

- **Bile acids** act to emulsify lipids, which increases the surface area on which the lipolytic enzymes may act. Once a high enough concentration is reached, the bile acids can induce the lipids to form **micelles**.
- **Lecithin** increases the amount of cholesterol that can be solubilised within the micelles.
- **Bile pigments** are excreted products of haem metabolism.

The formation of bile and its reabsorption form a cycle, allowing a large volume of bile to be secreted while the total pool of bile in the body is kept low, and little is lost in the faeces (Fig. 8.4).

Formation of bile acids

Bile salts and bile acids are synthesised by hepatocytes. Cholesterol derivatives may also be converted into bile acids, providing the major route for excretion of cholesterol from the body.

Bile pigments

Bile pigments are the excreted products of the breakdown of haem. The release of iron from the haem group of haemoglobin releases a carbon structure that is rapidly processed into bilirubin. The cytochrome P450 pathway and other pathways in the hepatocytes can conjugate bilirubin to other molecules, such as glucuronate. A variety of organic ions is also secreted into bile, in particular, anions, various prostanoids and derivatives of eicosanoic acid, as well as organic cations. Many antibiotics and other drugs are broken down by the liver, and the resulting components of breakdown are often secreted into the bile.

The storage and concentration of bile

The gallbladder stores bile and concentrates it for release during digestion. The Na^+/K^+ ATPase on the basolateral membrane of gallbladder epithelial cells draws H_2O out of the lumen by **transcellular** and **paracellular** routes. The net action of the transporters in the biliary epithelium leads to the progressive addition of H^+ into the bile, neutralising the HCO_3^- that is already present.

Liver

The liver is the major site of processing of bile. It is capable of producing bile from the cholesterol, as well as absorbing other cholesterol derivatives from the blood which, in turn, are converted to bile salts. Finally, those bile salts that have been reabsorbed from the intestines are returned to the liver through the portal circulation. Bile is secreted out of the bile ductal system and stored in the gall bladder until it is required for release to the intestines to aid the emulsification and absorption of fats.

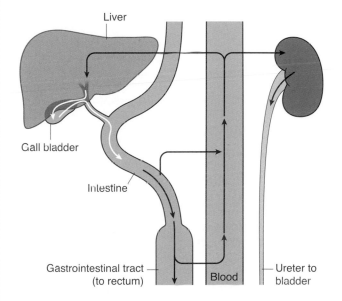

Kidney

Physiologically the vast majority of processing of bile is achieved by the liver, though a small amount can be processed and removed from circulation by the kidneys. The resulting metabolites are excreted within urine. If there is a defect in the GI processing of bile, the kidneys become the major route of excretion – as is reflected by the darkening of the urine associated within increased bile.

Gall bladder

The gall bladder Is located in contact with the liver and serves as a repository for bile, in between meals. Within the gall bladder, the epithelium aids the concentration of bile through the removal of water and ions from the fluid. Bile is released from the gall bladder and enter the intestine through the common bile duct into the second part of the duodenum.

Intestine

In the intestine, bile emulsifies ingested fats to aid their absoprtion. As a result a large proportion of the bile released through the bile duct is reabsorbed into the bloodstream, though a small proportion escapes and is excreted.

Blood

Bile and its precursor molecules are transported on the blood stream at low concentrations. In particular, those bile molecules reabsorbed from the gut reach the liver through the portal vessels. A small amount of bile will reenter the systemic circulation, where it can be excreted by the kidneys. In cases where is are defects in the excretion and processing of bile by the GI tract the body becomes more dependent on the kidney as a mechanism of bile excretion, and this is associated with jaundice, since the kidneys are less able to fulfil this function.

Figure 8.4 The enterohepatic circulation. The pool of bile salts is small; as a result several times the total volume is secreted and reabsorbed from the gut each day, with only a small proportion being excreted. This process occurs primarily in the gut, although a small amount of bile that is reabsorbed is also excreted by the kidneys.

DEFINITION Conjugated and unconjugated bilirubin

Bile pigments are categorised as conjugated and unconjugated, which affects their fat and water solubility:

- **Unconjugated bile pigment** is not joined to an acid. Haem released from the breakdown of senescent red blood cells is converted into unconjugated bilirubin. Unconjugated bile pigments are fat soluble and transported around the body bound to albumin. If the level of free unconjugated bile rises in the body **jaundice** may result.
- **Conjugated bile pigment** is attached to charged molecules such as taurocholate. These are water soluble, although they can be reclaimed from the gut by a Na^+-dependent transporter. This regulation and the inability to diffuse across lipids account for the preferential excretion of conjugated bile salts from the gut.

 CLINICAL Jaundice

Jaundice describes the yellow colour, particularly prominent in the eyes and the skin, that results from high levels of bile pigment present in the blood and extracellular spaces.

Bilirubin, the breakdown product of haemoglobin, is responsible for causing jaundice. Typically unconjugated bilirubin is present at <0.5 mg/L. Jaundice becomes apparent at levels around three times higher than this and often results from the destruction of red blood cells, leading to the rapid release of bilirubin from the breakdown of haemoglobin.

If there is damage to the liver or bile duct system, the excretion of conjugated bilirubin may not be possible, resulting in it entering the systemic circulation. In these cases, the soluble conjugated bilirubin can be filtered by the kidneys, causing urine to become very dark in colour, often accompanied by a light colour in the faeces. A measurement of the free and conjugated bilirubin in the blood allows determination of whether or not jaundice has an obstructive origin.

The circulation of bile

Only a small proportion of bile salts is excreted; most are reabsorbed in the terminal ileum and transported back to the liver, from where they are re-secreted by the hepatocytes. The total bile acid pool is relatively small, and may be secreted several times over during the course of a meal. Each day, around 20% of the bile acid pool must be replenished to make up for what has been excreted from the body.

The breakdown of fats

Lipids are hydrolysed in the gut through reactions catalysed by lipases, to generate fatty acids and glycerol, which can be readily absorbed in the intestines. The action of bile helps to maintain a stable emulsion, which prevents formation of micelles and coalescence of the lipid droplets. Bile acids are relatively insoluble in either lipids or water, although at the interface between the two they are very soluble. Lipases are secreted all along the GI tract to break down fats:

- **Gastric lipase** functions well at the low pH of the stomach and breaks down triglycerides into a fatty acid and a diglyceride. There is no absorption in the stomach, and the products of breakdown are transported to the small intestines.
- **Pancreatic lipase** is responsible for most lipid digestion outside the stomach. The gut mucosa releases CCK in response to fats entering the intestine, and this triggers the release of bile from the gallbladder and of pancreatic lipases from the pancreas.
- **Other lipases are secreted by the pancreas**, such as cholesterol esterases, which can hydrolyse lipid esters and phospholipase A_2; this can act against glycerophospholipids.

Absorption of nutrients

After ingestion and breakdown into its constituents, food must be absorbed into the body for processing and use in a variety of metabolic processes.

Absorption from the stomach

Water and ethanol and some other small molecules can be absorbed from the stomach itself. The stomach is also the site of absorption of some classes of drugs. However, for most substances, significant absorption does not occur until the small intestines where the surface area is vastly greater.

Absorption of carbohydrates

After the action of various amylases and other enzymes, saccharides must be absorbed from the gut. The rate-limiting step is the transport of the sugars, not the hydrolysis reaction to generate monosaccharides. As a result, there can be a build-up of monosaccharides in the lumen during digestion. There is a variety of transport mechanisms that absorb monosaccharides from the gut and transport them to the portal circulation (Fig. 8.5):

- **Glucose** and **galactose** compete for transport by the sodium–glucose transport proteins (SGLTs) expressed on the **brush border**. The SGLT1 transporter transports monosaccharides via secondary active transport as a result of the Na^+ gradient. The transport of glucose and galactose out of the cells across the basolateral membrane occurs in a Na^+-independent manner by the low-affinity GLUT2 transporter.
- **Fructose** transport from the gut lumen is achieved through Na^+-independent facilitated diffusion by the glucose transporter GLUT5. This transport does not compete with glucose across the luminal membrane, although transport across the basolateral membrane is competitive.

Absorption of proteins

A variety of different mechanisms of protein absorption occurs in the gut. Although, in most cases, the amino acids are required for the synthesis of new proteins, there are occasions when the absorption of a whole protein is crucial.

Pinocytic transport of proteins

In newborn babies, passive immunity in the gut and bloodstream is mediated by maternal antibodies carried in the milk. These antibodies can be transported intact across the gut mucosa by pinocytosis.

Peptide transport in the gut

There is a H^+-driven system of transport in the gut to allow the transport of small peptides across the enterocytes.

Amino acid transport system in the gut

The amino acids generated by the cleavage of peptides are transported across the brush border

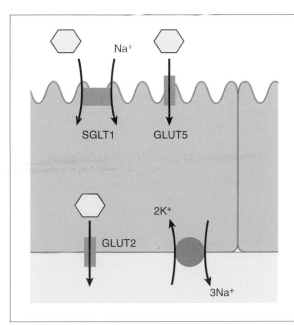

The three major monosaccharides – glucose, galactose and fructose – may be absorbed across the apical surface by one of two proteins. Glucose and galactose are transported into the cell by the SGLT1 transporter, where transport is driven by co-transport of Na^+ down its concentration gradient. Fructose is transported across the apical surface of the cells by the Na^+-independent GLUT5 transporter. All three monosaccharides leave the cell across the basolateral membrane through the Na^+-independent GLUT2 transport protein, which allows the sugars to enter the portal circulation from where they are transported to the liver and around the body.

Figure 8.5 **Carbohydrates**. These are broken down into small chains of saccharides. Enzymes on the epithelial surface further these oligosaccharides down break to single monosaccharide blocks.

by various proteins with overlapping specificities. These specificities ensure that all the required amino acids can be absorbed by the body.

There are both Na$^+$-dependent and -independent transporters. In particular, there are Na$^+$-independent transporters for cationic and large, branched-chain and aromatic amino acids, many of which are essential because they cannot be synthesised in the body. There are genetic defects that result from the absence of a functional version of one or more of these amino acids transporters. These disorders are often associated more with defects in the production of urine, because many of the same proteins are expressed in the gut and kidney.

 CLINICAL Hartnup's disease

Hartnup's disease is an autosomal recessive condition caused by a defect in the **neutral amino acid transporter**. This protein is expressed in the intestines and the proximal convoluted tubule (PCT) of the kidneys, and is particularly important in regulating the transport of tryptophan. Defects in this transporter result in increased excretion of tryptophan in the urine, because less is reclaimed from the nephron, which compounds the decreased absorption from the gut. There is still some uptake of tryptophan from the gut through oligopeptide transport systems – which function normally.

Tryptophan is an essential amino acid and the precursor for such molecules as serotonin and melatonin, as well as being a component of many proteins. Defects in its transport are detected early as a failure to thrive and photosensitivity. In addition, there are neural symptoms, particularly tremor, nystagmus and intermittent ataxia.

Treatment is through tryptophan supplements and a high-protein diet.

Absorption of lipids

Most lipids in the gut are found in a liquid phase. In the diet, lipids are made up of triglycerides, free fatty acids, cholesterol and cholesterol esters, as well as the fat-soluble vitamins (A, D, E and K). In the gut, the lipids are formed into micelles for absorption (Fig. 8.6):

- The effects of mechanical and enzymatic breakdown of lipids lead to the generation of a lipid droplet emulsion.

- Progressive addition of bile salts promotes the conversion of droplets into vesicles that contain many concentric lipid bilayers.
- These develop into single bilayer vesicles and finally into mixed **micelles**, made up of bile salts and mixed lipids.

Mixed micelles are able to diffuse close to the surface of the enterocytes, where they encounter an acidic environment generated by the **Na$^+$/H$^+$ exchanger**. The acidic environment is thought to help transport lipids into the cells. It is not clear which route is predominant in the transport of lipids out of the GI tract:

- Direct diffusion across the brush border
- Incorporation into the lipid bilayer
- Protein-mediated transport.

Processing of lipids in the enterocyte

The enterocytes absorb the components of lipid breakdown and package them with proteins to form **chylomicrons** – a large form of lipoprotein. Chylomicrons are released from enterocytes and enter the lymph because they are unable to pass through the windows/pores in the blood capillaries. They pass to the thoracic duct and re-enter the blood supply at the left subclavian vein from when they are taken up and absorbed by other tissues, in particular the **adipocytes**.

Essential fatty acids

Although the body can easily synthesis most lipids required for membrane structures, only limited fatty acids must be obtained from the diet. The body is unable to insert a double bond in a fatty acyl chain beyond carbon-9, which is required in some fatty acids associated with signal transduction, particularly the arachidonic acid metabolites. As a result, the precursor fatty acids, **linoleic acid** and **linolenic acid**, are essential components of the diet.

Absorption of vitamins

The transport of vitamins differs for those that are water soluble and those that are fat soluble.

- **Water-soluble vitamins** (B and C) are transported mainly by protein transporters although, if they are ingested in high enough doses, they may be absorbed by simple diffusion. Vitamin B$_{12}$ absorption requires the presence of intrinsic

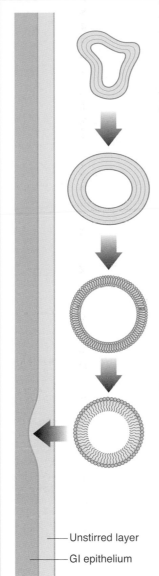

Emulsion

Ingested lipids are broken down to fatty acids and other derivatives by lipases. This, coupled with the mechanical action of the GI tract, results in the formation of an emulsion, where large droplets of lipids, consisting of several bilayers coating a lipid core, are produced.

Multilamellar vesicle

The progressive addition of bile salts to an emulsion produces multilamellar vesicles, which bud off from the larger droplets. They share a similar basic structure to the droplets, consisting of many concentric lipid bilayers surrounding a lipid core.

Unilamellar vesicle

Further addition of bile salts to the vesicles results in a 'thinning out' of the vesicle so that it consists of a single bilayer.

Micelle

The progressive addition of bile salts to a unilamellar vesicle produces a micelle, which consists of a single layer of lipids with the hydrophilic heads facing outwards, in contact with the water, whereas the hydrophobic tails all point inwards. Micelles are able to diffuse close to the epithelium. Here components may become protonated and enter the cell by carrier-mediated transport, or the micelle may enter the cell by diffusion and/or through incorporation into the cell membrane.

— Unstirred layer

— GI epithelium

Lipids

The lipids are not water soluble. As a result the body produces bile salts and other molecules that organise the lipids into small micelles in the gastrointestinal (GI) tract, which diffuse into the acid zone surrounding the epithelium. Here many components can be protonated and enter the cells through carrier-mediated transport. In addition the micelles may be absorbed by diffusion across the cell membrane, or incorporation into the cell membrane

Figure 8.6 Lipid absorption. These are hydrophobic, and must be emulsified into progressively smaller structures to allow absorption. This process is achieved in the gut by various emulsifying agents, which help to convert lipid aggregations from the large multilayered structures, which they naturally form in the stomach, into small micelles that can be readily absorbed.

factor, which protects the molecule from breakdown in the gut.

- **Fat-soluble vitamins** (A, D, E and K) are absorbed from mixed micelles. They are able to diffuse directly into the intestinal epithelial cells even in the absence of bile salts. The vitamins are then released into the portal blood for transport from the gut.

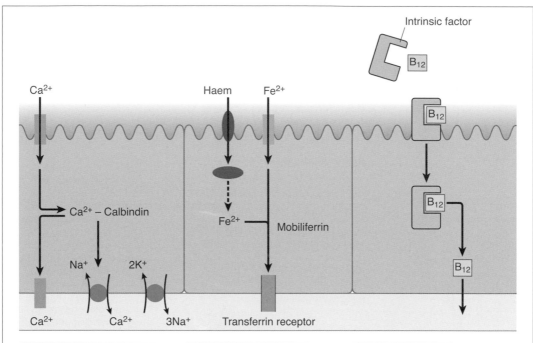

Ca²⁺

Ca^{2+} is absorbed across the apical surface of the epithelium through an intestinal epithelial channel. However, within the cell high levels of Ca^{2+} are highly toxic, due to its role as a major second messenger. To overcome this problem, high levels of the Ca^{2+}-binding protein, calbindin, are expressed to 'ferry' Ca^{2+} across the cell.

Transport across the basolateral surface is achieved both by the Ca^{2+} ATPase in an active transport mechanism, or through the Na^+/Ca^{2+} exchanger, which is driven by the presence of a Na+ gradient across the cell membrane. The transport of Ca^{2+} out of the cell generates a gradient between the intestinal lumen and cell interior that promotes the entry of Ca^{2+} into the cell from the gastrointestinal (GI) tract.

Iron transport

Iron can be obtained from the diet in two forms: as Fe^{2+} ions, or complexed within haem. In each case, there are specific proteins for the transport of the ion complex into the cell. Here the enzyme haem oxygenase promotes the breakdown of haem, to release Fe^{2+}. The Fe^{2+} must be complexed to calreticulin within the cell, because free Fe^{2+} is highly toxic. This mechanism allows transport across the cell for release into the bloodstream. Fe^{2+} is not transported within the blood as a free ion; rather it is release bound to the protein transferrin.

Vitamin B₁₂

Vitamin B_{12} is bound to intrinsic factor in the gut to prevent its breakdown, and it remains bound to this molecule on its passage through the GI tract, where it is absorbed into the cells through a receptor recognising the vitamin B_{12}–intrinsic factor complex. In the cytoplasm of the intestinal cells, the vitamin B_{12} and the intrinsic factor are separated, and the vitamin B_{12} molecule released into the portal circulation.

Absorption of minerals and water

The vast majority (around 99%) of the water and mineral present in food and gastrointestinal secretions is absorbed. Typically, around 2 litres of fluid is ingested each day, and about 7 L of secretions is released into the gut, yet only 100 mL water is lost in faeces each day. The remainder is absorbed along the GI tract (Fig. 8.7):

- The **duodenum** does not contribute much to reabsorption of water, because the fluid present is predominantly **isotonic**.
- The **jejunum and ileum** absorb a significant proportion of fluid.
- The **colon** accounts for most of the fluid reabsorption from the gut.

Reabsorption of Na$^+$

The net flow of Na$^+$ is out of the GI tract into the blood, although both secretion and reabsorption occur. Absorption occurs down an electrochemical gradient across the apical membrane of the intestinal epithelium. This electrochemical gradient is created by the Na$^+$/K$^+$ ATPase expressed in the basolateral membrane. The rate and mechanism of absorption vary along the length of the gut:

- The net rate of absorption of Na$^+$ is highest in the **jejunum**, where it is coupled to the transport of glucose, galactose and amino acids in Na$^+$-dependent secondary active transport.
- In the **ileum**, there is less absorption, due to the lower concentration of amino acids and sugars, as well as less Na$^+$ being present.
- In the **colon,** the Na$^+$ is reabsorbed against a large electrochemical gradient. Although plasma Na$^+$ is around 120 mmol/L, in the lumen of the colon Na$^+$ may be around 25 mmol/L.

Absorption of Cl$^-$ and HCO$_3$$^-$

Absorption of these anions occurs mostly in the jejunum. Although Cl$^-$ continues to be reabsorbed in the ileum, HCO$_3$$^-$ is secreted only when the concentration in the lumen is less than about 45 mmol/L, after which the net effect is reabsorption. Transport of anions in the colon is similar to that in the ileum.

Absorption of K$^+$

K$^+$ is reabsorbed partly by **solvent drag** in the jejunum and ileum, resulting from the reabsorption of H$_2$O, which generates a K$^+$ gradient. In the colon, there is usually net secretion of K$^+$ as a result of the negative electrical potential in the colon.

Absorption of Ca$^+$

Ca^{2+} can be rapidly absorbed in the duodenum and jejunum over a large concentration gradient, which is generated as a result of active transport of ions across the basolateral membrane. The Ca^{2+} is transported across the cells by the Ca^{2+}-binding protein **calbindin**, which allows the transport of high levels of Ca^{2+} across the cytosol, generating insoluble salts within the cell.

Transport of Ca^{2+} across the basolateral membrane is achieved by three mechanisms:

1 The **Ca^{2+}ATPase** transports Ca^{2+} across the basolateral membrane, using energy generated by the hydrolysis of ATP.
2 The **Na$^+$/Ca^{2+} exchanger** also removes Ca^{2+} from the cell.
3 Ca^{2+} contained in vesicles may be extruded across the basolateral membrane via **exocytosis**.

Ca^{2+} reabsorption is tightly regulated by vitamin D and parathyroid hormone; it forms part of a far larger and more complex system of calcium homoeostasis, including effects on Ca^{2+} absorption in the gut.

Absorption of iron

The level of iron in the body is regulated at the point of absorption. Although about 15–20 mg iron is ingested per day, only about 0.5–1 mg of this is absorbed by normal men. Iron depletion, such as

Figure 8.7 The transport of many essential molecules and ions across the gut wall is achieved through a variety of transport mechanisms, requiring specialised transporters and channels. Carbohydrates need transport by a variety of mechanisms, some of which are driven by a Na^{2+} gradient. Many ions present a problem because they are toxic to cells in high concentrations; in the case of calcium, this problem is overcome by a transport protein in the cells and, in the case of iron, by a blood-borne transport molecule. Finally, vitamin B$_{12}$ needs the presence of intrinsic factor for its passage through the gut, to avoid degradation in the stomach.

from haemorrhage, promotes increased absorption of iron from the gut. Growing children and pregnant women, in particular, absorb greater amounts of iron than men.

Iron is ingested in inorganic iron salts or as part of haem groups. About 20% of the ingested haem iron is absorbed – enzymes in the gut can release the haem groups from their attached proteins, and haem is then taken up in the gut by **facilitated diffusion**. Iron is released from haem in the epithelial cells, so that no intact haem enters the bloodstream from the gut.

Absorption of haem

Haem (Fe^{3+}) iron can bind a specific transporter on the surface of the enterocytes, or alternatively may be absorbed by **endocytosis**. In the enterocyte, the Fe^{3+} ion is released by enzymatic cleavage of the haem ring and reduction to Fe^{2+}

Absorption of Fe^{2+}

Iron absorption is hindered because it tends to form insoluble salts and complexes, which are more soluble at lower pH, so the low pH of the stomach promotes iron absorption.

Vitamin C promotes the absorption of iron; it associates with Fe^{3+} and its acidic nature reduces Fe^{3+} to Fe^{2+}, which forms fewer insoluble complexes. There are two methods of absorption of Fe^{2+}:

1 **Transferrin** can bind to Fe^{2+} in the gut. The Fe^{2+}–transferrin complex can then be taken up into the enterocyte by receptor-mediated endocytosis. In the cell Fe^{2+} and transferrin dissociate and the Fe^{2+} (including that derived from haem degradation) is transported in the cell bound to the protein mobiliferrin.
2 A **divalent cation transporter** in the duodenum can transport free Fe^{2+} directly into the enterocytes.

Fe^{2+} ions are then transported across the basolateral membrane where they can bind plasma transferrin for transport around the body within the plasma.

Absorption of other ions

Other ions that are required body are obtained from the diet, in particular:

- **Magnesium** is absorbed along the length of the intestine. About 50% of the dietary intake is absorbed.

- **Copper** is absorbed in the jejunum, so that about 50% of the ingested amount is absorbed. Copper may also be secreted in the gut, bound to some bile acids.

Changes in ion transport along the villus

The nature of transport changes along individual villi in relation to the maturity of the epithelial cells:

- The mature cells towards the tips of the villi are net absorbers of ions and water.
- Immature cells nearer the crypts are net secretors of ions and water.

Processing by the liver

The liver is a major metabolic organ in the body, and at rest receives about a quarter of the total body's blood flow, accounting for about 20% of the total oxygen consumption of the body. The blood from the gut drains into the portal circulation, a series of veins that unite into the hepatic portal vein, which carries venous blood to the liver. Here it is processed by the hepatocytes before being released into the bloodstream for use elsewhere. The liver regulates the storage and distribution of a variety of substances absorbed from the gut:

- Glucose
- Proteins and amino acids
- Cholesterol
- Iron
- Triglycerides and lipids – although the liver regulates these, it is not the first site of processing after absorption from the gut.

Glucose

Glucose is an essential requirement of many cells in the body. Nevertheless, the level of glucose release must be regulated, particularly through coordinated action of the endocrine pancreatic hormones.

The liver expresses both **glucokinase** and **hexokinase**, allowing it to commit large amounts of glucose to glycolysis for the production of fatty acids; these can be stored in the adipocytes across the body. The liver can synthesise and store glycogen, which can be released into the bloodstream to supplement the blood glucose during periods of starvation.

Amino acids

The composition of the amino acids taken up by the liver differs markedly from amino acids released. The metabolic pathways regulating the processing of amino acids in the liver are discussed in Chapter 3. The liver is integral is ensuring that free amino acids in the blood are enough to supply the body with the necessary building blocks for protein synthesis, while helping process toxic amine derivatives produced during amino acid metabolism. The liver is also a major site of protein synthesis, producing many of the plasma proteins, including:

- Albumin
- Clotting factors
- Acute phase proteins
- Transport proteins, e.g. lipoproteins, transferrin.

Triglycerides and lipids

Triglycerides and lipids are not directly processed by the liver after their ingestion. Instead, they are packaged into **chylomicrons** and transported to adipose tissue, where the fatty acids are extracted and stored. The liver has three roles related to the processing and storage of fats:

- During periods of starvation, fatty acids from the adipocytes can be released and processed as an energy source. In the liver, the **breakdown of fatty acids can be used to generate ketones** which are released into the blood as a supplementary energy source in starvation.
- The liver is the site of **lipoprotein synthesis,** required in the transport of lipids. It takes up the remnants of chylomicrons after they have transported fatty acids to the fatty adipose tissue.
- Excess glucose can be taken up by the liver and converted to acetyl Co-A, from which **fatty acids can be produced**.

Cholesterol

The liver processes cholesterol, which can be obtained from the uptake of cholesterol-rich chylomicron remnants or through new synthesis in the liver. The key process in the synthesis of cholesterol is regulated by the enzyme 3-hydroxy-3-methylglutarate (HMG)-CoA reductase. It is this enzyme that is inhibited by the 'statin' class of drug, the standard therapy for reducing high cholesterol, a common risk factor of 'western diseases'. The liver produces cholesterol for a number of functions throughout the body:

- The liver produces **bile acids** from cholesterol. These are used for the emulsification of lipids and provide a mechanism for the excretion of cholesterol.
- Cholesterol can be **converted into vitamin D**, involved in the regulation of total body calcium in a process involving reactions in the skin, liver and kidneys.
- **Steroid hormones**, which have widespread effects throughout the body, are produced from cholesterol.

Iron

The liver produces **transferrin**, which binds iron in the intestines for absorption and is also responsible for iron transport via the bloodstream to tissues. The liver is capable of taking up and storing a limited amount of iron, most of which is retained bound to the protein ferritin.

Regulation of gastrointestinal function

Many organs and functions must be coordinated to allow the ingestion, digestion and absorption of nutrients followed by packaging and removal of waste from the body. This activity is controlled by a series of signals, which include neural and hormonal signals from both the gut and other sites in the body. There is also regulation of when and how much an individual ingests. This is the regulation of appetite and satiety, which happens in response to many different stimuli.

Control of appetite

The control of appetite, i.e. the desire to eat food, is complex. It integrates psychological cues, neural cues, olfactory and gustatory inputs, and hormones. Control occurs at three levels:

Short term – terminating eating when you are 'full'
Medium term – knowing when it is time for breakfast, lunch and dinner
Long term – adapting to the environment (e.g. temperature, amount of food available).

All the factors discussed interact to control appetite; it is not yet known which are most important and how exactly these interactions occur. The **mesolimbic reward system** is involved, and the desire to eat is thought to be processed in corticolimbic structures, e.g. the amygdala, prefrontal cortex and ventral striatum. Certain foods make you feel 'good' so you eat more of them, even if you are not physiologically hungry.

Control of appetite is thought to be integrated within the **hypothalamus.** The ventromedial nucleus is known as the 'satiety centre' (preventing excess intake of food) while the lateral hypothalamus is known as the 'feeding centre'. The major outputs controlling feeding behaviour are two sets of neurons in the arcuate nucleus:

1 **POMC/CART neurons** release pro-opiomelano-cortin (POMC), the precursor of α-melanocyte-stimulating hormone (α-MSH), which is known to be **anorexigenic** (i.e. decreases feeding behaviour).
2 **NPY/AgRP neurons** release neuropeptide Y, a potent **orexigenic** agent (stimulates feeding).

A number of factors come together in the hypothalamus and act to control feeding via these mechanisms.

Short-term control

The presence of food in the stomach leads to the release of hormones and results in stomach distension, both of which stimulate the vagus nerve. Oral factors also play a role:

- **Oral factors** related to feeding, e.g. chewing, salivating, swallowing and taste, have been shown to have short-term effects, reducing food intake.
- **CCK** is a peptide hormone released by the enteroendocrine cells of the gastrointestinal tract in response to lipid in the duodenum. CCK activates receptors on the afferent sensory fibres of the vagus nerve.
- The **presence of food in the stomach** leads to glucagon and insulin release, both of which decrease feeding signals.
- **Distension** of the GI tract sends stretch inhibition signals via the vagus to the hypothalamus to suppress the desire for food. This integrates with CCK signals.

Medium-term control

A number of molecules either released from the GI tract or found in the lateral hypothalamus act within the hypothalamus to control food intake.

Anorexigenic molecules

Peptide YY is released from L-enteroendocrine cells about 15 min after food ingestion, and levels remain high for about 6 hours. It is thought to have anorectic effects.

Orexigenic molecules

Ghrelin – secreted from the endocrine cells of stomach and GI tract – levels fall after a meal, although the stimulus for this is unclear. When body weight decreases, ghrelin production and plasma levels increase, which makes it difficult to diet!

Long-term control

Leptin is a protein hormone secreted by adipose cells responsible for the long-term control of appetite. It maintains body weight by ensuring that we increase food intake and decrease metabolism when faced with starvation.

Secretion

Levels of leptin correlate with body fat mass and do not seem to increase or decrease with food consumption. **Insulin** may also stimulate leptin production.

Action in appetite

Leptin is an anorectic and increases activity in brown fat adipose tissue, increasing metabolism; however its role is not to decrease food intake/stimulate weight loss.

A falling level of leptin promotes energy intake, decreases energy expenditure and promotes

 CLINICAL Leptin deficiency

Very rarely, leptin deficiency is responsible for obesity due to frameshift mutations in the leptin gene. In these cases, administration of leptin results in weight loss, mainly due to altered feeding behaviour. However, administration of leptin to obese individuals without this deficiency is ineffective due to leptin resistance.

partitioning of energy towards fat. When weight is increased, leptin levels rise until 'leptin resistance' occurs. This means that leptin is unable to have anorectic effects so body weight is maintained for future times of starvation.

Gastrointestinal hormones

Many regulatory processes in the intestines rely on chemical signals, allowing the coordination of a large portion of the GI tract, as well as supporting organs. GI hormones act primarily in the GI tract to coordinate motility, digestion, secretion and absorption. They are released from:

- the enteric nervous system
- enteroendocrine cells found throughout the GI tract in the crypts. Most of the cells have sensory microvilli open to the gut lumen, and the hormone is secreted basally.

There are two families of gut hormones, which act by different mechanisms:

1 **Gastrin-like hormone**s (gastrin, CCK) act via camp.
2 **Secretin-like hormones** (secretin, vasoactive intestinal peptide [VIP], gastric inhibitory polypeptide [GIP], glucagon) act via alterations in intracellular Ca^{2+} levels.

Release of these hormones is often in response to release of acetylcholine from the enteric nervous system (ENS). This is stimulated vagally in response to sight, smell and taste of food. Also distension of the stomach after eating triggers mechanoreceptors, resulting in vagal stimulation of ACh release from the ENS.

Histamine

This amine acts to increase HCl secretion.

Release

Secreted from **ECL cells** in the gastric mucosa in response to either ACh release from the ENS or gastrin.

Action

Histamine acts on H_2-receptors of the stomach's **parietal cells** to stimulate a rise in cAMP. This triggers an increase in K^+ channels, hyperpolarising the cell and increasing the driving force for Cl^- secretion. Histamine also increases the conduction and insertion of Cl^- channels. The result is increased HCl secretion.

Gastrin

This is a protein hormone that acts to increase HCl secretion, pepsin secretion and antral motility.

Release

Gastrin is produced from progastrin in the **G-cells** of the gastric antrum (some are also found in the duodenum). Release is stimulated by: protein digestion products, ACh release from the vagus nerve, gastrin-releasing peptide (released from the ENS) and distension of the stomach. Release is inhibited by stomach pH <2.5 (gastrin acts to increase H^+ secretion – so H^+ feeds back to inhibit gastrin secretion) and somatostatin.

Action

Gastrin acts on the CCK-B receptor of **parietal cells** to increase intracellular calcium so increasing K^+ channel insertion and resulting in increased acid production. It stimulates pepsinogen secretion from chief cells and histamine release from ECL cells, and acts on the smooth muscle cells of the stomach to increase antral motility.

Cholecystokinin

This is a protein hormone that acts to increase secretion of pancreatic enzymes and bile and triggers satiety.

Release

Enteroendocrine type I cells in the gut and jejunum, and **enteric nerves** can secrete CCK. Release is stimulated by the products of protein and fat breakdown in the duodenum.

Actions

CCK stimulates secretion of pancreatic enzymes and contraction of the gallbladder; it potentiates the actions of secretin and also has a role in satiety.

Other gastrointestinal hormones

There are several other GI hormones that have been identified, and more are continually being identified; their roles are being explored further. Other prominent gut hormones include the following:

- **Secretin** stimulates pancreatic and biliary secretion and neutralises stomach acid.
- **Somatostatin** has an inhibitory role.
- **VIP** is released from the gut, pancrease and hypothalamus, and has actions throughout the body. VIP acts in the GI system to relax the cardiac sphincter and stomach, and inhibit gastric acid secretion.
- **GIP (Gastric inhibitory polypeptide; also known as glucose-dependent insulinotropic peptide)** is released from neuroendocrine K cells in the duodenum and jejunum. It increases insulin release and at high levels inhibits gastric acid secretion.
- **Motilin** is produced by endocrine M cells (distinct from immune M cells) in the duodenum and jejunum. Motilin stimulates gastric acid secretion, production of pepsin, and contraction of the gallbladder and sphincter of Oddi.
- **Peptide YY** is a small peptide released by the ileum and colon in response to feeding and appears to reduce appetite.

→ RELATED CHAPTERS

9

Urinary system

The urinary system processes waste products from the blood and stores them for excretion. At rest, the kidneys receive around 25% of cardiac output, allowing them to filter large volumes of plasma. The large blood flow also allows the kidneys to sense changes in blood composition and trigger homoeostatic responses through the release of hormones.

Anatomy of the urinary system

The urinary system, located in the abdomen and pelvis, consists of four structures:

1 The **kidneys** are located in the abdomen and produce urine.
2 The **bladder** is located in the pelvis and stores urine.
3 The **ureters** drain urine from the kidneys to the bladder.
4 The **urethra** links the bladder to the external environment for the removal of urine.

The gross anatomy and relations to other organs are covered in Chapter 14.

Kidneys

The kidneys are located retroperitoneally on the posterior abdominal wall, in the paravertebral gutters on either side of the spine. The adrenal glands are located on the upper pole of the kidneys, although separated by a thin fascial layer.

The kidneys are surrounded by fat and a fascial layer that is continuous with the interior surface of the diaphragm. This attachment accounts for the slight movement of the kidneys (about 2.5 cm) during breathing.

The kidneys are bean-shaped and approximately 10 cm from pole to pole. The hilum in the medial aspect is the site where three vessels supplying and draining the kidney enter its interior (Fig. 9.1):

- The renal artery
- The renal vein
- The ureter.

Segmental organisation of the renal pelvis

The nephrons drain urine into the collecting ducts, which progressively unite into larger vessels. The branching structure of the ureter and its tributary vessels follows a segmental organisation:

- Urine from the **collecting ducts** drains into the minor calyces.
- There are about 12–14 **minor calyces** in the kidney, which fuse to form 2–4 major calyces.
- The **major calyces** drain directly into the renal pelvis.

In a healthy individual, urine drained from the collecting duct system flows rapidly into the bladder; the collecting ducts are usually in a collapsed state in the kidney.

Biomedical Science Lecture Notes, First Edition. Ian Lyons.
© 2011 by Ian Lyons. Published 2011 by Blackwell Publishing Ltd.

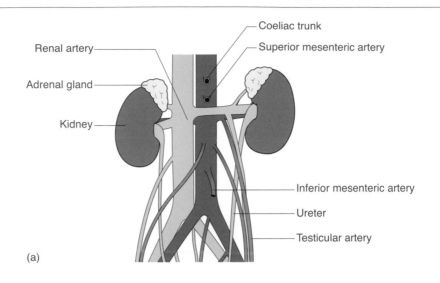

(a)

Coeliac trunk
Renal artery
Superior mesenteric artery
Adrenal gland
Kidney
Inferior mesenteric artery
Ureter
Testicular artery

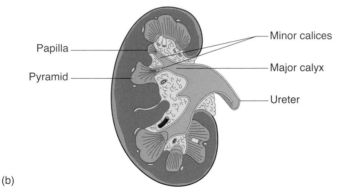

(b)

Papilla
Pyramid
Minor calices
Major calyx
Ureter

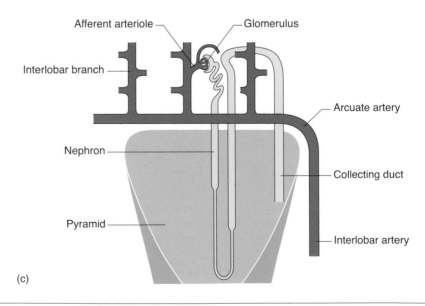

(c)

Afferent arteriole
Glomerulus
Interlobar branch
Arcuate artery
Nephron
Collecting duct
Pyramid
Interlobar artery

Kidney vasculature

The renal arteries

The renal arteries arise from the abdominal aorta at the level of L1–2 and branch as they enter the hilum; each is an end-artery to a separate renal lobe:

- The **segmental arteries** are the initial branches of the renal artery. They are short and divide immediately into interlobar arteries, which pass between the lobes of the kidney.
- The **interlobular arteries** supply the cortex and project towards the surface of the kidney, at right angles to the arcuate.
- The **arcuate arteries** arise from the interlobar arteries and course along the boundary the cortex and the medulla, roughly parallel to the kidney surface.
- The **afferent arterioles** are branches of the interlobular arteries, each forming a bundle of capillaries, the **glomerulus**, which is the site of blood filtration into the nephron.

The kidneys contain a **portal system**, because the vessels draining the glomeruli are **efferent arterioles**. These supply a second capillary bed in the renal cortex, which carries the fluid reabsorbed from the nephron. A few capillaries enter the renal medulla as the **vasa recta**. The medulla of the kidney receives only about 10% of the total blood flow to the kidney, all of which is derived from the efferent arterioles.

The vasa recta

The vasa recta carry fluid from the renal medulla. These capillaries are derived from the efferent arterioles, forming a series of loops that descend into the medulla of the kidney, and remove water and solutes from the tissue. The cross-sectional area of the vasa recta as they leave the medulla is much larger than the area as they enter the medulla, because a volume of fluid is recovered from the interstitium.

The renal vein

Several veins are produced from the vessels draining the peritubular capillaries and vasa recta. These progressively unite to form the renal vein, which lies anterior to the renal artery and drains into the inferior vena cava. The left renal vein is longer than the right, passing across the aorta to reach the inferior vena cava. The left renal veins accept branches from other structures, reflecting the comparatively long course that this vessel must take to reach the inferior vena cava:

- The **left suprarenal vein** drains the adrenal glands.
- The **left inferior phrenic vein** drains parts of the diaphragm.
- The **left testicular (or ovarian) vein** drains the gonads.

Lymphatic drainage of the kidney

The renal lymphatic vessels follow the course of the renal veins and drain into the aortic lymph nodes. Lymph from the upper part of the ureters also drains with the renal lymph.

Figure 9.1 (a) The kidneys are located retroperitoneally in the abdomen at the level of T11–12 and are attached to various fasciae. At the hilum of the kidney three vessels can be located. The renal artery is a branch of the abdominal aorta and enters the kidney, splitting into many branches to feed the various regions. The renal vein is located anterior to the renal artery and drains into the inferior vena cava. The final vessel found at the hilum is the ureter, which drains urine to the bladder. In addition, the suprarenal gland is located on the posterior aspect of the kidney and receives blood derived from the renal, suprarenal and inferior phrenic arteries. Its drainage is directly to the inferior vena cava on the right-hand side, and via the renal vein, on the left-hand side. (b) The interior of the kidney can be divided into two areas – the inner medulla and the outer cortex. Within the kidney a segmental series of pyramids can be identified, where the apex is within a minor calyx. These represent the sites where urine from the collecting duct drains into the ureteric system. The minor calyces coalesce to form major calyces; these drain into the renal pelvis which is continuous with the ureter. (c) The arterial supply to the kidneys reflects its formation by branching morphogenesis. Each renal pyramid is supplied by an interlobar artery, which branches to give off arcuate arteries. These in turn branch to interlobular arteries, which give rise to numerous afferent arterioles. The afferent arterioles supply the glomeruli of the nephron. A single nephron is demonstrated in the figure, although each kidney contains around 1 million of them. The nephron tubule descends into the renal medulla, before returning to contact the glomerulus. The nephron terminates in the collecting ducts which drain into the renal calyces.

Innervation of the kidneys

The kidneys have sensory and sympathetic innervation, although they receive no direct parasympathetic innervation:

- **Sensory innervation** is through the lower thoracic nerves, accounting for the referred pain to T11–12. Pain tends to radiate from the small of the back around to the front of the body in the region of the groin.
- **Sympathetic innervation** is via the renal plexus of nerves that branches around the renal artery. It is a continuation of the coeliac plexus and also receives innervation via the **least splanchnic nerve**.

The ureters

Urine drains to the bladder via the ureters. These muscular tubes run inferiorly from the renal pelvis across the anterior surface of the psoas major muscles to enter the posterior surface of the bladder. The muscular layers contract around every 30 s to propel urine into the bladder. The openings of the ureters into the bladders are slit like and at an angle, which helps them act like valves preventing urine from refluxing to the kidneys, particularly when pressure in the bladder increases during voiding. The precise course varies in men and women due to the differences in pelvic anatomy and reproductive organs. The ureters are made up of three tissue layers:

1 The **mucosal layer** is innermost and contains urothelium and lamina propria.
2 The **muscularis mucosa** contains longitudinal and circular muscle layers.
3 A **fibrous connective tissue layer** is outermost and continuous with the peritoneum and renal capsule.

 CLINICAL Renal colic and blockage of the ureters

Occasionally a ureter may become blocked, resulting in a sharp pain in the lower abdomen, often radiating into the groin and upper thigh. The pain has a colicky nature, getting progressively weaker and stronger with contraction of the ureters.
Blockage of the ureter can lead to an increase in pressure, causing severe pain and impeding renal filtration, because the hydrostatic pressure increases within the collecting ducts and the nephron as a whole.

The bladder

The bladder (Fig. 9.2) is a highly distensible sac with strong muscular walls. It lies on the pubic floor surrounded by fatty tissue and its superior surface is covered by a layer of peritoneum. In children, the bladder may protrude into the abdomen, but in adults the bladder is located entirely in the pelvis. The epithelium and muscular layers of the bladder are specially adapted to allow storage and expulsion of urine; their detailed histological structure is discussed later in Chapter 14.

Gross anatomy of the bladder

When empty, the bladder is tetrahedral in shape, with the apex facing downwards. The **trigone** is a triangular region of the bladder wall located posteriorly, with the ureteric and urethral openings at

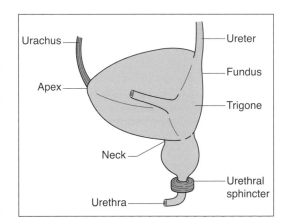

Figure 9.2 The bladder is located posterior to the pubic bone, such that the apex is superior to the pubis. The superior surface of the bladder is covered by the peritoneum, which continues posteriorly to intestines, also covering the uterus in females. Below the apex of the bladder is the body and the fundus, which leads to the neck of the bladder – the site of the urethra. The bladder is divided into many distinct regions. The ureters and the urethra enter at the corners of the trigone, which is found on the posterior wall. The urethra flows directly through the neck of the bladder, which is surrounded by the prostate in males. The flow of urine out of the bladder is regulated by the urethral sphincters. The urachus at the apex of the bladder is an embryological structure that has no function in the developed bladder.

the three corners. The trigone is derived from the mesonephric ducts, whereas the rest of the bladder is derived from the urogenital sinus, and cannot expand and contract in the same way as the rest of the bladder.

The superior surface of the bladder is covered in a layer of **peritoneum**, which is continuous with the anterior abdominal wall, although its course posterior to the bladder varies between the sexes:

- In **males** the peritoneum passes over the superior surface of the bladder and the seminal vesicles before forming the rectovesical pouch and covering the superior part of the rectum.
- In **females** the peritoneum extends from the bladder to the uterus, forming the vesicouterine pouch, and then from the uterus to the rectum, forming the rectouterine pouch.

Vasculature of the bladder

The bladder, as with other pelvic organs, receives its blood supply from the internal iliac arteries. The precise course and nature of the arteries vary between the sexes, as they do that for the veins draining the bladder.

Arterial supply of the bladder

The main arterial supply of the bladder is derived from branches of the internal iliac arteries, which supply the pelvic organs:

- The **superior vesical arteries** supply the superior part of the bladder.
- The fundus and neck of the bladder are supplied by the **inferior vesical arteries** in males and the **vaginal arteries** in females.

Venous drainage

The venous drainage of the bladder broadly follows the arterial supply:

- In **males**, the vesical venous plexus drains the bladder and combines with the prostatic plexus. The venous blood drains into the internal iliac veins via the inferior vesical veins.
- In **females**, the vesical venous plexus also drains the pelvic part of the urethra and the neck of the bladder, and communicates with the vaginal and uterovaginal venous plexus.

Lymphatic drainage

Lymphatic drainage of the bladder is to three different sets of lymph nodes:

- The **superior part of the bladder** passes to the external iliac nodes.
- The **fundus** is drained by the internal iliac nodes.
- The **neck of the bladder** drains to the sacral lymph nodes.

The urethra

The urethra connects the bladder to the external world for the voiding of urine. The urethra starts at the neck of the bladder. Its course varies considerably between the sexes and is discussed in Chapter 14.

Urine production in the kidneys

The **nephron** is the functional unit of the kidney. In each kidney there are approximately 1 million nephrons which perform two major homoeostatic functions:

- The **removal** of waste products
- The **regulation** of many homeostatic processes, including total fluid volume, ion content and acid-base balance.

The formation of urine is intrinsically linked to regulatory and excretory functions of the nephron and four distinct processes can be identified:

1 **Glomerular filtration** removes fluid and solutes from the blood into the kidney nephron.
2 **Tubular reabsorption** allows total reclamation of many essential molecules from the tubular fluid. Other components are reabsorbed under the influence of hormones to maintain homoeostasis.
3 **Tubular secretion** of some compounds into the tubule increases their removal from the body.
4 **Hormonal production** to maintain homoeostasis can be triggered by the nephron in response to changes in the composition of the tubular fluid.

Each nephron consists of five distinct regions, which are involved in performing these functions:

1 Renal corpuscle
2 Proximal convoluted tubule (PCT)
3 Loop of Henle
4 Distal convoluted tubule (DCT)
5 Collecting duct.

The renal corpuscle

The **renal corpuscle** is the first stage of the nephron. It is made of a cluster of capillaries – the glomerulus – surrounded by the start of the nephron tubule, a structure known as Bowman's capsule. The interface between the glomerulus and Bowman's capsule filters the components of blood into the nephron (Fig. 9.3).

Some parts of the renal corpuscle are directly involved in the process of **ultrafiltration**; additional cell types regulate the flow of blood through the glomerulus and the rate of filtration of the fluid into Bowman's capsule, including:

- Cells at the filtration barrier
- Supporting cells
- The juxtaglomerular apparatus.

 DEFINITION Ultrafiltration

This is the process by which fluid is filtered from the blood under high pressure in the glomerulus. As a result, around 20% of the plasma delivered to the kidney is forced into the nephron. Components with a molecular weight <7 kDa can cross, whereas the cells and protein components cannot cross the filtration barrier.

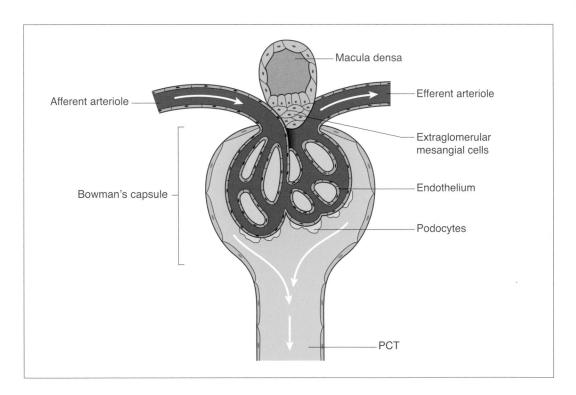

Figure 9.3 The renal corpuscle: this is the first structure in the nephron, and is responsible for ultrafiltration. The blood flows from the afferent to the efferent arteriole at high pressure, through the glomerular capillaries. The high pressure forces the soluble components of plasma out into Bowman's capsule. The layers contributing to the filtration barrier are the endothelium of the glomerular capillaries, the basement membrane and the podocytes, which are derived from the visceral layer of Bowman's capsule. The filtrate flows into the proximal convoluted tubule (PCT) of the nephron. The more distal region of each nephron feeds back to its glomerulus through the juxtaglomerular region, where it is in contact with the macula densa and the extraglomerular mesangial cells. These regulate function through hormonal release. Mesangial cells in the glomerulus can regulate blood flood to help control ultrafiltration.

Supporting cells in the renal corpuscle

Mesangial cells may be found between the glomerular capillaries.

These cells are responsible for producing components of the extracellular membrane and have contractile properties that may allow the regulation of blood flow through the capillaries. Other roles of the mesangial cells are not clear, although it is thought that they may function as scavengers in the glomerulus, to remove matter that gets stuck in the basement membrane during filtration.

The juxtaglomerular apparatus

The juxtaglomerular apparatus (JGA) is formed from cells of both the DCT and the afferent arteriole supplying the glomerulus of the **same nephron**. This apparatus has important roles in the regulation of flow rate within the nephron and blood pressure, and in Na^+ reabsorption. Three cell types are particularly prominent in the JGA:

1 The **macula densa** is a region of tightly packed cells of the DCT that are directly associated with the afferent arteriole. These cells detect changes in both the composition and the flow rate of the fluid – a decrease in the flow rate of the filtrate results in a decrease in the Na^+ ions reaching the JGA, providing direct feedback of the tubular flow and composition downstream of the glomerulus.
2 **Juxtaglomerular (granular) cells** are specialised smooth muscle cells that are found around the afferent arteriole. These cells respond to signals, including those from the macula densa, to release renin, which is involved in the regulation of Na^+ and fluid balance.
3 **Extraglomerular mesangial cells** (sometimes called Lacis cells) are found in contact with the glomerular mesangial cells between the arterioles. They are thought to aid transmission of signals from the macula densa to the mesangial cells within the glomerulus, which may contract to alter the blood flow.

Glomerular filtration and the filtration barrier

Blood flow and pressure regulate the rate of renal filtration. The kidneys can adjust their vascular resistance to allow a relatively constant glomerular filtration rate. This is regulated by the two arterioles between which the glomerulus is located.

There are three layers that water and solutes must cross to reach the interior of the nephron; they are responsible for the selectivity of ultrafiltration:

1 **Endothelial cells** are primarily responsible for preventing cells from leaving the capillaries. The capillaries are **fenestrated**, allowing many protein molecules to leave the vessels easily and, as such, they do not contribute to filtration of protein constituents of the plasma.
2 The **basement membrane,** composed mainly of collagen, contains many negatively charged molecules, particularly **glycosaminoglycans**. As many protein constituents of the blood are also negatively charged, this barrier restricts their movement into the nephron.
3 **Podocytes** envelope the endothelial cells and possess large projections (trabeculae), and many smaller projections (pedicles), which are interlaced, producing a series of narrow 'slit pores'. These are the final barrier before the fluid enters the nephron tubule.

At some points in the glomerulus, particularly the neck, the endothelium is surrounded by **mesangial cells** instead of podocytes. The mesangial cells may contract to alter filtration area, and hence the filtration rate.

Selectivity of ultrafiltration

Selectivity of the molecules filtered depends on the properties of the molecule and how they interact with the filtration barrier components:

- **Size**: molecules up to 7 kDa, are freely filtered. Those greater than around 70 kDa and of a molecular radius >4 nm are not filtered.

 CLINICAL Nephrotic syndrome

Nephrotic syndrome is defined as the loss of more than 3.5 g protein/day in the urine and occurs as a result of damage to the glomeruli; this permits larger molecules (i.e. proteins) to escape into the nephron. Common causes are minimal change disease and membranous glomerulonephritis.

Symptoms result from the loss of protein within the urine, which alters the oncotic pressure of the blood. As a result, systemic oedema occurs, particularly in the legs and around the eyes. Fluid may also build up in the lungs or peritoneum. Urine may become foamy in cases where protein loss is particularly high.

- **Charge**: negatively charged molecules located in the basement membrane particularly restrict the passage of negatively charged large molecules (>7 kDa) into the nephron.

CLINICAL Glomerulonephritis

Glomerulonephritis is an inflammation of the glomeruli which leads to a decrease in the function of the ultrafiltration barrier. The condition usually presents as protein in the urine (proteinuria) or nephrotic syndrome. There are a variety of causes of glomerulonephritis (e.g. some infection, or autoimmune conditions such as systemic lupus erythematosus) and the precise treatment varies with the underlying cause.

Forces driving ultrafiltration

Ultrafiltration is driven by **Starling's forces**, and depends on the balance between the forces favouring filtration and those opposing it. The strong driving force of ultrafiltration is maintained by the balance of Starling's forces – the high hydrostatic pressure in the glomerulus forces fluid and solutes into the nephron. This high glomerular capillary hydrostatic pressure is opposed by the oncotic pressure of the glomerular capillary protein and the hydrostatic pressure in Bowman's capsule. As negligible amounts of protein are filtered, there is normally no protein oncotic pressure in Bowman's capsule.

DEFINITION The coefficient of filtration

The coefficient of filtration (K_f) is an indication of the permeability of a structure to water. It is determined by two variables:

1 The surface area of the capillaries
2 The conductance by the capillaries of water.

A high K_f indicates that the vessels in question are highly permeable to water.

Renal clearance

Renal clearance allows assessment of whether a substance is being excreted or reabsorbed into the tubule, and can be an important

indicator of renal function. It is given as an idealised value – the minimum volume of plasma from which the amount of substance could have been obtained. It can be an important indicator of renal function.

DEFINITION Glomerular filtration rate

This is the amount of a substance that passes into the nephrons from the glomeruli in a given length of time.

CLINICAL Measurement of glomerular filtration rate

The rate with which a substance is removed from the blood can be used to assess the glomerular filtration rate (GFR) which, in turn, provides an assessment of the state of the kidneys. Historically, inulin was used to assess GFR, because it is neither secreted nor reabsorbed. It provides very accurate readings of GFR but has to be injected into the patient. Currently in the clinic, glomerular filtration is typically assessed through **creatinine** levels in the urine. This is a natural metabolite that enters the blood at a relatively constant rate. There is a small amount of active secretion of creatinine that can result in an overestimation of renal function (by about 10%).

Regulation of glomerular filtration

Although renal blood flow is variable, GFR remains almost constant over a wide range of arterial blood pressures. This regulation is possible because the glomerular pressure can be controlled by both afferent and efferent arterioles, e.g. if the afferent arteriole constricts and reduces the renal blood flow, constriction of the efferent arteriole can nevertheless maintain GFR. Two mechanisms are postulated to account for this regulation:

1 **Myogenic regulation**: increased pressure causes stretching of the capillary smooth muscle. This stretch triggers contraction of the smooth muscle to reduce flow.
2 **Juxtaglomerular feedback**: the JGA detects the NaCl delivery rate by the nephron at the

macula densa in the DCT, so that filtration can be altered to accommodate changes. Increased NaCl triggers the JGA to release **adenosine** which causes constriction of the afferent arteriole.

The proximal convoluted tubule

The PCT is responsible for the reabsorption of approximately two-thirds of the glomerular filtrate and reclamation of many essential molecules from the fluid.

It is made up of a single type of simple epithelium that possess **microvilli** to increase the surface area in contact with the lumen; it contains many vesicles, which are involved in transport, and many mitochondria, reflecting the high energy usage within the cells. The tubule cells rest on a thin basement membrane, outside of which are many peritubular capillaries. The junctions between the epithelial cells are 'leaky', allowing movement of fluid and some solutes by the paracellular pathway.

Transport within the PCT

Reabsorption in the PCT occurs isotonically – the osmolality of the tubular fluid does not change, although the volume decreases by about 70%. The major substances that the PCT reabsorbs are (Fig. 9.4):

- Na^+, Cl^-, HCO_3^-, glucose and amino acids via specific transport mechanisms
- Water, through osmosis
- K^+, Ca^{2+} and Mg^{2+} and many other substances by movement down their concentration gradient.

Na^+ ion gradient drives reabsorption in the PCT

Na^+, Cl^- and HCO_3^- account for about 90% of the osmotically active particles in the filtrate. Their reabsorption is essential to absorb the large volumes of fluid that are filtered and would otherwise be lost from the body. The high energy requirement of PCT cells is largely a result of the active transport of Na^+ by the Na^+/K^+ ATPase on their basolateral membrane. Transport of Na^+ from the cell to the blood establishes a concentration gradient between the cell and the lumen, which aids facilitated diffusion. It is the coupling of Na^+ reabsorption to other transport

mechanisms that allows the reuptake of a range of solutes:

- In in the first part of the PCT **organic solutes** (glucose and amino acids), phosphate and HCO_3^- transport are coupled to Na^+.
- In the later parts, **Cl^- reabsorption** occurs with Na^+ uptake.

Many other molecules are also reabsorbed by secondary active transport driven by the Na^+ gradient.

Reabsorption of bicarbonate

The reabsorption of bicarbonate within the nephron is essential to maintain pH balance in the blood. The reabsorption occurs in two stages:

1 In the **tubular lumen** secreted H^+ combines with filtered HCO_3^- to form H_2O and CO_2, both of which may diffuse freely into the epithelial cells.
2 In the **cells** the reverse reaction can be catalysed by **carbonic anhydrase** and the resulting HCO_3^- is returned to the plasma. By the cooperative actions of two transporters:
   (a) the **Na^+/H^+ exchanger** in the apical membrane which transports a single H^+ ion into the tubule while reabsorbing a Na^+ ion
   (b) the **Na^+/HCO_3^- symporter**, located in the basolateral membrane, which transports one Na^+ out of the cell (against its chemical gradient) with the transport of three HCO_3^- out of the cell.

Chloride reabsorption

Chloride ions are reabsorbed by two different mechanisms:

1 **Paracellular route:** Cl^- reabsorption occurs in the last parts of the PCT (S2 and S3) due to movement down its concentration gradient, because the absorption of Na^+ and HCO_3^- has caused H_2O reabsorption in the S1 segment.
2 **Transcellular route:** Cl^- reabsorption across the epithelium is through a Cl^-/anion exchanger in the apical membrane and a K^+/Cl^- symporter in the basolateral membrane.

Calcium reabsorption

Ca^{2+} is an essential ion in cell signalling and makes up the matrix of the bone. As with Cl^-, Ca^{2+} may

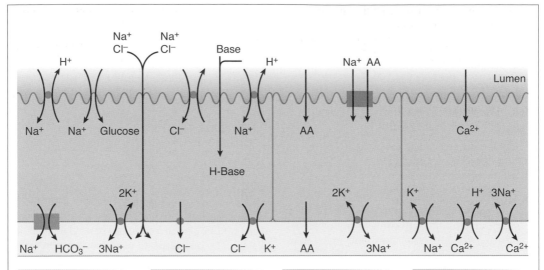

Sodium (Na⁺)

The reabsorption of sodium within the proximal convoluted tubule (PCT) is driven by the Na^+/K^+ ATPase in the basolateral membrane, generating a Na+ gradient. Transport of Na^+ across the basolateral membrane can also occur through the transport of Na^+ with HCO_3^-. The transport of Na^+ across the apical surface occurs through the Na^+/H^+ exchanger and co-transport with other molecules, such as glucose and amino acids. Finally, a large proportion of Na^+ can be transported between cells, being drawn out of the tubule down its electrochemical gradient.

Chloride (Cl⁻)

The transport of Cl^- across the apical surface occurs through a Cl^-/base exchanger. This base (e.g. HCO_3 or formate) is effectively recycled, because it can combine with H^+ in the tubule and diffuse back into the cell as a non-polar compound; there it becomes deprotonated once again and is used to reabsorb another chloride molecule. At the basolateral membrane, Cl^- transport can occur through a channel or through co-transport with K^+. In the early parts of the PCT, a large proportion of Cl^- is reabsorbed through solvent drag.

Amino acids

Amino acids are rapidly reabsorbed from the tubule, through either their own specific transporters or co-transport that is driven by the Na^+ gradient. Transport of the amino acids out of the tubule cells is through a specific transporter. In addition, significant metabolism of some amino acids occurs within the tubule cells such that the composition of amino acids entering the tubule cell will differ from that released into the bloodstream.

Calcium (Ca²⁺)

Ca^{2+} transport occurs due to the concentration gradient between the lumen and the epithelium, which is set up through the Na^+/Ca^{2+} exchanger in the basolateral membrane and the Ca^{2+}/H^+ exchanger. In turn, these gradients are driven, in part, by the Na^+/K^+ ATPase present on the surface of the epithelial cells.

Figure 9.4 The reabsorption of ions in the proximal convoluted tubule occurs through a variety of different processes. In addition, much of the reabsorption can occur through the transcellular pathway between cells. In this diagram, the reabsorption of each molecule is represented as it occurs in distinct cells, although in reality each cell in the epithelium expresses the transporters to reabsorb all the compounds detailed, as well as those discussed in this chapter.

be reabsorbed by both paracellular and transcellular routes:

- **Paracellular (between cells) reabsorption** occurs through movement down its concentration gradient and accounts for most Ca^{2+} reabsorption.
- **Transcellular (through cells) reabsorption** occurs at the apical membrane through the epithelial Ca^{2+} channel (ECaC), and the basolateral membrane by a Ca^{2+}/Na^+ antiporter protein which moves Ca^{2+} out as Na^+ enters the cell, driven by the Na^+ gradient.

Phosphate reabsorption

Phosphate (P_i) is required for the production of nucleotides and contributes to the bone matrix. Its transport is regulated by the **Na/P$_i$** symporter in the apical membrane, which transports two Na^+ with each P_i molecule. Approximately 80% of the filtered phosphate is reabsorbed in the PCT and about 10% in the DCT; the remainder is excreted. P_i is hormonally regulated by parathyroid hormone (PTH) which inhibits its reabsorption.

Glucose reabsorption

Reabsorption of glucose occurs through the $Na^+/glucose$ (SGLT) symporter found at the apical membrane of PCT cells. The SGLT transporters have a maximum rate of transport, which can be saturated if the filtered load of glucose is too high – as may be seen in diabetes mellitus. A failure to reabsorb glucose can lead to problems in the regulation of fluid levels, because it results in a tubular fluid with increased osmolarity, so causing 'osmotic diuresis'. Two types of SGLT exist, both specific for D-glucose:

1 **SGLT2** is found in the proximal parts of the PCT, and transports a single glucose molecule per Na^+ ion.
2 **SGLT1** is in the more distal part of the PCT and requires two Na^+ ions for the transport of a single glucose molecule. The use of two Na^+ ions increases the driving force of transport, allowing greater scavenging of glucose.

Reabsorption of amino acids

Amino acids are reabsorbed with Na^+ by one of at least four different symporters, each with a relatively broad specificity.

Defects in each of these transporters have been identified and that of **cystinuria** is particularly well studied.

Reabsorption of energy metabolites

Many intermediates of glycolysis and the tricarboxylic acid (TCA) cycle (e.g. acetoacctate, pyruvate and lactate) are filtered out of the blood. These molecules must be reclaimed to prevent the loss of a potentially crucial source of energy.

Reabsorption of water

About two-thirds of water is reabsorbed in the PCT. As a small osmotic gradient is sufficient to drive huge water flows, any gradient is rapidly collapsed by osmotic flow:

- **Transcellular flow** of water accounts for most reabsorption. The epithelial cells in the kidney tubule express **aquaporins**, specialised water channels. **Aquaporin I** is constitutively expressed on both the apical and the basolateral cell membranes in the PCT.
- The **paracellular** pathway also contributes to the reabsorption of water, although to a lesser extent than the transcellular pathway.

Secretory mechanisms in the PCT

Many waste products bind to plasma proteins and are not readily filtered; most of the removal of such compounds occurs through active secretion. Two distinct secretion systems exist in the PCT – one secreting anions and the other secreting cations.

The stereotypical example of active secretion is that for organic acids. An example of such an acid is p-aminohippuric acid (PAH). In a single pass

DEFINITION Osmolarity and osmolality

These are often referred to interchangeably, although there are potentially large differences between them:

- **Osmolarity** refers to the concentration of a molecule within a given total volume of solution, typically expressed in the units **osmol/L**.
- **Osmolality** is defined as the concentration of a substance in a defined weight of water and is expressed as the units **osmol/kg**.

The volume of a given weight of solute changes with temperature, so the osmolarity of a solution is also temperature dependent. Osmolality is the preferred measurement, because it is temperature independent and relates to a specific amount of water.

through the kidneys, about 90% of the PAH is removed from the blood.

The systems employed for the excretion of PAH are used for the excretion of a wide variety of anions including:

- naturally occurring metabolites, e.g. oxaloacetate.
- many drugs, e.g. penicillin
- conjugates of sulphates and glucuronate.

Back diffusion

Some substances are secreted in the PCT but reabsorbed to varying degrees in the more distal regions of the nephron. This occurs through simple diffusion that is not mediated by carrier proteins. In cases where compounds have both neutral and charged species, the rate of back diffusion can be influence by pH.

The loop of Henle

In humans only about 15% of the nephrons have significant loops of Henle. The loop of Henle protrudes into the medulla of the kidneys and is responsible for generating an extremely hypertonic environment in the interstitium to aid antidiuretic hormone (ADH)-driven reabsorption of H_2O from the collecting duct. In addition, some direct water reabsorption occurs in the generation of the gradient. Three distinct parts can be identified in the loop of Henle:

1 Thin descending limb
2 Thin ascending limb
3 Thick ascending limb.

The hypertonic environment generated by the loop of Henle occurs through a countercurrent multiplier, which generates hypertonicity. The medulla of the kidneys contains many **vasa recta** which carry reabsorbed fluid to ensure that it does not dilute the medulla.

Structure and function of the loop of Henle

The tubule cells in the loop of Henle have different structural features related to their function. The differential movement of H_2O and Na^+ in particular are discussed below (Fig. 9.5):

- The concentration of the fluid in the nephron is achieved by the **thin descending limb**, because it allows the movement of H_2O into the medulla, while being relatively impermeable to both Na^+ and urea. As the medulla is highly concentrated for both Na^+ and urea, it provides a concentration gradient that draws H_2O out of the descending limb into the medullary interstitium. Some Na^+ diffuses from the interstitium into the tubule.
- The **thin ascending limb** is impermeable to H_2O. The cells of the thin ascending limb are extremely thin and lack the large numbers of mitochondria seen in much of the rest of the tubule. This is reflected in their absorption of Na^+ which is entirely by **passive transport**. This movement relies on the high concentration of Na^+ in the tubular fluid which is the result of movement of H_2O into the medulla in the descending limbs of the loop.
- The cells of the **thick ascending limb**, which are impermeable to H_2O, help generate a hyperosmolar medulla by transporting NaCl, driven by the Na^+/K^+ ATPAse in the basolateral cell membranes. The main transporter in the apical cell membranes is the **$Na^+/K^+/2Cl^-$ co-transporter** (NKCC). This transporter is the target of loop diuretics.

The countercurrent multiplier

Although the PCT reabsorbs large amounts of water and solutes, the filtrate leaving the PCT is **isotonic**. The generation of hypertonic urine is achieved by the loop of Henle's functions, which

Descending limb

The descending limb is permeable to water, but only slightly permeable to Na^+; the water removed increases the osmolarity of the tubular fluid. The water that is removed is drained from the medulla by the vasa recta to prevent a loss of the high osmolarity in the interstitium.

Thin ascending limb

The thin ascending limb is permeable to Na^+ although not to water. This allows Na^+ to flow into the medulla, down its concentration gradient, to contribute to the high osmolarity there.

Thick ascending limb

As in the thin ascending limb, the thick portion is impermeable to water although transport of Na^+ occurs further, contributing to the high salt concentrations in the medulla.

Collecting duct

ADH released from the posterior pituitary triggers the expression of aquaporin II in the surface of the collecting duct epithelium; this allows the flow of water into the cells as a result of the high osmolarity of the medulla, which has been generated by the loop of Henle. This water reabsorption allows regulation of the fluid balance.

Medulla

The Na^+ that enters the medulla from the ascending limbs contributes to the high osmolarity of the interstitial fluid. This allows the flow of water from the collecting duct under the influence of antidiuretic hormone (ADH). The reabsorbed water from the collecting duct and the thin ascending limb is removed by the vasa recta to prevent dilution of the high osmolarity in the medulla.

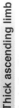
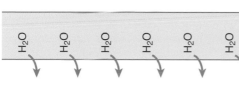
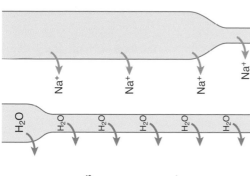

Figure 9.5 Countercurrent multiplier.

cause the interstitial fluid to be highly concentrated. The different permeabilities and transport processes of the ascending and descending limbs of the loop of Henle allow the concentration of solutes in the medulla. This concentration occurs in a series of steps, which progressively increase the concentration towards the tip of the loop of Henle:

1 The **ascending limb is impermeable to water** and (the thick part) transports Na^+ and urea to the medullary interstitium, to increase the osmolarity in the interstitium.
2 The **descending limb is permeable to water**, although relatively impermeable to Na^+ and urea, resulting in the movement of water from the descending limb to the medulla. This fluid is removed from the medulla by the vasa recta. The net result is a concentration of the fluid in the interstitium and the descending limb.
3 The cycle of movement of solutes from the ascending limb, movement of water from the descending limb and its subsequent removal from the medulla by the vasa recta causes a **progressive concentration of the medulla** towards the tip of the loop of Henle.

The contribution of urea to the concentration gradient

Na^+ and urea are the two main molecules responsible for the hypertonicity of the medulla. The role and transport of Na^+ have been discussed earlier.

Handling of urea in the glomerulus and PCT

The handling of urea by the nephron varies along its length:

- The **glomerulus** freely filters urea.
- The **PCT** reabsorbs about half the filtered urea.
- In the **thin ascending limb** and most distal portions of the descending limb of the loop of Henle, urea moves from the interstitium into the tubule, down its concentration gradient.
- The **collecting ducts** reabsorb urea in the inner medulla, raising the medullary interstitial osmolality.

Urea handling in the collecting duct is regulated by the ADH. High levels of ADH trigger the reabsorption of H_2O and urea into the medulla interstitium. Although H_2O is removed rapidly by the vasa recta, much of the urea remains in the medulla – it can account for up to 50% of total osmolality.

The high osmolality of the interstitium results in urea transport from the interstitium into the descending and thin ascending limbs, which contributes to the high concentration in the collecting duct. In conditions where there is less water reabsorption, the concentration of urea in the nephron is lower due to the presence of more water. In turn, this results in less reabsorption and a decrease in the osmolality of the loop of Henle. As a result, where there is little reabsorption of water, there is a lower interstitial urea concentration and more urea is excreted in the urine.

Recycling of urea

The urea in the collecting duct is processed and moved by three routes, which vary in relation to the homoeostatic needs of the body:

- A proportion of the urea (about 40%) is **not reabsorbed from the collecting duct** and is excreted in the urine.
- Urea is **removed from the collecting duct fluid**, regulated by ADH. This urea is dealt with by two distinct mechanisms:

  – some of the urea is **re-secreted into the loop of Henle** in the descending and thin ascending limbs and carried back to the collecting duct
  – some of the urea is **reabsorbed by the vasa recta** and returned to the circulation.

The distal convoluted tubule

The early DCT is a continuation of the thick ascending limb of the loop of Henle and is found in the renal cortex. The DCT and the collecting ducts are important in fine tuning reabsorption to maintain homoeostasis. The major function of the DCT is the reabsorption of Na^+ from the tubules, which is coupled to the secretion of K^+ and H^+.

Morphology of the DCT

The **macula densa** is found in the first part of the DCT, closely related to the glomerulus of the same nephron. It allows the tubule to feed back to the glomerulus, which, in turn, allows rapid responses to changes in the flow rate or composition of the tubule.

The cells in the DCT resemble those in the thick ascending limb of the loop of Henle. They have numerous tight junctions between them and many mitochondria located towards the basolateral aspect to power the active transport processes. As the net movement of ions is comparatively smaller than in the PCT, there are fewer microvilli.

Ion transport in the DCT

The distal tubule still plays a significant role in the reabsorption of Na^+ ions through a Na^+/Cl^- co-transport, which is responsible for around 7% of Na^+ reabsorption and is the target of thiazide diuretics.

Collecting ducts

Distal tubules converge to form collecting ducts, which merge to form progressively larger ducts, eventually draining into the minor calyces. The main function of the collecting duct is to concentrate urine by passive reabsorption, which is promoted by the concentration gradient set up by the loop of Henle.

Structure and morphology of the collecting duct

Two main cell types are found in the collecting duct, which are responsible for the reabsorption that occurs there:

1 **Principal cells** are responsible for Na^+ reabsorption, accounting for about 5% of the Na^+ reabsorbed. Principal cells also express selective aquaporins, under the control of ADH, for the reabsorption of H_2O to regulate fluid levels.
2 **Intercalated cells** play a role in the regulation of pH, being capable of active secretion of H^+ or HCO_3^-.

Concentration of urine

The daily amount of urine produced by an individual and its osmolality can vary enormously. The volume of urine is related to the fluid intake of the individual, as well as to fluid loss through other routes. When fluid intake is low, the fluid volume of the urine is small, resulting in the formation of concentrated urine. In contrast, when water intake is high, large amounts of hypotonic urine are produced to remove the excess fluid from the system.

The body regulates a portion of the fluid loss from the body such that total intake and output of water are balanced. In a typical individual, both the intake and output of water per day are normally around 2500 mL (Table 9.1).

The production of concentrated urine is related to **fluid homoeostasis.** Changes in osmolality in

Table 9.1 The daily intake and output of water

Route	Amount (mL/day)	Route	Amount (mL/day)
Intake:		Output:	
Fluid	1200	Insensible	700
Within food	1000	Sweat	100
Metabolically generated from food	300	Faeces	200
		Urine	1500
Total	**2500**	**Total**	**2500**

To ensure fluid balance is maintained the amount of fluid taken in and lost from the body must be equal. The figures in the table represent the approximate fluid balance in a normal adult at room temperature. The temperature will alter the fluid balance enormously: in hot conditions a larger volume of fluid will be lost through sweating, resulting in a relative decrease in the volume of urine produced. Insensible fluid loss is that which we are not consciously aware of, such as the water that evaporates from the lungs. This fluid loss is not regulated and, as a result, represents a volume of fluid that must always be recovered each day. In addition, there is a minimum volume (around 500 mL) of urine that must be produced each day to allow the body to remove solutes. This minimum volume is governed by the body's ability to concentrate urine.

the blood are sensed by cells in the supraoptic and paraventricular nuclei of the hypothalamus. The detection of blood becoming hypertonic triggers the release of ADH to reduce water loss.

The kidneys are the target organ for many hormones involved in the regulation of fluid and solute balance. Fluid resorption in the proximal parts of the tubule is under limited hormonal control, because it follows Na^+ absorption, which is regulated by angiotensin II. Most of the regulation occurs in the DCT and collecting duct.

Water reabsorption and ADH

The regulation of fluid balance is achieved within the collecting ducts in response to ADH (Fig. 9.6).

Synthesis and secretion

ADH, also known as arginine vasopressin (AVP), is a small peptide hormone (nine amino acids). It is produced in the neuronal cell bodies in the supraoptic and paraventricular nuclei of the hypothalamus and released from the axons of these cells, which terminate in the **posterior pituitary gland**.

Kidney

The kidney is both the start and the end-point for the renin-angiotensin-aldosterone axis. It secretes renin to trigger retention of Na+ and fluid, and is the end-target of the cascade, receiving and integrating inputs from the brain (ADH) and adrenal gland (aldosterone) as well as from angiotensin II. This pathway allows cross-communication of the many different regulatory systems, providing net control of the regulation of ion and fluid levels within the body.

Angiotensinogen

Angiotensinogen is a plasma protein formed in the liver; it is cleaved into angiotensin I by the enzyme renin, which is produced by the kidney in response to either a fall in Na+ in the tubular fluid at the macula densa or a decrease in perfusion. Renin secretion is also increased in response to sympathetic stimulation of the kidneys. The production of renin to cleave angiotensin I is the rate-limiting step of the axis.

Angiotensin I is subsequently cleaved to angiotensin II through the actions of the angiotensin-converting enzyme (ACE) which is expressed in many capillary beds, in particular the lungs. Angiotensin II acts on a variety of targets to aid fluid and Na+ retention. In particular, it causes systemic vasoconstriction and acts on the kidneys, adrenal gland and lungs.

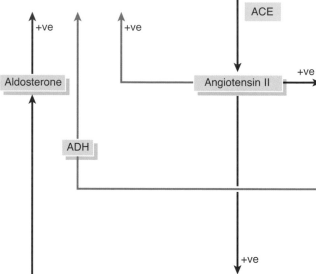

Brain

Angiotensin II provides a link with the control of fluid volume through stimulation of ADH secretion by the hypothalamus. ADH secretion is also directly stimulated by changes in the blood osmolarity, or a significant decrease in the circulating blood volume. These changes trigger the release of ADH from the posterior pituitary.

Adrenal

Angiotensin acts on the adrenal gland to stimulate the production of aldosterone, which promotes reabsorption of Na+ via the modulation of gene expression in the nephron, increasing the expression and activity of Na+ transporters.

Blood

The blood and the extracellular fluid surround almost all the cells of the body, making it essential that the osmolarity remain constant. In addition, the blood must maintain adequate volume to support perfusion. To ensure this the blood osmolarity and effective circulating volume are monitored by the hypothalamus. Increases in osmolarity, or significant decreases in the effective circulating volume can trigger ADH release.

The secretion of the ADH is triggered by the two major factors:

1 **Osmolality of the blood**: the osmoreceptors in the supraoptic and paraventricular nuclei of the hypothalamus are extremely sensitive to changes in blood osmolality.
2 **Volume of blood**: the loss of significant (>5%) amounts of the effective circulating blood volume is a powerful stimulus for ADH release. Changes in effective circulating volume are detected as a result of a change in blood pressure by the baroceptors in the aortic arch and carotid sinus, and the low-pressure receptors in the atria of the heart, These receptors signal to the hypothalamus.

Other factors may also act to modulate the release of ADH:

- **Pregnancy** is associated with decreased osmolality, as a result of the action of gonadotrophins. These appear to modulate the sensitivity of the osmoreceptors.
- Many **drugs** (e.g. morphine, barbiturates and nicotine) are associated with triggering ADH release. Other drugs, such as alcohol and those drugs that antagonise the action of morphine, can reduce ADH secretion.

Osmoreceptor cells also act on other cells in the hypothalamus to stimulate **thirst**, triggering a greater intake of water, to further **regulate fluid balance**. Decreased effective circulating volume will also stimulate thirst.

Actions of ADH on the nephron

Water crosses the collecting ducts of cell membranes through special water channels called **aquaporins**. ADH acts on the cells of the collecting duct by binding to V_2 receptors which are G-protein-coupled receptors on the basolateral cell membrane:

- Water transport across the **apical membrane** is mediated by **aquaporin II**, which is incorporated into the apical membranes in response to ADH binding to V_2 receptors on the collecting duct cells.
- The **basolateral membrane** of the collecting duct cells expresses **aquaporin III** channels constitutively.

Short-term expression of aquaporin II is triggered through the fusion of vesicles expressing the channel to the apical membrane, allowing rapid increases in permeability. In the **longer term** expression of aquaporin II is achieved through increased gene expression.

Due to the high osmolality of the renal medullary interstitium, water flows out of the collecting duct through the aquaporin channels. The amount of water reabsorbed by the ADH-dependent mechanism is relatively small (about 25 L/day) compared with what is reabsorbed in the PCT (>100 L/day), although it is crucial to maintain fluid balance. Its importance is highlighted in **diabetes insipidus**. ADH also acts on the collecting duct cells in the inner medulla to increase their permeability to urea, which aids the generation of a more hypertonic environment in the medulla, further aiding water reabsorption from the collecting duct.

 CLINICAL Diabetes insipidus

Defects in the ADH pathway, through a lack of production of ADH, or a defect in its receptors or in the collecting duct cell response to receptor binding, can lead to significant production of dilute urine, and this is known as diabetes insipidus. Diabetes insipidus resulting from damage to the neurons in the brain, which secrete the molecule, can be treated by intravenous administration of desmopressin, a form of ADH that acts only on the V_2 receptors and not the V_1 ones (which promote vasoconstriction). This treatment is not effective in those forms of diabetes insipidus that result from mutations in the ADH receptors or aquaporin II in the kidneys.

Figure 9.6 The renin–angiotensin–aldosterone pathway. The kidney plays a crucial role as a regulator of fluid balance and blood pressure through both the production of hormones and its end-organ effects. The key hormonal pathway is instigated by the production of renin, which activates the production of angiotensin from angiotensinogen. The subsequent production of angiotensin II leads to widespread effects on blood vessels and adrenal glands, as well as the kidneys, which lead to increased fluid and sodium retention and (both directly and indirectly) an increase in blood pressure.

Metabolism of ADH

ADH has a relatively short half-life in the circulation (<20 min), allowing rapid responses to changes in osmolality. It is broken down rapidly in the kidney and the liver.

Regulation of Na$^+$ and the aldosterone axis

This feedback pathway is responsible for maintaining the effective circulating volume in response to loss of salt and water, e.g. as a result of diarrhoea, vomiting, excess sweating, haemorrhage, heart failure. The major mechanism for Na$^+$ reabsorption is regulated by the renin–angiotensin–aldosterone system, which is also crucial in the regulation of fluid volume. The axis is complex, as a result of the many different signals that it integrates, and is centred on three distinct factors:

1 **Renin**
2 **Angiotensin II**
3 **Aldosterone**.

Renin

Renin is produced in the kidney in response to changes in the composition of the nephron's fluid in the DCT.

Synthesis

Renin is an enzyme produced by the granular cells of the afferent arteriolar component of the JGA. It is not strictly a hormone because it acts by cleaving another protein in the bloodstream, instead of directly binding to a cellular receptor.

Mechanism of action

Renin acts on the plasma protein angiotensinogen (also called α_2-globulin or renin substrate), and cleaves a 10-residue peptide (Angiotensin I [ATI]) from it. ATI is the rate-limiting step for the production of angiotensin II (ATII).

Regulation of renin secretion

Release of renin is regulated by the following:

- β-**Adrenergic stimulation** via the renal sympathetic nerves which increases renin production and release.
- **Pressure changes in the afferent arteriole,** detected by the smooth muscle cells of the JGA. Decreased pressure (and hence decreased wall tension) *increases* renin release.

- **Cl$^-$ and Na$^+$ concentration in the distal tubule** detected by the macula densa – decreased NaCl delivery to the macula densa will cause increased renin secretion

Angiotensin II

ATII acts on a variety of receptors to regulate further hormone release and act on the central nervous system (CNS) and vasculature.

Production of ATII

The starting point for ATII production is the molecule **angiotensinogen**, a globular protein produced by the liver. Renin cleaves angiotensinogen, to produce the molecule **ATI**. **ATI is the direct precursor for ATII**, which is generated by the removal of two amino acids by **angiotensin-converting enzyme** (ACE). ACE is expressed on the surface of endothelial cells, in particular in the lungs, which are an important site of conversion, due to its large surface area.

Function of ATII

ATII has many effects related to the regulation of fluid balance and Na$^+$ regulation at many different sites in the body:

- There is **generalised constriction of vascular smooth muscle** in response to ATII to **increase blood pressure**. However, this does not normally decrease GFR because ATII preferentially constricts the efferent arterioles.
- **Increased reabsorption** in the PCT occurs due to increased activity of the Na$^+$/H$^+$ exchanger in the cells' apical membrane.
- **In the adrenal cortex,** ATII triggers the release of **aldosterone**
- **At the hypothalamus** ATII increases thirst and promotes release of **ADH**.

Metabolism of ATII

The metabolism of ATII occurs in a series of steps that alter and eliminate its biological activity:

- **ATII is converted to ATIII**. This seven-amino acid molecule is produced by the enzyme angiotensinase on the endothelial and red blood cells. It has less activity on vascular smooth muscle although it has a similar potency in triggering aldosterone production.
- **ATIV is produced by the cleavage of ATIII**. This six-amino acid peptide has little biological activity.

Aldosterone

Aldosterone is a steroid hormone secreted by the adrenal cortex. It acts by modulating gene expression in the DCT and collecting ducts, which promotes the retention of Na^+, thus increasing water reabsorption. Aldosterone also acts within the parotid glands and the colon to modulate gene expression and promote retention of Na^+ within the body. The synthesis of aldosterone is covered with that of other steroid hormones in Chapter 10.

Function of aldosterone

Aldosterone acts to increase the reclamation of Na^+ from the DCT, and promotes the secretion of K^+ or H^+. The mechanisms by which this is achieved include altering the expression of specific genes to:

- **increase ENaC** expression in the luminal surface of the collecting duct cells
- **increase the number of Na^+/K^+ATPases** in the basolateral membrane of tubular epithelial cells
- **increase production of ATP** in the tubular epithelium and so increase active transport
- **increase expression of the thiazide-sensitive Na^+/Cl^- transporter** in the DCT.

Aldosterone can act through more rapid mechanisms that do not alter gene expression, in particular by increasing the activity of the Na^+/H^+ antiporter (NXH) protein.

Regulation of aldosterone secretion

Aldosterone secretion is stimulated by a number of stimuli:

- ATII which is the most potent stimulator of secretion
- Increased plasma K^+ concentration
- Increased adrenocorticotrophic hormone (ACTH)
- Decreased atrial natriuretic peptide
- Decreased plasma Na^+ concentration.

Modulation of systemic pH by the kidneys

Plasma pH must be maintained within a very narrow range, ideally between 7.35 and 7.45. The ingestion of acids and alkalis from the diet has the potential to seriously compromise this balance. Although buffering and respiratory correction can regulate pH in the short term, any change in the production of H^+ must result in an equivalent change in regulation by the kidneys. The total systemic regulation of pH is discussed in Chapter 11.

H^+ handling by the kidneys

H^+ handling in the kidneys contributes to the regulation of pH in two manners:

1 Much of the H^+ is recycled in the reclamation of HCO_3^-.
2 H^+ is secreted into the tubule fluid and excreted in the urine to remove acid from the system.

Removal of H^+ by the kidneys

H^+ is removed from the kidneys through the excretion of the ammonium ion (NH_4^+) and acid phosphate (HPO_4^-). Ammonium may be either produced in the tubules as part of the ornithine cycle or generated in the nephron itself from ammonia:

- NH_4^+ is primarily produced as part of the ornithine cycle. Glutamine metabolism in the kidney tubule cells results in the production of: $2HCO_3^- + 2NH_4^+$. The retention of the two HCO_3^- molecules is equivalent to the extrusion of two H^+ molecules. NH_4^+ is transported into the tubule by the NXH – where it can substitute for the H^+

 DEFINITION Diffusion trapping

Weak acids and bases may exist in equilibrium between charged and uncharged states. This equilibrium is governed by the H^+ concentration (pH). Although the uncharged variant of a molecule may readily diffuse across the tubule membrane, its charged variant may not. This difference can be accentuated by the more acid nature of the nephron tubule, in relation to the blood, which traps substances in one or other compartment. This can occur physiologically, as in the handling of ammonia, or, clinically, as in the treatment of aspirin overdose.

ions. This process occurs mainly in the PCT, although a proportion of NH_4^+ is reabsorbed in the loop of Henle.

- **Ammonia (NH_3)** can also be produced in the nephron. As it is not charged, NH_3 freely diffuses into the tubule, where it is protonated to NH_4^+, allowing H^+ removal by **diffusion trapping**.
- **HPO_4^-** is mainly filtered in the form of alkaline phosphate (Na_2HPO4). Absorption of Na^+ and secretion of H^+ into the lumen converts this into acid phosphate (NaH_2PO_4), allowing H^+ removal.

CLINICAL Pharmacological modulation of urinary pH

The pH of urine can be modulated to promote or reduce the excretion of drugs, as a result of **diffusion trapping**. The modulation of pH results in different proportions of the drugs existing in protonated or unprotonated forms. Clinically, the modulation of pH can be used to treat **aspirin overdose**. Bicarbonate is used to increase urinary pH, because it increases the trapping of **salicylate** from the urine, through eliminating H^+ ions donated by aspirin (**salicylic acid**).

CLINICAL Renal tubular acidosis

Renal tubular acidosis (RTA) is a syndrome characterised by **metabolic acidosis** resulting from a defect in acid handling by the nephron. This can be the result of:

- **insufficient recovery of HCO_3^-**
- **insufficient secretion of H^+**.

There are a variety of causes of RTA, including:

- Genetic defects, such as a mutation of the H^+ ATPase
- An autoimmune condition
- Some toxins.

The symptoms of RTA include a metabolic acidosis, hypokalaemia and kidney stones. Treatment is by giving bicarbonate to correct pH, and addition of potassium to correct the hypokalaemia.

Kidney hormones

The high blood flow in the kidneys allows it to sense any changes in blood composition very rapidly and release hormones in response. Other than renin, which has been previously covered, two factors are produced by the kidneys:

1 **Erythropoietin** which regulates production of red blood cells
2 **Vitamin D** which is involved in the regulation of Ca^{2+}.

Erythropoietin

Erythropoietin (EPO) regulates red blood cell production, and therefore the oxygen-carrying capability of the blood.

Synthesis and secretion

EPO is a glycoprotein that, in adults, is produced almost exclusively by fibroblast-like cells in the kidney interstitium, although small amounts are also produced in hepatocytes. In the fetus the liver is the major source of EPO.

Functions and regulation

EPO is a **mitogenic** growth factor and induces proliferation of red blood cell precursors in the bone marrow. Production of EPO is stimulated under hypoxic conditions and in response to anaemia – where there will be a lower O_2-carrying capability. Excess EPO production can result in **polycythaemia**, whereas failure to produce EPO occurs in chronic renal failure and causes anaemia. Patients with chronic renal failure need to be treated with recombinant human EPO.

Vitamin D

The kidneys form part of the series of organs that process vitamin D into its active form. In the kidney 25-hydroxyvitamin D from the liver is hydroxylated by **1α-hydroxylase** to **calcitriol** (active vitamin D), 1,25-dihydroxy- vitamin D_3 ($1,25(OH)_2$-vitamin D_3). Calcitriol, a steroid hormone, increases total body calcium; the mechanism of action and its role in calcium homoeostasis are covered in Chapter 10.

Pharmacological modulation of kidney function

The reabsorption of fluid by the nephron is tightly coupled with reabsorption of ions, in particular Na^+. When the body retains too much fluid, pharmacological diuretics can be used to modulate reabsorption of water, to reduce the total body fluid load, in particular to treat heart failure or hypertension. Although diuretics reduce the symptoms of both diseases, they do not actually treat the underlying cause. The three main classes of diuretic that are routinely used act on different regions of the nephron, through inhibition of ion transport, which subsequently hinders the reabsorption of H_2O:

1 Loop diuretics
2 Thiazides
3 Potassium-sparing diuretics.

Two other classes of drug have diuretic effects, although due to side effects they are rarely used clinically:

1 Carbonic anhydrase inhibitors
2 Osmotic diuretics.

Loop diuretics (e.g. furosemide)

Loop diuretics are the most powerful form of diuretic, targeting the loop of Henle to mediate their actions in the kidney.

Mechanism of action

Loop diuretics are actively secreted into the lumen of the tubule, from where they act. They have both a rapid onset of effect and a short half-life. A variety of different actions contributes to the effectiveness of loop diuretics, although the first is the most significant:

- **Inhibition of the $Na^+/K^+/2Cl^-$ co-transporter** on the thick ascending limb of the loop of Henle. This reduces the concentration gradient generated within the medulla of the kidney, restricting the reabsorption of fluid from the collecting duct.
- **Vasodilatation of the vasa recta** increases the blood flow entering the medulla, and is thought to further hinder the generation of a concentration gradient, because it increases solute 'washout' from the renal medulla.
- **Systemic vasodilatation** leads to an increased cardiac output, which increases renal perfusion, particularly in individuals with cardiac failure, and reduces the stimuli for fluid retention.

Side-effects of loop diuretics

The side-effects of loop diuretics may be quite severe, and affect a variety of processes:

- **Hypokalaemia** occurs due to the body's attempts to reclaim the extra Na^+ reaching the DCT. The elevated Na^+ leads to increased activity of the Na^+/K^+ ATPase in the basolateral membrane. This pumps Na^+ out of the cells and recruits K^+ from the interstitial fluid into the cells, from whence it is transported to the tubular lumen. The rate of K^+ secretion is also enhanced by the high tubular flow rate.
- **Postural hypotension** may occur as a result of the decrease in systemic fluid and also the vasodilatory effects of loop diuretics.

- **Loss of Mg^{2+} and Ca^{2+}** may result from loss of the lumen-positive electrochemical gradient across the cells of the thick ascending limb, which drives the reabsorption process.
- **Secondary hyperaldosteronism** may result from the activation of the renin–angiotensin–aldosterone axis, which also further increases the loss of K^+.
- **Carbohydrate intolerance** may result from the loss of K^+, on which insulin is dependent for its action.

Thiazide diuretics (e.g. hydrochlorothiazide)

These have a weaker action than loop diuretics, inhibiting the reabsorption of Na^+ from the DCT.

Mechanism of action

Thiazides inhibit the Na^+/Cl^- co-transporter in the DCT. Similar to loop diuretics, thiazides cause vasodilatation, which is beneficial in their use to treat heart failure and hypertension.

Side-effects

The side-effects of thiazides are very similar to those of loop diuretics, although milder, because the loss of K^+ is less severe.

- **Hypokalaemia** may occur, although less extreme than in loop diuretics, because fewer Na^+ ions enters the DCT for reabsorption. Similarly, secondary hyperaldosteronism and carbohydrate intolerance may also occur, as seen in loop diuretics.
- **Gout** may result because thiazides can compete with the uric acid transporter.
- **Ca^{2+} retention** is associated with the use of thiazides, although the mechanism is not clear.

 CLINICAL Gout

Gout results from the deposition of uric acid crystals within the tissues. These crystals form as a result of high levels of uric acid in the blood and cause a variety of symptoms, including arthritis, tenosynovitis, kidney stones and hypertension.

Potassium-sparing diuretics

The loss of K^+ ions through the use of loop and thiazide diuretics can lead to many side effects. In particular, K^+ loss may be potentiated by the actions of the **renin–angiotensin–aldosterone axis** to reclaim the excess Na^+ in the distal parts of

the nephron. Two classes of K^+-sparing diuretics with different mechanisms of action have been identified:

1 Direct aldosterone antagonists (e.g. spironolactone)
2 K^+ channel blockers (e.g. amiloride).

Both drugs act at the more distal regions of the DCT and have a relatively weak effect when used alone, although they both act well to oppose high aldosterone levels. K^+-sparing diuretics are often used in combination with loop or thiazide diuretics, which indirectly cause increased aldosterone levels as a result of the high Na^+ levels passing through the DCT.

Side-effects

By acting to inhibit the loss of K^+, the major side effect that may be caused is **hyperkalaemia**.

Other classes of diuretic

Although loop, thiazide and K^+-sparing diuretics are the main classes of diuretic used clinically, two other types are used in specific situations:

- Osmotic diuretics
- Carbonic anhydrase inhibitors.

Osmotic diuretics (e.g. mannitol)

Mannitol is freely filtered by the kidneys but cannot be reabsorbed. As fluid is reabsorbed from the PCT, the concentration of mannitol in the lumen increases and osmotically opposes water reabsorption (and therefore the absorption of many ions). Osmotic diuretics are rarely used as a result. However, they may be used in:

- the treatment of cerebral oedema
- patients who have not responded to other classes of diuretic.

Carbonic anhydrase inhibitors (e.g. acetazolamide)

Carbonic anhydrase catalyses the formation of H^+ and HCO_3^- from H_2O and CO_2 in the nephron cells, as part of the reclamation of bicarbonate. The H^+ produced in this process enters the filtrate to react with H_2O and CO_2 and generate further bicarbonate. Secretion of H^+ is balanced by the reabsorption of Na^+ down its concentration gradient, which promotes the reabsorption of H_2O. Thus, inhibition of carbonic anhydrase reduces

H^+ secretion, leading to reduced Na^+ absorption from the PCT and reduced fluid reabsorption.

Carbonic anhydrase inhibitors are no longer commonly used because their inhibition of HCO_3^- formation severely affects the pH balance within the body, where HCO_3^- is a major buffer. Thus, a common side effect of carbonic anhydrase inhibitors is metabolic acidosis. The decreased reabsorption of Na^+ in the PCT may lead to increased reabsorption within the DCT, and can potentiate the development of **hypokalaemia**.

Transport, storage and expulsion of urine

The kidneys constantly produce urine, although the body expels it infrequently. In the meantime, it is stored in the bladder. As the osmolality of urine may be quite variable, the bladder is adapted to accommodate this and the varying volumes of urine stored within it, and also develop sufficient pressure for urine expulsion. The adult bladder is capable of storing around 500 mL of urine, though this varies with the individual. Three structures are involved in the storage and expulsion of urine:

1 The ureters
2 The bladder
3 The urethra.

The gross anatomy has been discussed earlier, although their morphology and function are discussed below.

The ureters

The ureters are muscular tubes that exit from the hilum of the kidney. They are retroperitoneal and adhere to the posterior peritoneum within the abdomen.

Histology of the ureters

The ureters contain three layers of particular functional significance:

1 The **urothelium** (transitional epithelium) is in contact with urine, and protects the underlying cells from potentially harmful substances within the urine and prevents movement of water if the urine is hypertonic.
2 The **inner muscular layer** is made up of longitudinal smooth muscle.
3 The **outer muscular layer** is made up of circular smooth muscle.

The muscular layers of the ureters are a **functional syncytium**, allowing the coordinated contraction of the muscle cells, forcing urine from the kidneys into the bladder. These peristaltic waves occur around every 10–30 s. The contraction of the ureters is triggered intrinsically by the smooth muscles cells at the proximal end of the ureter, although they may be modulated by autonomic innervation. Sensory pain fibres also innervate the ureters, and can be stimulated by blockages, such as kidney stones. Such blockages trigger more violent contractions in an attempt to force the stone out of the ureter, and are associated with severe pain.

 CLINICAL Kidney stones

Kidney stones are crystals that form from high levels of minerals in the urine. This is typically the result of an underlying pathology which determines their composition. Stones may range in size from minute, which are passed without the individual being aware, to much larger stones that may be many centimetres in size.

Large stones may become lodged in the renal pelvis, bladder, or the ureters or urethra. The resulting referred pain depends on the location where the stone becomes lodged. The location may also account for other symptoms, e.g. a urethral kidney stone is likely to decrease urine flow, because it blocks the outflow, whereas ureteric stones are associated with renal colic, linked to peristaltic contraction of the ureters.

Stones much larger than 5 mm require intervention for their removal. This typically involves ultrasonic waves, or another form of stimulation, to break down the stone. Particularly large stones may require surgical removal.

The bladder

The bladder wall is made up of two main tissues:

1 The inner surface is lined with specialised **urothelial cells** which can tolerate the wide range of osmolalities found in the bladder.
2 The rest of the bladder wall is made up of the **detrusor muscle**.

The **trigone** is a triangular region on the posterior part of the bladder, which has a different embryological origin to the rest of the bladder, and does not expand.

The urothelium

The urothelial (or umbrella) cells must be resistant to the hyperosmolarity of the urine and maintain this resistance as the bladder expands and contracts. They are characterised by a plasma membrane which contains a series of plaques that are folded within the surface membrane; this leads to the presence of a series of vesicles in the apical surface that can unfold and become incorporated into the membrane to increase the surface area on expansion of the bladder. The urothelial cells are connected to each other by many junctional complexes to maintain cohesion.

The detrusor muscle

The detrusor muscle in the wall of the bladder is spontaneously active, such that the fibres can alter their length as the bladder fills. The cells of the detrusor muscle are highly innervated and connected by many gap junctions, allowing the rapid conduction of an impulse to maintain contraction. The length of the muscle fibres may change by about four times between an empty and a full bladder. This constant changing of fibre length ensures that the bladder remains compact without the internal pressure being too high, which could potentially allow urine to pass back to the kidneys.

Innervation of the bladder

The walls and sphincters of the bladder receive sensory and autonomic motor nerve fibres that sense filling of the bladder and regulate voiding. The innervation of the walls ensures that the bladder remains contracted around the fluid such that it does not take up too much space within the body. Contraction of the bladder must be even during voiding to ensure that other regions of the bladder do not expand under the increased intravascular pressure. The different nervous fibres have different roles in regulating the bladder:

- **Sympathetic innervation** is mainly to the neck of the bladder, where it regulates the contraction of the urethra and internal urethral sphincter. This may prevent voiding of urine and prevents entry of seminal fluid into the bladder during ejaculation. The sympathetic innervation of the bladder is carried by the **hypogastric nerves**.
- **Parasympathetic innervation** from S2–4 to the bladder walls mediates contraction of the bladder, particularly during voiding.

- **Sensory innervation** is predominantly to the fundus, to detect filling of the bladder.
- **Somatic motor innervation** is carried by the pudendal nerves, and innervates the external urethral sphincter, which provides voluntary control of voiding.

Regulation of bladder tone

When the bladder is relatively empty, the detrusor muscle has little tone, so that pressure within the bladder is relatively low. At the same time, the internal and external bladder sphincters are contracted to prevent the unintentional expulsion of urine into the urethra.

The trigone

The trigone is a triangular region found at the posterior aspect of the bladder. Unlike the rest of the bladder it is derived from the mesonephric ducts, as opposed to the urogenital sinus. The ureters and urethra enter the bladder at the corner of the trigone. In particular, the ureters enter at an oblique angle which acts as a one-way valve to prevent reflux of urine at higher bladder pressures – in some individuals this angle is not present, predisposing the affected individual to reflux of urine to the kidneys, and infection.

The urethra and the control of micturition

The urethra links the bladder to the external environment and its course varies between the sexes. Micturition is unusual in that it is an autonomic process under a significant degree of voluntary control. As the bladder fills, sensory neurons report the filling to centres within the brain stem which reduce the signals, inhibiting contraction of the detrusor muscle. Higher cortical centres are required to act to allow relaxation of the external sphincter, which is required for the bladder to empty at low pressure. This relaxation of the sphincter and the simultaneous contraction of the detrusor muscle trigger the expulsion of urine.

During filling, the bladder neck, which is made up of circular smooth muscle, is closed. In addition, the urethra is kept closed by voluntary sphincters made up of striated muscle:

- In males the membranous part of the urethra is covered with striated muscle.
- In females the shorter urethra is covered in striated muscle across its length.

Urinary sphincters

Two sphincters separate the urethra from the bladder:

1 The **internal urethral sphincter** is made up of cells that form part of the syncytium of the bladder walls. These muscle fibres are arranged in a radial pattern, so contraction causes opening of the neck of the bladder.
2 The **external urethral sphincter** lies distal to the internal sphincter. This band of muscle, which surrounds, the urethra is under voluntary control and is innervated by the pudendal nerve. Voluntary relaxation of the external sphincter is required to allow micturition to occur.

The micturition reflex

Bladder function is regulated by the micturition reflex, although this is inhibited by higher centres to ensure that voiding occurs only when there is a suitable opportunity. As a result, the control of urination has two stages:

1 Autonomic control – the micturition reflex
2 Somatic control learned during infancy.

Autonomic regulation of urination

As the bladder fills, it expands such that the pressure within it increases only when it is relatively full. Increase in pressure is detected by stretch receptors in the detrusor muscle. Sensory impulses are carried to the spinal cord, where they trigger parasympathetic outflow to the bladder:

- The detrusor muscle contracts to increase the pressure.
- The internal urethral sphincter relaxes to allow expulsion of urine.

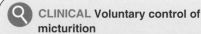

CLINICAL Voluntary control of micturition

Voluntary control of bladder function has to be learnt at an early age. In infants, the voiding of the bladder is regulated solely by the autonomic reflexes that are in place. In individuals with spinal injuries, particularly to the sacral region, elements of the micturition reflex may be eliminated and can trigger forms of incontinence.

The contraction of the detrusor muscle further increases the pressure detected by the stretch receptors in the detrusor muscle, stimulating contraction of the detrusor until the urine is voided.

Somatic control of the urination

Control of urination can be learnt, to override the autonomic reflex. There are two major points that allow regulation of the micturition reflex:

1 **Control of the external urethral sphincter** – this sphincter is made up of skeletal muscle, which is under voluntary control. Contract of the external sphincter prevents expulsion of urine regardless of the state of the internal sphincter.
2 **Higher centres** can suppress the autonomic micturition reflex. When voiding becomes possible, this inhibition is relaxed to allow the autonomic micturition relaxation to proceed as normal.

CLINICAL Urinary incontinence

Urinary incontinence is relatively common in older patients, particularly those aged >75. There are various causes of incontinence and these can be categorised. Of particular significance is overflow incontinence, which is due to an underlying obstruction of the urethra. This often occurs in older men as a result of prostate hypertrophy obstructing the urethra. Urge incontinence may result from pathology of the detrusor muscle.

CLINICAL Prostatic hypertrophy

The prostate gland is part of the male reproductive system and is located around the neck of the bladder. In older men hypertrophy of the prostate gland is particularly common, which can constrict the neck of the bladder and the urethra, resulting in difficulty in urinating. Prostatic hypertrophy may be treated by drugs to relax the neck of the bladder, or in more extreme cases through surgery.

 RELATED CHAPTERS

10

Endocrinology

The endocrine system is network of multiple organs that release hormones to maintain homoeostasis.

These chemical messengers are typically released into the bloodstream and influence many cells of the body to induce a desired response. Although they do not provide the same speed of response as the nervous system, hormones can travel throughout the body and trigger responses in many different tissues – resulting in widespread effects. In addition, many induce changes at a genetic level.

Overview of endocrinology

Hormones

Hormones are chemical signals secreted into the bloodstream which act on distant tissues that express hormone specific receptors. Effects of hormones can be classified depending on the site of action relative to where the hormone was released:

- **Endocrine** – travels in blood to distant target organ
- **Paracrine** – hormone released from one cell has a biological effect on a neighbouring cell
- **Autocrine** – hormone has a biological effect on the cell from which it was released.

Hormones themselves can be classified into amines, peptides and steroids.

Amines (e.g. adrenaline)

- They are synthesised from the amino acid tyrosine.
- They act via receptors on the surface of cells.
- They are stored as granules in the cytoplasm until release is triggered by stimuli.
- Their effects are short term and they act within minutes.

Peptides (e.g. insulin)

Peptides are lipophobic and bind to receptors on the surface of cells:

- Formed from pre-prohormones which undergo post-translational processing (e.g. pre-proinsulin is converted to proinsulin and then insulin).
- Secretion can be constitutive or regulated. In constitutive secretion, the hormone is secreted as it is synthesised; in regulated secretion the hormone is stored within the cell in secretory granules and released in response to stimuli.
- Their effects are mainly short term and they act within minutes. They may also trigger longer-term effects within the cell, e.g. upregulating transcription.

Steroids (e.g. cortisol)

- They are lipophilic: they can cross cell membranes and act on intracellular receptors.
- They are synthesised from cholesterol in the adrenal cortex, gonads and placenta.

Biomedical Science Lecture Notes, First Edition. Ian Lyons.
© 2011 by Ian Lyons. Published 2011 by Blackwell Publishing Ltd.

- Once secreted, steroid hormones are rapidly released and not stored within the secretory cells.
- In general their effects are more long term; the effects are seen after a few hours and may last for days. More recently, it has also been demonstrated that steroid hormones may have some more rapid effects via action on cell surface receptors.

Hormones are either transported freely (hydrophilic hormones) or bound to **carrier proteins**. These proteins are mostly globulins synthesised in the liver, acting to prolong the half-life of the hormone and allowing regulation of the activity of the hormones through regulation of the levels of free hormone.

Hormones are removed from the circulation either by **inactivation in the liver** (followed by excretion by the liver or kidneys) or **degradation** at the target cell, via internalisation of the hormone–receptor complex followed by lysosomal degradation.

Hormone receptors

The site of action of hormones is determined mainly by the chemical properties of the molecule – those hormones that are lipid soluble can diffuse through the cell membrane to act directly on intracellular receptors, whereas those which are not must bind to cell membrane receptors.

Cell membrane receptors

Hormone binding to cell membrane receptors triggers an intracellular signalling cascade. There are two types of these receptors:

1 **Ligand-gated ion channels**: binding stimulates opening of ion channels and consequent ion fluxes
2 **Receptors that regulate the activity of intracellular proteins**, e.g. G-protein-coupled receptors or receptor protein tyrosine kinase.

Generally amines and peptide hormones act via these receptors, and the effects are mediated very quickly (within minutes). Recent evidence has shown that some steroid hormones may act via cell membrane receptors, in addition to their better understood intracellular effects.

Intracellular receptors

These are transcription factors that have binding sites for the hormone. They bind lipid-soluble hormones (which can pass freely through the cell membrane) in the cytoplasm and migrate to the nucleus, where they regulate transcription by binding to hormone response elements. Generally, steroid hormones act via these receptors and the effects take longer (hours to days) to be mediated.

The pituitary gland

The pituitary gland is the major homoeostatic gland, releasing hormones that can modulate every system and process in the body. It integrates hormonal signals in the blood from the hypothalamic capillary beds with neural signals from the brain, and releases hormones which enter the systemic circulation through the jugular vein.

Development of the pituitary gland

The anterior and posterior parts of the pituitary gland have different embryological derivations, which fuse to form the pituitary gland during weeks 4 and 5 of gestation:

- The **anterior pituitary** is formed from the ectodermal tissue in the roof of the mouth which grows upwards to form Rathke's pouch.
- The **posterior pituitary** is formed from a downward process of the forebrain vesicle, known as the infundibulum.

The fusion of the anterior and posterior pituitary is followed by the anterior pituitary budding off from the ectoderm, leaving the entire gland supported by the stalk of the posterior pituitary.

The anterior pituitary

The anterior pituitary gland contains many distinct types of **endocrine cells**, which secrete hormones, and **folliculostellate** cells, which have a glial type of supporting function. Five different types of endocrine cell are found in the anterior pituitary, each associated with a distinct regulatory axis:

1 **Thyrotrophs** release thryotrophin (also known as thyroid-stimulating hormone or TSH). This hormone regulates the release of thyroid hormones through its actions on the follicular cells in the thyroid gland.

2 **Corticotrophs** release adrenocorticotrophic hormone (ACTH), which stimulates the release of cortisol, a steroid hormone, from the adrenal cortex.
3 **Somatotrophs** release growth hormone, which regulates tissue growth. This is via direct effects on the tissues, or through the release of insulin-like growth factor 1 (IGF-1) from the liver
4 **Gonadotrophs** release **luteinising hormone** (LH) and **follicle-stimulating hormone** (FSH), which are involved in the regulation of the reproductive system. In women, the cyclic release of these hormones is responsible for controlling the menstrual cycle.
5 **Lactotrophs** regulate the production of milk in breastfeeding women, and are also important in breast development through the production of prolactin. It is not clear if this hormone has a significant function in men.

Control of anterior pituitary hormones

The anterior pituitary integrates signals from the body and the brain to regulate the release of hormones. The major inputs are received from three sources:

1 The **hypothalamus** releases neurohormones into the **portal vessels** between the hypothalamus and the anterior pituitary.
2 **Systemic hormones** released by other tissues in the body may feed back to modulate the secretion of signals from the pituitary.
3 The cells in the pituitary gland may act in a **paracrine** manner to regulate each other.

The posterior pituitary

The posterior pituitary contains the ending of the nerves cells located in the **supraoptic** and **paraventricular** nuclei of the hypothalamus which directly release the hormones from their nerve terminals:

1 **Oxytocin** regulates contractions during labour and the production of milk by the breast. These processes are discussed in the reproduction chapter.
2 **Antidiuretic hormone** (ADH), also known as vasopressin, is crucial for the regulation of systemic fluid volume. The role of ADH in discussed in more detail in relation to kidney function and fluid balance.

The thyroid axis

The thyroid axis regulates the basal metabolic rate of an individual and is important in the young to regulate growth and development. The crucial end hormones are the thyroid hormones (triiodothyronine or T_3 and thyroxine or T_4). Their widespread effects are evident by the expression of the thyroid hormone receptor in almost every cell in the body.

Structures in the thyroid axis

Three main glands are involved in this axis, each releasing a specific hormone (Fig. 10.1):

1 The **hypothalamus** releases thyrotrophin-releasing hormone (TRH).
2 **Thyrotroph** cells in the anterior pituitary release TSH in response to TRH.
3 The **follicular cells** in the thyroid gland produce T_4 in response to TSH. T_4 is the end-hormone of the pathway, and also suppresses secretion of TRH.

Structure of the thyroid gland

The thyroid gland contains two prominent groups of cells involved in the secretion of hormones:

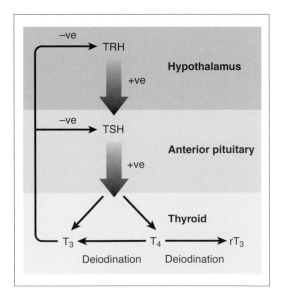

Figure 10.1 Schematic representation of the control of thyroid hormone production and the role of negative feedback.

1 The **follicular cells** are crucial for the release of T_4. These are arranged to form spheres (follicles) which contain thyroglobulin, a precursor to T_4.
2 The interstitial **C cells** are sparsely distributed between the follicles and responsible for the release of **calcitonin** – a hormone involved in the regulation of calcium and phosphate.

There are also many interstitial cells between the follicles. The thyroid gland contains many capillaries and lymphatic vessels. The gross anatomy of the thyroid gland is discussed in Chapter 14.

Synthesis and secretion of thyrotrophin-releasing hormone

TRH is a tripeptide molecule released by the paraventricular nucleus of the hypothalamus as a regulator of metabolism, through stimulation of the release of TSH from the pituitary gland which, in turn, acts on the release of thyroid hormones.

Thyrotrophin (thyroid-stimulating hormone)

TSH is the major stimulus to act on the thyroid gland triggering production and release of the thyroid hormones.

Synthesis and secretion

TSH is a glycoprotein made in the thyrotroph cells of the anterior pituitary, which make up about 10% of the cells. The hormone is made up of an α subunit, common to TSH, FSH and LH, and a unique β subunit. TSH is stored in granules in the cytoplasm of the thyrotroph cells.

Regulation of secretion

Release of TSH is triggered by TRH. TSH, in turn, stimulates the production of thyroid hormones, which act to negatively inhibit the production of TRH and TSH. It is thought that the major mechanism of this negative feedback is through down-regulation of TRH receptors on the thyrotroph cells, in response to increased levels of thyroid hormones. TSH production is also reduced by **somatostatin** from the anterior pituitary.

Actions on target organs

TSH acts on the thyroid gland where it is the major factor stimulating release of thyroid hormones.

TSH binds a G-protein-coupled receptor which promotes the production of the second messenger, cAMP.

 CLINICAL Prenatal hypothyroidism (formerly called cretinism)

Thyroid hormones are crucial to ensure correct neural development. Thus, prenatal thyroid deficiency can lead to severe defects. This includes learning disability, general poor neural development, stunted growth and a protruding tongue. The effects of deficiency are quite reversible if identified at birth (using the Guthrie test). Treatment is through giving thyroid hormones.

Synthesis and secretion of thyroid hormones

There are two main thyroid hormones – T_4 and T_3 – both of which are produced and released by follicular cells in the thyroid gland.

Structure of thyroid hormones

A variety of thyroid hormones exists. Each shares the same basic structure but varies in terms of the number and location of sites that have been iodinated. There are four important variants of thyroid molecules (Fig. 10.2):

1 **Thyronine** is the carbon skeleton that is common to all the thyroid hormones. The varying thyroid hormones consist of a thyronine skeleton, which possess iodine at up to four distinct sites on the molecule.
2 T_4 is the **major product** of the thyroid gland. It consists of a thyronine skeleton iodinated at all four available sites. It is relatively inactive as a hormone, and serves primarily as a reservoir for T_3, a far more active variant of the hormone.
3 T_3 is the **major active** thyroid hormone and contains three iodinated sites. It is primarily produced by deiodination of T_4 in tissues, although in times of low iodine levels it may also be produced at high levels by the thyroid.
4 **Reverse T_3 (rT_3)** is an inactive thyroid hormone that is produced by the deiodination of T_4. The deiodination of an alternative site yields rT_3 which is incapable of binding the thyroid hormone receptor.

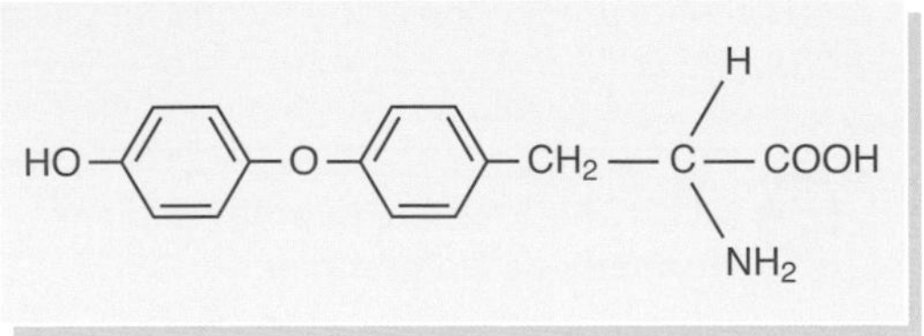

Thyronine

Thyronine is the skeleton that forms the basis of all thyroid hormones, it is formed within the thyroglobulin protein and the thyroid hormones vary, depending on whether they are iodinated at four specific locations on the thyronine skeleton.

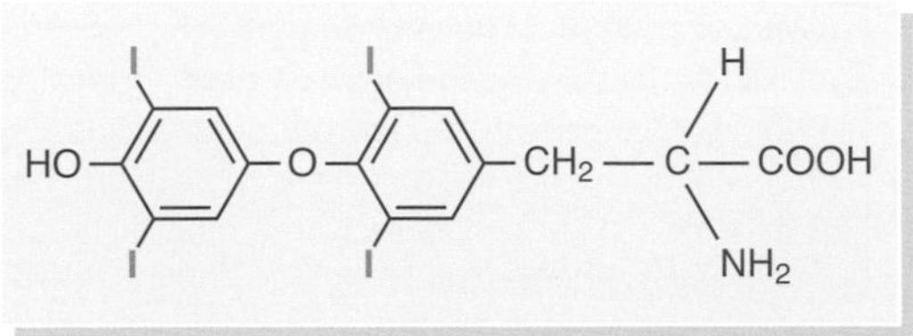

Thyroxine

Thyroxine (T_4) is the major product of the thyroid gland, and is iodinated at all four available locations. It has little direct biological activity, although it acts as a precursor to triiodothyronine (T_3).

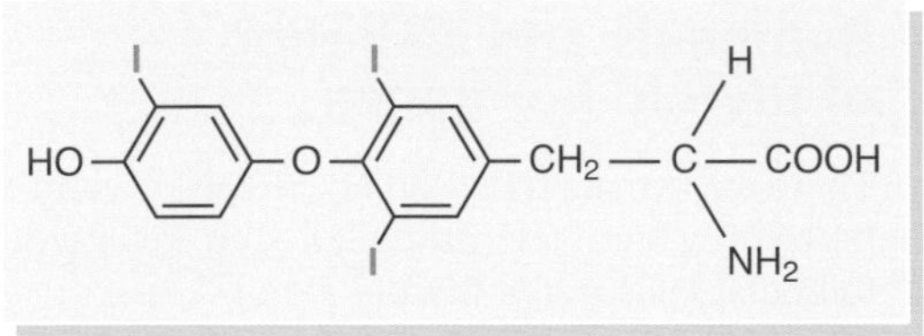

Triiodothyronine

T_3 is the most biologically active thyroid hormone although it is present in much lower concentrations in the blood than T_4. The thyroid gland usually releases 20-fold more T_4 than T_3. It is mainly formed in the periphery by the deiodination of T_4.

Reverse triiodothyronine

Reverse T_3 (rT_3) is a non-active isomer of T_3 and differs in the sites at which it is iodinated. It can be produced from T_4 through a different set of deiodination reactions. In particular, when there is an excess of cortisol (e.g. under stressful conditions), the inhibited conversion of T_4 to T_3 results in shunting towards rT_3, slowing metabolism and potentially producing features of hypothyroidism.

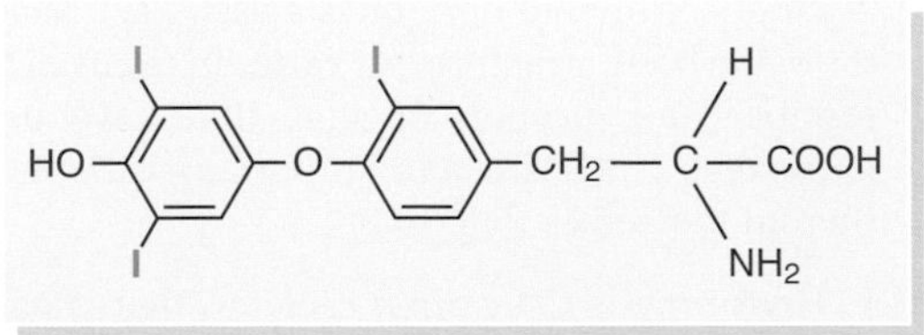

Figure 10.2 The thyroid hormones all follow the same basic structure, made up of two conjugated tyrosine residues. They vary in the number of sites of iodination (in blue), and the positions in which they have been iodinated. There are three significant structures – thyroxine (T_4) which is the most commonly produced form, triiodothyronine (T_3) which is the most metabolically active, and reverse T_3, which is a non-active form produced from T_4.

Specific tissues, such as the placenta and the brain, express deiodinase enzymes themselves, allowing them to regulate the relative proportions of T_3 and rT_3 produced from T_4. This allows those tissues to control the amount of T_3 that binds the receptor, relatively independent of the circulating levels of T_4 and T_3.

Synthesis and storage

The production of thyroid hormones is reflected in the histological organisation of the gland. The follicular cells are arranged in large spherical sacs surrounding a fluid suspension containing the glycoprotein thyroglobulin, which is produced and secreted by the follicular cells.

Active thyroid hormones are iodinated after the transport of iodine from the blood into the follicles. Once in the follicle, the iodine binds to specific tyrosine residues in thyroglobulin catalysed by **thyroid peroxidase**. After the addition of iodine, the iodotyrosine residues become coupled to form T_3 or T_4. Each thyroglobulin molecule produces up to four thyroid hormone molecules.

Thyroid hormones are stored in an iodinated form as an integral part of the thyroglobulin molecule, until they are required for release. This is achieved through endocytosis of thyroglobulin into follicular cells. Lysosomes then fuse with the thyroglobulin-containing vesicles and are enzymatically cleaved to release T_3 and T_4, in response to TSH.

Regulation of thyroid hormone release

The main stimulus for the release of thyroid hormones is the TSH. Regulation of the hypothalamic–pituitary–thyroid axis is by **negative feedback**, because T_3 and T_4 act on the pituitary and the hypothalamus to reduce the release of TRH and TSH, respectively, so that during adult life the levels of each are maintained relatively constant.

Actions on target organs

Thyroid hormones bind strongly to serum proteins, T_4 binding slightly more strongly than T_3. Less than 0.5% of thyroid hormones are found free in the plasma. As most cells do not take up bound hormones, most of the effects of thyroid hormone are mediated by free hormone.

Thyroid hormones are transported into cells by a membrane-bound transport system (although due to their lipid-soluble nature some movement into the cell may occur through simple diffusion) and bind to thyroid hormone receptors, which are nuclear receptors. T_3 binds more effectively than T_4. Activated thyroid hormone receptors bind to specific DNA sequences – thyroid response elements (TREs) – which modulate the expression of a variety of genes resulting in an increase in the basal metabolic rate. Specific actions of thyroid hormones include increases in:

- **expression of Na^+/K^+ ATPase**
- **protein production through increases in RNA polymerases**
- **protein and carbohydrate metabolism**
- **breakdown of lipids and cholesterols**.

Metabolism

T_3 and T_4 are inactivated through deiodination, and then excreted. T_4 can be converted into the more pharmacologically active T_3 through the activity of deiodinase enzymes. T_4 is converted into both T_3 and inactive rT3. This reaction is responsible for production of about 75% of the T_3 in circulation. There are a variety of locations where these enzymes are expressed:

- The **liver** and **kidneys** deiodinate the majority of T_4, to produce T_3 or rT_3.
- Cells in the **pituitary gland** are able to deiodinate T_4, which is important for the negative feedback regulation of this axis.
- The **brain** and **placenta** express deiodinases which directly inactivate T_3 and T_4, to prevent the brain and fetus from excessively high thyroid hormone levels.

Whether T_3 or rT_3 is produced is regulated by the needs of the body:

- In **starvation**, a lower basic metabolic rate is advantageous and is reflected in the increased proportion of T_4 being converted to rT_3.
- In **chronic stress**, rT_3 is preferentially produced in response to increased cortisol levels, to maintain energy stores.

Final processing of the hormones is through the complete deiodination to thyronine. The iodide is reabsorbed by the kidneys for use in generating future thyroid hormones.

Role of thyroid hormones in development

Thyroid hormones are crucial for early development, regulating a number of processes:

- **Stimulating myelination** and the production of neurotransmitters
- **Promoting the growth of axons**
- **Promoting the action of chondrocytes** and thus promoting the growth of long bones

 CLINICAL Iodine deficiency and goitre

In much of the world iodine deficiency is a serious problem. In children, iodine deficiency can be particularly severe because thyroid hormones are crucial for development. Where there are low levels of iodine in the body the thyroid gland compensates and secretes T_3 in preference to the less active T_4. In an attempt to scavenge more iodine, the gland tissue enlarges, producing a goitre. Treatment of iodine deficiency has been achieved in many cases through the supplementation of food with iodine, particularly by the spraying of salt with iodine solutions

- Glucocorticoids act with thyroid hormones to **promote surfactant production** to mature the lungs.

 CLINICAL Adult hypothyroidism

Hypothyroidism, where there is a failure to produce thyroid hormones, may occur as a result of:

- absence of TSH
- absence of TRH
- a mutation resulting in resistance to thyroid hormone
- autoimmune destruction of the thyroid gland.

Typical symptoms of hypothyroidism reflect the decreased metabolism due to the absence of the hormones. In particular, there is a general apathy, reduced pulse rate, weight gain, intolerance to cold and muscle weakness.

 CLINICAL Hyperthyroidism

Hyperthyroidism, or thyrotoxicosis, results in symptoms mainly reflecting an increased metabolism. These include loss of weight, restlessness and diarrhoea due to increased GI activity.

The major cause of thyrotoxicosis is the autoimmune condition **Graves' disease**, in which an antibody that activates the TSH receptor is produced. In addition, thyroid tumours may occur – the tumour consists of complete follicles.

The adrenal hormones

The adrenal gland can be divided into two parts with different roles:

1 The inner **medullar region** is responsible for the production of **catecholamines**, which contribute to the sympathetic response.
2 The outer **cortical region** is responsible for the production of the **steroid hormones**.

The adrenal cortex is responsible for the production of three main hormones, by modification of cholesterol. Although the pathways by which these hormones are regulated differ, they share many common enzymes. The major rate-limiting step in the production of these hormones is the production of pregnenolone from cholesterol by the cytochrome P450 pathway, which is regulated by the pituitary hormone ACTH. Each hormone is produced by a different layer of cells within the cortex of the adrenal gland (Fig. 10.3):

- **Aldosterone** is associated with regulating Na^+ levels within the body. It is produced by cells in the zona glomerulosa of the adrenal cortex, the outermost layer of the cortex.
- **Cortisol**, responsible for the stress response, is produced within the middle group of cells, the zona fasciculata.
- **The androgens** are produced by the innermost layer of cells, the zone reticularis.

The hypothalamic–pituitary–adrenal axis

The hypothalamic–pituitary–adrenal axis regulates the stress response. The adrenal cortex is the end-effector organ through its production of cortisol in response to ACTH. Although the other steroid hormones also require ACTH, they are further regulated at other points in their synthetic pathways.

Structures in the axis

Three main secretory structures are present in the hypothalamic–pituitary–adrenal axis:

1 The **hypothalamus** releases corticotrophin-releasing hormone (CRH) which flows to the anterior pituitary gland
2 The **corticotroph cells in the anterior pituitary** release ACTH in response to CRH.
3 The **adrenal cortex** is the main target of ACTH, and stimulates synthesis and release of cortisol by the adrenal cortex cells.

Corticotrophin-releasing hormone

CRH is a polypeptide released by the paraventricular nucleus of the hypothalamus. It may also be produced by the placenta during pregnancy, and is thought to partially regulate the duration of pregnancy. Although CRH acts mainly on the pituitary, receptors have been found in other areas of the brain including the amygdala and the hypothalamus itself.

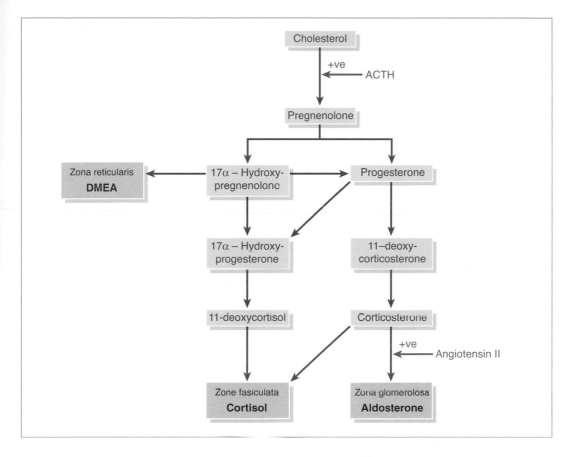

Figure 10.3 The synthesis of steroid hormones in the adrenal cortex involves many common steps. In particular, the production of pregnenolone from cholesterol is required for the synthesis of all the hormones, and is regulated by adrenocorticotrophic hormone (ACTH). The cells of the different zones of the adrenal cortex express unique enzymes that govern whether they produce dehydroepiandrosterone (DHEA), aldosterone or cortisol as an end-product.

ACTH

Synthesis and secretion

ACTH is a peptide produced from **pro-opiomelanocortin** (POMC).

 DEFINITION Pro-opiomelanocortin

POMC is a large precursor protein produced in the pituitary gland. It can be cleaved to yield a number of different proteins for release, in addition to ACTH. The sequences encoding different proteins are overlapping, with POMC producing vastly different proteins in the anterior and intermediate lobes of the pituitary, reflecting different cleavage patterns.

Function and regulation of ACTH

ACTH stimulates the conversion of cholesterol to **pregnenolone**, a crucial precursor in steroid hormone synthesis. The major influence on ACTH release is the secretion of CRH from the pituitary gland, although other stimuli, in particular the posterior pituitary hormone **vasopressin** (AVP; also known asanti-diuretic hormone [ADH]), can promote its release.

ACTH release follows a circadian rhythm. The highest levels are found in the morning, around the time of waking, and then slowly decrease during the day until around midnight, at which point levels start to increase towards the morning peak. Other stimuli can alter the levels of ACTH, in particular signals of starvation (e.g. hypoglycaemia) and cues for psychological stress (e.g. fear and pain).

CLINICAL ACTH-secreting tumours

Hormone-secreting tumours related to the hypothalamic–pituitary–adrenal axis disrupt the usual regulatory systems. The presence of an ACTH-secreting tumour triggers excessive production of cortisol from the adrenal cortex, resulting in Cushing's syndrome.

 CLINICAL ACTH deficiency

A deficiency in ACTH may occur through a tumour or infection, or as a result of radiation treatment – the hypothalamic–pituitary axis is very susceptible to radiation damage. This deficiency affects all steroid hormone production in the adrenal cortex, because ACTH regulates the rate-limiting step of hormone synthesis common to all hormones. As a result, affected individuals have the defects associated with loss of cortisol, and in addition have low androgen levels.

Synthesis of steroid hormones

The adrenal cortex hormones are derived from cholesterol, which is stored in lipid droplets. On stimulation cholesterol is converted to pregenolone by enzymes expressed on the smooth endoplasmic reticulum (ER). Pregnenolone is subsequently converted to the different steroid hormones by specific enzyme pathways within the different cells of the adrenal cortex, to yield the various steroid hormones.

Synthesis of cortisol

After the generation of pregnenolone, the next stages of cortisol synthesis are specific for androgens and cortisol, and are mediated by **7α-hydroxylase**. There are then two further hydroxylation reactions specific to cortisol production. As the hormone is lipid soluble, little is stored in the cells and secretion is the result of new synthesis. Transport of cortisol around the body is achieved by the transport protein, **transcortin**.

Regulators of cortisol secretion

ACTH signals through a G-protein-coupled receptor to stimulate cortisol production in the zona fasiculata. A prolonged elevation in levels of ACTH results in a generalised increase in the size of the zona fasiculata to cope with the increased requirements.

Cortisol itself acts as part of a **negative-feedback** loop. It acts directly on the pituitary gland to inhibit the production of ACTH, and on the hypothalamus to inhibit the release of CRH. The regulation of ACTH is linked to a diurnal pattern with a large variation in the hormone levels. This is reflected in the large changes seen in the levels of cortisol as well.

Actions on target organs

Cortisol diffuses directly across the cell membrane and binds to the intracellular glucocorticoid receptor that is found in almost every cell in the body. Cortisol is associated with prolonged stress, and it induces changes in gene expression to maintain vital functions and energy reserves. Cortisol counters stress by providing the metabolic substrates required for the body as well as retaining essential ions (e.g. Na^+) to promote the body's readiness for a flight-or-fight response. Non-essential processes that are likely to increase burden on the body are suppressed:

- The capacity for pregnancy, which would drain metabolic resources, is reduced.
- Wound healing is suppressed, because this requires materials that may be needed to maintain the fight-or-flight response.

The major effects of cortisol are shown in Table 10.1.

 CLINICAL Cushing's syndrome and disease

Cushing's syndrome refers to the abnormalities resulting from chronic excess of glucocorticoids. There may be many causes for this; if it is due to inappropriate ACTH secretion, it is called **Cushing's disease**. This is generally due to an ACTH-secreting tumour in the pituitary, although it may be caused by ectopic ACTH-producing tumours in adrenal adenomas or adrenal carcinomas. For both, symptoms are similar to the normal stress response but much more extreme. In particular, the syndrome is characterised by a change in fat deposition around the trunk and back, hypertension, a 'moon-face' (as a result of tissue oedema), osteoporosis, and poor wound healing and infertility.

Table 10.1 The major effects of cortisol

Increased metabolic substrates	Increased oxygen-carrying capacity	Decreased non-essential processes
↑ retention of Na⁺ and ↑ glucose concentration in blood, ↑ gluconeogenesis, ↑ glycogen production	↑ vascular tone	↓ immune response
↑ breakdown of proteins to supply substrates for gluconeogenesis	↑ cardiac contractility	↓ repair mechanisms
↓ use of glucose by other tissues	↑ red blood cell production	↓ LH and PRL release (reduces risk of pregnancy)
↑ generation of ketone bodies		
↑ breakdown of fats		

LH, luteinising hormone; PRL, prolactin.

CLINICAL Addison's disease

Addison's disease is the opposite of Cushing's syndrome – an absence of cortisol production, typically resulting from autoimmune destruction of cortisol-secreting cells. It is characterised by general weakness and is associated with high levels of ACTH, due to the aberrant regulation of the axis. Patients with Addison's disease are often highly pigmented because the α-Melanocyte-stimulating hormone (α-MSH) is secreted with ACTH.

Although cortisol is noted for its role in regulating the stress response, its secretion occurs even without prolonged stress and has essential homeostatic function, e.g. vascular tone maintained by the sympathetic nervous system requires low levels of cortisol.

Metabolism of cortisol

Cortisol is inactivated in the liver where **11β-hydroxysteroid dehydrogenase** converts it to **cortisone**. As it can bind to, and activate, the aldosterone receptor, cells that are responsive to aldosterone also express 11β-hydroxysteroid dehydrogenase.

Aldosterone

Aldosterone is produced in the zona glomerulosa of the adrenal cortex and is responsible for the regulation of Na⁺. Aldosterone and its effects in the regulation of Na⁺ are discussed in Chapter 9, although its synthesis and triggers are outlined below.

Synthesis and secretion of aldosterone

Aldosterone production does not require hydroxylation by the 17α-hydroxylase enzyme needed for the synthesis of cortisol and the androgens. After the production of **pregnenolone**, a separate enzymatic pathway synthesises aldosterone.

Aldosterone is transported around the body in the circulation, although only a small proportion is bound to plasma proteins, resulting in it being cleared more rapidly than cortisol from the system. In addition, it is present in far lower concentrations (around 100-fold lower) than cortisol.

Triggers and inhibitors of aldosterone secretion

The secretion of aldosterone is tightly regulated, with three major factors having been identified to promote aldosterone secretion:

1 **Angiotensin II** is the major stimulator of aldosterone secretion.
2 **ACTH** is essential for the production of aldosterone because it promotes the formation of the precursor molecule.
3 **Plasma potassium** is linked to the secretion of aldosterone.

There are two major inhibitory factors to the release of aldosterone:

1 **Atrial natriuretic peptide** is produced in response to high fluid levels and antagonises the production of aldosterone.
2 **Somatostatin** inhibits aldosterone production.

Adrenal androgens

The zona reticularis produces low levels of androgens, in particular the hormone dehydroepiandrosterone (DHEA), which is converted to testosterone in the tissues. DHEA is also an intermediate in the production of oestrogen:

- In men, DHEA has relatively little effect due to the larger amount of testosterone produced by the testes.
- In women, adrenal DHEA production accounts for around 50% of the sex steroid requirements.

Androgens in growth and puberty

Just before puberty the level of DHEA secretion increases rapidly, and is associated with the growth spurt seen around that time. DHEA secretion also promotes the development of pubic and axillary hair.

The adrenal medulla

The medulla of the adrenal gland is richly innervated by preganglionic fibres of the sympathetic nervous system. This neural crest-derived structure can supplement the production of noradrenaline, released by the sympathetic neurons with adrenaline, which it releases directly into the bloodstream.

Synthesis and secretion

The major catecholamine released from the adrenal gland is adrenaline, which accounts for around 80% of the release, although the remainder is made up of noradrenaline. Both compounds are produced in the cytoplasm of the chromaffin cells of the adrenal medulla from the amino acid tyrosine (Fig. 10.4):

- **Tyrosine** is converted to dopa (L-3,4-dehydroxyphenylalanine) and then to **dopamine** in the cytoplasm.
- **Dopamine** is pumped into granules in the cytoplasm and converted to **noradrenaline**.
- **Noradrenaline** can be stored in the granules or returned to the cytoplasm where it is converted into **adrenaline**.
- **Adrenaline** is then pumped into granules and progressively acidified and concentrated. The granules also contain high concentrations of ATP, which is a **co-transmitter**.

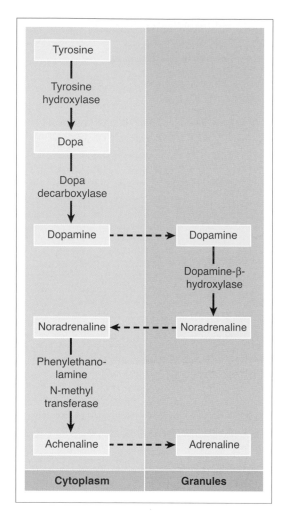

Figure 10.4 The synthesis of adrenaline in the chromaffin cells occurs through a variety of enzymatic reactions, which occur either in the cytoplasm or in the granules that are eventually released from the cells. The production of noradrenaline from dopamine must occur within the granules, before noradrenaline is pumped out into the cytoplasm for conversion to adrenaline. After its production in the cytoplasm, adrenaline is pumped back into the granules, together with ATP, which acts as a co-transmitter.

Regulation of catecholamine release from the adrenal gland

The preganglionic sympathetic neurons that synapse with the chromaffin cells release acetylcholine. Binding of acetylcholine to its receptors on the chromaffin cells triggers cell depolarisation and degranulation in a Ca^{2+}-dependent manner to release the granule's contents.

Function of adrenaline

Adrenaline acts to supplement the sympathetic response. As a result of its different affinity to the receptors and its differential access to the tissues, it produces a different response to that seen with noradrenaline.

 CLINICAL Phaeochromocytoma

This adrenaline-secreting tumour can arise from the chromaffin cells. Typical features include hypertension, headache, tachycardia, tremor and anxiety, due to uncontrolled secretion of catecholamines. Treatment involves surgical removal of the tumour.

Growth hormone axis

Growth hormone promotes tissue growth in the body. It can act directly as an effector of the growth hormone axis, or through stimulation of the production of IGF-1 in the liver (Fig. 10.5).

Three organs form the growth hormone axis:

1 The **hypothalamus** regulates growth hormone through positive and negative signals through growth hormone-releasing hormone (GHRH) and somatostatin, respectively.
2 The **pituitary gland** releases human growth hormone (hGH) from the somatotrophs in the anterior pituitary gland.
3 The **liver** releases IGF-1 in response to hGH.

Growth hormone-releasing hormone

GHRH is a polypeptide released by the hypothalamus in response to the integration of signals from the body and those from the centre of the brain. In addition, IGF-1, the secretion end-product of the axis, suppresses the secretion of GHRH. GHRH acts to increase GH synthesis through increasing intracellular cAMP.

Growth hormone

Synthesis and secretion

Growth hormone (hGH) is a protein that is released by the somatotroph cells of the pituitary gland. It is secreted in larger amounts than any other pituitary hormone.

Regulation of growth hormone

Control of hGH secretion is primarily by the two hormones, **GHRH** and **somatostatin**, both of which are released from the hypothalamus. The release of GHRH and somatostatin is tightly regulated, integrating stimuli from the body (such as the level of IGF-1) with signals such as stress, which can modulate the release of hGH.

hGH secretion is closely associated with sleep; in deep sleep, bursts of hGH release are commonly seen at 1- to 2-hour intervals. In addition, fat, carbohydrate and protein metabolites suppress the secretion of hGH. Other hormones are also crucial in the regulation of hGH secretion:

- Cortisol inhibits hGH secretion to prevent the extra strains of growth under prolonged stress.
- Sex hormones are associated with increased hGH secretion.

Actions on target organs

As the name suggests human growth hormone promotes the tissue growth. Much of this is achieved through the actions of IGF-1, although

 CLINICAL Growth hormone-secreting tumours

Growth hormone-secreting tumours result in excessive tissue growth, although the nature of this growth varies with the age of the individual. There are some common symptoms of a growth hormone-secreting tumour at any age, e.g. blurred vision as a result of pressure on the optic nerve, headaches and excessive sweating. The presence of the tumour may displace cells secreting other pituitary hormones, leading to mild deficiencies. The presence of hGH increases glucose in the blood and leads to prolonged elevated insulin levels that promote the development of type 2 diabetes.

In a pubescent individual, a growth hormone secreting tumour can lead to continued growth of the long bones, such that affected individuals may be over 7 feet tall.

In the adult, as the growth plates have fused, lengthening of the long bones cannot occur, although the soft tissues become enlarged and the bones of the hands and feet thicken. This condition is known as **acromegaly**.

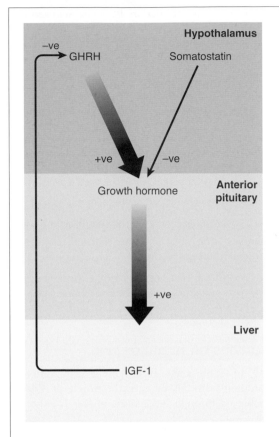

Hypothalamus

GHRH   Somatostatin

−ve

+ve   −ve

Growth hormone   **Anterior pituitary**

+ve

Liver

IGF-1

GHRH

The hypothalamus produces two signals that influence the growth hormone axis. Growth hormone-releasing hormone (GHRH) is negatively related to insulin-like growth factors (IGFs). Somatostatin can also be released by the hypothalamus to modulate the growth hormone cycle. Both GHRH and somatostatin release can be modulated as a result of activity in other centres of the brain, reflecting circadian rhythms and stress, for example.

Growth hormone

Growth hormone (hGH) is released from the anterior pituitary in response to GHRH; it is inhibited by somatostatin. In addition, IGFs can act directly on the anterior pituitary to reduce hGH release. hGH is carried around the body with around 50% bound to growth hormone binding protein. This reduces its excretion by the kidney, pronging its half-life. hGH may act directly to increase blood sugar and promote tissue growth.

IGF-1

Growth hormone acts on the liver to promote the release of IGFs. These act with hGH to promote tissue growth and increase blood glucose. IGFs also promote cartilage growth; they regulate the growth hormone axis by negatively inhibiting its activity at all levels.

Figure 10.5 Schematic representation of the control of growth hormone and insulin-like growth factor 1 (IGF-1) production and the role of negative feedback.

there are also direct actions of hGH, many of which are basically antagonistic to insulin:

- **Increased breakdown of fatty acids**, to release energy stores from adipose tissue for use
- **Increased transport of amino acids** to muscle and liver for increased protein synthesis
- **Reduction in the transport and metabolism of glucose** through reducing insulin receptor expression
- **Increased fibroblast differentiation** into adipocytes and chondrocytes to promote the growth of bone.

hGH receptors are single-chain protein molecules on the surface of the cell membrane which dimerise and bind a hGH molecule. On binding a molecule of hGH, the receptors recruit the tyrosine kinase JAK2, which triggers a cascade of phosphorylation reactions within the cell.

 CLINICAL Loss of growth hormone

hGH levels decrease with age, and produce few obvious symptoms. In younger individuals loss of hGH can lead to a decrease in growth rate and decrease in metabolism, causing increased body fat and decreased muscle strength. This leads to a characteristic short, fat appearance. Treatment of hGH deficiency is through giving hGH by injection.

Insulin-like growth hormone

Synthesis and secretion

IGF-1 is a polypeptide hormone with a high degree of homology with insulin. It is produced by the liver and exists in equilibrium in the blood between free hormone and those molecules bound to plasma protein, with the free unbound form being responsible for the activity of the hormone. There are also IGF-binding proteins in the tissues that maintain high local concentrations.

Actions on target organs

IGF-1 binds to a receptor that is closely related to the insulin receptor – insulin and IGF-1 can bind and weakly activate each other's receptors. The IGF-1 receptor signals through tyrosine kinase activity. IGF-1 acts on almost every tissue in the body to stimulate proliferation and differentiation. Major mechanisms by which this occurs include:

- **increases in glucose intake** into the tissues (in particular, the muscles)
- **stimulation of protein synthesis** within the muscles
- synergy of IGF-1 with hGH to **promote long bone growth** within children
- after puberty stimulation by IGF-1 of **appositional growth** of the long bones.

IGF-1 has many insulin-like effects, partly through actions on its own receptor, but also through partial activation of the insulin receptor.

Prolactin

Prolactin is secreted by the mammotroph cells of the pituitary. It is important in breast development and regulating milk production. In men and non-pregnant women prolactin appears to have little function. There are three major structures involved in the regulation and function of prolactin:

1 Hypothalamus
2 Mammotrophs of the anterior pituitary
3 Breasts.

Dopamine

The regulation of prolactin is through the release of dopamine from the hypothalamus. Unlike other pituitary hormones, prolactin is under a **dominant negative control** by dopamine. Stimuli such as suckling and pregnancy trigger prolactin release through inhibiting hypothalamic dopamine production. Prolactin acts through a tyrosine kinase-linked receptor, triggering development of breast

tissue and milk production. Prolactin also acts on the pituitary gland and the gonads to reduce the probability of pregnancy.

 CLINICAL Prolactinoma

Prolactin-secreting tumours are the most common form of pituitary tumour. They often present with vision problems, due to impingement on the optic nerves, as well as headaches. The high secretion of prolactin may lead to unwanted milk production in both sexes, and irregular menstruation in women and impotence in men.

Treatment is usually with bromocryptine, a dopamine agonist that inhibits the secretion of prolactin. If drug treatment fails, a surgical or radiological intervention is usually required.

The pancreas and diabetes

The pancreas is a large secretory gland in the abdomen, having both exocrine and endocrine functions:

- Most pancreatic cells have an **exocrine** function. They produce digestive enzymes that enter the duodenum at the ampulla of Vater. The exocrine pancreas is discussed in Chapter 8 in relation to digestion.
- Some 3–5% of cells have an **endocrine** function. These cells aggregate around capillaries, forming islets of Langerhans. A delicate connective tissue capsule surrounds each islet, which can contain up to 3000 cells.

The endocrine pancreas

The major endocrine function of the pancreas is the control of glucose hom0eostasis. Glucose in the body is derived from three sources:

1 **Intestinal absorption** as the result of carbohydrate digestion
2 **Glycogenolysis** – the release of glucose by the breakdown of glycogen
3 **Gluconeogenesis** – the formation of glucose from precursors such as lactate.

The pancreas detects the levels of glucose in the blood and produces insulin, a glucose-lowering hormone, or glucagon, a glucose-raising hormone, as necessary. If levels of glucose are not controlled, as in diabetes mellitus, this can result in **hypo-** or **hyperglycaemia**. The islets compose only 3–5% of the mass of the pancreas, but receive 10–15% of the blood supply. Venous drainage is via the hepatic portal vein, which means that the liver is the major target for the endocrine products of the pancreas and they will reach the liver at much higher concentrations than for the rest of the body.

 CLINICAL Hypoglycaemia

In hypoglycaemia there is an abnormally low level of glucose in the blood. This is due to either:

- excessive use of glucose/external losses or
- deficient endogenous production when there is lack of exogenous delivery, i.e. not making enough glucose when the person hasn't eaten.

Clinically, this results in sweating, hunger, tremor, drowsiness, seizures and eventually coma.

 CLINICAL Diabetic ketoacidosis

This occurs in patients with previously undiagnosed type 1 diabetes, or patients with diabetes who do not comply with their treatment or have an intercurrent illness. Due to insulin deficiency there is **hyperglycaemia** (>11.1 mmol/L) which causes osmotic diuresis, and increased catabolism of fatty acids, resulting in uncontrolled production of ketones. The combination of these two things results in metabolic acidosis. Patients present with symptoms of acidosis – hyperventilation, nausea, vomiting, abdominal pain and eventually coma. They are severely dehydrated. This is a medical emergency and treatment is with urgent fluid and electrolyte replacement as well as insulin.

The islets of Langerhans are made up of four main cell types, each associated with production of a different hormone, which is secreted directly into the bloodstream:

1 **β cells** – make up 60% of the islet mass and produce **insulin**
2 **α cells** – make up 20% of the islet mass and produce **glucagon**
3 **δ cells** – make up <10% of the islet mass and produce **somatostatin**
4 **PP cells** – make up <2% of the islet mass and produce **pancreatic polypeptide.**

Insulin

Synthesis and secretion

Insulin is a polypeptide, produced as the result of the cleavage of proinsulin by prohormone convertase in the β cells and packaged into secretory granules that are stored in the cytoplasm. About 5% of these granules are stored as a readily releasable pool. Insulin secretion occurs in two phases: the first phase is due to stimulation of the readily releasable pool of granules; in the second phase, more granules are recruited and then released. Glucose can also stimulate proinsulin gene transcription.

Triggers and inhibitors of release

Glucose and amino acids stimulate release of insulin. β Cells have a K^+_{ATP}-dependent channel that needs a high ratio of ATP:ADP to open:

- High glucose levels in the blood result in increased glucose uptake into β cells.
- Increased cellular levels of glucose result in increased metabolism, producing ATP.
- Increased levels of ATP causes the K^+_{ATP}-dependent channels to close.
- The decrease in K^+ entering the cells causes depolarisation, triggering the opening of voltage-gated calcium channels.
- Entry of calcium increases exocytosis of the secretory granules containing insulin.

Amino acids act similarly by increasing the ratio ATP:ADP. Other factors sensitise β cells to the levels of glucose in the blood to stimulate the release of insulin. These include **acetylcholine, cholecystokinin** (CCK) and **glucagon-like peptide** (GLP).

Actions on target organs

Insulin has a wide range of actions, all of which work to promote anabolism and lower plasma glucose levels (Table 10.2).

Diabetes mellitus

Diabetes mellitus refers to the illness resulting from inappropriate blood glucose control. This

Table 10.2 The range of actions of insulin

Insulin	Carbohydrate metabolism	Lipid metabolism	Protein metabolism
Increases uptake	Glucose uptake into adipose tissue and muscle	Triglyceride uptake into adipose tissue and muscle	Amino acid transport into tissues
Increases synthesis	Glycogen in adipose tissue, muscle and liver	Fatty acids and triacylglycerols	Protein in muscle
Increases rate	Glycolysis in adipose tissue and muscle	Cholesterol synthesis in liver	
Decreases rate	1 Glycogen breakdown 2 Rate of gluconeogenesis	1 Lipolysis in adipose tissue 2 Fatty oxidation in muscle and liver 3 Ketogenesis	1 Protein degradation in muscles 2 Urea formation

differs from diabetes insipidus, which is due to a defect in ADH signalling. Diabetes is chronic hyperglycaemia as the result of either deficient insulin production (type 1) or resistance to the actions of insulin at the target organs, potentially with some impaired production (type 2). Deficient levels of insulin mean that plasma glucose levels are high and the body is unable to adequately store glucose or decrease the production of glucose. It can be divided into **type 1** and **type 2 diabetes** which have common symptoms:

- **Polyuria** (increased urination): blood glucose levels exceed the renal threshold (9–10 mmol/L), resulting in loss of glucose in the urine and therefore osmotic diuresis.
- **Polydipsia** (increased thirst) due to the loss of fluid and electrolytes in the urine.
- **Weight loss** due both to fluid depletion and to increased breakdown of fat and muscle.

Patients with diabetes are likely to experience chronic hyperglycaemia. This increases the risk of staphylococcal infections, retinopathy, polyneuropathy, erectile dysfunction and arterial disease.

 CLINICAL Type 1 diabetes

This normally presents in younger patients around the time of puberty (it is therefore also known as juvenile-onset diabetes). It occurs as a result of an autoimmune reaction against the pancreatic β cells, and has a genetic predisposition. Patients present with polyuria, polydipsia and weight loss, and may present acutely with **ketoacidosis**, because they are using fatty acids as an alternative energy source.

 CLINICAL Type 2 diabetes

This normally presents in patients over the age of 40, but is being diagnosed in increasingly younger people and is associated with obesity and a family history. Insulin can bind normally to target cells, but abnormal cell signalling (possibly partly as a result of obesity) means that the cells are insulin resistant. Eventually, the pancreas is unable to secrete enough insulin to overcome this resistance, resulting in loss of β cells and insulin deficiency. Insulin resistance in these patients means that treatment with insulin will eventually have no effect; the first-line treatment is with oral hypoglycaemics, such as metformin, sulphonylureas and glitazones).

 CLINICAL Hyperosmolar non-ketotic state (HONK)

Severe hyperglycaemia that develops without ketosis can typically occur in type 2 diabetes – this is probably because, in these cases, insulin levels are sufficient to inhibit hepatic ketogenesis. Patients present with dehydration, confusion or coma.

Glucagon

Glucagon is a polypeptide produced by α cells in the islets, and has antagonistic effects to insulin.

Synthesis and secretion

Proglucagon in the pancreas is cleaved to produce glucagon. In the intestine it is cleaved to produce **GLP-1**.

CLINICAL Treatment of diabetes

- **Diet**: patients should eat complex carbohydrates (e.g. potatoes, pasta) which are absorbed relatively slowly, so that there aren't rapid fluctuations in blood sugar. For the same reason meals should be spread equally throughout the day. In other respects the diet should be similar to a normal healthy diet. Dietary regulation is important in both forms of diabetes, and in type 2 may be sufficient in itself to provide adequate glucose control.
- **Sulphonylureas** act to close the K^+_{ATP}-sensitive channels in the β cells, stimulating insulin release, and can be used in patients who still have functioning β cells (i.e. some patients with type 2 diabetes). Sulphonylureas are well tolerated although they can cause hypoglycaemia.
- **Metformin** acts to decrease gluconeogenesis and also to increase insulin sensitivity; it is useful in patients with type 2 diabetes. It also lowers levels of low-density lipoproteins (LDLs) and very-low-density lipoproteins (VLDLs). There are few side effects, although there is a risk of gastrointestinal (GI) disturbance and lactic acidosis.
- **Insulin** injections can be long acting or short acting depending on the preparation. In type 1 diabetes insulin replaces that produced by the β cells. In type 2 diabetes it supplements the natural release from the remaining functional β cells.
- **Thiazolidinediones** (glitazones) act on the peroxisome proliferator-acitvated receptor-γ (PPARγ) and trigger increased glucose uptake in muscle and decreased hepatic glucose output. They also trigger increased expression of insulin-signalling genes.

Triggers and inhibitors of release

In contrast to insulin, which is stimulated by high blood glucose, glucagon production is **stimulated by low levels of glucose**.

Actions at target tissues

Glucagon acts mainly in the liver and adipose tissue, with effects directly opposite to those of insulin. In the liver it acts via cAMP to stimulate gluconeogenesis and glycogen breakdown, and decreases glycolysis, so hepatic glucose output is increased. In adipose tissue it increases lipolysis.

Somatostatin

This inhibitory hormone is produced by the δ cells in the islets. In the pancreas it acts to suppress the release of insulin, glucagon and exocrine secretions. Somatostatin is also secreted by the stomach, intestine and hypothalamus, although the precise roles are not well understood.

Triggers of secretion

Secretion is stimulated by meals with high protein, fat and carbohydrate content, and inhibited by insulin.

Action at target organs

Somatostatin has different roles when secreted in different organs:

- In the **pancreas**: inhibits both endocrine and exocrine function
- In the **stomach**: inhibits gastrin release and secretion of acid by the parietal cells
- In the **pituitary**: inhibits the response of somatotroph cells to GHRH.

Pancreatic polypeptide

Pancreatic polypeptide is secreted from the PP cells. This hormone is thought to antagonise the effects of insulin.

Triggers of secretion

Food, exercise and parasympathetic stimulation all trigger release pancreatic polypeptide.

Actions at target organs

PP stimulates production of glucocorticoids (thus antagonising the effects of insulin) and GI motility. It may have similar effects on appetite to neuropeptide Y (NPY) and peptide YY (PYY). It inhibits pancreatic exocrine secretion and gallbladder contraction.

Calcium, phosphate and bone

Calcium is an essential mineral in the body. It has roles including maintenance of membrane stability and regulation of Na^+ permeability of cells, intra- and intercellular signalling, and skeletal mineralisation with phosphate to maintain bone structure.

The adult human body contains approximately 1100 g calcium, 99% of which is deposited in bones and teeth, complexed with phosphate to form hydroxyapatite. The remaining 1% is found mainly in the blood, with a minute amount located intracellularly (in both the ER and the cytoplasm). In normal individuals the range of **serum total calcium is 2.12–2.62 mmol/L**. The concentration of intracellular calcium is much less than this, approximately 0.1 μmol/L. Peak bone mass occurs at about 30 years in women and is then lost at approximately 3% per decade. This increases to 9% per decade postmenopausally. In men, peak bone mass occurs at about 40 years and is lost at approximately 3% per decade throughout the rest of life.

In the blood calcium is found in three forms:

1 **Ionised** (50%) – calcium unbound in the blood
2 **Protein bound** (40%) – of this 80–90% is bound to albumin and the rest to globulins; binding to albumin is sensitive to pH changes
3 **Complexed to citrate and phosphate-forming soluble complexes** (10%).

The regulation of bone is achieved by two cells:

1 **Osteoblasts** are responsible for laying down bone, and as such are associated with locking calcium into the bone matrix.
2 **Osteoclasts** are involved in the breakdown of bone for remodelling and may be responsible for the release of calcium from the bone matrix.

 CLINICAL Hypercalcaemia

The symptoms of hypercalcaemia can be divided into four organ systems:

1 **Nervous system**: fatigue, lethargy, coma, depression, psychosis, decreased concentration
2 **Musculoskeletal**: weakness, bone/joint pain, fractures
3 **Gastrointestinal**: polydipsia, anorexia, nausea, emesis, weight loss, constipation, abdominal pain
4 **Kidneys**: polyuria, nocturia; kidney stones resulting in haematuria and dysuria (this occurs after long-term hypercalcaemia).

 CLINICAL Hypocalcaemia

Hypocalcaemia is clinically a more serious problem than hypercalcaemia. It alters neuromuscular excitability resulting in paraesthesia, seizures and smooth muscle spasm (such as bronchospasm and laryngospasm), and, if severe, may cause confusion and psychosis.

As **phosphate** combines with calcium to form hydroxyapatite, hyperphosphataemia results in decreased levels of ionised calcium. Phosphate is also an essential component of DNA, RNA, ATP, phospholipids and many metabolic intermediates; hypophosphataemia can limit ATP production and cause muscle weakness.

Regulation of calcium and phosphate relies on three hormones, the coordinated action of which regulates both the total body levels and the concentration of those ions present in the blood (Fig. 10.6):

- **Parathyroid hormone** increases Ca^{2+} in the blood.
- **Vitamin D** increases total body Ca^{2+} levels.
- **Calcitonin** decreases Ca^{2+} in the blood.

Parathyroid hormone

This is the principal hormone involved in calcium homoeostasis, acting to normalise low plasma calcium.

Synthesis and secretion

PTH is a polypeptide secreted by the cells of the **parathyroid glands,** which sit posterior to the thyroid. The glands contains chief cells, which secrete PTH. PTH is preformed in the cells and stored until release is triggered through changes in levels of plasma calcium.

Triggers and inhibitors of release

Release of PTH is mainly controlled by the levels of ionised calcium, which are detected by the calcium-sensing receptor (CaSR) in the parathyroid glands:

- Low levels of **ionised calcium** inhibit the CaSR, resulting in secretion of preformed PTH, upregulation of PTH synthesis and decreased

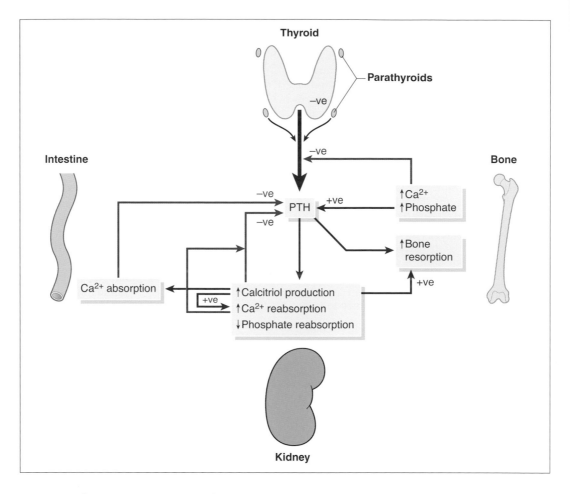

Figure 10.6 Schematic representation of calcium homoeostasis.

intracellular PTH degradation. There is therefore biphasic PTH secretion.

- High levels of **phosphate** increase PTH secretion. This also occurs indirectly as high levels of phosphate will buffer calcium, decreasing calcium levels.
- **Magnesium** regulates PTH secretion in a similar manner (though to a lesser extent) to calcium.

Actions on target cells

PTH has two main target organs:

1 **Bone**
2 **Kidneys**.

Actions of PTH on bone

PTH acts to increase bone resorption for release Ca^{2+} into the blood. Osteoblasts express PTH receptors. Binding of PTH stimulates production of the **RANKL** receptor (also known as the osteoclast differentiating factor or osteoprotegerin ligand). RANKL binds to the **RANK** receptor found on the precursors of osteoclasts, stimulating their differentiation into functional osteoclasts.

At the same time PTH inhibits the production of **osteoprotegerin** by osteoblasts. This soluble protein competes with RANKL to bind to RANK, although it has no effect on binding. The increase in osteoclasts results in increased bone resorption, leading to increased levels of free calcium and phosphate.

Actions of PTH in the kidneys

PTH increases transcellular calcium reabsorption in the distal tubule of the nephrons, through three main actions it:

1 Stimulates insertion and opening of apical calcium channels
2 Decreases renal reabsorption of phosphate by decreasing the expression of a Na^+/phosphate co-transporter
3 Increases 1α-hydroxylase activity, thus upregulating levels of active vitamin D. As vitamin D acts to alter calcium absorption and secretion in the gut, leading to increased absorption, PTH therefore has indirect effects in the gut.

 CLINICAL Hyperparathyroidism

Hyperparathyroidism leads to **hypercalcaemia**:

- **Primary hyperparathyroidism** – inappropriate levels of PTH, commonly due to hyperplasia, adenoma or carcinoma of the parathyroid glands, result in excess secretion of PTH.
- **Secondary hyperparathyroidism** – often occurs in chronic renal failure. Phosphate cannot be excreted renally, so levels of phosphate rise and buffer calcium, resulting in decreased levels of calcium and therefore increased PTH. At the same time renal failure results in loss of 1α-hydroxylation of inactive vitamin D, so calcium levels fall even lower and PTH levels are even more raised. Over time this results in resistance to the effects of PTH and loss of sensitivity of PTH secretion to hypercalcaemia.
- **Hypercalcaemia of malignancy** – PTH-related peptide is secreted by tumours such as breast or lung carcinomas, and mimics the effects of PTH.

CLINICAL Hypoparathyroidism

Hypoparathyroidism – a deficiency in PTH – leads to **hypocalcaemia** and may result from a variety of different causes:

- Acquired (post-thyroidectomy)
- Hereditary (congenitally absent parathyroids, e.g. DiGeorge syndrome)
- Autoimmune destruction
- Hypomagnesaemia (may cause resistance to, and eventually decreased secretion of, PTH).

Pseudohypoparathyroidism can also occur, where there are normal levels of PTH but an inability to respond due to a genetic defect in the PTH receptor.

Vitamin D

Vitamin D and its related molecules are responsible for regulating total body calcium and promoting the mineralisation of bone, to store calcium and phosphate in hydroxyapatite. The active form of vitamin D is **calcitriol**.

Synthesis and secretion

Calcitriol is synthesised in a series of stages:

- **Ergocalciferol** which is obtained either from plants, fatty fish and fortified milk, or as a result of the action of UV light on **cholesterol-derived precursors** in the skin
- This inactive precursor is transported to the **liver** where it is 25-hydroxylated by 25-hydroxylase to **25-hydroxyvitamin D or 25(OH)-vitamin D_3**. This is the major circulating form of vitamin D.
- In the **kidney** this is hydroxylated to **calcitriol** (active vitamin D) – $1,25(OH)_2$ vitamin D_3 – by **1α-hydroxylase** which is regulated to control calcitriol levels.

Triggers and inhibitors of release

An increase in ionised calcium inhibits the second hydroxylation step, blocking calcitriol production. Conversely **low levels of ionised calcium stimulate PTH production**, which in turn increases the activity of 1α-hydroxylase. Calcitriol feeds back to depress 1α-hydroxylase activity.

Actions on target cells

Calcitriol acts via altering gene expression to:

- **stimulate calcium reabsorption** from the intestine and kidney distal tubules
- **stimulate bone resorption** (via osteoblastic production of RANKL)
- repress transcription and secretion of PTH.

Calcitonin

Calcitonin is a peptide hormone that acts to normalise **high** levels of ionised calcium in the blood.

Secretion

Calcitonin is produced by the parafollicular cells (C-cells) of the thyroid gland.

CLINICAL Vitamin D deficiency

Vitamin D deficiency may be due to poor diet, lack of sunlight, malabsorption or liver/renal disease, and results in hypocalcaemia. Patients have vague symptoms of bone pain and muscle aches, as well increased susceptibility to fractures, high bone turnover and bone loss or deformity. The deficiency has different names (and different features) depending on the age of onset:

- If this occurs **before the epiphyseal plates** fuse (i.e. in childhood) it is called **rickets**
- In **adults** it is **osteomalacia**.

Osteomalacia may also result from calcium or phosphate deficiency.

CLINICAL Excess vitamin D

Excessive intake or excess production (rarely by lymphomas, or in granulomatous disease) of vitamin D results in hypercalcaemia, calcification of soft tissues and renal impairment.

Triggers and inhibitors of secretion

Increases in plasma calcium act on the CaSR of the parafollicular cells to stimulate the release of calcitonin.

Actions on target organs

Calcitonin acts on osteoclasts to inhibit motility, differentiation and secretory activity, thus decreasing bone resorption. The **role of calcitonin has been shown not to be essential**; total removal of the thyroid does not alter calcium homoeostasis. Similarly, calcitonin-secreting tumours have no major effect on calcium levels.

Other hormones

- **Androgens and oestrogens** decrease bone resorption and increase osteoprotegerin synthesis.

- **Growth hormone** stimulates proliferation and differentiation of osteoblasts and bone protein synthesis.
- **IGF-1** increases proliferation of osteoblast precursors.
- **Thyroid hormone** increases bone resorption.
- **Glucocorticoids** increase bone resorption and decrease bone synthesis, possibly by inhibition of **osteoprotegerin**.

CLINICAL Paget's disease

Paget's disease is a localised disease of bone that results in an imbalance between bone formation and resorption, occurring mainly in the pelvis, vertebrae, skull, mandible and tibia.

Treatment aims to relieve bone pain and gives drugs such as bisphosphonates, which prevent bone resorption. Finally, diet is monitored to ensure that the patient is receiving adequate calcium.

CLINICAL Osteoporosis

Osteoporosis is a condition in which there is decreased bone mass and deterioration of bone tissue resulting in increased bone fragility and fracture risk.

Osteoporosis most commonly occurs in ageing women, as a result of decreased oestrogen levels. Other endocrine disorders may also result in osteoporosis (e.g. Cushing's disease) and giving corticoids can induce osteoporosis.

Treatment uses the administration of drugs to reduce bone resorption (e.g. bisphosphonates) and those to stimulate bone formation, most commonly oestrogen.

 RELATED CHAPTERS

Chapter 4   Physiology
Chapter 5   Pharmacology
Chapter 11 Integrative physiology

Integrative physiology

The organ systems function in concert to maintain homoeostasis. Disturbance of a single variable typically results in a complex and coordinated response involving many systems to regulate the change. Different systems use varied mechanisms to regulate this change, with different time courses of response.

Blood serves as the unifying factor in many regulatory systems; it provides a reservoir of nutrients and a site to remove waste, and it can be altered by all the organ systems in the body.

The individual organ systems and their physiology have been discussed previously. This chapter discusses the control of responses requiring the coordinated and integrated function of several organ systems.

Blood pressure

Blood pressure must be regulated: if it is too high, there is serious risk of damage to the cardiovascular system due to the additional strain imposed; if it is too low, adequate perfusion of the organs becomes impossible. The mechanisms regulating blood pressure respond to both changes in the requirements of the tissues and the total work imposed on the cardiovascular system, while ensuring that appropriate perfusion is maintained. Two circulatory systems exist in the body, arranged in series:

1 The systemic circulation
2 The pulmonary circulation.

This arrangement ensures that blood oxygenated in the pulmonary capillary beds is carried to the systemic circulation. Changes in the perfusion of one circulatory system directly impact on the performance of the other.

In each circulatory system, almost all capillary beds are arranged in parallel. A single red blood cell passes through one capillary bed in a circulatory system before entering the other circulation (the exception being the portal systems and shunt vessels). Each capillary bed is afforded some independent control of its perfusion, over which systemic regulation is imposed. The blood flow through each capillary bed is regulated by two major factors:

1 **Local control mechanisms** responding to the needs of the tissue
2 **Systemic regulation of circulation** to ensure that there is adequate pressure in the whole circulation so that all tissue beds can be perfused.

The effects of local changes on cardiac output

Independent of systemic factors controlling the blood pressure, the cardiac output of the two sides of the heart is intrinsically linked. The heart receives the total blood which flows through all the capillary beds of the systemic circulation. This return must be pumped by the right-hand side of the heart to the pulmonary circulation. Starling's law ensures that the heart pumps all the venous return to the pulmonary arteries – the volume of blood expelled in a single contraction increases as venous return

Biomedical Science Lecture Notes, First Edition. Ian Lyons.
© 2011 by Ian Lyons. Published 2011 by Blackwell Publishing Ltd.

increases. In normal people, this effect is a relatively minor mechanism of regulating blood pressure, because neurological mechanisms ensure that the dominant effect of increased venous return is through an increase in cardiac output.

Short-term regulation of systemic blood pressure

The systemic blood pressure is regulated by a variety of mechanisms, which control it in the short and long term. There are three steps in the short-term regulation of blood pressure (Fig. 11.1):

1 Detection of changes in blood pressure, volume and composition
2 Central control and processing
3 Effector mechanisms.

Detection of changes in blood pressure and composition

Blood pressure is determined through a series of different factors:

- **Total peripheral resistance** is determined by the contraction of the arterioles.
- **Cardiac output** is governed by the force generated by the heart

Three types of receptor have been identified providing information on the volume and pressure of the blood:

1 High-pressure receptors
2 Low-pressure receptors
3 Chemoreceptor: these are involved in the regulation of blood pressure through sensing the

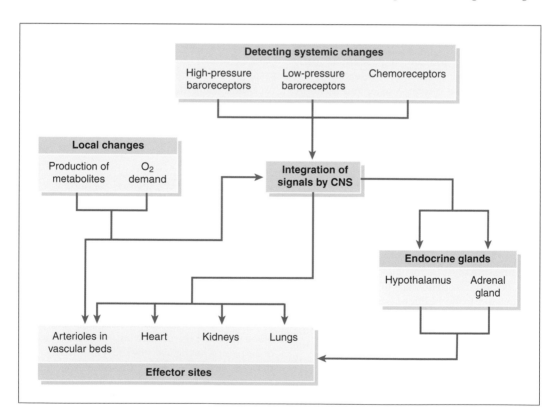

Figure 11.1 Blood pressure is regulated as a result of sensing both local and systemic changes. The local changes in the tissue beds can directly alter their perfusion, and contribute to a change in blood pressure. Systemic changes, in terms of pressure and composition of the blood, are detected at various sites and integrated in the central nervous system (CNS). The CNS innervates many organs that modulate their function to alter blood pressure directly or, in the case of the lungs, can modulate ventilation to alter O_2 and CO_2; this, in turn, can alter the composition of blood. The CNS can also stimulate the hypothalamus and adrenal gland, modulating the behaviour of the various effector systems.

composition of blood gases; it is used as a measurement of the metabolic demands of the tissues.

High-pressure arterial baroceptors

Arterial baroceptors are the major detectors of systemic changes in blood pressure. These clusters of nerve fibres fire in response to stretch of the blood vessels to which they are attached. They are extremely sensitive and discharge with each heart beat, detecting both changes in the blood pressure and the rate at which this change occurs. High-pressure baroceptors are found in two locations:

1 The **carotid sinus**, at the bifurcation of the common carotids to the internal and external vessels. Innervation is through a branch of the glossopharyngeal nerve and the fibres project to the nucleus tractus solitarius in the brain stem.
2 Those at the **arch of the aorta** are innervated by the vagus nerve. The nerve fibres project to the nucleus tractus solitarius.

Low-pressure baroceptors

These receptors can, in effect, detect the effective circulating volume of the blood. This is achieved through a series of low-pressure baroceptors located in the atria and the pulmonary circulation. The best understood low-pressure receptors are those found in the right atrium. These are made up of two types of fibre derived from the vagus nerve (cranial nerve X) which are found within the walls of the right atrium. The 'A' and 'B' fibres respond to different stimuli:

- **'A' fibres respond to contraction of the atrium**, providing a measure of heart rate
- **'B' fibres respond to distension of the atrium**, providing a measure of the venous return to the heart.

Chemoreceptors in the regulation of blood pressure

Peripheral and central chemoreceptors detect changes in the composition of blood gases and act to stimulate an increase in blood pressure and heart rate, to maintain adequate perfusion of the tissues with oxygenated blood, while removing CO_2 to the lungs so that it can be removed from the body.

Peripheral chemoreceptors sense changes in blood pH, CO_2 and O_2, and project this information to the medulla. Peripheral chemoreceptors are especially sensitive to low O_2 and are found in two locations:

1 The **carotid bodies** are found at the bifurcation of the internal and external carotids, innervated by cranial nerve IX.
2 **Aortic bodies** are found in the aortic arch at the angle between the right subclavian and carotid arteries, and under the concavity of the aortic arch, innervated by cranial nerve X.

The **central chemoreceptors** are located in the medulla of the brain and primarily detect changes in pH in the cerebrospinal fluid (CSF), which are associated with changes in PCO_2.

Central areas regulating blood pressure

The inputs from the high- and low-pressure baroceptors project to the nucleus tractus solitarius (NTS) in the brain stem. The cardiovascular centres are located in the ventrolateral part of the medulla, where they receive interneurons from the NTS, as well as signals from the hypothalamus to provide information on the internal state of the body, and from higher centres as well. Many regions can be determined in the cardiovascular centres, in particular:

- The **vasomotor area** is concerned with the regulation of vasoconstriction. The neurons fire tonically to maintain normal vessel tone; as a result, inhibition of the vasomotor centre can trigger vasodilatation.
- The **cardioinhibitory area** of the medulla decreases the heart rate when stimulated.
- The **cardioacceleratory area** increases heart rate.

Effector mechanisms

The neurons projecting from the cardiovascular centres send efferent signals through the sympathetic and parasympathetic nervous systems; these systems focus on short-term regulation through upregulation of the heart rate and contraction.

Sympathetic output occurs through the sympathetic chain and the prevertebral ganglia and produces a number of responses:

- Vasoconstriction of the arterioles, via noradrenaline release

- Increase in cardiac contraction and rate, via noradrenaline release
- Release of adrenaline from the adrenal medulla.

Parasympathetic output produces the opposite effect to that of the sympathetic nervous system. It acts through fibres in the vagus nerve to decrease cardiac rate and contraction.

Vascular reflexes regulating blood pressure

Many processes may secondarily alter the blood pressure. In particular, changes in posture can markedly alter the distribution –and therefore the pressure – of blood. About two-thirds of the blood volume is found in the veins. On standing, venous pooling in the lower limbs will occur unless there is compensation. Venous return will fall, consequently leading to a decrease in arterial blood pressure. The pooling of blood in the limbs would lead to less being returned to the heart, preventing atrial filling. A number of factors mediate this **orthostatic response**:

- The **blood vessels are not uniformly distensible**. The small veins are less distensible than the larger veins. The stiffness of the blood vessels is further regulated by the contraction of smooth muscle in the venous walls to improve venous return.
- **Venous blood pools in the legs** under the influence of gravity. The contraction of the skeletal muscles in the limbs, coupled to the valves present in the veins, promotes return to counteract this. Further movements result in further action of the muscle pumps helping venous return.
- **Autonomic reflexes**: cardiac output tends to fall by around 20% when one stands, decreasing right atrial pressure and also stroke volume. This is, in turn, detected by the high-pressure baroceptors as a decrease in arterial pressure. The resulting response triggers a generalised sympathetic output that raises the vascular tone throughout the body (including venous tone) and increases heart rate and contraction. The net effect is a return of the mean arterial pressure.

Long-term regulation of blood pressure

There are two major factors that regulate blood pressure in the long term:

1 Vascular tone
2 Fluid balance.

Regulation of vascular tone

A variety of signals act in paracrine and endocrine manners to regulate the tone of smooth muscle:

- **Adrenaline** released from the adrenal medulla, in the sympathetic response, acts predominantly on the β_2-receptors found on skeletal smooth muscle to trigger vasodilatation. However, through its actions on α-adrenoceptors on the splanchnic blood vessels, it has the opposite effect, triggering vasoconstriction
- **Angiotensin II** is produced as part of the renin–angiotensin–aldosterone pathway and is a powerful vasoconstrictor. Angiotensin II also modulates fluid balance.
- **Atrial natriuretic peptide** (ANP) is released from the atrial cells in response to stretch. It acts as a vasodilator, in addition to its role in reducing fluid volume by promoting Na^+ and water excretion.
- **Antidiuretic hormone** (ADH; also known as Arginine Vasopressin [AVP]) has vasoconstrictive effects, at very high concentrations.

Regulation of fluid volume

Many signals provide information on the circulating volume of blood in the body: the high- and low-pressure baroceptors. As fluid volume is regulated by the actions of the kidneys, they are the major site of long-term regulation of blood pressure.

The primary effector mechanism by which the kidneys regulate fluid volume is through modulating the excretion of Na^+. Four systems are predominantly involved in this regulation, and have been discussed in Chapter 9:

1 The renin–angiotensin–aldosterone system
2 Autonomic stimulation of the kidneys
3 Antidiuretic hormone
4 Atrial natriuretic peptide.

Pharmacological control of hypertension

There are a number of sites that can be targeted to manage blood pressure (although most current therapies target three and four):

1 The **baroceptors** sensing changes in blood pressure
2 The **central areas** coordinating the cardiovascular response
3 The **effector mechanism** of the heart and vasculature
4 Regulation of **blood fluid volume**.

1 Inhibition of the sympathetic response
2 Mimicking and promoting the actions of the parasympathetic response
3 Direct antagonism of the intracellular calcium or prevention of Ca^{2+} entry into cells.

CLINICAL **Hypertension**

Hypertension is a chronically high blood pressure – typically described as a pressure higher than 140/90 mmHg. It is associated with a number of pathological changes. In particular, the additional stress can damage the endothelium and promote arteriosclerosis. Furthermore, hypertension predisposes to myocardial infarction, heart failure, stroke and coronary artery disease.

In most cases, people have 'primary (essential) hypertension' when there is no identifiable specific cause. In rare cases there is 'secondary hypertension', when an underlying cause for the hypertension can be identified and correction of the underlying pathology results in correction of the blood pressure. A major cause of secondary hypertension is **renal artery stenosis**, where there is reduced perfusion of the kidneys, due to a blockage of the renal artery. This triggers the kidney to increase the blood pressure because it is unable to distinguish the localised loss of perfusion from a systemic loss of pressure.

Modulation of baroceptor function

To date there are no therapies that modulate the behaviour of the baroceptors to regulate blood pressure.

Modulation of central coordinating areas

The cells in the central cardiovascular areas are rare targets of antihypertensive medication: cells in these regions express presynaptic α_2-adrenoceptors, which inhibit vasomotor function. Administration of the α_2 agonist, **clonidine**, can be used to reduce blood pressure.

The cells in the vasomotor areas express **imidazoline** receptors which, when activated, inhibit vasomotor areas. The I_1-receptor agonist **moxonidine** can be used as a treatment for hypertension. Moxonidine has fewer side effects than α_2-adrenoceptor agonists.

Regulation of mechanisms of the heart and vasculature

Pharmacological modulation of blood pressure can be divided into three areas of treatment:

Inhibition of the actions of the sympathetic nervous system

The catecholamines released by the sympathetic nerves and the adrenal gland cause constriction of the blood vessels and increase heart rate and contraction. In addition, activation of β_1-adrenoceptors in the kidneys promotes renin release to activate the renin–angiotensin–aldosterone system. Two main classes of adrenoceptor antagonist are used to treat hypertension:

β Blockers

β Blockers (e.g. propanolol) antagonise the β-adrenoceptors found in the heart. At rest, they have little effect, although the reduce the ability of the sympathetic system to increase heart rate. β Blockers have a gradual effect on the cardiovascular system, leading to a **reduction in cardiac output and blood pressure**, and on the kidney to **reduce the production of renin**. As β-adrenoceptors are not involved in regulating the orthostatic reflex, postural hypotension is not seen in patients on β blockers.

β Blockers are not without side effects. **Fatigue** is common and in patients with heart failure the sympathetic drive may be essential to maintain cardiac output. There is also some **bronchoconstriction**, which can be problematic in people with severe asthma because the β blocker may antagonise the action of bronchodilators (e.g. salbutamol).

α_1-Adrenoceptor antagonists

α_1-Adrenoceptor antagonists (e.g. prazosin) inhibit the noradrenaline-mediated contraction of the arterioles, which occurs through α_1-adrenoceptors on vascular smooth muscle. These drugs also decrease LDL levels and increase high-density lipoprotein (HDL) levels, reducing the risk of atherosclerosis.

There are some side effects of α_1-antagonists: the inhibition of vasoconstriction promotes the occurrence of **postural hypotension**. **Impotence** is another side effect.

Mimicking the parasympathetic response

The parasympathetic response that triggers vasodilatation is complex. Parasympathetic fibres innervate the endothelial cells of some blood vessels. They release acetylcholine (ACh) which binds muscarinic (M_3)-receptors on the muscle cells to trigger an increase in Ca^{2+}. This stimulates the production of a variety of endothelial factors. Of particular importance is the gaseous mediator nitric oxide (NO) which diffuses to nearby vascular muscle cells, where it triggers a cGMP-mediated pathway activating the PKG (cGMP-dependent protein kinase), which, in turn decreases Ca^{2+} in the muscle cells, reducing contraction.

NO donors are a common treatment of hypertension; both glycerol trinitrate and sodium nitroprusside release NO into the body to stimulate vasodilatation. It is also thought that the coronary arteries are particularly dilated to increase the perfusion of the cardiac tissue.

Direct antagonism of intracellular calcium

Contraction of muscle is linked to increased intracellular calcium levels and many therapies target this effect. They act to inhibit the L-type Ca^{2+} channel on the cell surface, reducing calcium entry into the cell and limiting induced calcium release from the sarcoplasmic reticulum. Targeting different tissues lowers blood pressure by different mechanisms:

- Antagonism of intracellular Ca^{2+} in the heart reduces contraction and work done.
- Antagonism of intracellular Ca^{2+} in the arterioles reduces vascular tone and directly reduces blood pressure.

Different classes of Ca^{2+} antagonists favour different tissues:

- **Dihydropyridines** (e.g. nifedipine) act predominantly on the vascular smooth muscle.
- **Phenylalkylamines** (e.g. verapamil) act predominantly on the heart tissue.
- **Benzothiazepines** (e.g. diltiazem) has an effect on both tissues.

Calcium antagonists may have antiarrhythmic effects although they are also linked to atrioventricular block, because they can act on conducting tissues in the heart. Despite inhibition of contraction in the heart, the total cardiac output is relatively unchanged due to the decreased resistance against which the heart must work.

Reducing fluid volume

The volume of fluid in the cardiovascular system can vary; greater volumes of fluid place additional demands on the heart. Fluid volume is regulated by the kidneys, which sense changes in the composition of the blood and respond to direct measures of fluid volume through the release of circulating hormones such as ADH and ANP. It the **effective circulating volume**, and not the actual blood volume, that is regulated.

In individuals with hypertension, the renin–angiotensin–aldosterone system is often targeted because it not only reduces fluid volume, but also decreases vasoconstriction. The major pharmacological target in this pathway is the angiotensin-converting enzyme (ACE).

Heart failure

Heart failure occurs when cardiac output is no longer sufficient to supply the metabolic demands of the body. Failure begins with insufficiency during exercise, although it progresses so that the heart is unable to meet demand during rest. Heart failure may be caused by pathology in the myocardium (usually ischaemic heart disease), or circulatory defects. The prognosis for those with heart failure is poor. Those with serious heart failure are unlikely to survive more than 6 months and 50% of individuals with milder heart failure may be dead within 5 years.

Progression of heart failure

As cardiac output decreases in the affected side of the heart, it causes a backlog of fluid to build up in the venous system of the opposite circulation: serious failure of the left side of the heart may result in **pulmonary oedema** because the left heart is unable to clear the venous return quickly enough. Increased fluid volume may occur as a result of the reduced renal blood flow, stimulating the **renin–angiotensin–aldosterone axis** to retain Na^+, with consequent retention of H_2O.

Classification of heart failure

The severity of heart failure can be classified with regard to the physical limitations of the patient; the New York Heart Association (NYHA) classification is used for heart failure because it is a good indicator of prognosis:

- Class I – no physical symptoms and no apparent limitation of physical exertion. Symptoms of heart failure are diagnosable by imaging (e.g. chest radiograph).
- Class II – symptoms present during physical activity, not affected under ordinary activity.

- Class III – symptoms manifest under ordinary activity.
- Class IV – unable to perform any activity without symptoms.

Treatment of heart failure

Treatment of heart failure is through the management of symptoms. The therapies used do not have a significant effect on correcting the underlying pathology:

- **Diuretics** reduce fluid volume.
- **Vasodilators** reduce the resistance against which the heart must pump. Nitrates donate NO to trigger vasodilatation whereas ACE inhibitors act through both inhibition of vasodilatation and reduction in fluid retention by the renin–angiotensin–aldosterone axis.
- **β Blockers** may be added to reduce the work that the heart does, limiting the damaging effects of sympathetic stimulation on the failing heart.
- **Cardiac glycosides** increase the contractile force of the heart without significantly increasing its metabolic demands. These are often used in patients with chronic atrial fibrillation or who have not responded sufficiently to treatment with ACE inhibitors and diuretics. Although cardiac glycosides do little to improve mortality, it improves the symptoms and reduces hospital admissions.

Shock

Shock is inadequate perfusion of the body's organs. It is a medical emergency with a high mortality, even at specialist centres. In a normal physiological response, the vasculature supplying essential organs will dilate to increase blood flow if they are inadequately perfused. In shock, this response can contribute to a further lowering of the blood pressure – the hypoxia of the tissues leads to the release of many vasodilatory mediators which cause both capillary dilatation and increased vascular permeability. There are many causes of shock and they share similar symptoms:

- Shortness of breath and oedema
- Fatigue
- Cyanosis
- Enlarged heart
- Low blood pressure.

Shock may have one of many underlying causes, including:

- **Cardiogenic shock** results directly from defective surgery of the heart so that it cannot generate sufficient contractile force, despite adequate filling of the ventricles. The treatment of cardiogenic shock depends on the underlying cause.
- **Hypovolaemic shock** results from an insufficient vascular volume, although significant loss of the circulating blood volume (around 10%) is required. Treatment of hypovolaemic shock focuses on restoring the circulating volume, and repairing the underlying cause (e.g. surgery to repair trauma).
- **Anaphylactic shock** results from the widespread vasodilatation that occurs in a severe allergic (anaphylactic) reaction. Treatment depends on managing the underlying causes, while adrenaline stabilises the blood pressure in the interim.
- **Septic (toxic) shock** results from bacterial infection causing a widespread vasodilatory response. Antibiotics are crucial to clear the infection that causes septic shock; activated protein C also appears to be effective

The response to exercise

Increased physical activity dramatically increases the metabolic demands of the tissues. This exertion requires changes in the distribution and circulation of blood and thermoregulation of the body, as well as greater ventilation to supply sufficient oxygen to the blood and tissues and to clear metabolic products. Exercise can be divided into two types based on the utilisation of oxygen:

1 **Anaerobic respiration** utilises the muscles stores of ATP. Additional ATP can be generated through **use of phosphocreatine** and **glycolysis of glucose** to produce lactate. Fast twitch muscle fibres generate force rapidly through anaerobic respiration and are unable to maintain contraction for more than a few seconds, because their energy stores are rapidly depleted.
2 **Aerobic respiration** is a more efficient means of generating ATP, allowing prolonged exercise, although at a lower rate than is generated from phosphocreatine stores. Aerobic respiration is the dominant form of ATP production in skeletal muscle over prolonged exercise, because it produces fewer toxic by-products.

During exercise, skeletal muscle must use large amounts of ATP for contraction. At rest, skeletal muscle typically uses less than $2\,mL\ O_2/min$, whereas at maximal exercise it can require more than $150\,mL\ O_2/min$. The dominant mechanisms of ATP production during muscle contraction are initially anaerobic:

- Stores of **phosphocreatine** in the muscle are used to regenerate ATP without the need for respiration, although these are very limited and exhausted within seconds.
- **Anaerobic generation of ATP through glycolysis** is also possible in small amounts. The process is extremely inefficient and can be sustained only for a short while, due to the build-up of **lactate** as a by-product.

Longer periods of activity require the generation of ATP by aerobic respiration:

- **Glycogen stores** can be used to generate glucose for aerobic respiration (as well as anaerobic glycolysis). This pathway occurs rapidly through the breakdown of glycogen stores in the muscle.
- **Energy supply during long-term exercise** is through glucose release from the breakdown of glycogen in the liver and fatty acids released from the adipose tissue.

Fatigue in exercise

Over long periods of exercise muscles become fatigued, and are incapable of generating a consistent contractile force. This fatigue results from a decrease in the level of glycogen in the muscle fibres, although the reasons for this leading to fatigue are not entirely clear. Athletes often eat carbohydrate-rich meals before exercise to increase stores of glycogen within the muscle, thus delaying the onset of fatigue. During exercise there are also changes that occur to the plasma levels of lactate and potassium, which can limit exercise:

- **Lactate levels** are low at rest and mild exercise, but rise during intense exercise through anaerobic respiration. Lactate limits exercise because it lowers the pH of the blood and contributes to the pain in fatigue. Training can reduce the amount of lactate produced during exercise, reducing fatigue.
- **Potassium** is released due to the continued cycles of depolarisation of muscle cells. As a result, potassium levels may reach $6-7\,mmol/L$, a level that would be seen as very dangerous at rest. However, the heart appears to be protected during exercise.

Changes in the demands for oxygen during exercise

Oxygen supply to the tissues usually limits the rate of exercise in the long term. Increasing intensity beyond the threshold to where anaerobic respiration predominates rapidly leads to intolerable increases in lactate and potassium. At rest, oxygen consumption is about $250\,mL\ O_2/min$, increasing to more than $3000\,mL/min$ at maximal exercise. Three changes occur to provide the additional oxygen required by the muscle:

1 **Cardiac output increases** so that more oxygenated blood reaches the tissue during a given time period.
2 **Ventilation increases** to allow more oxygen into the blood.
3 **Venous O_2 saturation** falls as the tissue removes more O_2 from the blood. Arterial O_2 saturation is almost maximal at rest, so there is little scope to increase O_2 in the blood by this means.

Changes to the cardiovascular system during exercise

About a fourfold increase in cardiac output can be achieved during exercise through increases in both heart rate and stroke volume. Although heart rate can rise significantly (to around $200\,beats/min$), stroke volume rapidly reaches a maximum (around $130\,mL$) at about a third of maximum ventilation. The cardiac output and the total peripheral resistance are responsible for determining systemic blood pressure:

$$Cardiac\ output \times Total\ (systemic)\ peripheral\ resistance = Blood\ pressure.$$

During exercise, mean blood pressure does not change significantly. Although the cardiac output increases, there is a corresponding decrease in the total peripheral resistance (as a result of the dilatation of the vascular beds in the skeletal muscle). The changes that occur in the vasculature system are twofold, both due to the effects of the sympathetic nervous system:

1 **The vessels in the respiring skeletal muscle dilate** to allow increased blood flow and therefore increased oxygen delivery. Circulating adrenaline and sympathetic stimulation will trigger vasodilatation of the skeletal muscle capillaries through β_2-adrenoceptors.

2 **The vessels in the viscera contract** to maintain some peripheral resistance and an adequate blood pressure through activation of the α_1-adrenoceptors expressed on the vascular smooth muscle.

The effects of sympathetic stimulation on the skeletal muscle capillaries is accentuated by the dilatation induced by local metabolic signals. In exercise the blood passing through the skeletal muscle may increase 20-fold to meet demand.

Changes in the respiratory system

Ventilation increases rapidly with exercise, reflecting increased oxygen usage. At low-intensity exercise additional ventilation is achieved through increases in the tidal volume, whereas at higher-intensity exercise the rate of ventilation also increases significantly. At rest, a blood cell spends about 0.8 seconds in the alveolus. However, during exercise this may be as low as 0.2 seconds (as a result of the fourfold increase in cardiac output). The time taken to equilibrate O_2 between the blood cell and the alveolus is around 0.25 seconds, causing a slight discrepancy in alveolar and arterial PO_2 at high exercise.

In tissues, the additional oxygen gained is O_2 extracted from the red blood cells by the tissue, which is reflected in the lower venous O_2 seen during exercise. At rest:

- PaO_2 is about 100 mmHg (13.3 kPa) and it is similar at exercise
- PvO_2 is about 40 mmHg (5.3 kPa) and will decrease further during exercise.
- $PvCO_2$ is about 50 mmHg (6.7 kPa) and increases during exercise, reflecting the increased respiration in the muscles.
- $PaCO_2$ is about 40 mmHg (5.3 kPa) and decreases during exercise due to the increased ventilation.

Regulation of exercise

Respiratory and cardiovascular systems are controlled by changes detected through the chemoreceptors and the baroceptors, yet in exercise rapid changes are seen faster than would be detected by these systems. This has lead to the definition of three phases in exercise:

1 **Phase I** is characterised by increases in both ventilation and heart rate. This process is centrally controlled and may precede the initiation of exercise.

2 In **phase II** there is a gradual increase in both ventilation and cardiac output to reach a maximum. The responses appear to be driven by the peripheral chemoreceptors and also through afferent signals from the muscles and their release of K^+ and H^+.
3 **Phase III** reflects steady-state exercise where constant high levels of ventilation and cardiac output are seen.

Regulation of pH

All the enzymatic processes in the body require very specific pH values to function optimally. Blood pH is maintained at about 7.4 and must remain between 7.35 and 7.45. Typically, 50 mmol of H^+ is ingested per day and is closely related to the protein (amino acids) ingested. Around 70 mmol of H^+ and 20 mmol of alkali are excreted per day, predominantly through the kidneys and the gut, respectively.

Acids produced in the body can be classed as volatile and non-volatile:

- **Volatile acids refer to CO_2.** This acidic gas is carried in the blood as H_2CO_3 and can be excreted in the lungs by ventilation, without the loss of HCO_3^-.
- **Non-volatile acids are those non-gas-derived acids** produced in metabolism. These are typically through the metabolism of amino acids, leading to the production of H_2SO_4 and HCl. Buffering of non-volatile acids uses HCO_3^- which must be replaced by new production of HCO_3^-.

Three different mechanisms can compensate for changes of pH over different timescales:

1 Buffering of H^+
2 Respiratory regulation of pH
3 Metabolic (renal) regulation of pH.

Buffering reduces the pH change seen through the addition of acid, by reducing the number of free H^+ ions present. However, H^+ must be removed or the buffering becomes progressively less effective.

Buffering of H^+

In the blood H^+ is buffered by bicarbonate. The addition of H^+ leads to the production of H_2O and

CO_2. As a result of this buffering, H^+ can be tightly controlled, although the pH of the blood is also affected by PCO_2 and the concentration of HCO_3^-.

$$H^+ + HCO_3^- \leftrightarrow H_2CO_3 \leftrightarrow H_2O + CO_2.$$

The buffering reaction for H^+ takes place in two stages:

1 The first stage of this reaction, the conversion of H^+ and bicarbonate to carbonic acid, occurs spontaneously and does not require enzymatic catalysis.
2 The second reaction, converting H_2CO_3 to CO_2 and H_2O, is catalysed by the enzyme **carbonic anhydrase**, which is found on the surface of red blood cells.

In addition to bicarbonate, there are other molecules that contribute to a lesser extent to pH buffering, through similar reversible reactions:

• Inorganic phosphate:
$$H^+ + HPO_4^{2-} \leftrightarrow H_2PO_4^-$$

• Ammonia
$$NH_3 + H^+ \leftrightarrow NH_4^+.$$

Regulation of intracellular pH

Intracellular pH is maintained through two processes:

1 **Buffering** by weak acids and proteins similar to that seen in the blood
2 H^+ **transport** across the cell membrane.

Buffering of intracellular pH

Buffering of intracellular pH is similar to that which occurs in the blood, although the actual buffers and their contributions vary slightly. The major molecules accounting for buffering intracellularly are:

• Bicarbonate
• Phosphate
• Amino acids (predominantly histidine).

H^+ transport across the cell membrane

Two transporters contribute to the regulation of H^+ movement across the cell membrane:

1 The **Na^+/H^+ exchanger** extrudes an H^+ ion across the cell membrane by **secondary active transport**, powered by the Na^+ gradient across the membrane.

2 The **HCO_3^-/Cl^- exchanger** is powered by the Cl^- gradient across the cell membrane to extrude HCO_3^-, allowing the retention of H^+ in the cell as an acid-loading mechanism. Furthermore, H^+ inhibits the function of the exchanger, reducing its action in lower pH conditions.

Respiratory regulation of pH

The respiratory system aids regulation of pH through alteration of the CO_2 levels. Removing CO_2 from the blood allows more H^+ to be drawn into the reaction, thus correcting, to some extent, the pH. Although such compensation does not replenish the HCO_3^-, it allows for rapid compensation of pH to a greater extent than if there were a closed buffering system, i.e. one where CO_2 could not be removed from the system.

Regulation of ventilation by pH

As a result of the equilibrium reaction between H^+ and HCO_3^-, which produces CO_2 and H_2O, a lower pH increases ventilation, by increasing CO_2 in two locations, stimulating the respiratory drive:

1 The **central chemoreceptors,** which detect an increase in CO_2 in the CSF
2 The **peripheral chemoreceptors** in the carotid and aortic bodies.

 CLINICAL Respiratory acidosis

Respiratory acidosis results from an inability of the lungs to remove sufficient amounts of CO_2 from the blood. It is associated with **hypoventilation**, either through a decreased respiratory drive or through obstruction of the airways or lung disease. The body can compensate for a respiratory acidosis through the actions of the kidneys, which extrude the additional H^+, although such compensation occurs over several hours or days.

Renal regulation of pH

Although volatile acids can be removed from the blood without using up bicarbonate, non-volatile acids require bicarbonate to neutralise H^+. New bicarbonate must be produced to replace that which is lost, or reclaimed by moving H^+ directly out of the body. The kidneys perform two functions related to the acid–base balance:

1 Reabsorption of filtered HCO_3^-
2 Production of HCO_3^- which is used to buffer non-volatile acids.

Different processes occur in different sections of the nephron tubule:

- HCO_3^- is released into the nephron by ultrafiltration of the blood in the **glomerulus**.
- In the **proximal tubule** most of the HCO_3^- is reabsorbed – about 80%. This is accomplished by H^+ secretion into the nephron (mainly by countertransport with Na^+).
- The **distal tubule** and collecting duct make a smaller contribution to the reabsorption of HCO_3^-, but are important for the secretion of non-volatile acids.

Reabsorption of filtered HCO_3^-

HCO_3^- combines with H^+ in the nephron to form carbonic acid. This is converted to H_2O and CO_2, catalysed by **carbonic anhydrase IV** which is found on the luminal surface of the nephron cells. The resulting H_2O and CO_2 diffuse into the cell where they are reconverted to H^+ and HCO_3^-. The HCO_3^- enters the bloodstream, whereas the H^+ can be reused to reabsorb more HCO_3^- from the lumen. The reabsorbed HCO_3^- is transported across the basolateral membrane, mainly through the actions of the HCO_3^-/Cl^- anion exchanger (Fig. 11.2).

There are three transporters that transport H^+ to the lumen of the nephron for the reabsorption of HCO_3^- or the excretion of H^+:

1 **The Na^+/H^+ exchanger** transports H^+ into the nephron lumen, driven by the Na^+ gradient from the lumen to the cell cytoplasm. In

particular, the NHE3 isoform of the transporter is responsible for most H^+ transport in the kidney.
2 **H^+ATPase** is found mainly in the distal nephron, and can move H^+ against a significant concentration gradient using the energy generated by hydrolysis of ATP. H^+ATPase function and expression appear to be regulated, in part, by aldosterone, which promotes its expression.
3 The **H^+/K^+ exchanger** is mainly found in the collecting duct and extrudes H^+ ions while re-absorbing K^+ ions.

Regeneration of HCO_3^-

HCO_3^-, which neutralises H^+ derived from non-volatile acids, must be regenerated, so that the excess H^+ is retained in the urine and excreted from the body. H^+ is secreted by the same process used in the reclamation of filtered HCO_3^-. However, instead of combining with HCO_3^-, the H^+ combines with either HPO_4^{2-} or NH_3. This occurs mainly in the distal parts of the nephron, where much of the HCO_3^- has already been reclaimed.

Regulation of H^+ secretion

Much of the net acid–base balance in the body can be regulated by the secretion of H^+. This is controlled by intercalated cells, which are classified by the arrangement of their transporters (and hence the direction in which they transport H^+ and HCO_3^-), although they can alter the polarity of

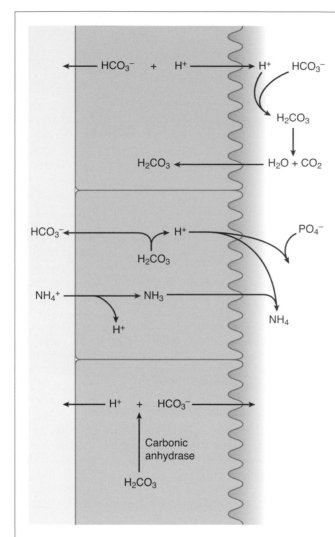

Reabsorption

H_2CO_3 is produced in the tubule from H^+ and HCO_3^- and is converted to CO_2 and H_2O catalysed by carbonic anhydrase. CO_2 can freely diffuse into the cell where it is returned to H^+ and HCO_3^- by an intracellular carbonic anhydrase. While HCO_3 is returned to the bloodstream to replenish the buffering potential, the H^+ can be re-extruded to the tubules, primarily through Na^+/H^+ exchange proteins on the cell surface.

Neutralisation

To remove H^+ from the system it must combine with a urinary buffer other than HCO_3. Typically, H^+ combines with NH_3 or H_2PO_4, because the resulting ions are trapped in the tubule and not transported back into the epithelium. The majority of H^+ from non-volatile acids is processed in this way.

Type B cells

Type B cells possess the same protein systems as found on type A cells but in reverse. This allows removal of HCO_3^- into the urine, and corresponding secretion of H^+ into the blood to lower the blood pH, counteracting alkalotic changes.

Figure 11.2 Non-volatile acids are removed from the body through the kidneys. This process requires the tubular reclamation of bicarbonate (HCO_3^-) filtered by the glomeruli, as well as the removal of H^+ through its tubular secretion and binding to buffers in the tubular fluid. Finally, type B cells excrete HCO_3^- and return H^+ to the blood.

expression of proteins to suit the needs of the nephron:

- **Type A intercalated cells** transport H^+ across their luminal surface and HCO_3^- from their basolateral surface, following generation of both species by the cytoplasmic carbonic anhydrase. This allows them to increase the pH in the blood through the removal of H^+ from the body and the addition of HCO_3^-.
- **Type B intercalated cells** possess the same machinery for acid transport as seen in the type A

cells, although reversed so that the H^+ is transported into the blood, whereas HCO_3^- is transported into the tubule.

The synthesis of ammonia is altered to maintain a steady acid–base balance, through modulation of the amount of H^+ excreted, which alters the pH of the blood.

Diffusion trapping

Diffusion trapping is the mechanism by which H^+ ions are retained in the nephron so that they can be excreted. Ammonia (NH_3) is released into the nephron by diffusion because it is uncharged. In the nephron, it combines with H^+ to form the charged NH_4^+, which cannot diffuse out of the nephron. At physiological conditions, the equilibrium of the reaction is such that more than 99% of ammonia in the nephron exists as NH_4^+ allowing the removal of H^+ from the body. This trapping increases down the nephron, because the decreasing pH drives more generation of NH_4^+, further shifting the equilibrium.

 CLINICAL Metabolic alkalosis

Metabolic alkalosis results from a loss of volatile acid or acquisition of HCO_3^-. This may be caused by loss of acid through vomiting, or as a result of some diuretics or excessive consumption of antacids. As with metabolic acidosis, compensation is through the lungs, although again it is limited due to the lungs' inability to synthesise or remove HCO_3^- directly.

Regulation of potassium

Most K^+ is found intracellularly and results in a gradient that has important physiological roles:

- It accounts for much of the resting membrane potential.
- Movement of K^+ is the driving force behind membrane repolarisation in the action potential.

Intracellular K^+ ions regulate important cellular variables:

- The **osmotic potential of the cell**, and hence the cell volume
- **Enzyme function**
- **Intracellular pH**.

At rest, plasma potassium is typically 4 mmol/L, whereas intracellular K^+ is around 140 mmol/L. The exclusion of Na^+ from cells as a result of the **Na^+/K^+ ATPase** is essentially the cause of the high intracellular K^+.

Normal potassium balance

Potassium is ingested in the diet and absorbed by the gut – around 80 mmol/day is ingested, of which 70 mmol is absorbed. The major loss of K^+ is through the kidneys, where it is used by exchange proteins. K^+ can also be found in many of the

secretions in the body, and a small amount may be lost in sweat, through shedding of skin and through secretion of K^+ in the distal sections of the gut.

 CLINICAL Hyperkalaemia

Hyperkalaemia is defined as a resting plasma potassium concentration >**5 mmol/L**. It is typically caused by renal failure, preventing normal secretion of K^+. Acidosis can also trigger hyperkalaemia (as increased H^+ excretion can result in retention of K^+). The abnormal levels of K^+ in the blood affect many different systems. They:

- **promote cardiac arrhythmia** – prolonged QRS complex and a peaked T wave
- **reduce reabsorption of NaCl** by the kidneys
- **reduce ammonia production**, promoting acidosis
- **increase vasodilatation** leading to hypotension
- **promotes paraesthesia and muscle paralysis**.

Treatment of high K^+ is initially to stabilise the heart through administration of calcium gluconate, and then administration of insulin with glucose and β blockers, both of which promote uptake of K^+ into the tissues. Finally a K^+-binding substance can be used to sequester the K^+ from the blood.

Short-term regulation of K^+

In the short term, K^+ plasma levels can be 'buffered' by movement of K^+ into or out of cells by the concentration gradient, and to some extent by the Na^+/K^+ ATPase, which many hormones regulate:

- **Insulin** increases intracellular potassium through stimulating the function of the Na^+/K^+ ATPase. Related to this, increased extracellular K^+ stimulates insulin release from the β cells.
- **Catecholamines** have differing effects on K^+ handling depending on the receptors through which they act. The $β_2$-receptors stimulate Na^+/K^+ ATPase promoting uptake of K^+, whereas α-adrenoceptors trigger release of K^+ from the liver, which may lead to a transient **hyperkalaemia**. Infusing adrenaline is likely to trigger a mild hyperkalaemia first, as a result of the effects on the α-adrenoceptors, and then a longer hypokalaemia, as a result of the actions on the $β_2$-adrenoceptors.

CLINICAL **Hypokalaemia**

Hypokalaemia is a resting K^+ of **<3.5 mmol/L** which may result from a lack of K^+ in the diet. Many diuretics can trigger loss of K^+ secondary to increased reabsorption of Na^+. Hypokalaemia can have particularly severe consequences on the heart because it hyperpolarises the sinoatrial node cells, resulting in a bradycardia. This hyperpolarisation may also reduce cardiac contraction and result in the heart stopping in diastole. Treatment of hypokalaemia is through increasing K^+ in the diet and, if necessary, infusing K^+-containing solutions.

Processes modulating the regulation of the K^+ balance

There are a number of systems that modulate K^+ levels to maintain the homoeostasis of other variables. As a result, there can be considerable alterations in K^+ levels due to many different factors:

- The **acid–base balance** regulates pH level through the movement of H^+ ions; this often involves movement of K^+ in the opposite direction, particularly in response to inorganic acids. In general, an increase in H^+ results in a decrease in K^+, although the precise mechanisms are not fully understood.
- **Cell volume** is regulated by the distribution of K^+ and other ions across the cell membrane, which triggers osmosis to maintain an osmotic equilibrium.
- **Cell lysis** causes release of intracellular K^+ to the plasma. Severe trauma can cause hyperkalaemia through the release of K^+ from the ruptured cells.
- **Exercise** can lead to a transient increase in K^+. Although the hyperkalaemia is marked, it does not appear to have effects associated with a similar hyperkalaemia at rest.
- **Diarrhoea** prevents the absorption of K^+ from the gut.

Long-term regulation of K^+

Although the short-term regulation of K^+ is achieved by movement into and out of cells, the longer-term regulation is through the **kidneys**. On average, 100 mmol K^+ is taken up by the body each day; a similar amount must be excreted each day from the kidneys, as a result of three processes:

1 **Filtration**: about 800 mmol K^+ enter the nephrons through glomerular filtration each day. A large proportion of the filtered K^+ must be reabsorbed.
2 **Reabsorption**: in normal conditions, K^+ is rapidly reclaimed in the early segments of the proximal convoluted tubule. This occurs predominantly through the setting up of a concentration gradient by Na^+ (and fluid reabsorption). To ensure K^+ absorption, K^+ channels are rapidly upregulated in response to upregulation of Na^+/K^+ ATPase.
3 **Secretion**: with normal diets, there is some secretion of K^+ in the distal convoluted tubule and collecting ducts. This secretion is through K^+ channels and expressed in the apical membrane, powered by the Na^+/K^+ ATPase in the basolateral membrane of principal cells. In **low-K^+** diets, cells may reabsorb K^+ to further reduce K^+ loss; this is achieved by intercalated cells, which obtain K^+ from the lumen via the K^+/H^+ exchanger.

Regulation of renal K^+ handling

Renal K^+ handling is associated with the reabsorption of Na^+ from the nephron. Three major hormone pathways modulate K^+ handling in the kidneys:

1 **ADH** promotes the uptake of Na^+, thus increasing the electrochemical gradient between the cell membrane and the nephron, by making the interior of the cell less negative. This change increases K^+ excretion from the cells, to offset the decreased excretion resulting from the decrease in tubular flow – allowing greater exchange of K^+ for Na^+ by the Na^+/K^+ ATPase.
2 **Aldosterone** promotes K^+ excretion by Na^+/K^+ ATPase activity in the principal cells of the nephron. Unsurprisingly, hyperkalaemia stimulates aldosterone secretion from the adrenal glands.
3 **Glucocorticoids** increase flow through the nephron, therefore indirectly increasing K^+ excretion.

Temperature

Core body temperature is typically maintained close to 37 °C, although during sleep it may drop markedly. If body temperature changes much from 36–37.5 °C, it is a serious clinical problem. Both hypothermia and hyperthermia are dangerous.

 CLINICAL Hypothermia

Hypothermia is defined as a core body temperature **below 35 °C**; as body temperature falls, there is progressive loss of CNS function. At around 30 °C, loss of consciousness occurs and ventricular fibrillation is likely at around 27 °C. Nevertheless, should these risks be avoided, people may survive low core temperatures without circulation and be revived.

 CLINICAL Hyperthermia

Hyperthermia is associated with a core body temperature **greater than 40 °C**. Elevations in temperature may be caused by fever and exercise, and illness may induce hyperthermia. The body is less able to withstand increases in temperature – at 42 °C there is a risk of death.

Regulation of body temperature

The ambient temperature is usually lower than that of the body. As a result, there is a general loss of heat from the body to its surrounding environment. The body aims to regulate its heat loss within the thermoneutral zone, where the heat loss from the body is roughly equal to the basal metabolic rate, ensuring that the core body temperature remains constant. The thermoneutral zone is dependent on the regulation of three factors:

1 The **basal metabolic rate**
2 The **heat lost by the body**
3 The ambient temperature.

Regulation of metabolic rate

The production of heat by the body is related to the metabolic rate. Although heat production is related to body mass, heat loss is related to the surface area, which increases more slowly. As a result, smaller individuals need a higher basal metabolic weight to account for their proportionally larger surface area related to their body mass.

The basal metabolic rate is regulated by many factors. In particular, thyroid hormones play a key role. Babies and children tend to have a higher metabolic rate which is further accentuated by the presence of brown fat, a tissue that is specialised for heat generation. Metabolic rate may also be upregulated during exercise and fever. In exercise, the increased metabolism reflects the increased activity of the body, whereas during fever it is a systemic response to infection.

 DEFINITION Basal metabolic rate

The basal metabolic rate (BMR) is the energy expended to maintain function of the vital organs at rest. The BMR makes up a large proportion of the energy expenditure in a normal day – it is usually quoted as around 2000 calories/day, although it varies due to a number of factors:

- **Decreases in BMR** can occur with increasing age and loss of muscle mass.
- **Increases in BMR** can occur with exercise and increased muscle mass, as well as during infection, changes in environmental temperature, stress, and ingestion of food and drink.

Heat loss

There are four processes by which heat can be transferred to the external environment:

Radiation is usually the major source of heat loss. The body also can absorb radiant heat, e.g. from direct sunlight.

Evaporation results from the heating of water, causing it to evaporate, thereby removing heat. This form of heat loss accounts for around 20% of the total. Sweating, as occurs during exercise, can increase heat loss to around 20 times that of the BMR, although it can also account for the loss of up to 3 L of water/hour.

Convection is responsible for around 15% heat loss. It results from heating of the air, which rises and is replaced by cooler air. Forced convection, as occurs in strong winds, can increase the loss of heat by this means.

Conduction accounts for very little heat loss in still air (around 5%). However, the conductivity of water is more than 20 times greater than that of air; this can account for hypothermia resulting rapidly from cold water immersion.

> **DEFINITION Thermoneutral zone**
>
> The thermoneutral zone is the band of environmental temperature in which the heat lost to the environment is balanced by the basal metabolic rate. Although the body remains in the thermoneutral zone, the core body temperature is maintained.

Regulation of the heat loss

Although core body temperature must remain within a very narrow range, the skin itself is not similarly constrained and acts as a heat exchanger to ensure that heat lost maintains the body in the **thermoneutral zone**. The skin alters how close the blood flows to the skin through modulation of the distribution of blood flow between the two plexus (Fig. 11.3):

1 The **dermal plexus** is found at the dermal–epidermal boundary so that much of the heat from the blood can be transferred to the ambient environment.

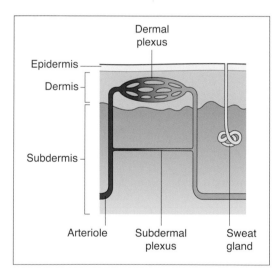

Figure 11.3 The skin is the major site of temperature regulation by balancing blood flow through plexus located at different depths in the skin. Blood flow through the dermal plexus allows a greater loss of heat, whereas opening of arteriovenous shunts in the subdermal plexus retains blood deeper in the tissue to reduce heat loss. The arterioles supplying the skin are particularly muscular and can reduce the net flow of blood to further limit heat loss. In times when greater heat loss is required, the sweat glands in the skin can be stimulated to promote evaporation.

2 The **subdermal plexus** is found much further from the surface of the skin and can act as a shunt to reduce heat loss through the opening of arteriovenous (AV) anastomoses.

The blood flow through the skin can be varied markedly to affect heat loss:

- In the **thermoneutral** zone, around 5–10 mL/min of blood flows through every 100 g of skin.
- At **maximal vasodilatation**, blood flow may be as high as 100 mL/min per 100 g of skin.
- To **retain body heat**, AV shunts in the skin can open, reducing blood flow near the surface of the skin to as low as 1 mL/min per 100 g of skin.

Temperature receptors

The main site of temperature regulation is the **hypothalamus**:

- **Cells in the anterior region** directly sense the temperature in the blood itself. Stimulation of this region triggers a response to increase heat loss.
- **Cells in the posterior region** receive information about temperature changes in the skin and other distant sites. Stimulation triggers a response to conserve heat, although the region itself contains no thermosensitive areas.

Similar to pain stimuli, temperature stimuli are carried on the thin $A\delta$- and C-fibres. The skin contains two types of receptor:

1 **Cold receptors** detect decreasing temperatures, with a peak response at around 30 °C.
2 **Hot receptors** have an increasing response, which peaks at around 40 °C.

At higher temperatures (>42 °C), heat can be sensed as a painful stimulus through the activation of the pain receptors. The conscious sensation of temperature is adaptive: water in a swimming pool initially feels very cool but rapidly becomes comfortable.

Responses to high temperature

Three mechanisms can be used to accommodate high temperatures:

1 **Reduced heat production** by reducing activity and intake of food; this decreases heat generation through the breakdown of substrate to ATP. Foods with high water content become favoured.
2 **Increased heat loss** is promoted through the vasodilatation of the skin. Sweating is also increased to promote heat loss by evaporation. In

humans, behaviour is also altered, e.g. varying the clothes worn.

3 **Increase in body temperature** does not appear to play a significant role in humans, although it occurs in many animal species.

It appears that some adaptation occurs to high temperatures. After 1 month in a high temperature environment, the amount of sweat produced has markedly decreased.

Responses to low temperature

Many of the responses to low temperature are the opposite of those seen at high temperature:

- **Increased heat production** is achieved by increasing muscle activity. This may be voluntary, as in hand rubbing or stamping, or involuntary such as shivering. **Thermogenesis** can also be achieved through the presence of brown fat, and regulation of the thyroid hormones can alter metabolic rate. Food intake is also increased – particularly protein – to provide a source of chemical energy.
- **Decreased heat loss** is achieved through vasoconstriction of the vessels at the surface of the skin and erection of the hairs to trap a layer of insulating air. Also, behavioural changes include wearing more clothes and turning up the heating indoors.
- **Reduction of body temperature** is seen in some individuals – particularly the Kalahari Bushmen, who can allow their body temperature to drop at night.

Unlike high temperatures, the body appears to be unable to adapt to low temperature and is just as sensitive after some 60 days of acclimatisation.

Regulation of external environment

Humans have been able to vary their external environment to match the thermoneutral zone, effectively increasing the climates in which they can live. The major mechanism by which this is achieved is through **wearing clothes**. Humans can also **modulate the ambient temperature** of their environment, through the use of central heating and air conditioning.

Response to high altitude

At high altitudes the amount of oxygen available decreases, due to both the lower amounts present and the low gradient to drive diffusion from the air

to the blood to the tissues. A series of changes occur that lead to a long-term acclimatisation to altitude-induced hypoxia.

Detection of hypoxia

The major sensors of O_2 change are the peripheral chemoreceptors:

- The **peripheral chemoreceptors** in the carotid bodies can detect hypoxia and stimulate ventilation.
- The **central chemoreceptors** detect changes in CO_2 and H^+ levels and are not driven by pure hypoxia.

Changes induced by hypoxia

A number of body systems are involved in compensating for hypoxia:

- **Ventilation increases in hypoxia** to ensure that enough O_2 is taken up in the lungs, resulting in reduced alveolar and arterial PCO_2. This decrease in CO_2 acts on the chemoreceptors to suppress ventilation; there is then a gradual increase in ventilation as the set point of the peripheral chemoreceptors changes during acclimatisation.
- Hypoxia induces a **respiratory alkalosis** through the removal of CO_2. To compensate, the kidneys excrete HCO_3^-, although this is a relatively slow process. In addition, higher levels of **2,3-diphosphoglycerate** are produced in the red blood cells, to promote dissociation of O_2 from haemoglobin in the tissues.
- **Haematocrit** is increased in chronic hypoxia due to elevated erythropoietin (EPO) production, restoring potential O_2 availability.

 CLINICAL **Acute mountain sickness**

Acute mountain sickness can develop after ascents of more than around 3000 m, particularly in those undertaking strenuous physical activity shortly after reaching high altitudes, and may be fatal, because of the potential for cerebral and pulmonary oedema. The symptoms include severe headache, insomnia, rapid breathing (tachypnoea) and nausea, which result from the oedema caused by respiratory alkalosis which in turn results from hyperventilation induced by hypoxia.

Symptoms may last for around a week, although they may be reduced by giving **acetazolamide**, which can oppose the alkalosis and promote bicarbonate loss in the kidneys.

- **Cardiac output increases** transiently at high altitude to aid the transfer of O_2 to the tissues from the lungs. However, this is limited by the necessity for diffusion in the alveoli to load the blood cells with O_2. During long-term acclimatisation, cardiac output returns to normal values, ensuring sufficient time for diffusion to be completed.

 CLINICAL Chronic mountain sickness (Monge's disease)

During the long-term acclimatisation to high altitude the haematocrit may increase, to help the oxygen-carrying potential of the blood. A haematocrit >60% causes a marked increase in the amount of cardiac work required per millilitre of O_2 delivered due to the greater blood viscosity.

Monge's disease occurs when the haematocrit increase becomes detrimental. It is thought that this is caused by a decrease in the sensitivity of the ventilatory system to hypoxia without a similar loss of sensitivity in the EPO system.

Stress

Stress is any change or event capable of disrupting homoeostasis to an unusual degree. Humans are unusual in that they can be stressed by anticipation of future difficulties – such as exams – and respond to these.

The nature of stressors and the stress response

Stresses affecting the body may be acute or chronic. Any sufficiently strong stressor invokes a general response that affects many different systems and is largely independent of the stimulus:

- **Acute stressors** can include trauma and the resulting effects, extreme environmental conditions (hot or cold), as well as infection and sleep deprivation.
- **Chronic stressors** include many of the above stimuli, although triggers can be more complex and subtle, such as social problems. Such stresses may affect people differently (e.g. phobias).

Initiation of stress response

The stress response is initiated by the hypothalamus in response to three main sources of information:

1 The **hypothalamus** provides information on the state of the body, receiving sensory nervous input from tissues throughout the body.
2 The **higher centres of the brain** provide information on the state of the mind. Much stress is the result of a perceived, and not necessarily physical, stimulus.
3 The **external environment** can be detected by the senses (e.g. touch, hearing, sight) to trigger an appropriate stress response.

Three potential phases can be identified in a stress response:

1 An **acute response** characterised as an 'alarm' reaction, associated with upregulation of the sympathetic 'fight-or-flight' response.
2 A **long-lasting resistance reaction** regulated predominantly by the hormone cortisol.
3 If the stressor is not eliminated **exhaustion** can result, which may be terminal.

Acute stress response

The acute stress response prepares the body for immediate activity in a 'fight-or-flight' response. It can be divided into three interrelated components:

1 **Effects on the CNS**
2 **Effects on the sympathetic nervous system**
3 **Effects on the adrenal medulla**.

Effects on the CNS

The acute stress response in the CNS is activated by the hypothalamus. It induces the sympathetic response, as well as promoting the activity of the necessary cortical regions:

- **Increases in heart rate and ventilation** are triggered by stimulating the medullary control centres.
- The **cerebral cortex is stimulated** by the release of noradrenaline from the locus ceruleus.
- **The release of endorphins** is triggered to blunt the pain response.

- **Release of ACTH (adrenocorticotrophic hormone)** from the anterior pituitary gland is triggered by **corticotrophin-releasing hormone** (CRH) released from the hypothalamus. This system is activated at the same time as the acute response, although it is associated with the chronic response due to the longer time that it takes to reach a significant effect.
- **Release of ADH** is stimulated in the posterior pituitary gland to reduce water loss and trigger glycogenolysis by the liver.

Activation of the sympathetic nervous system

The sympathetic nervous system is activated to ready the body for physical activity:

- **Blood pressure, heart rate and force of cardiac contraction** are increased to aid oxygen and glucose delivery to the tissues.
- **Release of energy substrates** is triggered. In particular, glycogen is broken down to glucose in the liver and lipid stores from the adipose tissue are also mobilised.
- The **blood vessels in the skeletal muscle and skin dilate** to increase flow to the muscles and remove potential heat from the body, respectively. Vessels to non-essential tissues are constricted to divert blood to the muscles.

Effects on the adrenal medulla

Preganglionic sympathetic fibres synapse with chromaffin cells in the adrenal medulla. These fibres release acetylcholine to trigger **release of adrenaline** and **noradrenaline**.

The chronic stress response

Long-lasting stress results in a prolonged 'resistance response' that is distinct from the acute 'fight-or-flight' response. This resistance response has evolved to conserve essential functions, allowing the body to continue counteracting a stress long after the acute response would have been exhausted. The elements of this 'resistance reaction' are triggered at the same time as the acute phase of the stress response, although they take far longer to manifest themselves.

The role of the sympathetic nervous system in the chronic response

The sympathetic nervous system plays a smaller part in the chronic stress response. It is responsible for stimulating the juxtaglomerular apparatus of the kidney to activate the renin–angiotensin–aldosterone axis. The resulting angiotensin triggers retention of both Na^+ and H_2O (via aldosterone) as well as an increase in blood pressure, all of which maintain the effective circulating volume.

The role of cortisol in the chronic stress response

Cortisol, a glucocorticoid, is the major hormone in the chronic stress response. It has a variety of effects that preserve the body's integrity and function:

- Stimulates release of lipids and catabolism of protein for energy
- Increases blood vessel sensitivity to constrictors and reduces capillary permeability
- Maintains cardiac contractility
- Increases erythrocyte production.

Although glucocorticoids maintain body function, they also suppress repair because it is a costly process in terms of materials. As a result, cortisol triggers:

- **reduced inflammation** to avoid disruption of the tissue function.
- **decreased production of fibroblasts** to suppress repair.
- **inhibition of the immune response**.

 CLINICAL Stress-related illness

The stress response evolved to counter a physical threat. As many of the stressors affecting us in modern society are not physical, the stress response is often counterproductive. High levels of psychological stress may cause a mild physical stress response, which may contribute to the development of many 'stress-related' illnesses, such as type 2 diabetes and heart disease. Treatment of such conditions can involve blunting of the stress response (e.g. β blockers and ACE inhibitors).

Effects of stress on the regulation of other hormone pathways

Although the adrenal gland is the major regulator of the stress response, under the control of the pituitary gland and the sympathetic nervous system, other pathways are also important in the regulation of the stress response:

- **Thyroid hormones** are elevated in the stress response, as a result of increased release of thyrotrophin-releasing hormone (TRH) from the hypothalamus. The thyroid hormones increase the metabolic rate and breakdown of glucose and proteins and fats, to ensure that there is a readily available energy source. In prolonged stress, glucocorticoids reduce the conversion of thyroxine (T_4) to the more active triiodothyronine (T_3), reducing the catabolic response to lengthen survival by conserving energy stores.
- **Growth hormone** (GH) levels are increased during the stress response, due to increased hypothalamic release of GH-releasing hormone (GHRH). Prolonged secretion of growth hormone increases the release of glucose and fatty acids into the circulation, to provide energy, and also reduces the use of glucose by the tissues, conserving it for the brain and blood where it is an essential energy source.

Exhaustion

If the stress response continues without resolution, the body or the CNS may no longer be able to sustain it, resulting in exhaustion, which may be fatal and manifests in obvious illness due to depletion of the body's resources. Although exhaustion of the stress response is not well understood, there are thought to be two major causes of exhaustion:

1 **Excessive prolonged aldosterone activity** may lead to the loss of K^+ through prolonged attempts to conserve Na^+. This progressive depletion can lead to a wide number of hypokalaemic problems and be fatal. High levels of cortisol may exceed the activity of the deactivating enzymes present in cells expressing the aldosterone receptor with which it can bind. As a result, cortisol may potentiate excessive activation of the aldosterone response, and further loss of K^+.
2 **Adrenal medullary exhaustion** results from depletion of the catecholamine stores in the adrenal gland. This leads to a sudden fall in blood glucose and loss of blood vessel tone and renal function, associated with the sudden withdrawal of adrenaline. The resulting hypotension can rapidly cause death. The standard treatment is stabilisation by treatment with adrenaline to restore blood pressure.

→ RELATED CHAPTERS

12

Reproduction

In humans, the sex chromosomes define the two sexes. Males and females develop different sexual organs to produce the **gametes**, and in the female to allow the development of a baby from the single fertilised cell, the **zygote**.

Following puberty, an individual becomes sexually mature and capable of reproducing, which is associated with a growth spurt, and the development of mature gametes and the characteristic differences between the sexes. The sex cells are regulated by the production of sex hormones, which stimulate continuous production of sperm in men. In women, the sex hormone levels vary in a cyclic fashion to coordinate maturation and release of an egg, with preparation of the lining of the uterus.

Advances in medicine have allowed individuals to control their fertility through contraception or sterilisation, and also allowed the induction of abortion to prevent an unwanted pregnancy. In addition conception through *in vitro* fertilisation is possible.

Sexual differentiation

Sexual differentiation is the process by which the undifferentiated fertilised egg (zygote) is committed to becoming either male or female. Sexual differentiation can be categorised into three different types:

1 **Genetic sex** is determined by the presence or absence of a Y chromosome.

2 **Gonadal sex** is determined by the presence of ovaries or testes.
3 **Phenotypic ('legal') sex** is determined by the external genitalia.

Male sex is determined by the presence of a Y chromosome, more specifically the **SRY** region; female sex is the default pathway in the absence of a Y chromosome.

Gonadal development

Until week 6, **gonadal** development is the same for both sexes. **Primordial germ cells** (the cells that give rise to the gametes) are formed within the primary ectoderm in week 2; in week 4 they detach and move into the yolk sac. During weeks 5–6, they migrate to form **genital ridges** – these are swellings medial to the developing mesonephroi (Fig. 12.1). The genital ridges consist of:

- **Primordial germ cells** which will develop into **oogonia** or **spermatogonia**
- **Primitive sex cords** which are supporting cells, stimulated by germ cells to form the adjacent tissue. They are split into **medullary** and **cortical** regions.

Adjacent to the genital ridges are the **mesonephric (wolffian) ducts**, which will develop into the ducts of the male reproductive system, and the **paramesonephric (müllerian) ducts**, which will develop into the uterus, fallopian tubes and vagina in females.

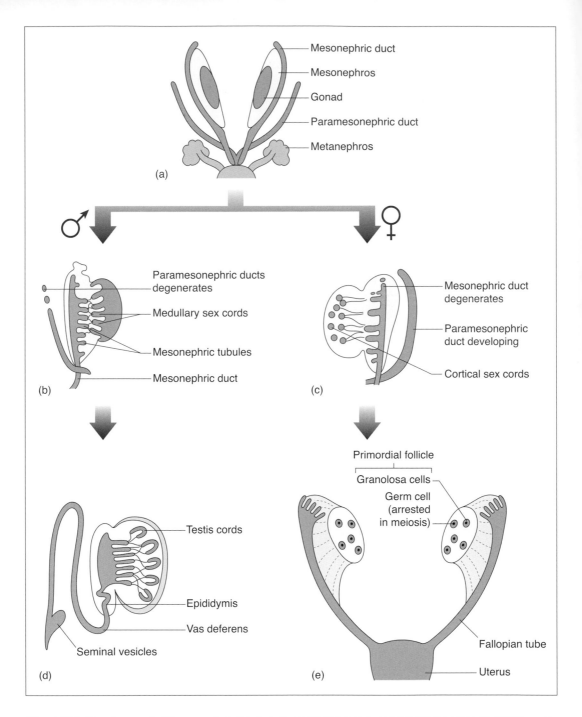

Figure 12.1 Development of the gonads. (a) Early on the male and female gonads are the same. (b,d) In the male the paramesonephric ducts degenerate, the medullary cells differentiate into Sertoli cells which form the testis cords, and the mesonephric ducts form the epididymis, vas deferens and seminal vesicles. (c,e) In the female the mesonephric ducts degenerate and the cortical sex cords differentiate into granulosa cells which, along with the germ cells, form primordial follicles. The paramesonephric ducts form the fallopian tubes and fuse to form the uterus and top of the vagina.

DEFINITION Gametes

The gametes are the **haploid** reproductive cells that fuse at fertilisation to produce a diploid **zygote**. The gametes develop from the **oogonia** and **spermatogonia** in women and men, respectively. They are produced by mitotic division of the **primordial germ cells**.

DEFINITION The gonads

The gonads are the reproductive organs that support the **gametes**:

- In men, the **testes**
- In women, the **ovaries**.

Development of the male gonads

The presence of the *SRY* gene stimulates development of **Sertoli cells**, which form the **testis cords** and release **anti-müllerian hormone** (AMH), causing the paramesonephric ducts to regress. **Leydig cells** develop and secrete testosterone, stimulating the mesonephric ducts to form the vas deferens, epididymis and seminal vesicles.

Week 7

- **SRY protein production** stimulates the medullary sex cord cells to differentiate into **Sertoli cells**, and the **cortical** sex cord cells to degenerate.
- The **Sertoli cells** form the testis cords. At puberty the testis cords differentiate into **seminiferous tubules** and **rete testis**.

Weeks 8–10

- **Sertoli cells secrete AMH** causing the paramesonephric ducts to regress. Sertoli cells also inhibit germ cell development before meiosis can occur.
- **Leydig cells** develop from the mesenchymal cells in the genital ridge; these produce

testosterone, which promotes survival of the mesonephric ducts. At this stage maternal **human chorionic gonadotrophin (hCG)** controls secretion of testosterone, although this is later controlled by the pituitary gonadotrophs of the male fetus.

Weeks 8–12

The mesonephric ducts differentiate into the vasa deferentia and the epididymis.

Week 10

Seminal vesicles form from the mesonephric ducts, near the attachment to the pelvic urethra.

The prostate is formed from endodermal evaginations budding from the pelvic urethra.

DEFINITION Anti-müllerian hormone (AMH)

AMH is a glycoprotein produced by **Sertoli** cells of the male fetus. It suppresses the generation of the **paramesonephric (müllerian) ducts** in the male fetus during the first 8 weeks, to ensure that female genital structures do not develop.

Development of the female gonads

In the absence of the Y chromosome, development of male gonads is not stimulated, resulting in a female developmental pathway (see Fig. 12.1).

Week 7

The **medullary** sex cords degenerate and the **cortical** sex cord cells differentiate into **granulosa cells**.

Weeks 8–10

- The germ cells enter their first meiotic division and are surrounded by granulosa cells to form **primordial follicles**. The granulosa cells subsequently arrest germ cell development until puberty.
- The lack of testosterone results in **regression of the mesonephric ducts**, whereas the **absence of AMH allows paramesonephric** ducts to develop and fuse at their caudal end to form

the uterus and the superior end of the vagina. The unfused, superior portion of the paramesonephric ducts forms the fallopian tubes.

- The inferior end of the vagina is formed from the **sinuvaginal bulbs,** a pair of swellings on the posterior wall of the **urogenital sinus**.

Development of the external genitalia

Development of external genitalia in the first 12 weeks follows the same course in both sexes (Fig. 12.2). At week 5, the **cloacal folds** develop on either side of the **cloacal membrane**. These folds

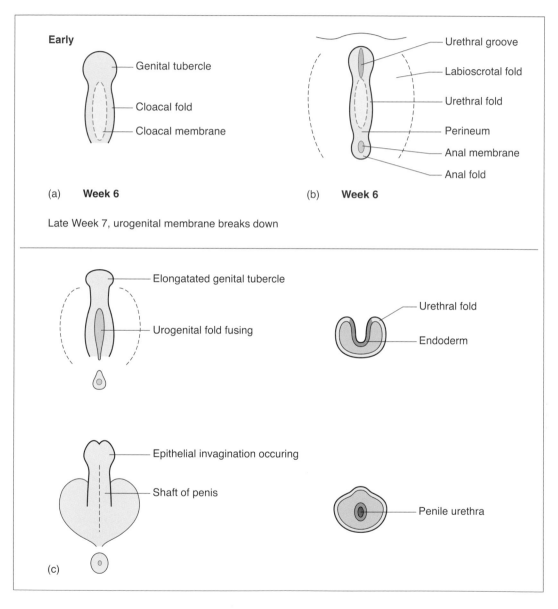

Early

— Genital tubercle

— Cloacal fold

— Cloacal membrane

(a) **Week 6**

— Urethral groove

— Labioscrotal fold

— Urethral fold

— Perineum

— Anal membrane

— Anal fold

(b) **Week 6**

Late Week 7, urogenital membrane breaks down

— Elongatated genital tubercle

— Urogenital fold fusing

— Urethral fold

— Endoderm

— Epithelial invagination occuring

— Shaft of penis

— Penile urethra

(c)

Figure 12.2 **Development of the external genitalia**. In the early stages the male and female do not differ. The urorectal septum fuses with the cloacal membrane to form the perineum and the anal fold. The urogenital membrane breaks down. In the male, the urethral folds fuse, forming the penile urethra. The genital tubercle forms the shaft and glans, and the urethral folds form the scrotum.

meet anteriorly to form a midline swelling – the **genital tubercle**. At week 7, the **urorectal septum** fuses with the cloacal membrane to form the **perineum**, dividing the cloacal folds into the anterior urogenital membrane and the posterior anal membrane. The area of cloacal fold flanking the urogenital membrane is now called the urethral fold, whereas that flanking the posterior anal membrane is now called the anal fold:

- **Labioscrotal folds** form either side of the cloacal folds.
- The **definitive urogenital sinus** extends on to the surface of the genital tubercle as the urethral groove. In the male this is long and broad, whereas in the female it is shorter and tapered.
- The **urogenital membrane** ruptures so that the cavity of the urogenital sinus is open to the amniotic fluid, and the genital tubercle elongates to form the **phallus**.

Male external genitalia

From week 12, high levels of **dihydrotestosterone**, converted from testosterone, trigger the development into male genitalia.

- The **definitive urogenital sinus** forms the penile urethra.
- The **urethral fold** fuses to enclose the urogenital sinus, forming the penile urethra.
- The **genital tubercle** elongates to form the glans and shaft of the penis.
- The **labioscrotal folds** fuse to form the scrotum.

 DEFINITION Dihydrotestosterone

Dihydrotestosterone (DHT) is a metabolite of testosterone that is produced mainly in the testes and adrenal glands by the action of the enzyme **5α-reductase**. DHT is far more potent than testosterone, and responsible for development of male characteristics *in utero*.

Female external genitalia

In the absence of DHT, the primitive perineum does not lengthen and the labioscrotal and urethral folds do not fuse. The phallus bends inferiorly to form the clitoris:

- The **definitive urogenital sinus** forms the vestibule of the vagina.

- The **urethral fold** forms the labia minora.
- The **labioscrotal fold** forms the labia majora.
- The **genital tubercle** forms the glans and shaft of the clitoris.

Migration of the gonads

The gonads descend from their original position at the level of T10 due to shortening of the **gubernacula**. The arterial supply to the gonads does not migrate, accounting for why the blood supply to the testes (and the ovaries) is at the level of T10.

 DEFINITION Gubernaculum

The gubernaculum is a ligamentous cord connecting the gonads to the fascia by the labioscrotal folds. The shortening of the gubernacula mediates the descent of the testes in males, whereas it develops into the round and ovarian ligaments in women.

Migration of the male gonads

Between weeks 7 and 12 the gubernaculum shortens (by getting larger at the bases), pulling the testes down to the level of the deep inguinal ring. They remain there until month 7, when testosterone and other androgens cause further reduction and regression, pulling the gonads into the scrotal sac.

 CLINICAL Hermaphroditism

Defects in the development of the sexual organs can result in individuals with both male and female sexual tissue, or ambiguous genital organs.

True hermaphrodites have both ovarian and testicular tissue. Most commonly this occurs in mosaics.

Pseudohermaphrodites have the external genitalia of one sex and the gonads of another:

- Male pseudohermaphrodites are XY with feminized genitals.
- Female pseudohermaphrodites are XX with masculinised genitals.

Pseudohermaphroditism may occur as a result of either abnormal levels of sex hormones **or** defects in sex hormone receptors.

In female pseudohermaphrodites, virilising androgens cause clitoral hypertrophy and fusion of the urethral and labioscrotal folds.

Migration of the female gonads

In week 7, the gubernaculum becomes attached to the paramesonephric ducts. As the ducts fuse to form the uterus, they sweep out peritoneal folds (the **broad ligaments**) and pull the ovaries into these folds.

Puberty and sexual maturation

Puberty is the series of events that occur during the transition from childhood into adulthood and sexual maturity. Puberty occurs at about 8–13 years in girls and 9–14 years in boys. It is characterised by physical growth and pronounced accentuation of sexual characteristics. The sexual organs mature and become functional during puberty, although the order and timeframe of these events may differ considerably and can take many years.

Hormonal changes during puberty

The developmental and physical changes that occur during puberty are the result of hormonal changes. Three major events occur:

1 The **hypothalamus** increases the production of gonadotrophin-releasing hormone (GnRH).
2 The **anterior pituitary** becomes more sensitive to GnRH, triggering increased release of luteinising hormone (LH) and follicle-stimulating hormone (FSH).
3 The **ovaries** and **testes** become sensitive to FSH and LH. As a result, the gametes begin to develop and the sexual organs produce the sex hormones in large quantities, triggering a growth spurt and other changes.

Changes during puberty

The chronology of the changes that occur during puberty varies greatly between individuals. The production of sex hormones results in a number of changes:

- Development of the genitalia
- Development of the secondary sexual characteristics

- Actions of the central nervous system (CNS)
- Changes to the musculoskeletal and cardiovascular systems.

Development of the genitalia

In **men**, the production of testosterone stimulates the function of the prostate gland and seminal vesicles. Testosterone promotes the growth and development of the penis and testes, and initiates **spermatogenesis**.

In **women**, the increased levels of oestrogen stimulate development of the muscular tissue of the uterus and increase development of the blood vessels to the endometrium, as well as stimulating cervical mucus production. The oestrogen surge stimulates follicular development and the menstrual cycle, although the initial cycles are not associated with ovulation.

Development of secondary sexual characteristics

The development of secondary sexual characteristics of men and women differs due to the different hormones released, as well as the different tissues present. However, there are some common events. For example, the growth of thick hair around the external genitalia and under the axillae occurs in both sexes:

- In **men,** testosterone triggers lengthening of the vocal folds which is associated with deepening of the voice. In addition, testosterone stimulates the production of thick terminal hairs on the face and chest.
- In **women**, puberty also results in the development of the breast tissue.

Actions on the CNS

At puberty the sex hormones activate the centres in the CNS that regulate sex drive and sexual behaviour. These centres differentiate during the second and third trimesters as a result of fetal secretion of testosterone or oestrogen.

Development of the musculoskeletal system

Puberty is associated with a marked increase in height because the sex hormones increase bone deposition and the growth of the long bones at the epiphyseal plates. The sex hormones also promote closure of the growth plates, effectively limiting the height that can be reached:

- **In men**, growth is associated with broadening of the shoulders and development of a male skeletal frame.
- **In women**, oestrogen accounts for the growth of the female frame, in particular the widening of the pelvis. Oestrogens cause more rapid closure of the growth plates, accounting for the shorter height of women in adulthood.

The sex hormones also stimulate development of the skeletal muscle fibres to become stronger and more durable, and lead to an increase in muscle mass. As the effects of testosterone are greater than those of oestrogen, the increase in muscle mass is greater in males.

Effects of sex hormones on the cardiovascular and respiratory systems

Testosterone stimulates red blood cell formation in the bone marrow and accounts for the increase in blood volume and the haematocrit. Once menstrual cycles have started, iron loss is associated with menstruation, increasing the risk of iron-deficiency anaemia in women.

 CLINICAL Precocious puberty

Precocious puberty is the onset of puberty at an extremely early age. This may be the result of disease (e.g. a sex hormone-secreting tumour), although in some very rare cases the individuals may be otherwise medically normal. As well as premature development of the sexual characteristics, precocious puberty causes a decrease in eventual height, due to early closure of the epiphyseal plates.

Generation of the male gametes

There are two main processes in generation of the male gametes:

1 **Spermatogenesis** is the process by which spermatid cells develop from the germ cells.

 CLINICAL Delayed puberty

Puberty may be delayed for many reasons, including malnutrition, a systemic disease (e.g. inflammatory bowel disease) and a development defect (e.g. pituitary or gonadal abnormality), or the individuals may be medically normal.

If an underlying defect is detected, treatment of this will often allow the onset of puberty (e.g. redressing malnutrition). Puberty can also be induced hormonally, if there is such a deficiency. If the individual appears healthy and normal but with delayed puberty, no intervention is warranted.

2 **Spermiogenesis** is the series of remodelling processes that occurs without cell division, resulting in the production of a mature spermatocyte from a spermatid.

Cells of the male sexual system

The seminiferous tubules are made up of a series of distinct populations of cells:

- **Sertoli cells** are tightly apposed cells that form the tubules.
- **Leydig cells** are found in the interstitium between seminiferous tubules and regulate spermatogenesis through secretion of hormones.
- **Germ cells** are found in the basal compartment; through differentiation and proliferation they give rise to the mature sperm.

Sertoli cells

Sertoli cells enclose and support all the cells undergoing **spermatogenesis**. These cells have a large cytoplasm and an ovoid nucleus. They contain large numbers of mitochondria as well as lipid droplets and small amounts of rough endoplasmic reticulum (ER). Sertoli cells are connected by a series of tight junctions found close to the basal aspect of the epithelium, regulating the movement between the two compartments. In addition, Sertoli cells secrete a number of factors:

- Those that regulate spermatogenesis and spermiogenesis
- Those that regulate hormone production – in particular **inhibin**
- Factors that phagocytose excess spermatid cytoplasm.

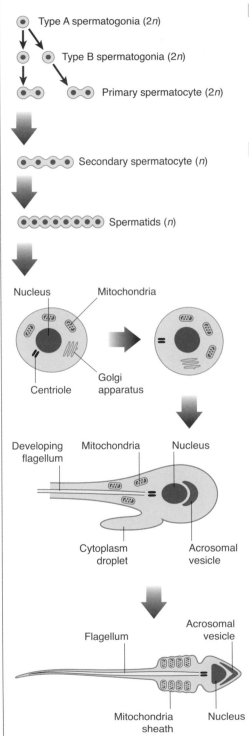

Type A spermatogonia (2n)

Type B spermatogonia (2n)

Primary spermatocyte (2n)

Secondary spermatocyte (n)

Spermatids (n)

Nucleus   Mitochondria

Golgi
Centriole   apparatus

Developing   Mitochondria   Nucleus
flagellum

Cytoplasm   Acrosomal
droplet   vesicle

Acrosomal
vesicle
Flagellum

Mitochondria   Nucleus
sheath

Spermatogenesis I

The Type A spermatogonia cells are found in the basolateral compartment of the seminiferous tubules. These cells proliferate mitotically to give rise to many diploid Type B spermatogonia. During these divisions the cells make their way to the adluminal compartment of the seminiferous tubules. The subsequent divisions of the cells are not complete – the cells retain a cytoplasmic connection between each other until they mature.

Spermatogenesis II

The primary spermatocytes develop from the Type B spermatocytes as they enter into the prophase of the first meiotic division . The resulting secondary spermatocytes are haploid cells, containing only 23 chromosomes. The second meiotic division results in the production of spermatids, the end product of spermatogenesis, which are sculpted through the processes of spermatogenesis to produce functional spermatozoa.

Spermiogenesis I

The spermatids develop specific characteristics in becoming spermatozoa. The first stage requires the centrioles, which will organise the development of the flagellum migrating to one end of the cells, whilst the Golgi apparatus – which will develop into the acrosomal vesicle - migrates to the opposite end of the cell.

Spermiogenesis II

The centrioles organise the generation of the flagellum and the mitochondria migrate around the first section of the flagellum. In addition the nucleus progressively condenses and the acrosomal vesicle fills with enzymes and sits around the nucleus. The volume of cytoplasm progressively decreases and buds off as a cytoplasmic droplet, which is removed by the Sertoli cells.

Spermiogenesis III

The complete spermatozoa consist of a tightly condensed nucleus surround by the acrosomal vesicle. A mitochondrial sheath develops around the first part of the flagellum containing the numerous mitochondria to generate sufficient energy. The complete spermatozoa have yet to be fully functional, they develop motility as they pass through the epididymis.

Figure 12.3 **The generation of male gametes**. The male gametes develop in Sertoli cells through a number of stages to form spermatids, which are progressively remodelled to form the mature spermatozoa.

Leydig cells

Leydig cells in the interstitial tissue synthesise and secrete the male sex hormones. The main hormone that is produced is testosterone, secretion of which is regulated by LH released from the pituitary gland. Leydig cells have large nuclei and extensive cytoplasm with eosinophilic granules and lipid droplets. Their hormone-secreting function is reflected in the rich plexus of blood and lymph that spreads throughout the cells.

Spermatogenesis

To ensure continuous production of sperm, different parts of a single tubule are involved in different points of spermatogenesis (Fig. 12.3):

- Undifferentiated germ cells are termed **type A spermatogonia** and are characterised by a large oval nucleus containing condensed chromatin with large nucleoli and a nuclear vacuole.
- **Type B spermatogonia** develop from the division of Type A spermatogonia. They have undergone several mitotic divisions and have migrated to the adluminal compartment of the tubules, to commence meiosis.
- The **first meiotic division** takes around 3 weeks to produce **secondary spermatocytes** which are rarely seen as they divide rapidly to form spermatids.
- **Spermatids** mature to produce sperm through spermiogenesis. They progressively form **spermatozoa** as the cytoplasm is progressively removed and the nucleus condenses.

Spermiogenesis

Spermiogenesis is the process by which spermatids develop into mature spermatozoa. This process occurs in the seminiferous tubules and is regulated and supported by Sertoli cells.

- The **acrosomal vesicle** develops from the Golgi apparatus.
- The **centrioles migrate** opposite to the acrosomal vesicle and form the flagellum.
- The cytoplasm and the **mitochondria migrate** to the first part of the flagellum.
- The **flagellum elongates** and the excess cytoplasm in the cell is progressively removed by supporting Sertoli cells.

 DEFINITION Acrosomal vesicle

The acrosomal vesicle is a specialised structure that develops from the Golgi apparatus in spermatozoa. This structure contains various enzymatic secretions to help sperm penetrate the ovum for fertilisation.

Maturation of sperm and the production of semen

Developed spermatozoa are continuously released from the tubules and pass through the rete testis to the epididymis, where sperm are concentrated by reabsorption of fluid. In the epididymis further secretions are added, in particular fructose and carnitine, which act as energy sources, and various glycoproteins, which coat the sperm.

The passage of the sperm through the epididymis takes approximately 6–12 days, during which they begin to acquire the ability to move. After maturation, the fully activated sperm pass into the vas deferens.

Semen

The combination of sperm and other secretions released into the female reproductive tract is known as **semen**. Although sperm taken from the vas deferens are capable of fertilisation, the secretions in semen help the sperm:

- They act as a fluid vehicle for transport of the sperm.
- They provide nutrition to the sperm.
- They act as an alkaline buffer to protect sperm from the vagina's acid environment.
- Enzymes trigger coagulation and decoagulation of the semen in the vaginal tract.

Development of the female gametes

A woman is born with a limited number of follicles containing oocytes, the female gametes, which mature progressively throughout her reproductive life. At each stage of maturation only a small proportion of follicles successfully progresses, ensuring that only the most viable can be released at ovulation. There are several distinct stages of development:

- The **primordial germ cells** give rise to the primary oocytes in the fetus and develop into **primordial follicles**.
- **Growing follicles** develop after puberty. Groups of primordial follicles begin to mature in a 3-month cycle under the influence of hormones, in preparation for one to mature sufficiently for ovulation.
- A single **mature follicle (secondary** or **graafian follicle)** develops from each group of growing follicles; this follicle develops completely and the oocyte is released.
- After release of the oocyte, the follicle becomes the **corpus luteum**, which, should fertilisation occur, regulates the early stages of pregnancy through hormonal secretion.

Primordial germ cells and the development of primordial follicles

The primordial germ cells migrate to the ovarian tissue in early fetal development. Unlike the development of sperm, which occurs throughout life, there are a finite number of follicles that mature progressively.

Primordial germ cells mature in the fetus during months 4 and 5, developing into primary oocytes, which start the first stage of meiotic division. During month 7 of fetal development, primary oocytes becoming encapsulated by a single layer of follicular cells, which stops meiotic division of the primary oocyte until after puberty.

Growing follicles

During each menstrual cycle, coordinated secretions of FSH and LH from the pituitary gland trigger the maturation of about 20 primordial follicles, although typically only one will mature to release an oocyte (Fig. 12.4). Follicular growth results in development of both the follicular cells and the primary oocyte itself:

- The **single matured oocyte** rapidly enlarges, the nuclear volume increases and the number of mitochondria increases. The oocyte becomes surrounded by a thick coat, the **zona pellucida**.
- The **follicular cells** develop and proliferate to form the granulosa layer.
- The **stromal cells** surrounding the follicle differentiate to form the theca folliculosa, which

itself develops into the theca interna and theca externa.

 DEFINITION Zona pellucida

The zona pellucida is a glycoprotein membrane surrounding the oocyte, which is produced by the oocyte and follicular cells. The major components of the zona pellucida are involved in binding sperm and triggered the acrosome reaction.

As the follicle develops, fluid accumulates within a cavity known as the antrum. The antral fluid contains steroid-binding proteins and high concentrations of steroids. In the granulosa layer cells accumulate around the oocyte, forming the **cumulus oophorus**. Expanding follicles will die unless they receive a coordinated release of an LH surge simultaneous with their expression of high levels of LH receptors on the cell surfaces. LH acts on both granulosa and thecal cells, leading to a variety of changes to allow ovulation and the subsequent generation of the corpus luteum.

Growth preovulation

The LH surge reactivates meiosis, allowing completion of the first meiotic division. The cytoplasm is divided extremely unevenly; the secondary oocyte retains almost all the cytoplasm, whereas the **first polar body** is produced which contains almost no cytoplasm.

The secondary oocyte immediately enters the **second stage of meiosis** though arrests in metaphase. It is not clear how this process is directly regulated – although the oocyte matures after the LH pulse, it does not directly express LH receptors, relying instead on signals from the surrounding cells. The changes in the oocyte are accompanied by changes in the follicular cells, in particular they produce large amounts of extracellular fluid, resulting in an increased follicle size.

 DEFINITION Polar body

The polar body is a structure that results from asymmetrical portioning of cytoplasm during divisions of the ovum. These cells contain chromosomes and very little cytoplasm. They serve no function other than to allow the extrusion of chromosomes during meiosis.

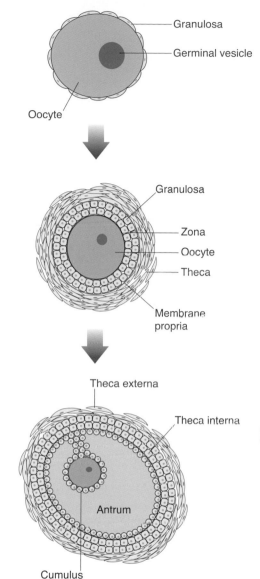

Primary follicle

The follicles present before puberty are the primary follicles, made up of the oocytes surrounded by a thin layer of granulosa cells. These follicles are surrounded by the stromal cells of the ovaries.

Preantral follicle

During the menstrual cycle the sex hormones stimulate cohorts of follicles to develop. These growing follicles have a developed zona separating the oocyte from its supporting granulosa cells. In addition, the thecal cells that surround the granulosa are separated by a basement membrane.

The dominant follicle in a cohort expresses increased numbers of luteinising hormone receptors, which allow them to further develop, while preventing the maturation of other follicles within the cohort. As a result the increased stimulation triggers secretion of fluid and development of a graafian, or secondary, follicle.

Graafian follicle

The mature follicle that releases its oocyte has a specialised structure. Distinct layers of the theca interna and externa can be found surrounding the membrane propria. The granulosa cells form a thin layer around a fluid filled cavity and a stalk of cells connects the oocyte to the sides of the follicle. The oocyte itself is surrounded by a layer of granulosa cells forming the cumulus.

Figure 12.4 **Development of the female gametes**. The female gametes develop by a very different process to the male ones. There are a limited number of follicles, containing an oocyte, present in each female at birth. This results in a finite number of cells that can be fertilised. Indeed, only a limited number of follicles ever mature to the point where the oocyte is released.

Mature follicles and ovulation

Mature (Graafian) follicles are large structures – about 2.5 cm in diameter – which can be found as a large vesicle forming a bulge on the surface of the ovary. The follicular cavity contains a large volume of fluid, and the oocyte is attached to the wall of the follicle by a pedicle of granulosa cells.

The rapid growth of the follicle immediately before ovulation leads to a bulge forming on the surface of the ovary. The epithelial layer that separates the follicle from the abdomen starts to thin and degenerate. Ovulation results from the rupture of this layer. The fluid and cells supporting the oocyte leak out of the ovary and bring with them the oocyte, surrounded by cumulus cells.

In humans, the surface of the ovary is directly exposed to the peritoneal cavity. The ovary is swept up into the fallopian tubes by the **fimbriae** and transported towards the uterus for fertilisation. The remainder of the follicle in the ovary collapses and becomes engorged by a blood clot to form the **corpus luteum**.

Corpus luteum

The corpus luteum is approximately 1.5–2.5 cm in diameter, and forms from the remainder of the follicle not released during ovulation. It functions transiently as an endocrine organ to support the embryo:

- The **granulosa cells secrete progesterone** under the influence of LH, which stimulates proliferation of the uterine endometrium, to prepare it for implantation.
- The **theca interna cells secrete oestrogen** to maintain the mucosa of the female reproductive tract.

Progesterone production by the corpus luteum is regulated by LH secretion from the anterior pituitary. Without continued LH, the corpus luteum degenerates after 12–14 days, and production of oestrogen and progesterone ceases. This cessation secretion results in the collapse of the endometrium and the onset of menstruation. The degenerated corpus luteum forms the **corpus albicans**, which has no function.

If implantation of a fertilised ovum occurs, the uterine cycle becomes interrupted. The developing placenta begins to secrete **hCG**, which has an analogous function to LH, maintaining the viability of the corpus luteum until around week 12 of pregnancy. After week 12, the placenta takes over the secretion of oestrogen and progesterone, and the corpus luteum regresses.

Atresic follicles

Follicular development may cease at any stage, which could reflect the fact that only the most viable follicles develop to ovulation. The precise appearance of atresic follicles varies enormously, depending on stage of development before atresia occurs, developing into a collagenous structure known as a **corpus fibrosum**.

Menstruation

The menstrual cycle is the series of cyclic hormonal changes that regulate the development of follicles and the uterus, to coordinate them for release and implantation of a fertilised oocyte (Fig. 12.5). The menstrual cycle can be divided into four phases:

1 Menstruation
2 Follicular phase
3 Ovulatory phase
4 Luteal phase.

The development of each group of follicles takes about 3 months, whereas development of the uterine lining occurs in a monthly cycle. There are four hormones that regulate each other's secretion and control the menstrual cycle (Fig. 12.6).

Menstruation

The first day of menstruation defines the first day of the menstrual cycle. The **decrease in progesterone secretion**, following degeneration of the corpus luteum, results in the shedding of the endometrial lining of the womb.

Follicular phase

The follicular phase (and, thus, the whole menstrual cycle) starts on the first day of menstruation, when the levels of **oestrogen, progesterone** and **inhibin** all fall after collapse of the corpus luteum. The absence of these luteal hormones promotes an increase in FSH, and then LH, levels, which stimulates the antral growth in the follicles; this results in release of oestrogen and progesterone. In the uterus, the oestrogen released by the new cohort of follicles stimulates the generation of the endometrium and also promotes generation of mucus in the cervix.

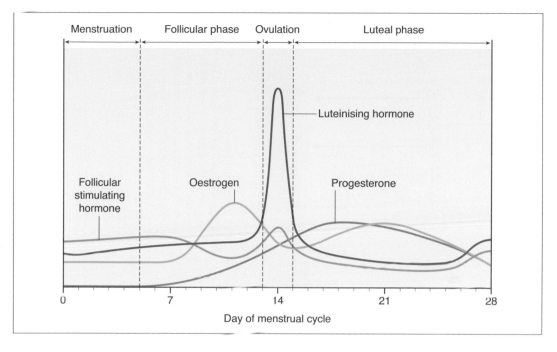

Figure 12.5 The hormonal regulation of the menstrual cycle. The four phases of the menstrual cycle are regulated by the varying secretions of the sex hormones. Follicle-stimulating hormone (FSH) and luteinising hormone (LH) are responsible for regulating the development of the follicles, and the marked 'spike' in concentration is crucial for triggering rupture of the Graafian follicle and release of the oocyte. After ovulation, the production of progesterone is responsible for promoting preparation of the endometrium in case fertilisation should occur. In the absence of implantation, the corpus luteum degenerates and ceases to produce progesterone, triggering breakdown of the endometrial lining and the onset of menstruation.

 DEFINITION Inhibin

Inhibin is a hormone produced by the granulosa of ovarian follicles in women and by Sertoli cells in men. It is of particular importance in suppressing FSH secretion and is regulated by GnRH, which suppresses secretion, whereas insulin growth factor 1 (IGF-1) promotes inhibin secretion. Decrease in **inhibin** secretion after collapse of the corpus luteum promotes a rise in FSH levels to stimulate follicular development.

Ovulatory phase

In the ovulatory phase the production of FSH and LH is triggered by the positive feedback of progesterone and oestrogen, leading to a surge in the concentration of both hormones, which triggers ovulation.

Luteal phase

After ovulation the luteal phase occurs, when androgen and oestrogen production falls. The phase is characterised by a gradual increase in progesterone, which peaks around 8 days after the LH surge. Progesterone inhibits LH and FSH production, suppressing the development of the antral follicles, and acts on the uterus, triggering a change in the endometrium so that it can accept a fertilised egg for implantation. Should implantation occur, the release for hCG from the embryo maintains the corpus luteum, halting the menstrual cycle. Otherwise, the corpus luteum rapidly degenerates and menstruation starts.

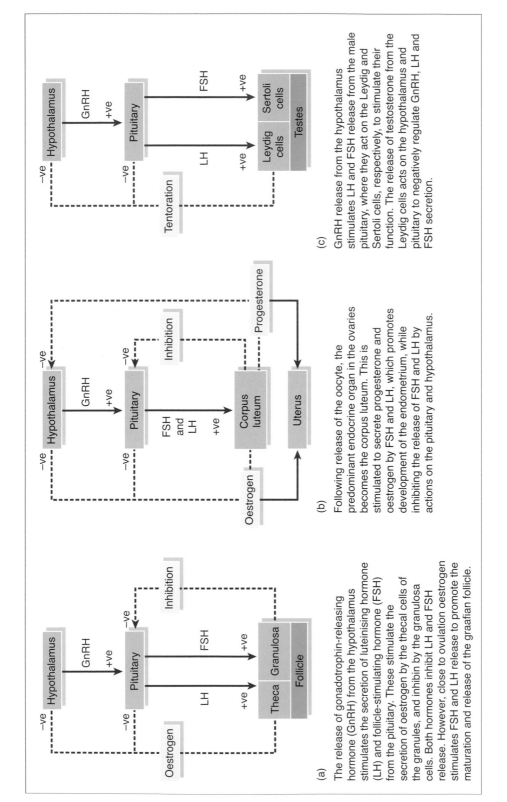

(a)

The release of gonadotrophin-releasing hormone (GnRH) from the hypothalamus stimulates the secretion of luteinising hormone (LH) and follicle-stimulating hormone (FSH) from the pituitary. These stimulate the secretion of oestrogen by the thecal cells of the granules, and inhibin by the granulosa cells. Both hormones inhibit LH and FSH release. However, close to ovulation oestrogen stimulates FSH and LH release to promote the maturation and release of the graafian follicle.

(b)

Following release of the oocyte, the predominant endocrine organ in the ovaries becomes the corpus luteum. This is stimulated to secrete progesterone and oestrogen by FSH and LH, which promotes development of the endometrium, while inhibiting the release of FSH and LH by actions on the pituitary and hypothalamus.

(c)

GnRH release from the hypothalamus stimulates LH and FSH release from the male pituitary, where they act on the Leydig and Sertoli cells, respectively, to stimulate their function. The release of testosterone from the Leydig cells acts on the hypothalamus and pituitary to negatively regulate GnRH, LH and FSH secretion.

Figure 12.6 Regulation of the sex hormones.

Coitus

During coitus sperm are released into the female reproductive tract. The process of coitus involves physiological changes in both individuals.

Coital changes in the male

In the male the penis becomes erect as a result of both physical and psychological stimuli. Three nervous outflows influence erection:

1 The **pelvic nerve** carries parasympathetic fibres.
2 The **pudendal nerve** is a somatic nerve.
3 The **hypogastric nerve** carries sympathetic fibres.

There are three processes culminating in the release of semen:

Erection, largely mediated by parasympathetic stimulation
Emission, mediated by sympathetic stimulation.
Ejaculation, largely controlled by somatic stimulation.

Throughout this process there are simultaneous changes in the rest of the body's physiology. Heart rate and blood pressure both increase. Just before ejaculation, skin rashes may appear. At ejaculation, the cardiovascular changes become more pronounced and hyperventilation occurs.

Erection

Erection is achieved by the vasodilatation of arterioles to allow filling with blood of the corpus cavernosa of the penis. The parasympathetic stimulation triggers dilatation of the vessel walls to allow filling of the corpus cavernosa. This is further augmented by closure of arteriovenous shunts to divert blood into the sinus beds within the corpus cavernosum. As a result of the increased pressure, the venous vessels in the penis become compressed, reducing venous outflow from the penis and further promoting the erection.

Emission

Emission results from the contraction of the prostate, seminal glands and vas deferens to release all the components of semen into the urethra. As ejaculation approaches, erection of the penis increases and the circumference at the glans may increase. The testes are also drawn into the perineum and may enlarge due to vasoconstriction.

Ejaculation

Ejaculation is the final release of sperm from the urethra, as a result of contraction of the smooth muscle of the urethra and the striated muscles enclosing it. To prevent the release of semen into the bladder, the sphincter at the entrance of the bladder contracts.

Orgasm is associated with ejaculation and releases sexual tension and arousal, resulting in a feeling of intense sexual pleasure. After ejaculation the man enters an absolute refractory phase where re-arousal and orgasm are impossible. This is accompanied by loss of erection due to the decline in vasodilatation.

Coital changes in the female

Many of the changes seen in the man during coitus are mirrored in the women. Tactile and psychological stimulation reinforce frictional stimulation provided by the movement of the penis against the walls of the vagina and the external genitalia. A vascular response is evoked causing engorgement of the cavernous tissue in the clitoris. Furthermore, the vagina and labia become engorged and expand. Similar to men, women experience increases in heart rate and blood pressure, as well as skin flushes. In addition, there are rhythmic contractions of the pelvic muscle. After orgasm, clitoral erection is lost, and the uterine and vaginal walls relax to their original positions. Women do not generally experience an absolute refractory phase and can therefore be repeatedly aroused.

During coitus, semen is ejaculated into the vagina. The semen rapidly coagulates immediately after deposition, as a result of the interaction of prostatic enzymes with various components of the seminal vesicle secretion. This process is thought to aid retention of the sperm in the vagina and protect against the vagina's acidic environment. In normal circumstances the coagulum rapidly dissolves after around 20 min through the activation of proenzymes excreted in the semen.

Fertilisation

Fertilisation is the process where the two haploid germ cells – the sperm and the ovum – fuse to form a diploid zygote.

This can be divided into four stages:

1 **Motility**
2 **Activation**
3 **Acrosome reaction**
4 **Meiosis and fusion**.

Motility

The ovum and sperm must meet in the female reproductive tract so that fertilisation can occur:

- **Ovum**: at the time of ovulation the ciliated fimbria at the end of the fallopian tube transport the cumulus oophorus into the oviduct. The cumulus oophorus is then transported down the fallopian tubes to the ampullary–isthmic junction where it remains for 1–2 days, and where fertilisation takes place.
- **Sperm**: approximately 250 million sperm are released into the vagina at ejaculation. Only about 50 of these will reach the oviduct. Sperm motility depends on flagellar movement, which is helped by the increased fluidity of cervical fluid around the time of ovulation. Ideally sperm should reach the ampullary–isthmic junction at the time of ovulation, but they can remain at the isthmus for several days.

Activation ('capacitation')

Sperm are capable of fertilisation only when they have been exposed to the female tract. Interaction with the female tract triggers a series of changes in the sperm membrane that increase its affinity for the **zona pellucida**, and may also increase its motility.

Acrosome reaction

The sperm penetrates the cells of the cumulus oophorus to reach the zona pellucida. The head of the sperm binds to the zona pellucida glycoprotein ZP3, stimulating the acrosome reaction. The release of the contents of the acrosome causes an increase in extracellular calcium and release of proteins from granules in the oocyte, which hardens the zona pellucida to prevent a second fertilisation of the egg (polyspermy).

Meiosis and fusion

Fusion of the sperm with the oocyte membrane triggers the **second stage of meiosis in the oocyte**, resulting in formation of a mature oocyte and second polar body. The **second polar body** is extruded from the egg and a haploid number of chromosomes is present in both the egg and sperm pronuclei. The two pronuclei fuse to form the **zygote**.

 CLINICAL **Ectopic pregnancy**

An ectopic pregnancy is one that occurs outside the uterus. This is usually in the fallopian tubes, and occurs when there is a delay in the progress of the ovum from the fallopian tubes to the uterus. As the muscular walls of the fallopian tube are not adapted for embryonic growth, the trophoblast gradually erodes the tubal wall, resulting in damage to blood vessels. Tubal rupture may occur, resulting in intraperitoneal haemorrhage from erosion of an artery. This is a clinical emergency.

Ectopic pregnancies may be absorbed naturally, or tubal abortion may occur (where the products of conception are expelled from the tube into the peritoneal cavity). Ectopic pregnancies may also occur in the ovary or cervix. Very rarely they may occur in the abdominal cavity, and this can occasionally proceed to a full-term pregnancy.

 DEFINITION **Zygote**

The zygote is the cell formed by the fusion of the male and female haploid pronuclei, generating a single diploid cell. It is the cell from which all structures in the embryo and placenta are derived, and has the potential to differentiate into any tissue. It is **totipotent**.

Implantation

Initial divisions of the zygote occur in the fallopian tube. The embryo enters the uterine cavity as a **morula** (16–64 cells) on days 3–4. At this stage the embryo has differentiated into two different groups of cells: an outer cell mass and an inner cell mass. The inner cell mass is called the embryoblast; it gives rise to the embryo and the amnion. The outer cell mass is called the trophoblast and is the main source of placenta; on days 5–6 a cavity forms within the morula and it is now called a blastocyst.

On day 7, the blastocyst implants on the endometrial lining:

- Contact with the endometrium causes the trophoblast at the embryonic pole to differentiate into a **syncytiotrophoblast** and a **cytotrophoblast**.
- The **syncytiotrophoblast** cells secrete proteolytic enzymes such as heparin sulphate, proteoglycans, integrins and selectins, which erode the endometrium to allow implantation.
- **Progesterone** and **hCG** induce the differentiation of endometrial epithelial cells into **decidual cells**, the cells that line the uterus during pregnancy.
- **Corticotrophin-releasing hormone** (CRH) produced by the trophoblast also promotes implantation, and may have a role in immune tolerance in early pregnancy.

There are only 4 days (days 20–24) of the menstrual cycle when the blastocyst is able to implant into the endometrial lining of the uterus.

 DEFINITION Syncytiotrophoblast

The syncytiotrophoblast is made up of many fused cells containing many nuclei. This component of the placenta secretes hCG in the early stages of pregnancy to maintain the corpus luteum. In addition, it contributes to the chorionic villi, which allow nutrient exchange between the mother and fetus. Syncytiotrophoblast cells secrete proteolytic enzymes to allow them to invade the uterine walls for implantation.

 DEFINITION Cytotrophoblast

The cytotrophoblast is the precursor layer to the syncytiotrophoblast, and also makes up an interior layer of the placenta. There cells contribute to the placenta, playing a role in nutrient exchange and also releasing CRH.

The placenta

The placenta is developed from trophoblast tissue (Fig. 12.7). Lacunar spaces that are in immediate contact with the maternal circulation form in the syncytiotrophoblast. Within the lacunar spaces, chorionic villi develop – these provide a large surface area for nutrient and gas exchange. The villi are bathed in maternal blood. The placenta has three main roles:

1 **Exchange**: transport of nutrients and oxygen from the mother to the fetus, and removal of waste products from the fetus into the maternal bloodstream. There is exchange of gases and molecules, but not of cells.
2 **Endocrine**: hormone synthesis, transport and metabolism.
3 **Immune**: the placenta acts to prevent immunological rejection of the fetus (which is an allograft), possibly via secretion of hCG.

Pregnancy

The maintenance of pregnancy and the process of parturition (birth) depend on complex maternal–placental–fetal interactions. The structural development of the fetus, which occurs particularly during the first trimester, is discussed in detail in Chapter 13. The main hormones regulating pregnancy are progesterone, oestrogen, hCG and human placental lactogen (hPL).

Hormonal regulation of pregnancy

Many hormones are involved in regulating the growth of the fetus and placenta, as well as triggering changes in the maternal body to support the fetus during its growth and shortly after birth.

Progesterone

In the first 6–8 weeks of pregnancy the corpus luteum is the main source of progesterone; after 8 weeks the developing trophoblast takes over, and levels increase throughout pregnancy. Progesterone acts to:

- **inhibit smooth muscle contractility** and thus prevent uterine contraction
- **inhibit prostaglandin (PG) formation**, which is thought to be involved in parturition
- **stimulate maternal appetite** and alter the deposition of fat reserves
- **inhibit oxytocin release** and **downregulate oxytocin receptor expression** on uterine muscle, preventing parturition.

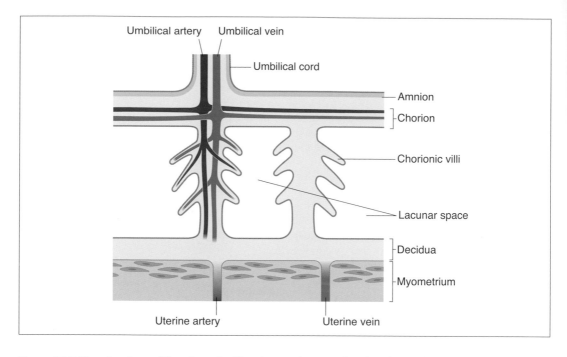

Figure 12.7 The structure of the placenta. The placenta forms an interface for exchange between the mother and fetus. In particular the placenta invades the uterine tissue and projects chorionic villi into the lacunar spaces of the endometrial tissue. These spaces form in response to the placental formation and bathe the chorionic villi in maternal blood, allowing exchange by diffusion. The lacunar spaces receive blood from the uterine vessels, which supply the myometrium.

Oestrogen

Levels of oestrogen increase throughout pregnancy. The **corpus luteum** is the primary source of oestrogen during the first few weeks. After this the fetoplacental unit is responsible for the production of oestrogen, because neither the fetus nor the placenta expresses all the enzymes necessary for oestrogen production:

- The fetal adrenals synthesise dehydroepiandrosterone sulphate (DHEA-S) from cholesterol.
- The fetal liver hydroxylates **DHEA-S** which passes to the placenta as **16α-OH-DHEA-S**.
- The placenta processes **16α-OH-DHEA-S** into **oestrogen**.

Oestrogen acts to:

- stimulate uterine growth
- stimulate prostaglandin synthesis
- thicken the vaginal epithelium
- stimulate growth and development of mammary epithelium
- inhibit milk production.

Human chorionic gonadotrophin

This hormone is a glycoprotein hormone, similar to LH in structure and action, binding to the LH receptor. It is secreted by the syncytiotrophoblast into the fetal and maternal circulations. Levels are high in early pregnancy (hCG is used in pregnancy tests and levels can be detected 6–8 days after ovulation) peaking at 9 weeks, then declining.

Human chorionic gonadotrophin acts to:

- maintain the corpus luteum in early pregnancy to ensure production of progesterone until the placenta takes over
- regulate testosterone production in fetal Leydig cells in the male fetus, which is important for fetal development.

Human placental lactogen

HPL is a **polypeptide hormone** secreted by the syncytiotrophoblast. Levels increase throughout pregnancy triggering changes related to milk production. It acts to:

- stimulate lipolysis, increasing availability of circulating free fatty acids
- inhibit glucose uptake in the mother
- inhibit gluconeogenesis in the mother; this favours transport of glucose and protein to the fetus.

Growth of the fetus during pregnancy

The development of the major structures in the fetus occurs early in development and is discussed in Chapter 13. The growth and development of the fetus can be in three 3 month phases or 'trimesters':

1 The **first trimester** starts with implantation of the embryo. During this phase, the growth and development of structures in the embryo are extremely rapid. Miscarriages are most common during the first trimester.
2 The **second trimester** occurs from month 4 to month 6 and is associated with growth and weight gain of the fetus. In addition, movement by the fetus in the womb may be detectable.
3 During the **third trimester** the fetus gains weight and the final development of the organ systems occurs to prepare for birth.

Parturition

During pregnancy, the myometrium of the uterus is inactive. At parturition, many factors act together to cause coordinated contraction of the myometrium, and remodelling and softening of the cervix. The control of parturition in humans is not well understood, although a number of contributing processes have been identified:

- The levels of **prostaglandins** in the uterus rise; this occurs before the onset of clinical labour and is thought to have a role in stimulating myometrial contractility.
- Other inflammatory mediators such as neutrophils and macrophages infiltrate the human myometrium – they may increase prostaglandin production and also facilitate tissue remodelling.
- **Gap junctions** form between the myometrial cells so that there is rapid spread of contraction.
- **Oxytocin** stimulates myometrial contraction. At term, **oxyntinergic** cells in the hypothalamus fire

synchronously and oxytocin receptors in the myometrium increase.
- **Relaxin** and **prostaglandins** act to soften the uterine cervix.

 CLINICAL Eclampsia and pre-eclampsia

Eclampsia is characterised by epileptiform fits and hypertension during pregancy. The patient develops cerebral ischaemia, leading to fits, as a result of cerebral oedema, vasoconstriction and hypoxia. Maternal mortality is rare but the fetus may die during the fit, or as a result of hypoxia or pre-term birth.

    Pre-eclampsia generally precedes eclampsia and is defined as a blood pressure of more than 160/110 mmHg and the presence of proteinuria. It usually presents in the third trimester.

Lactation

After birth the mother produces milk to feed the newborn baby. Milk is produced by the breast and performs different functions at different points; initially it has a primarily protective function, although later its function is nutritional.

Structure of the developed breast

The developed mammary gland is made up of a lobed mass of glandular and ductile tissue. There are two type of duct found in the breast:

1 The **lactiferous ducts** are made up of a series of ducts that converge at the areola. These ducts open on to the surface of the breasts at the nipple and expel milk for ingestion by the infant.
2 The **Montgomery glands** open on to the areola and secrete lubricating fluids during suckling.

The lactiferous ducts

The human breast is typically made up of 15–20 lobes; these contain lobules of milk-secreting alveoli draining into the lactiferous ducts which carry the milk to the nipple. The walls of the alveoli are made up of the single layer of epithelial cells, which synthesise milk and secrete it into the lumen. The alveoli are surrounded by a basement membrane and **myoepithelial cells** which contract to drive the milk into the ducts for ejection.

Development of breasts

The tissue of the breast is minimal at birth, consisting of very few lactiferous ducts. The breasts develop during puberty and then further during pregnancy, when they become functional and begin to produce milk for the first time.

Changes of the breast during puberty

At puberty, oestrogen stimulates the duct tissue to divide and develop functional alveoli. As menstrual cycles continue, the secretion of oestrogen and progesterone triggers further breast tissue development and promotes the growth of connective tissue and the deposition of fat. The ductal tissue also develops in response to corticosteroids.

Breast development during pregnancy

During pregnancy, development of the breast is stimulated under the control of a number of hormones. During early pregnancy, estradiol and progesterone act to mature the lactiferous glands and ducts. The breasts then develop the capacity to produce milk for the first time, providing nutrition to the newborn child. This is stimulated by prolactin, human placental lactogen (hPL), oestrogen, progesterone, insulin and glucocorticoids.

Milk
Synthesis of milk

In the last part of pregnancy **hPL** and **prolactin** stimulate milk. However, secretion of milk by the alveolar cells does not occur due to the inhibitory activity of progesterone and oestrogen. Milk fat is produced in the smooth ER of the alveolar epithelium, and develops into droplets in the cytoplasm, which move towards the luminal surface of the cell. Milk protein passes through the Golgi apparatus and is secreted by exocytosis. As the droplet moves towards the surface of the cell, it 'pinches off' as a membrane-bound droplet.

The composition of milk varies:

- Initially, **colostrum** is produced. This contains high amounts of proteins, in particular antibodies to provide protection before the infant's immune system develops.

- The composition of milk transitions during the first 2–3 weeks postpartum. Its production of proteins and antibodies decreases whereas nutrients in the milk, in particular lactose and fats, increase.

Prolactin

Prolactin is a peptide hormone produced by the anterior pituitary; it is primarily regulated by the release of dopamine, an inhibitory signal, from the hypothalamus. The main effect of prolactin is to stimulate milk production from the breast. Prolactin secretion increases during pregnancy, although milk is not released due to the inhibitory effects of progesterone. After birth, the levels of progesterone decrease to allow milk release. After parturition, levels of progesterone and oestrogen fall due to the loss of the placenta; continued milk production is due to high levels of prolactin which is stimulated by suckling.

Milk ejection

The milk ejection reflex (MER) moves milk from the glands to the surface of the nipple for ingestion:

- **Stimulation** of the nipple and the sensation of suckling are the most potent triggers of milk ejection. The sound of a baby crying can also act as a stimulus.
- The various stimuli are **integrated by the hypothalamic** neurons, which trigger **oxytocin** release.
- **Oxytocin acts on the mammary glands** to cause contraction of the myoepithelial cells that surround the alveoli. This results in expulsion of the milk into the ducts beneath the nipple and a build-up of intramammary pressure.

The suckling stimulus also reduces the pulsatile release of GnRH, which controls ovulation, from the hypothalamus, reducing the potential for a second pregnancy. However, it is still possible for a woman to get pregnant while she is breastfeeding.

Age and reproductive capacity

There is a limited period of time during which individuals are fertile; this fertile period starts with puberty, although towards the end of life fertility decreases. In women this cessation of fertility is determined by the menopause – the cessation of the menstrual cycle. In men, there appears to be some decrease in fertility with age, although it is not defined, nor as definitive as the menopause.

Women

The fertility of a woman begins and ends with defined events:

- The **menarche** – the first uterine cycle – which implies that a full oocyte development may also have occurred. Early menstrual cycles are not entirely regulated, often not associated with ovulation and have a shortened luteal phase.
- The **menopause** is the point at which menstrual cycles and ovarian function ceases, altogether typically occurring in the early 50s. The menopause is associated with mood changes, irritability, loss of libido and hot flushes, as a result of reduced sex hormones.

The fertility of a woman is highest in her early 20s and decreases gradually as she ages. This is thought to be associated with an increased risk of failed ovulation.

Men

Sperm can be continually produced by men into later life, although loss of libido and impotence do increase with age. Much of this is thought to be the result of other age-related factors and not directly through failure of the reproductive system.

Control of fertility

Sex has a role in society other than for reproduction. Mechanisms have been developed to reduce the potential for conception as a result of sexual intercourse. Three broad mechanisms of controlling fertility have been developed, although their acceptance in different societies varies, as does their effectiveness:

1 Contraception
2 Abortion
3 Sterilisation.

Contraception

Contraception is the prevention of fertilisation. This can be achieved by many different means: preventing ovulation, preventing the sperm from reaching the egg by altering cervical mucus or preventing the sperm from entering the uterus. The main methods of contraception are:

- barrier protection
- hormonal control
- intrauterine devices
- natural rhythm method.

Barrier contraception

Barrier methods physically prevent the sperm from getting through the cervix. They also protect against sexually transmitted infections:

- The **male condom** is a sheath (normally latex) which can be fitted onto the erect penis. If used correctly, around 3 pregnancies may result per 100 women per year.
- The **female condom** is a sheath that fits inside the vagina; failure rates are similar to a condom and it is less acceptable to females.
- **Diaphragms** and **caps** are inserted just before intercourse and fit over the cervix. A diaphragm, also known as a Dutch cap, is a flexible latex dome with a spring, which is held between the pubic bone and the sacral curve, covering the cervix. A cervical cap also fits over the cervix.
- **Spermicidal gels** are often used with caps and diaphragms to increase their success.

Hormonal contraceptives

These are contraceptives that use progestogen and/or oestrogen to create an artificial hormonal environment to prevent ovulation. The different types of hormonal contraceptive are:

- the combined oral contraceptive (COC)
- progesterone-releasing contraceptives.

The combined oral contraceptive ('the pill')

This contains oestrogen and progestogen, which negatively feed back on gonadotrophin release from the pituitary, inhibiting ovulation. The direct action of oestrogen and progesterone on the uterus causes the endometrium to atrophy and alters the cervical mucus, inhibiting the entry of sperm. The pill is extremely effective if used correctly.

Normally, the pill is taken daily for 21 days at approximately the same time each day. There is then a 7-day break, when there is a 'withdrawal bleed' (similar to a period) due to the withdrawal of progestogen. Most women find this reassuring to know that they are not pregnant, even though it is not a proper period. If a woman misses a pill by less than 24 hours, the last missed pill should be taken and the remaining tablets continued; she still has contraceptive protection. If a woman misses a pill by more than 24 hours, the last missed pill should be taken and the packet finished as usual. However, she is no longer protected and should use another form of contraception for the next 7 days. Moreover, if there were fewer than seven pills left, the next packet should be started without a break. The pill also has non-contraceptive benefits including regular, lighter and less painful periods.

Minor side effects include weight gain, nausea, headaches and breast tenderness. There may be breakthrough bleeding in the first month of taking.

Major side effects are very rare. The most important are venous thrombosis and myocardial infarction; the risk of these increases with increased age and smoking. Others include thromboembolic disease, and increased risk of liver, cervical and breast cancer. The pill is contraindicated in anyone with a history of any of the major side effects listed above, and in smokers aged more than 35 years.

Progestogens

Progestogens cause the cervical mucus to become hostile, and also prevent ovulation. In most women menstruation also ceases. Progestogens can be given in a number of forms:

- **The progestogen-only pill** (mini-pill) is taken at the same time of day, each and every day. If a pill is taken more than 3 hours late, it is necessary to use another form of contraception for 7 days.
- **Depot contraception** can be given by injection every 3 months – progestogens are released slowly, bypassing the portal circulation.
- **Implanon** is a single 6-cm rod containing progestogen, which is inserted subdermally in the upper arm using local anaesthetic. It lasts for 3 years.
- **Progesterone**-containing intrauterine devices (IUDs) – discussed below.

Side effects of progestogens include vaginal spotting, weight gain, mastalgia and premenstrual like symptoms. They do not have any of the contraindications associated with the COC.

Intrauterine devices

These devices are inserted into the uterine cavity in an outpatient setting and can be left in place for up to 5 years. Thin strings hang down from the opening of the cervix, which allow the woman to check that the IUD is still in place. IUDs are very effective forms of contraception, resulting in less than 0.5 preganancies per 100 women per year.

- **Copper-containing devices** are normally T-shaped and the copper has a toxic effect on sperm which prevents fertilisation. Copper devices can cause increased menstrual loss, more painful bleeding and increased risk of ectopic pregnancy (if pregnancy occurs).
- **Intrauterine system** (IUS): the **Mirena coil** is a T-shaped device containing progestogen that is released gradually over 5 years. It has progestogenic side effects. However, it decreases blood loss and painful periods.

Natural contraception

The theory behind natural contraception is that a couple will abstain from intercourse during a woman's fertile period, i.e. around ovulation. This is judged by changes in basal body temperature, cervical mucus and the cervix, and there are commercially available kits to detect these changes. However, failure rates are high because couples fail to abstain and as a result of inaccuracies in the mechanisms used to predict ovulation.

Therapeutic abortion

Therapeutic abortion is the medical termination of pregnancy – as opposed to a spontaneous abortion, known as a miscarriage. This is usually performed before the age at which the fetus is able to survive outside the womb, which is considered to be 24 weeks. In the UK, abortion is essentially offered 'on demand', although this is a contentious issue.

Surgical abortion

The patient is put under a general anaesthetic. The neck of the cervix is dilated and a small catheter inserted through the cervix. Suction is used to remove the fetal tissue from the uterus.

Medical abortion

Mifepristone, a drug that blocks progestogen receptors in the uterus, is given; 48 hours later a vaginal pessary of prostaglandins is given. As progesterone acts to inhibit smooth muscle contractility and decrease prostaglandin production, keeping the uterus quiescent, antagonism of the progestogen receptors removes this effect. The products of conception are passed as they would be during a spontaneous abortion. Ten per cent of midtrimester medical abortions require subsequent surgical evacuation.

Sterilisation

Sterilisation is generally regarded as an irreversible procedure and should be 100% effective.

In **men** sterilisation is through ligation or removal of a section of vas deferens – a **vasectomy**. As a result the ejaculate produced rapidly becomes aspermic. There are potential side effects of vasectomy as a result of the continuing build-up of sperm, as the seminiferous tubules remain effective:

- The **build-up of sperm and fluid** can cause chronic or periodic tenderness in the testes.
- **Leakage of sperm antigens** into the circulation may trigger an immune response. This can result in infertility even if the vasectomy is reversed.

In **women**, sterilisation is achieved through ligation or removal (either part or all) of the fallopian tubes. This is a much more major procedure than a vasectomy, requiring a general anaesthetic. Tubal ligation is, in most cases, reversible. Sterilisation may also be achieved through a hysterectomy – removal of the uterus.

Assisted conception

There are a number of reasons why a couple may not be able to reproduce. These can be best understood by looking at the requirements for conception:

- **An egg must be produced**. – the woman may not ovulate.
- **The sperm must have adequate function**. – sperm can have decreased motility, be abnormal in form or not be present (azoospermia).
- **The sperm must reach the egg**. – the fallopian tubes can be damaged, or there can be problems with the cervix or the mechanical act of intercourse.

- **The fertilised egg must implant**. – there can be problems with the uterus.

There are a number of options for assisted conception depending on what the problem is. The current methods are:

- *in vitro* fertilisation (IVF)
- intrauterine insemination
- intracytoplasmic sperm injection.

Assisted conception is often unavailable on the NHS and is very expensive. Other options are egg donation, surrogacy and adoption.

In vitro fertilisation

This is useful when there is anovulation or tubal blockage. Endogenous LH and FSH production is abolished and ovulation is induced with exogenous gonadotrophins. The eggs are then removed from the ovaries under ultrasound and incubated with paternal sperm. The embryo is transferred to the uterus 3–5 days later, and progesterone and **hCG** given to support the pregnancy for the first 10 weeks. The live birth rate is approximately 25%; more than one embryo may be transferred to the womb to increase the chance of implantation, although this increases the potential for multiple pregnancies.

Intrauterine insemination

As in IVF, ovulation is stimulated with exogenous hormones. A semen sample is taken and the best quality sperm are selected in a laboratory. The sperm are then placed in the uterus at the time of ovulation. Intrauterine insemination is often performed when there are moderate abnormalities of sperm, or when the cause of infertility is unknown.

Intracytoplasmic sperm injection

When there is male infertility with abnormal or immotile sperm, intracytoplasmic sperm injection may allow conception. Sperm is extracted from the testis or epididymis, and injected directly into the oocyte. The egg can then be implanted. The success rate is 20% per cycle.

➔ RELATED CHAPTERS

Chapter 10 Endocrinology
Chapter 11 Integrative physiology
Chapter 13 Embryology

13

Embryology

Each individual is created from a single cell – the zygote – formed by the fusion of an egg cell with a sperm. The zygote divides and differentiates into all the tissues in the body and the placenta. The developmental programme is immensely complex to allow for the formation of the many organs, some of which must continue to develop while remaining functional (Fig. 13.1). Four processes are crucial for the correct development of the embryo: division, differentiation, migration and apoptosis.

This chapter discusses the processes that follow implantation of the embryo into the lining of the uterus. The developmental process up to this point, and the formation of the placenta, are covered in Chapter 12.

Concepts of embryology

Implantation occurs at around day 5. At this point the embryo consists of a ring of cells, which contains a clump at one point, and is known as the **blastocyst**. From this structure, both the embryo and the placenta develop. The blastocyst rapidly grows to form the bilaminar germ disc – made up of two layers of cells with a fluid-filled cavity on each side (Fig. 13.2).

The bilaminar germ disc develops into a three-dimensional fetus. One of the crucial processes is that of **axis formation**, whereby three axes are generated in the embryo:

1 Rostrocaudal: head to tail
2 Dorsoventral: back to front
3 Left to right.

The first crucial stage in axis formation occurs with **gastrulation**. This provides the primitive streak along the rostrocaudal (head-to-tail) axis, and the primitive node is found at the rostral end, which develops into the head.

Potency

The potency of a cell refers to its ability to generate a range of tissues. In general the more differentiated a cell, the less potency it has and the smaller the range of cell types into which it is capable of differentiating:

- A **totipotent** cell can give rise to all structures in the embryo and placenta. Totipotent cells are found only before formation of the blastocyst.
- A **pluripotent** cell is capable of dividing into any cell. These embryonic stem cells are being investigated as a source of tissue for therapy.
- A **multipotent** cell is capable of dividing into tissues in a related line of cells. Many adult stem cells are multipotent, e.g. the haematopoietic stem cell can generate all the blood cells, but cannot contribute to nervous tissue.
- A **unipotent** cell is a fully differentiated cell, although it may be capable of renewing itself (e.g. the hepatocyte).

Formation of the amnion and chorion

The first significant structure that consists purely of embryonic (instead of placental) tissue is the bilaminar germ disc. It develops from the proliferation of both layers of the inner cell mass of the

Biomedical Science Lecture Notes, First Edition. Ian Lyons.
© 2011 by Ian Lyons. Published 2011 by Blackwell Publishing Ltd.

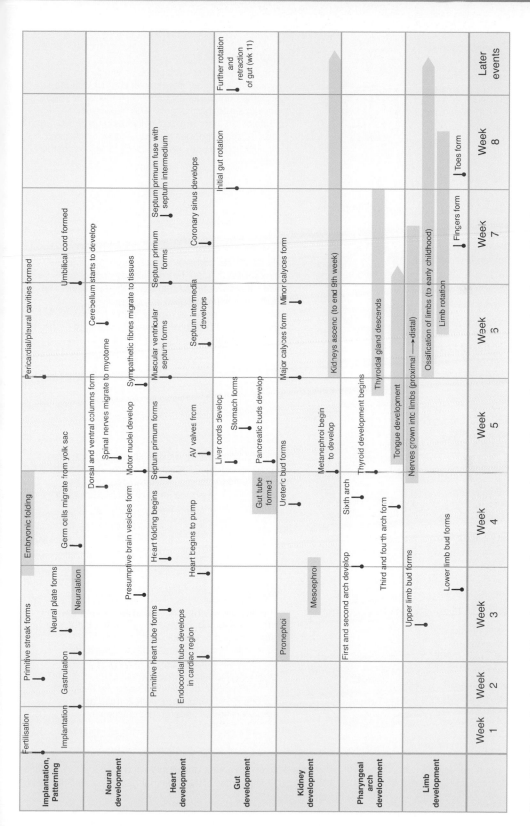

Figure 13.1 During development of the embryo several processes must occur at the same time – to pattern the embryo and then allow the simultaneous development of all the organ systems. The major features of the embryo develop in the first 8 weeks whereas other parts of development, such as formation of the alveoli and ossification of the bones, may continue until well past birth.

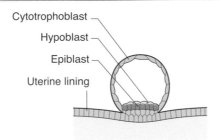

Day 7

The blastocyst implants at day 7, where the syncytiotrophoblast develops in contact with the endometrium; it rapidly penetrates this layer which develops into the placenta. The blastocyst contains an inner mass of cells made up of two layers – the hypoblast develops into the yolk sacs and the epiblast develops into the structures of the embryo.

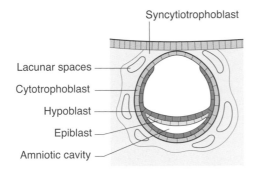

Day 9

By day 9, the embryo has fully implanted and the syncytiotrophoblast has developed spaces to allow the flow of maternal blood for exchange. The epiblast has proliferated and generated a small amniotic cavity that is rapidly filled with fluid, while the hypoblast proliferates around the edged of the cytotrophoblast.

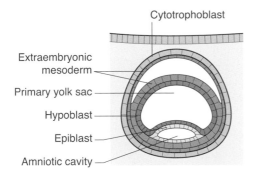

Day 12

The cytotrophoblast has proliferated to form two layers of extraembryonic mesoderm surrounding a loose acellular tissue, while the hypoblast has completely coated the inner of the two layers to form the primary yolk sac.

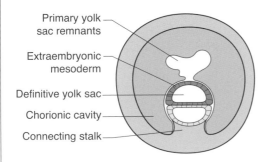

Day 13

The extraembryonic mesoderm has grown to surround the chorionic cavity, while the embryo is suspended in the middle of this cavity by a connecting stalk of extraembryonic mesoderm. The primary yolk sac rapidly degenerates and further proliferation of the hypoblast leads to the formation of the definitive yolk sac. By this point the bilaminar germ disc is fully formed and the embryo ready to undergo gastrulation.

Figure 13.2 Immediately after implantation, the placenta develops to nourish the embryo and the important cavities surrounding the embryo develop. These processes result in the formation of the bilaminar germ disc, definitive yolk sac, and chorionic and amniotic cavities by the end of week 2.

blastocyst, resulting in two layers of cell surrounded on either side by fluid-filled cavities (Fig. 13.3):

1 The **hypoblast** forms the yolk sac.
2 The **epiblast** gives rise to the structures in the embryo. It is the epiblast that undergoes gastrulation.

Formation of the amnion

The amnion begins to form at around day 8. This results from fluid accumulating between the cells of the epiblast. This cavity progressively grows throughout the embryo's development so that it encloses the entire embryo by the end of the second month. During this time it protects the embryo and provides it with a space in which to develop.

Formation of the chorion

The chorion is the cavity that develops to separate the **cytotrophoblast** from the yolk sac. It forms from the **extraembryonic mesoderm** cells arising from the **epiblast.** Two layers of mesoderm are separated by the extraembryonic reticulum, which is a large region of acellular matter. This reticulum then breaks down and fluid progressively accumulates between the layers to form the chorionic cavity.

Formation of the yolk sac

The yolk sac has several important functions in development:

- It gives rise to the germ cells that migrate into the gonads.
- It is an early site of haematopoiesis.
- It produces some serum proteins during development.
- It may have some role in the early nutrition of the embryo.

The yolk sac forms in two stages: there is production of the primary yolk sac through the migration of hypoblast cells over the interior of the cytotrophoblast. This is a transient structure that begins to break down by day 13, as the definitive yolk sac is produced by further proliferation from the hypoblast.

The **yolk sac** is a developmental structure that, in most cases, regresses before birth. However, it can persist as **Meckel's diverticulum**.

Gastrulation and patterning

In gastrulation the bilaminar germ disc structure develops into the three-layered **trilaminar germ disc**. The cells in each layer are derived from the epiblast, although they undergo different developmental programmes and give rise to different tissues. Gastrulation provides the first gross sign of orientation in the embryo.

Mechanism of gastrulation

- The bilaminar germ disc is fully formed by day 15, at which point a groove in the epiblast – the primitive streak – develops. This midline structure consists of a long depression with a mound of cells at the rostral end – the primitive mound. The first groups of cells that migrate differentiate to form the **definitive endoderm**.
- Later, cells migrating through the primitive streak migrate in between the endoderm and the ectoderm to form the **definitive mesoderm**.
- The epiblast cells that do not migrate through the primitive node develop into the **ectoderm**.
- The primitive streak regulates the development of the different cell layers through the release of signalling factors.
- Throughout most of the trilaminar germ disc the three layers are found.
- At the extreme ends of the disc, the endoderm and ectoderm are directly in contact; these sites will form the ends of the **gut tube**.

The primitive streak rapidly disappears by the middle of week 4.

Ectoderm

The ectoderm is the outermost layer of the embryo and generates three major tissue groups:

1 Most of the ectoderm remains on the outside of the embryo, and will give rise to the **skin**.
2 The ectoderm becomes folded during neurulation and is responsible for forming the **neural tube** which gives rises to the **nervous tissues** within the body.
3 During neurulation, the ectoderm gives rise to the **neural crest** cells, which contribute to specialised cells throughout the body, often those involved in pigmentation (e.g. melanocytes).

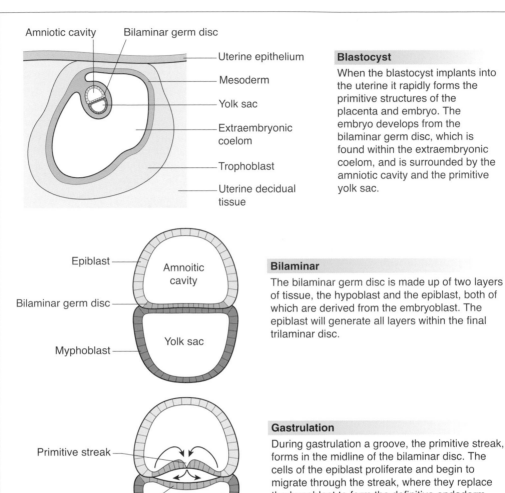

Blastocyst

When the blastocyst implants into the uterine it rapidly forms the primitive structures of the placenta and embryo. The embryo develops from the bilaminar germ disc, which is found within the extraembryonic coelom, and is surrounded by the amniotic cavity and the primitive yolk sac.

Bilaminar

The bilaminar germ disc is made up of two layers of tissue, the hypoblast and the epiblast, both of which are derived from the embryoblast. The epiblast will generate all layers within the final trilaminar disc.

Gastrulation

During gastrulation a groove, the primitive streak, forms in the midline of the bilaminar disc. The cells of the epiblast proliferate and begin to migrate through the streak, where they replace the hypoblast to form the definitive endoderm. Later cells migrate into a space between the two layers and form the mesoderm.

Trilaminar disc

The trilaminar disc consists of the endoderm and mesoderm, which have formed from the cells that migrated through the primitive streak during gastrulation. The epiblast cells that do not migrate give rise to the ectoderm of the trilaminar disc. Although the endoderm and ectoderm are epithelial layers made of tightly apposed cells, the mesoderm is a mesenchymal cell layer made of cells suspended in an extracellular matrix.

Figure 13.3 The first process in the embryo that demonstrates definite axes on a gross scale is gastrulation, by which the bilaminar disc is converted to a trilaminar germ disc. The three resulting layers have different developmental fates, each giving rise to specific lineages of tissue in the embryo.

Mesoderm

The mesoderm is the middle, non-epithelial, layer of the trilaminar germ disc; it forms much of the connective tissue. Through the various patterning that follows, the mesoderm becomes segmented, giving rise to the bones and muscles as well as the tissue of the internal organs. Although the epithelial layers are often endo- or ectodermally derived, the remainder of the organs are mesodermal in origin. Unlike the endoderm and ectoderm, the mesoderm is found in its own extracellular matrix and is not tightly apposed. This arrangement of cells is known as a **mesenchyme**.

Endoderm

The endoderm is the innermost cell layer in the embryo and is continuous with the **yolk sac**. Similar to the ectoderm it is an epithelial layer and will go on to generate the gut and related structures, including the lungs and biliary tree.

Neurulation

The spinal cord is the major structure that forms along the rostrocaudal axis. Developmentally, the vertebrae are derived from the mesoderm, although the cells that go on to form the spinal cord itself are derived from the ectoderm. This 'inside-out' structure is formed in neurulation (Fig. 13.4):

- Formation of the notochord.
- Development of the neural plate.
- Folding of the neural plate into the neural tube.

Formation of the notochord

Generation of the notochord is regulated by the primitive streak. As the primitive streak regresses, the primitive node migrates rostrally, and cells proliferating in this region form the hollow **notochord**. By day 20, this hollow tube structure is completely formed and begins to remodel itself into a solid rod in the mesoderm:

- The ventral surface of the tube fuses with the endoderm, and then opens ventrally to form a

flat bar of tissue in the midline – the **notochordal plate**.
- The plate detaches from the endoderm at the start of week 4 and becomes located within the endoderm and develops into a more cylindrical shape.

The notochord is thought to develop into the **nucleus pulposus**, located within the centre of the intervertebral discs.

Development of the neural plate

The neural plate is a thickened layer of ectoderm cells that forms in response to signalling factors released by the notochord and the underlying mesoderm. As with the other patterning mechanisms discussed so far, the neural plate starts to form at the rostral end of the embryo and migrates caudally. The neural plate starts to develop from the middle of week 4 of development and rapidly becomes expanded at the cranial end, where it will develop into the brain.

Folding of the neural plate into the neural tube

The final product of neurulation is the neural tube which lies entirely within the mesoderm along the rostrocaudal axis of the embryo. This structure will give rise to the central nervous system (CNS). The neural tube is crucial for the segmental organisation of the embryo and regulates the development of many of the mesoderm-derived structures found in the embryo. Its formation from the neural plate occurs in a series of steps:

1 The notochord acts as a hinge region for the folding of the neural plate and governs the process through the release of signalling factors.
2 The thickened neural plate tissue on either side of the groove folds up and fuses to form the neural tube.
3 The surface ectoderm also fuses above the neural tube, drawing the entire structure into the mesoderm. The resulting tube remains open at the rostral and caudal ends.

Neural tube closure is essential for proper formation of the spinal cord and vertebrae and other structures that surround it; failure of the neural tube to close can lead to **spina bifida**.

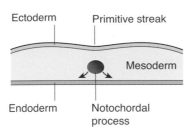

Notochord

During gastrulation, the primitive node at the head of the midline streak regresses caudally down the embryo. As this occurs, it signals to mesodermal tissue to proliferate and develop into a hollow tube – the notochordal process – which develops progressively along the length of the embryo. This tube briefly forms a plate on the endodermal surface before reorganising into the solid notochord in the mesodermal tissue.

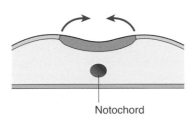

Ectodermal proliferation

The notochord secretes signalling factors that stimulate the ectodermal tissue in the midline to proliferate and thicken to form the neural plate. Growth of the embryo stimulates folding along the rostrocaudal axis, which is hinged at the notochord and allows fusion of the neural plate along the midline.

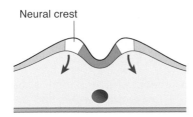

Neural crest

As the neural plate folds to fuse, the cells at the interface between the neural plate and the ectoderm proper detach and migrate around the body; these neural crest cells give rise to many structures throughout the embryo.

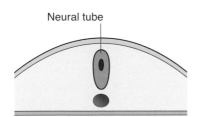

Neural tube

The folding of the neural plate leads to the edges of the neural plate fusing to form a cylinder through the midline – the neural tube. The neural tube remains open at both ends, although it migrates into the mesoderm of the embryo and will give rise to the structures of the central nervous system. In addition, the ectoderm fuses above the neural tube so that the ectoderm remains a continuous layer across the embryo's surface.

Figure 13.4 Neurulation results in the development of the neural tube, which gives rise to the central nervous system, and the neural crest, which gives rise to many structures throughout the embryo. Both these tissues are derived from the ectoderm and form from a variety of complex folding reactions and signals, primarily regulated by the notochord, a mesoderm-derived structure.

CLINICAL **Spina bifida**

A failure of neurulation can lead to the neural tube not closing completely. The defect may hinder the development of tissue within the spinal cord and, in severe cases, may be incompatible with life:

- **Spina bifida occulta** is the least serious defect and often goes undetected (occurrence may be as high as 10%). This is where there has been a failure in the formation of the vertebrae, typically resulting in the formation of a hemivertebra. This is often associated with the presence of a tuft of hair on the skin over the defect.
- **Meningocele** occurs where the neural tube has not closed; the dura and arachnoid of the spinal cord may protrude. This defect contains no neural tissue and is usually relatively easily repaired.
- A **meningomyelocele** is a serious defect, in which neural tissue protrudes from the defect. If this occurs in the cranial region, brain tissue may protrude from the defect. These defects are often not fatal; as a result of incomplete development, there are likely to be long-term motor and mental defects.
- Severe cases, in which the **neural tube fails completely to develop**, are associated with spontaneous abortion.

The neural crest

Those cells that exist at the interface of the ectoderm cells and future neural tube tissue develop into the **neural crest cells,** which contribute in a variety of manners to many different systems.

Neuronal tissue outside the CNS

Peripheral sensory neurons, which have cell bodies within the dorsal root ganglia, can be:

- Postganglionic sympathetic neurons
- Postganglionic parasympathetic neurons
- Neurons in the lower part of the enteric nervous system
- Sensory ganglia of cranial nerves V, VII, IX, X and XI.

Connective tissue structures

- Tissue in the spiral septum, which divides the heart outflow tract into aortic and pulmonary trunks

- Dermis of the head and neck
- Teeth
- Connective tissue of the head and neck glands, including the lacrimal, pituitary, thyroid, parathyroid and salivary glands.

Other structures

- Calcitonin-secreting cells of the thyroid gland (the C-cells)
- Chemoreceptor cells in the aortic and carotid bodies
- Melanocytes.

 CLINICAL **Hirschsprung's disease**

Hirschsprung's disease (frequency approximately 1/5000 births) is characterised by an enlarged bowel segment, arising from the absence of peristalsis in the more distal sections of bowel. This is a result of the absence of migration of neural crest cells to the gut, which contribute to the enteric nervous system. The enteric nervous system regulates peristalsis and other functions in the gut.

Segmentation in the embryo

Many of the axial structures in the body are organised in a segmental fashion, as illustrated by the peripheral nerves that leave the spinal cord regularly between the vertebrae. This segmental organisation is seen in development, particularly in the **somites** which form much of the connective tissue structures in the body (Fig. 13.5).

At the end of week 3, the paraxial mesoderm coalesces to form a series of compact groups of tissue on either side of the notochord, known as somitomeres, which contribute to two major sets of structures:

1 The **seven most cranial somitomeres** develop into the muscles found in the head and neck.
2 The **majority of the somitomeres** develop into 42–44 pairs of somites which form more rapidly at the cranial end of the embryo.
   - Additional caudal somitomeres regress.

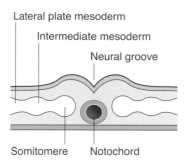

Lateral plate mesoderm
Intermediate mesoderm
Neural groove
Somitomere   Notochord

Mesoderm

The mesoderm differentiates into a series of regions, which give rise to different structures. The paraxial mesoderm will develop into the somites, which give rise to the vertebrae and much of the axial skeleton. The intermediate mesoderm contributes to the urogenital system. The lateral plate mesoderm of the embryo fuses in the midline, as a result of embryonic folding, and contributes to the body and gut walls.

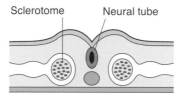

Sclerotome   Neural tube

Somitomeres

The paraxial mesoderm rapidly forms clusters arranged in pairs either side of the neural tube. These develop into hollow somites, which contain many mesenchymal cells in their interior. The somites rupture on their interior aspect and release the sclerotome.

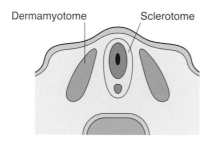

Dermamyotome   Sclerotome

Dermamyotome

The sclerotomal cells accumulate around the neural tube and develop into the vertebral body. The notochord becomes encased in the sclerotome and gives rise to the nucleus pulposus of the intervertebral discs. The remaining somite tissue coalesces into a band of tissue with each side of the future vertebral arch forming the dermamyotome, which differentiates into the dermatome and the myotome. These give rise to the dermis of the back and lateral trunk, as well as the musculature of the axial skeleton. At the site of the limb buds, the myotome cells migrate into the limb bud to contribute to the future connective tissue.

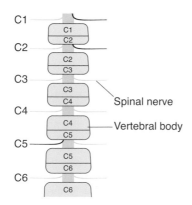

C1
C2
C3
C4
C5
C6
Spinal nerve
Vertebral body

Spinal nerve

The vertebral bodies develop from the sclerotome of two different somites. The rostral portion of each vertebral body is derived from its corresponding somite, while the caudal part is derived from a portion of the next somite. This splitting of the somites results from the migration of the spinal nerves, which must exit between the future vertebrae.

Figure 13.5 The mesoderm generates the connective tissue found in the embryo. It develops into different groups of tissue which give rise to different systems and structures. In particular, the somites contribute to many of the axial structures and, with the spinal nerves, give rise to the segmental organisation of the axial skeleton.

Table 13.1 Types of somites

Type of somite	Number of pairs	Structures generated
Occipital	4	Bones in the occipital part of the skull, bones around the nose, ears and eyes. Extrinsic ocular muscles and the muscles of the tongue
Cervical	8	Cervical vertebrae and associated muscles; the dermis of the neck
Thoracic	12	Thoracic vertebrae; dermis, muscles and bones of the thoracic and abdominal walls.
Lumbar	5	Lumbar vertebrae, parts of the abdominal wall muscles and dermis
Sacral	5	The sacrum and associated muscles and dermis
Coccygeal	3	The coccyx

The somites

The somites give rise to almost every structure in the axial skeleton, as well as generating parts of the overlying dermis. The somites can be classed into five groups, travelling caudally along the embryo. Each group gives rise to a different set of structures (Table 13.1).

Cells in the somites also migrate to develop into the limb muscles:

- The **upper limb musculature** is derived from the cervical and thoracic somites.
- The **lower limb musculature** is derived from the lumbar somites.

The development and differentiation of the somites

The somites rapidly divide into specific components. They form a hollow structure containing a central core of cells, and start to open on their medial side. Two main divisions of the somite can be identified (Fig. 13.6):

- The **sclerotome** is made of the cells that migrate to the notochord and neural tube and will develop into the vertebrae.
- The **dermamyotome** is made up of the remaining cells and rapidly differentiates into the dermatome and the myotome.

The **dermatome** contributes to the dermis of the neck, back and trunk, although most of the dermis is developed from the lateral plate mesoderm.

The **myotome** develops into muscle structures, after their division into two distinct groups of tissue:

- The **epimere** develops into the deep muscles of the back.

- The **hypomere** develops into the lateral muscles, such as the thoracic muscles.

Formation of the vertebrae

The vertebrae develop from the sclerotome of two separate segments. The development of the vertebrae occurs as the peripheral nerves migrate out of the spinal cord:

- The vertebrae form **intersegmentally**, each being made up of elements from two somites.
- Between the vertebrae, the axial skeleton is supported by fibrous **intervertebral discs**. The centre of these discs is made up of the jelly-like **nucleus pulposus**, derived from the notochord cells. These cells become surrounded by sclerotomal cells and develop into the **annulus fibrosus** – the tough outside layer of the intervertebral disc.

The development of the mesoderm

Although the paraxial mesoderm develops into the somites, the remaining portion of mesoderm forms many other structures. Two other groups of mesoderm tissue have particular developmental significance:

1 **Intermediate mesoderm** is located close to the somites and gives rise to the tissue forming much of the urinary and genital systems.
2 **Lateral plate mesoderm** is the most lateral of the mesoderm structures. It differentiates into two layers associated with the endoderm and ectoderm:
   (a) the **splanchnopleure** is the ventral of the two layers of lateral plate mesoderm and is associated with the endoderm,

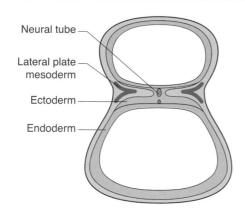

Neural tube

Lateral plate mesoderm

Ectoderm

Endoderm

Following neurulation, the embryo is a relatively flat structure. The lateral plate mesoderm, which will line the future body cavities, exists as two sheets at the extreme sides of the embryo – the somatopleure and the splanchnopleure.

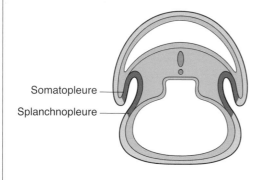

Somatopleure

Splanchnopleure

As the lateral sides of the embryo start to fold, the layers of the lateral plate mesoderm start to invaginate into the sides of the yolk sac. This process occurs as a result of the rostral and caudal folding of the embryo, as well as folding down the midline of the embryo, hinging at the neural tube and notochord. This folding progressively brings the edges of the lateral plate mesoderm on either side of the embryo together, as well as promoting the development of the gut tube from the endoderm.

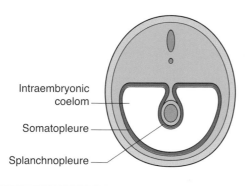

Intraembryonic coelom

Somatopleure

Splanchnopleure

After folding, the edges of the lateral plate mesoderm fuse such that the somatopleure lines the inside of the intraembryonic coelom, while the splanchnopleure lines the gut tube, which has formed from the endoderm. This structure remains entirely within the embryo, except at the point where it connects with the yolk sac, where the abdominal wall has not closed. Progressively, the abdominal wall closes such that the yolk sac becomes incorporated within the umbilical structures

Figure 13.6 The disc-like early embryo must develop into a three-dimensional structure. In this process the lateral edges of the embryo must fuse with each other, generating the gut tube from the endoderm. In addition, the layers of the lateral plate mesoderm fuse to form the tissue that lines both the interior of the abdominal cavity and the gut tube. It is this tissue that gives rise to many of the connecting tissues within the abdomen.

contributing to the walls of the viscera; the splanchnopleure also generates blood cells in the embryo

(b) the **somatopleure** is the more dorsal layer of lateral plate mesoderm and associates with the ectoderm, giving rise to the lining of the body walls.

Embryonic folding and organogenesis

The embryo starts development as a flat trilaminar disc, but it must develop into a three-dimensional

Table 13.2 The different types of embryonic folding

Type of folding	Cause	Effect
Rostral folding (days 22–28)	Growth of the brain in the embryo	Cardiogenic regions and the septum transversum fold from their rostral origin to their location in the abdomen as a result of growth of the primitive brain
Lateral folding (days 22–28)	Expansion of the amniotic cavity	Lateral plate mesoderm fuses to form body wall and intraembryonic coelom. Endoderm fuses to form primitive gut tube. The gut is in communication with the yolk sac and open at the ends
Caudal folding (days 24–28)	Lengthening of the neural tube and somites grow past end of the yolk sac	The cloacal membrane in the germ disc becomes part of the embryo; the connecting stalk merges with the neck of the yolk sac. The root of the connecting stalk develops a diverticulum within the connecting stalk – the allantois

structure as a result of differential growth and folding (Table 13.2). The process also converts the flat endoderm into the **primitive gut tube**:

- The trilaminar disc lengthens rapidly, although the yolk sac does not, leading to folding at the cephalic and rostral ends.
- The lateral edges of the embryo fold and fuse in the midline to form the intraembryonic coelom.

Formation of the body cavities

All the major cavities in the body are derived from the intraembryonic coelom. The **peritoneal**, **pericardial** and **pleural** cavities form as a result of two subdivisions:

1 The division of the intraembryonic coelom into the **abdominal** and **thoracic** cavities occurs through the **rostral folding of the embryo**, which brings the **septum transversum** into position, dividing the two cavities.
2 The **pericardium** forms from the outgrowth of folds of tissue in the lateral body wall. These folds

grow towards each other between the lungs and heart. Upon fusing in week 5, they form the pericardial cavity centrally and two pleural cavities laterally, into which the lungs will develop.

The development of the diaphragm

The diaphragm separates the thorax from the abdomen. Developmentally, it prevents the intestines from entering the thorax, affording the lungs sufficient space. Development of the diaphragm occurs from week 5 to week 7, starting with the caudal folding of the embryo. There are four origins to the tissue in the diaphragm shown in Table 13.3.

Innervation of the diaphragm

The motor and sensory innervation of the diaphragm develops differently:

- Myoblasts migrate into the tissue at the level of C3, -4 and -5, drawing their motor innervation with them. The diaphragm continues to migrate

Table 13.3 Origins of tissue in the diaphragm

Tissue	Source	Structures given rise to
Septum transversum	Mesenchymal tissue rostral to the cardiac regions, which divide the abdomen as a result of caudal folding	Central tendon of the diaphragm
Pleuroperitoneal membranes	Derived from the lateral body wall as the lungs and pleura expand	Connective tissue of diaphragm
Dorsal mesentery of the oesophagus	Part of the mesentery of the gut tube attached to the primitive oesophagus	The crura of the diaphragm
Lateral body walls	Fuse with the septum transversum	Muscular periphery of the diaphragm

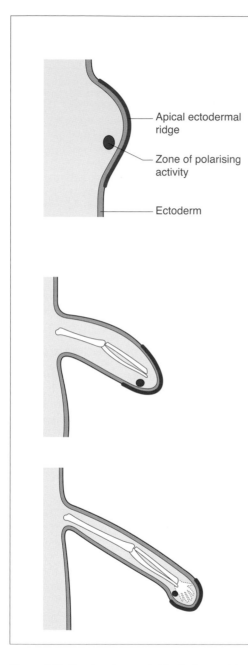

- Apical ectodermal ridge
- Zone of polarising activity
- Ectoderm

Patterning

The three axes of the limb bud must be patterned by the release of different signals. First, the proximal distal signals are the result of signalling between the ectoderm overlying the mesenchyme, in the apical ectodermal ridge, found along the tip of the limb bud. The rostral–caudal axis is patterned through the secretion of the morphogen sonic hedgehog (Shh) from the zone of polarising activity (ZPA). This high level of secretion from the ZPA results in the tissue differentiating into the more caudal structures – the fourth and fifth fingers. As the concentration of Shh decreases, the more rostral thumb and first finger form. Finally the dorsoventral axis is patterned through the secretions by the overlying epithelium.

Growth

It is thought that the length of time that cells spend close to the apical ectodermal ridge alters the structures into which they differentiate. The cells leaving the zone at a later point – as the limb has grown – result in the formation of more distal structures. Many different tissues types are found in the limb – as growth continues many tissues migrate in. The somatic mesoderm is recruited to give rise to the muscle and connective tissue structures in the limb, while the nerve cells migrate into the limb both to innervate the muscles and to provide sensory innervation.

Remodelling

After patterning and growth of the limb, there is a need for regulated cell death – the most prominent place being the tissue that exists between the digits in the developing limb. In addition, the limbs must rotate to reach their final orientation. In the upper limb this is a relatively small rotation, but in the lower limb a much more extreme rotation occurs.

Figure 13.7 The development of the limbs provides a prototype for the development of an organ. There are specific regions or structures that pattern each axis, and tissue is recruited to generate the limb. Finally, after development of the structure there is regulated growth and rotation of the organ to reach its final orientation. The developmental programmes of the limbs are very similar, although there are differences in the genes and signalling molecules involved that reflect the differences in the final structures of the organ.

to the level of the thoracic vertebrae, although innervation from the cervical region is retained. The **phrenic nerve** innervating the diaphragm may be more than 30 cm long in adults.

- The sensory innervation of the diaphragm migrates with the peripheral parts of the diaphragm and comes from a lower part of the spinal cord.

 CLINICAL Congenital diaphragmatic hernia

During development the pleuroperitoneal membranes may fail to fuse with the septum transversum, resulting in a patent pleurocardioperitoneal canal. As the thorax and abdominal cavities are not sealed off from each other, intestines may develop in the thorax and reduce development of the lungs.

Congenital diaphragmatic hernias occur in around 1 in 2500 births. They are more frequent on the left side of the diaphragm, because the pleuroperitoneal membranes close later and must seal a larger canal. The defect is corrected surgically at birth, although in particularly severe defects the damage during development may result in the death of the child even though the defect has been corrected. There are rare cases when surgery has been performed *in utero* to correct the defect.

Limb development

Limb formation is one of the best-understood developmental programmes. There are three basic requirements for the formation of any structure within the embryo and these occur in the formation of the limb:

1 The **specification** of a group of cells to build the organ
2 The **patterning** of the primitive structure to organise the processes required for correct development
3 The **differentiation and growth** of the correct cell types at the right time and location in the developing organ.

Specification of tissues to form the limbs

The limbs develop from the limb buds which form on the lateral walls of the embryo. These buds are derived from lateral plate mesoderm, covered in an overlying layer of ectoderm. Two paired limb buds form on the 'limb line', which is defined in the dorsoventral axis of the embryo:

1 The **upper limb** buds appear at around day 24 and are located at C5–8
2 The **lower limb** buds appear at around day 28 and are located at L3–5.

Patterning of the limb

The organisation of the limb requires patterning in three axes. Each axis is patterned in a different manner through different signalling molecules (Fig. 13.7):

- Proximal – distal (shoulder to fingers)
- Anterior – posterior (thumb to little finger)
- Dorsoventral (back of hand to palm).

Patterning of the proximal–distal axis

The mesenchymal tissue within the limb bud induces the ectodermal tissue to form the **apical ectodermal ridge** (AER), which lies along the edge of the limb bud. The signals from the AER maintain the mesenchymal cells beneath it in an undifferentiated, proliferating state. As the cells leave this region they progressively develop into more distal structures. The time spent in the proliferating region determines the structures developed on leaving the structure.

Patterning of the anterior–posterior axis

The crucial structure for patterning within the anterior–posterior axis is known as the **zone of polarising activity (ZPA)**. The ZPA is located on the posterior side of the limb bud close to the region that will develop into the bones and structures of the little finger. The ZPA releases the protein **sonic hedgehog** (Shh), which is a **morphogen** – a substance that influences development through the gradient of chemical release. High levels of Shh trigger the formation of the little finger and related structures, whereas lower levels of Shh trigger the development of the thumb and first finger.

Patterning in the dorsoventral axis

The patterning of the dorsoventral axis is achieved through signals released by the ectoderm. In particular, the product of the gene *Wnt7a*, which is produced by the dorsal ectoderm of the limb bud, has been implicated in the patterning.

 CLINICAL Thalidomide

Thalidomide was a drug used in the 1950s and 1960s to treat morning sickness. However, it was discovered that the drug was a teratogen and responsible for many defects in the developing embryo. The limb defect, phocomelia, was particularly common. The proximal structures of the limb fail to develop, although the hands and feet develop normally. It is thought that thalidomide may have reduced the rate of proliferation of the cells located underneath the AER, such that cells could not escape from the region to form the proximal structures, although, as the cells survived, the distal structures did form.

Specification of limb type

The developmental programmes that pattern the fore- and hindlimbs are very similar, although the limbs that they produce are crucially different. Although the upper limb is developed for range of movement and grabbing, the lower limb is adapted for load bearing.

The different development programmes are specified by the expression of limb-specific genes. It is thought that expression of the gene *Tbx5* triggers the development of upper limb structures, whereas expression of the gene *Tbx4* triggers the development of lower limb structures. The expression of these genes is induced through a signalling pathway involving fibroblast growth factor-related genes and other genes implicated in whole-body patterning, such as the *Hox* genes.

Development and differentiation of limb structures

Cells from the mesoderm must contribute to the bones, muscles, tendons, ligaments and vessels found in the limbs.

The **bones** of the limbs are produced by **endochondral ossification**. A cartilaginous template is first laid down, and then converted into bone. The ossification of the bones continues after birth, e.g. the carpal bones do not start to ossify until after the first year. The **muscles** of the limbs are derived from somite tissue that migrates into the limbs.

The somatic tissue enters in two groups, one dorsally and one ventrally, which generate the flexor and extensor muscle compartments, respectively. The muscle precursors develop around the skeletal tissue and initially divide into myoblast cells which fuse to develop into the long multinucleated myocytes seen in skeletal muscle.

Migration of the nervous tissue of the limbs

Innervation of the limbs is derived from the sites at which the limb buds developed. The nerves supplying the limbs are brought together from their spinal roots and form two large plexus, in which the nerve bundles are organised to the branches that innervate the limbs:

- The **brachial plexus** receives nerve fibres from C5 to T1 and innervates the upper limb
- The **lumbosacral plexus** receives nerve fibres from L2 to S2 and innervates the lower limb.

The segmental plan by which the limb is innervated is slightly confused by the rotation of both the limbs during development, particularly the lower limb in which the rotation is more pronounced and the plan of innervation varies between the sensory and motor neurons:

- The **motor neurons** migrate into the limb as it develops, and the more distal structures within the limbs are innervated by progressively more caudal spinal segments.
- The **sensory neurons** migrate into the limb at a later stage than the motor neurons, and hence follow a different plan of innervation.

Rotation of the limbs

The limbs in the embryo begin their formation on the same plane, and the developmental programme resembles that of a quadruped. The limbs rotate, reflecting our bipedal nature; if rotation did not occur, the knee and elbow joint would be identically oriented. Instead the upper limbs are slightly rotated, whereas the lower limbs undergo a pronounced rotation.

Sculpting of the limbs

In the following formation of required structures, there is a significant role for apoptosis in the development of the limbs (as well as in other organs). For example, webbing develops between the digits but this is removed through apoptosis before birth.

Development of the gut and lungs

The gut and lungs develop from the **primitive gut tube** which is contained mainly within the abdominal cavity. Throughout this process there are also complex interactions with the mesodermal tissue to form the many **glandular structures** associated with the gut. Finally, the **lungs** must also develop from the gut tube, again regulated through interactions with the mesodermal tissue.

Precursors of the gut

The gastrointestinal (GI) tract is derived from the endoderm, although regions of mesodermal and ectodermal tissue must also contribute:

- The **endoderm** develops into the mucosa of the GI tract.
- The **splanchnopleure** develops into the submucosal layers of the gut tissue. As a result of the embryonic folding the gut tube becomes surrounded by a thin layer of mesoderm, derived from the splanchnopleure.

The primitive gut tube itself can be divided into three sections which will contribute different sections of the mature gut. These different developmental sections are reflected within the vasculature supplying them, both in the embryo and in the adult (Table 13.4).

The furthest extremes of the GI tract do not originate from the primitive gut tube:

- The mouth, jaw and pharynx are derived from the pharyngeal arches.
- The lowest parts of the rectum and anus develop from ectodermal tissue.

Rotation of the gut tube

The gut tube starts as a single straight tube, running along the dorsoventral axis of the embryo, yet in the developed human it is convoluted and tightly folded into the abdomen as a result of a complex series of folds that occur outside the abdominal cavity.

Folding of the gut starts with the lengthening of the midgut at about week 6. This lengthening results as the gut projects into the umbilical cord and rotates in a series of continuous steps:

- As the gut lengthens it turns around 90° anti-clockwise if viewed from a dorsal aspect.
- As the gut rotates the gut tube continues to lengthen and form a series of folds.
- The gut tube continues to rotate as it returns into the abdomen. The small intestine returns first and then the large intestine is drawn round, resulting in the formation of the transverse and ascending colons.

Formation of the mesentery

The mesentery carries the blood vessels supplying the gut, as well as attaching it to the abdominal wall:

- As the **small intestine rotates**, the mesentery rotates around the origin of the superior

Table 13.4 The blood supply of different embryonic structures

Embryonic structure	Mature derivative	Blood supply
Foregut	Gastrointestinal tract up to the ampulla of Vater	Cranial region – pharyngeal arches
		Caudal region – coeliac trunk
Midgut	Ampulla of Vater to two-thirds of the way along the length of the transverse colon	Superior mesenteric artery
Hindgut	From transverse colon to rectum	Inferior mesenteric artery, except the lowest parts of the rectum, which are supplied by the middle rectal artery

mesenteric artery, to form a series of fan-shaped folds and fuses with the posterior abdominal wall. The mesentery runs from the left superior aspect to the right iliac fossa.

- In the **large intestine**, the ascending and descending colons become pressed against the posterior abdominal wall, resulting in absorption of the mesentery. As a result, the ascending and descending colons develop into **retroperitoneal structures** whereas the transverse and sigmoid colons retain mesenteries.

Development of the omenta

The omentum of the gut is derived from the dorsal mesentery, which suspends the gut from the body wall during development. This layer of tissue lengthens and twists as the stomach moves, so that it forms the division between the **lesser** and **greater sacs** of the peritoneum. The large growth of the mesentery results in a folded loop that hangs from the curvature of the stomach and lies over the intestines, forming the greater omentum.

Development of the supporting organs of the GI tract

The GI tract has many associated glands and organs that are related to its function or derived from the primitive gut tube. Developmentally, many of these organs form as a result of interactions of the mesoderm with the cells of the primitive gut tube. Four prominent organs form as a result of such actions:

- Liver
- Pancreas
- Spleen
- Lungs.

Development of the liver

The liver forms from a small diverticulum in the gut tube at about day 22, and rapidly has a role in haematopoiesis. The hepatic diverticulum projects into the septum transversum, and develops by **branching morphogenesis** to produce **liver cords** through interaction of the diverticulum with mesenchymal tissue within the septum transversum. The different tissues contribute different components of the liver:

- The **liver cords** develop into the hepatocytes and the biliary system.

- The **mesoderm** develops into the blood vessels and connective tissue within the liver.
- The **septum transversum** develops into the connective tissue of the liver and forms the falciform ligament and lesser omentum.

Development of the pancreas

The pancreas arises from the pancreatic buds. The dorsal and ventral buds form at the caudal part of the foregut, which will give rise to the duodenum. During the rotation of the small intestine, the buds fuse:

- The dorsal pancreatic bud contributes to most of the pancreatic tissue.
- The ventral pancreatic bud gives rise to the uncinate process of the pancreas.

Four different tissues are found in the pancreas – each with different developments:

- The **ductal system** throughout the pancreas forms through branching morphogenesis, although a great deal of the ductal system from the dorsal bud degenerates, so that the main duct from the ventral duct carries all the pancreatic juices to the duodenum.
- The cells surrounding the ductal system form the **acinar tissue** which makes up the **exocrine pancreas**.
- At the bifurcations of the ductal system, portions of tissue separate and develop into the **islets of Langerhans**. The endocrine tissue is functional by 20 weeks.
- The **connective tissue** within, and surrounding, the pancreas is formed from mesenchymal tissue into which the pancreatic buds grow.

Formation of the trachea and lungs

The trachea and lungs develop from a bud from the gut tube during week 4. The endodermal tissue of the GI tract gives rise to the respiratory epithelium and the alveoli, whereas surrounding mesenchyme is recruited to generate the connective tissue, including the cartilage and muscular layers.

As the trachea develops and lengthens, two buds arise at the end and begin to bifurcate, producing the respiratory tree. As the tissue bifurcates, it draws the surrounding mesenchyme to form the dividing septa between the bronchopulmonary segments. Development of the lung structure occurs throughout gestation and into infant life (Table 13.5).

Table 13.5 Development of the trachea and lungs

Stage	Period	Developmental processes
Embryonic	22 days–5 weeks	The trachea and lungs begin as a bud from the gut tube, which lengthens, and then three rounds of branching, to form the lungs and their segments
Pseudoglandular	6 weeks–4 months	Further division (14 rounds) develops the bronchiole tree into the terminal bronchioles
Canalicular	5–7 months	First stages of the respiratory portion of the bronchiolar tree develops; accompanying vasculature also develops
Saccular/Alveolar	7 months gestation–8 years postpartum	Alveoli continue to develop and mature

Development of the heart and vasculature

The formation of the heart and primitive vasculature occurs relatively early in embryo development, at the point where diffusion is no longer sufficient to meet the nutritional and excretory requirements – about **week 3**. The heart must continue to meet the supply demands that the embryo places on it as it develops; this results in a complex developmental programme to ensure that the heart remains functional as it develops.

Formation of the early heart tube

The tissue that develops into the heart is initially located at the rostral part of the embryo. This 'cardiogenic' region of tissue is rostral to the developing brain and is brought into its correct position in the embryo as a result of **rostral folding**, driven by the increased growth of the brain and the increasing size of the amniotic cavity.

At around 3 weeks, three separate processes lead to the formation of the primitive cardiovascular system:

1 **Pre-endothelial cells in the yolk sac** differentiate into **haematopoietic stem cells** that coalesce to form 'blood islands'. These groups of cells join up to form the early blood vessels, as well as to generate the blood cells required by the vascular system.
2 **Pre-endothelial cells in the embryo** are located on either side of the notochord. These cells develop into two tubular structures: the right and left dorsal aortas.
3 **Endocardial tubes** develop in the cardiogenic region at the rostral end of the embryo.

Through embryonic folding, the endocardial tubes fold down to the correct regions, and the septum transversum comes to rest to divide the intraembryonic coelom. The simplest form of heart is merely a tube with contractile activity, which can force blood to move in one direction; by week 4 the primitive heart tubes have fused to each other and with the aortas (Fig. 13.8). The myocardial cells in the heart tubes have intrinsic contractile activity that starts just before fusion.

The heart tube becomes surrounded by mesoderm cells that differentiate into the myocardium. The myocardial cells secrete an extracellular matrix – the cardiac jelly – which separates them from the heart tubes. Finally, a layer of splanchnic mesoderm encloses the heart tube, which forms the epicardium.

The structure of the early heart tube

The heart tube consists of four primitive different structures from inflow to outflow:

1 The left and right horns of the sinus venosus which receive venous blood
2 The primitive atrium
3 The primitive ventricle
4 The bulbus cordis, the outflow tract of the heart.

After leaving the bulbus cordis, the blood flows through the first aortic arch and then runs through the left and right aortas, either side of the notochord.

Development of the venous vessels

The sinus venosus receives three pairs of veins from different systems that drain blood from the embryo (Table 13.6).

Heart tubes

After the rostral folding of the embryo, the first structure that forms the heart is the paired dorsal aorta tubes. These are surrounded by a thick layer of cardiac jelly, which is crucial for the future development of the heart.

After the fusion of the dorsal heart tubes the heart tube is formed. This has contractile activity and is made up of four main regions. The sinus venosus receives blood from the embryo and placenta, from where it is pumped through the primitive atrium and ventricle before entering the aortic arches through the bulbus cordis.

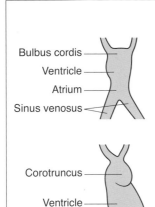

Bulbus cordis
Ventricle
Atrium
Sinus venosus

Deformation

As the embryo grows, the sinus venosus starts to alter, with the right side enlarging to accommodate the blood from the body – it develops into the future vena cava. The left venous sinus regresses and develops into the coronary sinus. The resulting changes in the flow of blood causes deformation of the heart tube into the soft cardiac jelly that surrounds it.

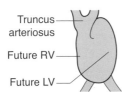

Corotruncus
Ventricle
Sinus venosus

Looping

The progressive lengthening and folding of the heart tube result in it starting to loop around, developing the future left and right ventricles. Within the heart tube, the wall septa in the heart start to develop.

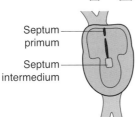

Truncus arteriosus
Future RV
Future LV

Septum primum

Septa must develop in the heart to separate the right and left sides of the heart. In the atria, this occurs by growth of the septum primum from the roof of the atria and fusion with the septum intermedium, which separates the atria from the ventricles. The septum primum then develops a perforation – the foramen ovale – towards its superior end to allow the flow of blood from the right to left sides of the heart to bypass the lungs.

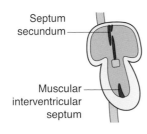

Septum primum
Septum intermedium

Septum secundum

When the baby is born there is an instantaneous need for the lungs to become functional. This results in a massive change in the nature of the circulation, such that blood is no longer shunted from the right to the left side of the heart. This is achieved by the growth of the septum secundum on the left side of the septum primum. With the change in fetal circulation the pressure in the left atrium increases, pushing the septum secundum against the septum primum to prevent flow of blood between the sides of the heart. As the growth of the atrial septa continues, the muscular part of the interventricular (IV) septum begins to grow to separate the ventricles.

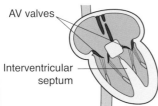

Septum secundum
Muscular interventricular septum

AV valves
Interventricular septum

The finally developed heart consists of two discrete ventricles and two atria that are linked by the foramen ovale – which will close at birth. The atria are separated from the ventricles by the atrioventricular valves, which develop from endocardial swellings on the wall of the heart and the septum intermedium. The ventricles expel blood out of the pulmonary arteries and the aorta, to allow it to flow through the pulmonary and systemic circulations, respectively.

Figure 13.8 The development of the heart: the heart undergoes a particularly complex development because it must continue to supply blood to an ever-growing fetus as it develops. As a result it undergoes a complex series of folding and remodelling throughout the pregnancy. In addition the fetal heart develops so that it can cope with the rapid changes in circulation after delivery.

Table 13.6 Development of the venous vessels

Venous system	Embryonic function	Adult derivatives
Vitelline system	Drains the yolk sac and developing gut structures	Left and right veins form anastomoses that develop into the liver sinusoids, the portal system. Much of the left vein regresses whereas the right develops into the portion of the inferior vena cava between the liver and heart
Umbilical system	Carries blood to and from the placenta	Right umbilical vein regresses during month 2. Left umbilical vein fuses with ductus venosus, which constricts at birth
Cardinal system	Drains the body and head of the embryo	Gives rise to the superior vena cava, and the azygos vein system

Cardinal vein system

The cardinal vein system is made up of three paired vessels:

1 The **anterior cardinal system** drains the head and neck of the embryo.
2 The **posterior cardinal veins** drain the body of the embryo and are progressively superseded by other vessels to develop into the system present at birth.
3 The **common cardinal veins** are formed by the fusion of the anterior and posterior cardinal systems. The common cardinal system enters the sinus venosus.

Development of the heart

The primitive heart tube must develop into a four-chambered mammalian heart. The heart tube grows and loops such that the precursors of the four chambers are brought into the correct position. This process occurs between weeks 3 and 5. The heart looping is the first process where asymmetry is seen in the embryo.

Looping and heart asymmetry

The initial stage is elongation of the heart tube, so that the primitive atrium moves dorsally and bulges to form the left and right atria. The primitive ventricle is displaced to the left and will develop into the left ventricle, whereas the right ventricle develops from the bulbus cordis.

Development of the heart chambers

The heart shape has developed by the end of week 5, although the chambers of the heart have not been divided. The blood draining into the right and left sides of the heart tube is at different pressures and deforms the heart into the **cardiac jelly** that surrounds it. At later stages in the development,

cells migrate into the cardiac jelly to form myocardium, and neural crest cells also migrate, and differentiate into postganglionic parasympathetic cells and the tissue that forms the septum.

The right and left bloodstreams flow through the heart in a spiral path, shaping the septum which divides the outflow tract of the fetal heart, to partition the great vessels. Abnormal blood flow through the heart tubes can influence septation, resulting in inappropriate division of the outflow tract, as seen in tetralogy of Fallot.

 CLINICAL Tetralogy of Fallot

Tetralogy of Fallot (3–5/10000 births) is a major cause of 'blue baby syndrome' and is caused by four main features resulting from inappropriate division of the outflow tract of the vessels:

1 Ventricular septal defect
2 Overriding aorta
3 Right ventricular hypertrophy
4 Pulmonary stenosis.

The resulting effect of these changes is that the blood leaving the heart becomes mixed, and insufficient blood from the heart travels to the lungs to become oxygenated. This syndrome can now be corrected surgically.

 DEFINITION Cardiac jelly

Cardiac jelly is a non-cellular matrix that is secreted by the primitive myocardium. It separates the endocardium from the developing myocardium and provides space into which the endocardial tube deforms during the looping and asymmetrical development of the heart.

Septation of the ventricles

The ventricles separate during weeks 5–7 as a result of the blood flow that deforms and enlarges the primitive ventricles. The interventricular septum contains both a muscular and a fibrous part:

- The muscular portion of the interventricular septum is formed between the enlarging ventricles as they both grow in size closely apposed to one another.
- The fibrous portion is produced by the lowest part of the outflow tract, which develops during weeks 5–8 and grows to fuse with the muscular portion of the septum.

 CLINICAL Ventricular septal defects

Ventricular septal defects (VSDs) are the most common form of congenital heart defect (6 in every 10 000 births). A VSD results from the failure of the ventricular septum to fuse; a connection between remains the two ventricles. This leads to two major problems:

1 The **left ventricle becomes overloaded** because it is unable to efficiently pump blood from the heart.
2 **Pulmonary hypertension** results from the movement of the high-pressure blood from the left ventricle into the right side of the heart.

Detection of a VSD is usually through detection of a heart murmur caused by the flow of blood through the defect. This finding can be confirmed by ultrasonography. Treatment of a VSD can be by surgery, although small defects often close as the heart grows, allowing more conservative management.

The septation of the atria

Septation of the atria occurs at the same time as septation of the ventricles, in a series of continuous steps:

- Septation starts with the formation of the **septum primum** which grows down from the roof of the atrium, forming a crescent-shaped sheet of tissue.
- The **septum primum becomes perforated** superiorly through apoptosis, allowing flow of blood between the atria to continue.

- A **septum secundum** forms to the right of the septum primum. This septum extends so that it overlaps the perforation in the septum primum, forming a valve that allows the flow of blood from the right atrium to the left, so bypassing the lungs.

 CLINICAL Atrial septal defect

Atrial septal defect (ASD): in about 6 in 10 000 live births there is a persistent shunt between the left and right atria. This results from the septum secundum being too short to cover the ostium secundum. As a result blood becomes shunted from the left atria to the lower-pressure right atrium.

Initially, this defect occurs without symptoms; however it causes progressive enlargement of the right ventricle and the pulmonary trunk, and can lead to development of heart failure.

An ASD is associated with many chromosomal defects and is often seen in trisomy 21. Detection of an ASD is by echocardiogram and it can be treated by surgery.

Formation of the heart valves

The formation of the valves occurs shortly after septation. The heart valves are all reinforced by collagen fibres, which are secreted by mesenchymal cells:

- The **aortic** and **pulmonary valves** form from swellings in the endocardium which develop at the distal parts of the ventricles. The swellings become hollowed out to form functional valves.
- The **tricuspid** and **mitral valves** form from the tissue in the atrioventricular canals and the endocardial tissue.

The development of the outflow vessels of the heart

In the primitive heart, blood exits the heart through the paired first aortic arches. As the embryo grows, the blood flows through the second, third, fourth and sixth aortic arches, although they are never all present at the same time within the embryo. The fifth aortic arch is not present in humans at any time during development.

Table 13.7 Aortic arches and their derivatives

Aortic arch	Adult derivative
First	Part of the maxillary artery
Second	Stapedial artery
Third	Internal and common carotid arteries
Fourth	Pulmonary arteries
	Right arch also contributes to the right subclavian
	Left arch contributes to the arch and part of the descending aorta
Sixth	Left: ductus arteriosus
	Right: regresses

The aortic arches in the embryo rapidly regress, although some of the arches contribute to arteries within the adult (Table 13.7).

By week 7 the separate aortic and pulmonary trunks have developed, although within the fetus the lungs are not required, resulting in most blood being shunted through the **ductus arteriosus** into the descending aorta.

The development of the circulation

During week 6 of development a shunt develops that links the left umbilical vein to the right vitelline vein. As a result, the right sinus venosum enlarges because it must accept most of the blood from the lower body, and will subsequently form the inferior vena cava. The right umbilical vein gradually regresses because it is not required to drain blood. By week 10 the left sinus horn has regressed to drain the heart tissue, forming the coronary sinus.

The left and right cardinal veins become linked by the left brachiocephalic vein, which results in blood being channelled to the right side of the heart into the superior vena cava, which derives from the right sinus horn.

Features of the fetal circulation

Before birth, there are sites of bypass in which little blood passes through the lungs or liver because they are not required. However, immediately after birth the neonate must breathe and develop liver function. This requires a rapid change.

Three prominent points of bypass exist within the fetal circulation (Fig. 13.9):

1 The **foramen ovale** in the atrial septum allows blood to pass from the right atrium to the left atrium down the pressure gradient between the two chambers.
2 The **ductus arteriosus** is a vessel that exists in the fetus connecting the pulmonary trunk to the aorta. This vessel allows blood pumped by the right ventricle to flow to the aorta, back round the systemic circulation, effectively bypassing the lungs and the right side of the heart.
3 The **ductus venosus** allows the umbilical blood from the placenta to bypass the liver.

The placenta is responsible for providing nutrients and oxygen to the body, while helping the removal of waste metabolites. After birth, the organs in the body must fulfil many of the functions of the placenta. The placenta is linked to the fetal circulation through the umbilical vessels:

- The **umbilical arteries** form as branches of the aorta, although they rapidly shift to originate from the internal iliac arteries.
- The **umbilical veins** form symmetrically and carry blood from the placenta to the sinus venosus. By month 2, the left umbilical vein remains whereas the right has regressed. The left umbilical vein drains into the ductus venosus, which drains into the sinuses of the liver.

Changes to the fetal circulation at birth

Several changes occur at birth to remove the placenta from the circulation and to ensure that the body's blood flows through the lungs to oxygenate it:

- **The baby tries to breathe**: the act of filling the lungs helps the opening of the alveolar vessel, reducing the pressure within the pulmonary circulation, and promotes blood flow through it.
- The walls of the **ductus arteriosus contract** to close the vessel. This prevents the right ventricular blood from passing straight to the aorta, rather forcing it through the pulmonary arteries to the lungs. The ductus arteriosus develops into the **ligamentum arteriosum** in the adult, which is clinically significant because the left recurrent laryngeal nerve passes around it on its course to the larynx.
- The **foramen ovale closes** as a result of the drop in the pressure of the pulmonary circulation, and the increased pressure of the systemic

Foramen ovale

The foramen ovale exists between the atria of the heart. In the fetus it allows blood to shunt from the right to the left atrium, to bypass the lungs. After birth, the foramen closes to allow adequate pulmonary circulation and sufficient oxygenation of the blood.

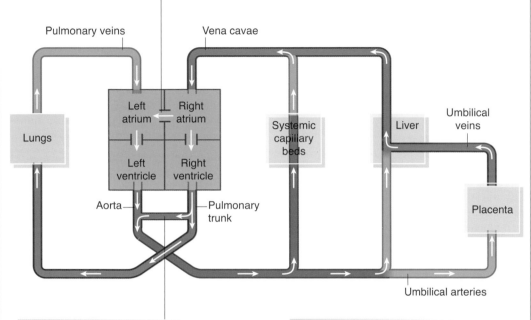

Ductus arteriosus

The ductus arteriosus is a conduit linking the pulmonary trunk the aorta. In the fetus it ensures that blood in the pulmonary circulation is transferred to the systemic circulation, bypassing the lungs, which have no function in the fetus. On birth, the lungs become essential for the oxygenation of the blood, and the ductus arteriosus rapidly closes to remove this shunt. The ductus arteriosus develops into the ligamentum arteriosum in the adult.

Umbilical cord

The umbilical cord connects the fetus to the placenta, and carries the umbilical vessels. These allow gas and nutrient exchange with the maternal circulation. In the fetus, the umbilical arteries arise from the internal iliac arteries and travel through the umbilical cord to the placenta; the nutrient- and oxygen-rich blood is then returned through the umbilical veins, which join the circulation at the liver through the ductus venosus. At birth the umbilical vessels rapidly contract to isolate the baby from the placenta; the umbilical arteries contract before the umbilical veins, to allow placental blood to return to the child's circulation. In addition, the ductus venosus closes, because it is no longer required, and develops into the ligamentum venosum.

Figure 13.9 Until birth the fetus depends on the placenta for its nutrition, removal of waste and oxygenation of blood. At birth rapid changes in the circulation occur so that the lungs are used for oxygenation, and the placenta is isolated from the child's circulation. This occurs by rapid changes at three points in the circulation: the foramen ovale, ductus arteriosus and umbilical cord.

circulation, due to the large volume of blood being received in the left atrium. This closure relies on the one-way valve nature of the foramen ovale, with the septum secundum being forced against the septum primum, to prevent flow through the foramen ovale.

- The **umbilical vessels close**: the umbilical arteries close rapidly to prevent loss of blood to the placenta; the umbilical vein closes more slowly, allowing placental blood to return to the body.
- The **ductus venosus closes** to prevent the blood from bypassing the liver. The ductus venosus develops into the **ligatmentum venosum** which helps tether the liver to the abdominal wall.

 CLINICAL **Patent ductus arteriosus**

The circulation required for the development of the fetus varies enormously from that needed for functioning in the outside world; as a result, failure of the body to make the necessary changes results in serious defects, which require rapid correction.

A **patent ductus arteriosus** (PDA) after birth reduces the blood entering the lungs. Such conditions must be corrected rapidly before the damage to the heart and the pulmonary system becomes too severe. This can be done by the administration of chemicals to promote closure of the ductus arteriosus or a plug may be inserted to block the vessel.

Development of the urinary system

Once the fetus develops to a certain size, it develops a urinary system, which has three roles during development:

1 Fetal urine contributes to the amniotic fluid surrounding the embryo. If kidney development is impaired, **oligohydramnios** may result
2 Portions of the urinary system contribute to the formation of the genital system.
3 The embryonic kidneys are functional *in utero* to help process waste although most waste removal is achieved by the exchange of toxic substances across the placenta.

Three kidney structures develop sequentially in the embryo from the intermediate mesoderm.

These form progressively in more caudal regions of the embryo, reflecting their evolutionarily later development:

1 Pronephroi
2 Mesonephroi
3 Metanephroi.

In addition, the bladder and the conduits linking the kidneys to the external environment must also develop. Although most of the pronephric and mesonephric structures regress, the mesonephric duct is also crucial to the development of the male reproductive system.

Development of the pronephroi

The **pronephroi** are the most primitive form of kidneys. They develop in **week 4** from around six paired balls of intermediate mesoderm, which form a hollow epithelial structure known as a nephrotome. Lines of nephrotomes are found in the cervical regions on both sides of the vertebral column. The pronephroi are not functional in the embryo and their development reflects the functional pronephroi seen in many lower vertebrates. The pronephroi regress during **week 5**.

Development of the mesonephroi

The **mesonephroi** are the first functional kidney structures found in the embryo. They also contribute to the development of other structures, particularly the male genital system.

The mesonephros system can be broken down into two regions that are distinct in terms of development, as well as their contribution to structures in the fully developed fetus:

1 Mesonephric tubules – the excretory units of the mesonephros
2 Mesonephric ducts, which drain the mesonephric tubules.

The formation of the mesonephric tubules

The intermediate mesoderm in the upper thoracic and lumbar regions condenses to form a mesonephric ridge on either side of the spinal column. This ridge coalesces to form about 40 tubules, which form sequentially so that, as the more caudal segments develop, the cranial tubules regress.

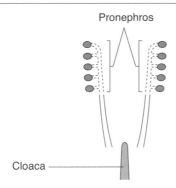

Pronephros

Cloaca

Pronephros

The first structures to form are the pronephroi, which form in the cervical region of the intermediate mesoderm. In humans, these are non-functional. The mesoderm medial to the pronephros begins to coalesce to form the mesonephric ducts – beginning at the rostral end of the mesoderm and progressing caudally.

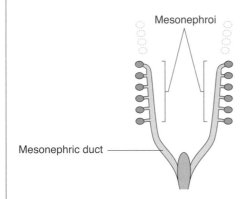

Mesonephroi

Mesonephric duct

Mesonephroi

The first functional kidney structures are the mesonephroi which form from the thoracic and abdominal intermediate mesoderm. These link up with the mesonephric ducts, which drain them; during the development of the mesonephroi, the ducts fuse with the cloaca to form the bladder.

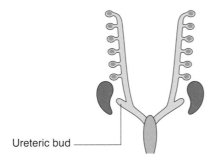

Ureteric bud

Metanephroi

The metanephroi develop from the interactions between a bud of the mesonephric ducts and the region of intermediate mesoderm in the pelvis. The ureteric bud rapidly undergoes branching morphogenesis in the mesoderm to generate the collecting tubules and nephron.

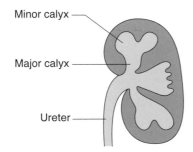

Minor calyx

Major calyx

Ureter

Calyces

The calcyces of the kidney are formed by the fusion of the early branches of the ureteric bud. This results in the formation of 2 or 3 major calyces and then around 8 minor calyces, into which the collecting ducts drain.

Each tubule is effectively an abbreviated version of the adult nephron. The mesonephric tubules drain into the mesonephric ducts after fusion of the lateral tip of the tubules with the mesonephric ducts.

Formation of the mesonephric ducts

The mesonephric ducts form as a pair of solid rods of intermediate mesoderm midway through week 4. The rods of tissue develop caudally into tubes and fuse to the walls of the cloaca. The site of fusion develops into part of the wall of the bladder in the adult.

The role of the mesonephric system in the developed infant

The mesonephric system is functional in the fetus until week 10, at which point it starts to regress. The contribution of the mesonephric system varies with the sexes:

- In the **male**, the mesonephric system develops into the bladder whereas the mesonephric ducts and a few modified tubules develop into parts of the male genital system.
- In the **female** almost the entire system regresses, except that which contributes to the bladder.

Metanephric system

The metanephroi develop into the functional kidneys in the adult. They develop through weeks 5–15 from the intermediate mesoderm within the sacral regions. This is induced by the **ureteric buds**, which develop from the mesonephric ducts (Fig. 13.10). The ureteric bud penetrates into the intermediate mesoderm and begins to bifurcate rapidly; the tubule structure that forms will develop into the nephrons. The growing tip of the ureteric buds acquires a cap of cells, which develops into the glomerulus. The neurons innervating the kidney are found in the tips of the metanephric tissue during induction of the nephrons.

Development of the ureteric buds

Initially, the tip of the ureteric bud expands to form a widened ampulla which forms the renal pelvis:

- During week 6 the bud bifurcates to form 16 branches, which give rise to the major calyces.
- The next set of branching develops into the minor calyces.
- Branching continues until week 32 when about 11 further generations of branching have occurred. This branching pattern results in the mature collecting duct organisation.

 CLINICAL Renal agenesis

Failure of the ureteric bud to develop prevents development of the metanephroi. Around 75% of cases occur in men. Typical occurrence is fewer than 9 in every 10 000 live births:

- **Unilateral renal agenesis** is around five times more common than bilateral agenesis. The single functional kidney usually undergoes compensatory growth. Afflicted individuals are often relatively healthy.
- **Bilateral renal agenesis** is invariably fatal.

Renal agenesis is associated with **oligohydramnios** due to the kidneys' *in utero* role in contributing to the amniotic fluid.

 CLINICAL Oligohydramnios

Oligohydramnios is when there is insufficient amniotic fluid, which restricts the space available for the fetus to grow. The resulting defects are known collectively as **Potter's syndrome,** and typically result from **bilateral renal agenesis**:

- Pulmonary hypoplasia caused by constriction of the thoracic cavity
- Deformed limbs
- Abnormal facial features – receding chin, wide-set eyes, deformed nose.

Figure 13.10 Three kidney structures form in the embryo, although only the latter two (the mesonephroi and metanephroi) function. These form in progressively more caudal regions of the intermediate mesoderm. The other prominent structures that form the urinary section are the mesonephric ducts, which drain both the mesonephroi and the metanephroi, and develop into the ureters. These ducts fuse with the cloaca, a remnant of the hindgut, to form the bladder.

The interaction between the ureteric buds and the mesodermal tissue surrounding the tip is responsible for formation of the glomerular structure. The mesodermal tissue surrounding the tip invaginates into the tip of the capsule and starts to differentiate into the glomerulus:

- The **mesodermal tissue** divides into a tightly knit group of capillaries that form the glomerulus.
- The **inner layer of the ampulla** thins and develops into the podocytes which surround the glomerular vessels.
- The **outer layer of the ampulla** is continuous with the tubular epithelial cells of the nephron.

As the glomerulus is developing, the remaining structure of the tubule lengthens and differentiates into its constituent regions.

Ascent of the kidneys

The metanephroi form in the pelvis, yet in the adult they are found in the abdomen. During weeks 6–9, the kidneys ascend either side of the abdominal aorta. During this process the blood supply of the kidneys also ascends.

 CLINICAL Ascent of the kidneys

There are several abnormalities related to the development of the kidneys or their vasculature which can lead to abnormal ascent of the kidneys:

- **Horseshoe kidney** results from the fusion of the inferior poles of the kidneys during their ascent. This prevents the kidneys ascending above the inferior mesenteric artery, where they become caught.
- **Pelvic kidney** occurs when the kidneys completely fail to ascend.

Changes in the function of the kidneys before and after birth

- The metanephroi are functional by week 12 and contribute to the formation of amniotic fluid. The fetus swallows amniotic fluid that is absorbed from the gut and the waste products are filtered by the placenta. **Before birth** the urine produced by the nephrons is dilute, due to

the small length of the loops of Henle in the immature nephrons.
- **After birth** the loops of Henle lengthen, allowing concentration of urine because there is now a need for the infant to retain fluid volume and so produce concentrated urine.

Development of the head and neck

The development of the head and neck is particularly complex because there are many organs present that have distinct developmental programmes and different embryological origins:

- The **brain and special sense organs** are formed from the neural tube and ectodermal placodes.
- The **face, palate, tongue, ear and neck structures** are formed from the neural crest cells.
- The **muscles of the head** are formed from the cranial paraxial mesoderm.

Much of the development of the structures in the head and neck occurs through the formation of the **pharyngeal arches**.

The pharyngeal arches

The pharyngeal arches develop during weeks 4 and 5 and form five pairs: one to four and six. The five pairs of pharyngeal arches are separated by four pharyngeal grooves. The pharyngeal arches each start with the same basic structure:

- The **outer surface** is made up of a layer of ectoderm.
- The **inner layer** is made up of endoderm.
- The **mesenchymal tissue** is primarily derived from neural crest tissue and gives rise to most of the connective tissue structures.
- **Paraxial mesoderm** is present in the mesenchyme and gives rise to muscular structures.

The pharyngeal arches are segmentally organised. This is reflected by the arch-specific arteries that supply the structures and the innervation of each arch by a distinct cranial nerve. The pharyngeal arches give rise to a variety of structures in the adult (Table 13.8).

Table 13.8 The pharyngeal arches and structures formed

Arch	Innervation	Arterial supply	Structures formed
First	Maxillary and mandibular branches of the trigeminal nerve (cranial nerve V_2 and V_3)	Maxillary artery	Muscles of mastication, anterior digastric, tensor tympani and tensor veli palatini
			Maxilla, zygomatic, squamous part of the temporal bone and the mandible
Second	Facial nerve (cranial nerve VII)	Stapedial artery	Muscles of facial expression posterior digastric, stapedius
			Upper rim of hyoid bone, styloid process, stapes
Third	Glossopharyngeal nerve (cranial nerve IX)	Common and internal carotids	Stylopharyngeus, lower rim of hyoid bone
Fourth	Superior laryngeal branch of vagus nerve (cranial nerve X)	Arch of aorta, right subclavian	Pharyngeal constrictor muscles, cricothyroid
			Laryngeal cartilages
Sixth	Recurrent laryngeal branch of vagus nerve	Roots of pulmonary arteries, ductus arteriosus	Intrinsic muscles of the larynx, laryngeal cartilages

Development of the thyroid

The thyroid starts to form in week 4 in the midline between the first and second pharyngeal pouches. The primitive structure enlarges and elongates to reach its final location at the level of T2–3 by week 7. The glandular duct structure forms through branching morphogenesis and secretion of thyroxine starts in month 4 of gestation.

 CLINICAL Thyroglossal cyst

The thyroglossal duct may persist in some individuals. This can result in the formation of a cyst, or occasionally a sinus, which communicates with the surface of the neck. The cyst is usually detectable as a lump in the neck that moves during swallowing. It is usually painless, although it can cause discomfort or difficulty swallowing, particular if the cyst swells as a result of infection.

Development of the tongue

The tongue develops from many of the pharyngeal arches, which is reflected in its complex innervation of the mucosa and musculature. Initially, the tongue develops from a series of tissue swellings in the pharynx. These are progressively overgrown:

- The first arch provides much of the musculature in the tongue.
- The second arch contributes to the midline region of the tongue.
- The third arch also provides musculature in the tongue.
- The fourth arch (with the third arch) gives rise to midline structures in the tongue.

Development of the face

The facial structure forms a series of facial swellings:

- Two maxillary swellings
- Two mandibular swellings
- A single frontonasal swelling.

The face forms through the fusion and moulding of these structures. In particular, the maxillary swellings produce palatine shelves on their interior, which develop into the hard palate of the mouth. The failure of these swellings to fuse correctly results in a **facial cleft**.

Development of the nervous system

The nervous system develops from the neural tube and the neural crest cells, both of which are formed during neurulation. The processes involved are complex and not fully understood, although the morphological changes and structure that develop from each major division of the neural tube are well established. Although the CNS is formed from the neural tube, many of the cells in the peripheral nervous system are derived from the neural crest.

Principles of axon growth

Nerves often have to grow a long distance to innervate their target tissue. The growth of the axon is guided through sensing substances secreted by the target tissue. The first neurons that successfully innervate their target tissue are thought to serve as a guide for further neurons travelling to the same tissue.

Growth of the CNS

The formation of the primitive CNS is marked by the process of neurulation to form the neural tube. By day 22, neurulation has been completed and, by day 24, the cranial neuropore has closed. Three primitive brain vesicles are then formed:

1 Prosencephalon – the primitive forebrain
2 Mesencephalon – the primitive midbrain
3 Rhombencephalon – the primitive hindbrain.

In week 5, the brain vesicles become further subdivided to give rise to five secondary vesicles which develop into the major divisions in the developed brain. The central cavity also develops into the ventricular system (Table 13.9).

Formation of the spinal cord

The spinal cord develops from the neural tube of the embryo. By day 26, the caudal neuropore has closed, generating a completely enclosed structure in the embryo. The cavity within the neural tube develops into the central canal of the spinal cord and the ventricular system of the CNS.

The tissue in the spinal cord become organised at the end of week 4 to form two paired columns that run along its length:

1 The **alar columns** will develop into the dorsal columns of the spinal cord, carrying the sensory tracts.
2 The **basal columns** will develop into the ventral columns of the spinal cord, developing into the motor neurons. The most dorsal cells within the basal columns develop into the intermediolateral cell columns at some levels. At T1–L3, these give rise to sympathetic fibres, whereas, at S2–4, they give rise to parasympathetic fibres.

The development of the peripheral nerves that communicate with the spinal cord is described below.

Table 13.9 Development of the ventricular system

Origin (primary vesicle)	Secondary vesicle	Structures developed	Fate of central cavity
Prosencephalon	Telencephalon	Cerebral hemispheres, olfactory bulbs and olfactory tracts (Cranial nerve I)	Lateral ventricles
Prosencephalon	Diencephalon	Thalamus, hypothalamus, epithalamus, posterior pituitary gland, optic vesicles	Third ventricle
Mesencephalon	Mesencephalon	The midbrain, nuclei to the oculomotor nerve (cranial nerve III)	Cerebral aqueduct
Rhombencephalon	Metencephalon	Pons and cerebellum	Fourth ventricle
Rhombencephalon	Myelencephalon	Medulla	Fourth ventricle

Growth of the peripheral nervous system

The peripheral nervous system can be divided into three portions, each of which develops differently:

- Motor fibres
- Sensory fibres
- Autonomic fibres.

As the fibres grow into and out of the spinal cord and associated ganglia, they form a complex arrangement of fibres. Initially, two bodies of fibres leave the spinal cord at each level:

1 The **dorsal root** contains the sensory fibres, the cell bodies of which are found outside the spinal cord in the dorsal root ganglion.
2 The **ventral root** carries the axons of the motor and autonomic neurons.

At the thoracic levels, the spinal nerves are connected to the sympathetic chain by two rami:

1 The **white ramus** carries preganglionic fibres (which are myelinated) to the sympathetic chain, where they may synapse in the ganglion, ascend/descend before ascending or pass directly through to for the splanchnic nerves.
2 The **grey ramus** carries the unmyelinated postganglionic fibres from the sympathetic chain to innervate the target organs.

The spinal nerve consists of motor, sensory and autonomic fibres, and rapidly splits into two primary rami:

1 The **dorsal primary ramus** migrates to innervate the epimere and the tissues that develop from it.
2 The **ventral primary ramus** migrates to innervate the hypomere and the tissues that develop from it.

Development of the motor fibres

Motor (ventral column) fibres are the first to grow out of the spinal cord, starting to emerge early in week 5. They migrate to the **sclerotome**, rapidly condensing into spinal nerves as they migrate.

Development of sensory fibres

Sensory (dorsal column) fibres are derived from the **neural crest**. The neural crest cells form ganglia that are segmentally organised. The ganglia form at every level from the second cervical level to the coccyx. The cells in the ganglion produce two axons: one migrates to the spinal cord, entering the dorsal column, whereas the other migrates to the periphery.

Development of the sympathetic neurons

Sympathetic neurons are produced from neural crest cells that condense to form the chain ganglia, segmentally organised along the spinal cord. Three larger ganglia form in the cervical region, and are the sympathetic outflow for the head and neck:

- The **preganglionic** sympathetic axons in the spinal cord migrate to the chain ganglia, where they synapse or may migrate up or down to different levels before synapsing. The preganglionic fibres originate from T1–L3.
- The **postganglionic** fibres, which are neural crest derived, migrate to the tissues with the spinal nerve.

Some fibres from the CNS enter the sympathetic chain ganglia and do not synapse but pass straight through the ganglia, and form the **splanchnic nerves** which provide sympathetic innervation to the structures in the GI tract.

Development of the parasympathetic fibres

Parasympathetic fibres are organised differently to the sympathetic system. The preganglionic neurons in the parasympathetic system are generally long, whereas the postganglionic neurons are very short. There are two sites of origin for the preganglionic neurons:

1 The motor nuclei (cranial nerves III, VII, IX and X)
2 The intermediolateral cell columns at S2–4.

In the cranial nerves the preganglionic fibres migrate to the parasympathetic ganglia, which are located close to the target organ, where they form a synapse with the second neuron. In particular, the fibres in cranial nerve X may be extremely long, because it is responsible for much of the parasympathetic outflow below the head, including the GI tract, heart, liver and gonads:

- The **preganglionic fibres** from the spinal cord arise in the sacral region and join to form the pelvic splanchnic nerves. They innervate ganglia embedded in the walls of the target tissue.

- The **postganglionic parasympathetic** cells are derived from the neural crest. Throughout the body, most of the cells are derived from the neural crest in the occipitocervical region (the vagal region). In the lowest parts of the gut there is some contribution from the sacral neural crest.

→ **RELATED CHAPTERS**

14

Anatomy

The body is built around a bony skeleton, which provides a framework to support the soft-tissue structures and allow movement. The skeleton is made up of bones that articulate at joints. The joints are surrounded by ligaments and other connective tissue providing a stable interaction. At those joints where movement is permitted, muscles cause movement of the joint through contraction. An understanding of the location of structures and their relations allows an appreciation of the origin of the symptoms and signs that help diagnosis of the underlying condition. In this chapter, the anatomy of the body is broken down into a series of regions for purely descriptive purposes. Specific regions are often associated with broadly related functions, as a result of their related developmental programmes.

The bony skeleton

The adult skeleton is composed of 206 bones. Bone is a rigid connective tissue made up of a collagen network strengthened by the presence of hydroxyapatite crystals, which generate the rigid structure.

The structure of bone

There are two cells that are found in bone and regulate and maintain it:

1 **Osteoblasts** lay down new bone, generating collagen and mineralising the extracellular matrix.

As bone is produced, osteoblasts may encase themselves inside the bone, where they become known as **osteocytes**.

2 **Osteoclasts** are responsible for the resorption of bone. They are related to macrophages and typically are found at sites of bone remodelling, particularly where growth occurs.

Bone is continuously remodelled in response to stresses on it and this requires the coordinated action of osteoblasts and osteoclasts. Bone acts as a store for calcium, which can be liberated from or trapped in bone, to regulate plasma calcium levels.

The osteoblasts and osteoclasts maintain bone in two different structural arrangements:

- **Compact bone** (or cortical bone) forms the protecting surface of bones and is extremely hard. It is also heavy, due to its dense nature, accounting for 80% of the weight of all bone within the body. It has an extremely organised structure (Fig. 14.1).
- **Cancellous bone** (or trabecular bone) is made up of a honeycomb structure known as **trabeculae**; this forms the interior of long bones and creates a relatively strong, but lightweight, structure. The cancellous bone in the long bone contains bone marrow, the site of **haematopoiesis**.

Organisation of the bony skeleton

The bony skeleton is often thought of in two parts:

1 The **appendicular skeleton** relates to the limbs, shoulder girdle and pelvis.

Biomedical Science Lecture Notes, First Edition. Ian Lyons.
© 2011 by Ian Lyons. Published 2011 by Blackwell Publishing Ltd.

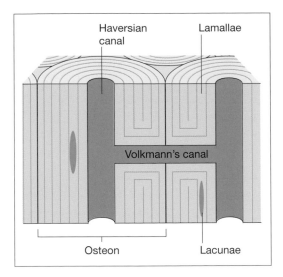

Haversian canal

Lamallae

Volkmann's canal

Osteon

Lacunae

Figure 14.1 Compact bone has an organised structure. The **osteon** (or haversian unit) is the functional unit of compact bone. It is made up of many concentric lamellae of bone, which are arranged around a central haversian canal. This canal carries the neurovascular bundle that innervates and vascularises the bone. The adjacent osteons are linked through Volkmann's canals which run perpendicular to the haversian canals. In between the lamellae are frequent spaces, lacunae, which contain osteoclasts. The lacunae are connected to the rest of the haversian channel by fine channels (not shown).

2 The **axial skeleton** consists of the skeletal components in the midline – the bones of the head, neck, chest and vertebral columns.

Types of bone and their articulations

Bones are grouped into five main classes:

- **Long bones** are the main levers of the appendicular skeleton; many of these bones contain bone marrow.
- **Short bones** resist deformation. They are found where heavy loads are normally applied, such as in the wrist and the foot.
- **Sesamoid bones** are found in tendons, usually where they pass over a joint. They enhance the mechanical effect by acting as a pivot.
- **The flat bones** either give extensive protection to an area (e.g. the cranial bones of skull) or provide a large surface area for muscle attachment (e.g. the scapula).

- **Irregular bones** are those that cannot be divided into any of the other subtypes.

Joints

The degree of movement and the stability of a joint vary with its function:

- **Synovial joints** are adapted for mobility (e.g. shoulder joint). The articulating parts of the bone are covered with smooth hyaline cartilage and encased in a capsule filled with a lubricating **synovial fluid**. Synovial joints are further divided according to the movement that they allow.
- **Cartilaginous joints** (e.g. pubic symphysis) allow less movement than synovial joints but are much more stable. In a child, the long bones contain 'growth plates' which are the site of growth and are effectively cartilaginous joints.
- **Fibrous joints** (e.g. skull sutures) link bones tightly with dense connective tissue. These joints are essentially **immobile**.

> ✓ **DEFINITION Growth plates**
>
> The bone continues to growth after birth. Growth in length of the bone occurs at the growth plates (also known as **epiphyseal plates**), which are cartilaginous joints located towards the end of the long bones. Growth is achieve by the generation of an extracellular matrix by the chondrocytes, which is then remodelled and converted to bone in a process known as **ossification**, similar to what occurs in development.
>
> The growth plates are particularly active during puberty, accounting for the 'growth spurt', although they fuse at the end of puberty, after which no more growth is possible.

Types of synovial joints

Synovial joints are adapted for movement and are classified by the movements that they allow as a result of orientation of the bones in the joints:

- **Hinge** joints (e.g. the phalangeal joints in the fingers) allow flexion and extension only.
- **Plane** joints (e.g. the patella joint) result from two flat bone surfaces interacting. The joint allows sliding movement, usually in a single direction.
- **Pivot** joints (e.g. the atlantoaxial joint) consist of a round process that fits into a socket, allowing rotation around a single axis.

- **Saddle** joints (e.g. the metacarpophalangeal joints) are made up of two saddle-shaped heads that interact to allow movement in two perpendicular planes.
- **Condyloid** joints (e.g. the wrist joint) are made up of a rounded process, which fits into a bony socket. Due to the shape of the joint it allows movement in two planes.
- **Ball-and-socket** joints (e.g. shoulder joint) are made up of a ball-shaped head that articulates with a round socket, to allow movement and rotation in several different planes.

Movement at joints

Different articulations of different bones enable different movements around joints; in relation to this movements relate to the anatomical position (Fig. 14.2):

- **Flexion**: a forward/anterior movement
- **Extension**: a backward/posterior movement
- **Abduction**: a movement away from the midline of the body (except the thumb)
- **Adduction**: a movement toward the midline of the body (except the thumb)
- **Rotation**: medial rotation is rotation of the joint or part of the body towards the midline; lateral rotation is movement away from the midline
- **Circumduction**: this is a complex circular movement combining flexion, abduction, extension and adduction without rotation.

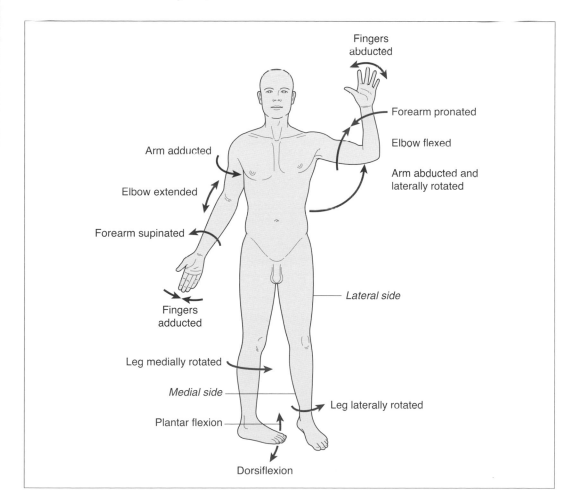

Fingers abducted

Forearm pronated

Elbow flexed

Arm abducted and laterally rotated

Arm adducted

Elbow extended

Forearm supinated

Fingers adducted

Lateral side

Leg medially rotated

Medial side

Plantar flexion

Leg laterally rotated

Dorsiflexion

Figure 14.2 The different movements possible at the different joints are given specific names, in relation to the type of movement (e.g. rotation or flexion) and, also, whether the movement is towards or away from the midline of the body.

DEFINITION The origin and insertion of muscles

The intricate control of the movement is due to the position of the 'origin', the most proximal attachment, and the 'insertion', the most distal attachment, of muscles to bones. Tendons join muscle to bone; the direction of force on these, as well as the fibrous tissue that holds them in place, contribute to the direction of the movement that occurs.

Fascia

Fascia are the layers of fibrous connective tissue which surround and seperate discrete tissues of the body. Muscles of the limbs are grouped into fascial compartments which are functionally associated with similar movements, in most cases. Fascia is further classified into deep and superficial subtypes.

Deep fascia

Deep fascia is a dense fibrous connective tissue responsible for dividing the limb muscles into functional compartments. The thickness of the fascial layer varies depending on its function. It is often thin in areas where it should allow expansion of an organ; however, it is thick in other areas to facilitate venous return.

Separation of muscles into compartments by the deep fascia determines the gross type of movement that they cause about a joint. The direction of force on the tendon, which joins the muscle to the bone, also influences the direction of movement. Muscles organised into the same fascial compartments are controlled by the same nerves.

Superficial fascia

Superficial fascia lies over the deep fascia. This layer of subcutaneous connective tissue fuses with the dermis and contains the superficial vessels and nerves. The connective tissue contains fibrous and adipose tissue in varying proportions.

In areas where there is a high concentration of fibrous tissue, the skin is more firmly attached to the underlying structures, e.g. the palm, to facilitate grip.

 CLINICAL **Compartment syndrome**

If the contents of a deep fascial compartment are placed under increased pressure, as may occur by haemorrhage, compartment syndrome may result. As the pressure increases, it compresses the low-pressure capillaries and veins compress first, further increasing the pressure because blood is unable to leave the compartment; finally the arteries are constricted. This decreases the supply of oxygen to the muscles and allows a build-up of waste products within the compartment. Compartment syndrome is a surgical emergency and must be treated by relieving the pressure, usually by a fasciotomy to open up the compartment. Compartment syndrome typically presents after a trauma (either accidental or surgical) and the key presentation is one of **pain** particularly on movement of the muscles of that compartment.

The appendicular skeleton

The appendicular skeleton consists of the upper and lower limbs, which have evolved distinct structures reflecting their different functions.

The upper limb

The upper limb is specialised to give the hand a free range of movement to complete highly technical manipulative tasks (Fig. 14.3). It consists of:

- The **shoulder girdle** which attaches the upper limb to the axial skeleton
- The **humerus** of the upper arm
- The **radius** and the **ulna** of the forearm
- The eight **carpal bones** of the wrist
- The five **metacarpal bones** of the palm and the **phalanges** of the fingers.

The shoulder girdle

Thus, the shoulder girdle (Table 14.1) has developed to give mobility to the hand relative to the trunk. This incomplete ring of bony structures offers stability to the upper limb, while maintaining a high degree of motility. Three major bones (in addition to the sternum and the vertebrae) make up the shoulder girdle (Fig. 14.4):

- **Clavicle**: a long bony strut that holds the scapula away from the chest. It articulates with the sternum to form the sternoclavicular joint.

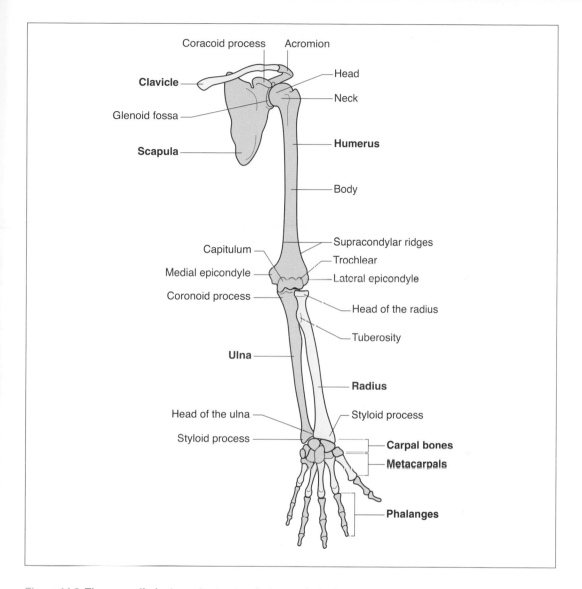

Figure 14.3 The upper limb: the main structure in the arm is the humerus, which connects to the scapula at the glenoid fossa and to the ulna and radius at the elbow. The elbow joint is formed by the trochlea and capitulum – cartilage-covered prominences of bone, which articulate with the radius and ulna, respectively. Above the trochlear and capitulum are the epicondyles and supracondylar ridges, which are important sites of attachments for ligaments and muscles. The ulna and radius form the forearm and form complex synovial joints at the elbow. The styloid processes of both bones form the wrist joint with the carpal bones, which connect the hand to the upper limb.

- **Scapula**: pushes the humerus away from the torso and is the site of attachment of the humerus at the glenoid fossa.
- **Humerus**: acts as a mobile lever, which directs the forearm and hand in most directions.

The glenohumeral joint

The glenohumeral joint is a ball-and-socket joint between the head of the humerus and the glenoid fossa of the scapula. The fossa is very shallow which allows the joint a wide range of movement,

Table 14.1 Joints of the shoulder girdle, their muscles and their movements. The sternoclavicular and acromioclavicular joints move in coordination to facilitate positioning of the scapula for movement at the glenohumeral joint

Joint	Structural and functional classification	Type and range of movements	Main muscle groups acting
Sternoclavicular	Plane, synovial joint	Elevation	Trapezius
Acromioclavicular	Plane, synovial joint	Depression	Trapezius and pectoralis minor
		Protraction	Serratus anterior and
		Retraction	Pectoralis minor
			Rhomboid muscles
Glenohumeral	Synovial ball and socket joint	Flexion	Muscles that pass across the anterior of the joint
		Extension	Muscles that pass across the posterior of the joint
		Abduction	Muscles that pass above the joint
		Adduction	Muscles that arise from the front or the back of the trunk and insert on the upper end of the humerus
		Medial rotation	Muscles that exert their pull anterior to the joint
		Lateral rotation	Muscles that act posterior to the joint and insert on to the upper end of the humerus

although it decreases the stability of the joint. Joint stability is enhanced by three features:

- The **rotator cuff** is made up of short muscles that secure the humerus to the scapula and are the major stabilising force of the joint. The rotator cuff comprises subscapularis anteriorly, supraspinatus superiorly, and infraspinatus and teres minor posteriorly (Fig. 14.5).
- The **glenoid labrum** is a ring of cartilage that effectively deepens the joint socket.
- A **fibrous capsule** surrounds the joint to stabilise it. The capsule is strengthened by the rotator cuff, except at its inferior aspect.

 CLINICAL Shoulder dislocation

The rotator cuff surrounds the glenohumeral joint in all but its inferior aspect. Dislocation of the head of the humerus most commonly follows a downward hit on the abducted humerus, dislocating the joint inferiorly and anteriorly due to the absence of a rotator cuff on its inferior aspect.

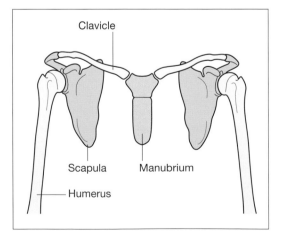

Figure 14.4 The **pectoral girdle** supports and attaches the upper limb to the rest of the body. Unlike the pelvic girdle, the pectoral girdle is an incomplete ring made up of the scapulae, clavicles and sternum. This structure allows a high degree of movement, although in turn it compromises some stability.

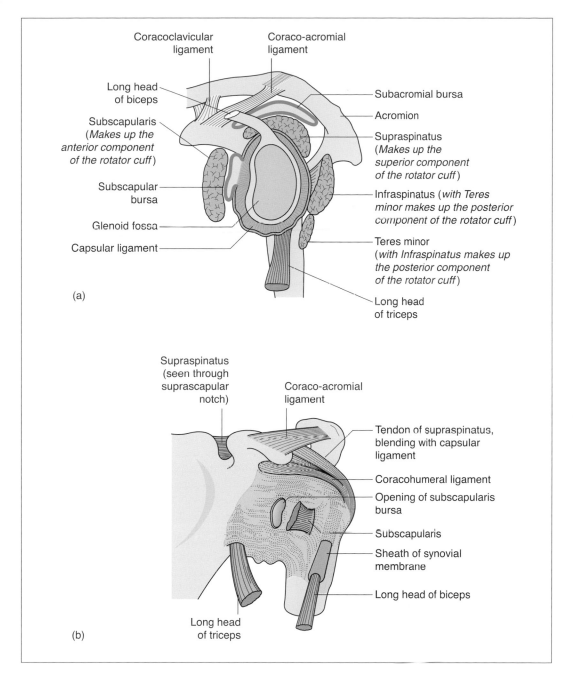

Figure 14.5 The **rotator cuff** is made up of four muscles –supraspinatus, infraspinatus, subscapularis and teres minor – which support the shoulder joint to increase its stability. The rotator cuff is incomplete inferiorly, which results in a weakness to dislocation in this direction. (a) A cross-section of the left glenoid cavity, detailing the orientation of the rotator cuff around the glenoid fossa. (b) An anterior view of the shoulder joint, detailing the arrangement of the rotator cuff in relation to the capsule.

Table 14.2 The elbow joint, its muscles and movements

Joint	Structural and functional classification	Type and range of movements	Main muscle groups acting
Elbow	Synovial, hinge	Flexion	Anterior compartment of upper arm
		Extension	Posterior compartment of upper arm
Radioulnar	Synovial, pivot	Pronation	Pronators – anterior compartment
		Supination	Supinators – posterior compartment

The elbow

The elbow is a complex joint (Table 14.2), made up of articulations of the humerus, radius and ulna (Fig. 14.6):

- The **synovial hinge joint** between the humerus and ulna allows **flexion** and **extension**.
- The **synovial plane joint** between the humerus and the radius allows rotation of the radius on the surface of the humerus, resulting in **pronation** and **supination** at the wrist. The **annular ligament** loops around the head of the radius, to retain its contact with the ulna and enable this rotation of the radius.

 DEFINITION Pronation and supination

The rotation of the radius allows pronation and supination to occur:

- **Pronation**: the forearm rotates so that the palm faces downwards. The ulna remains fixed while the radius rolls around it at both the elbow and the wrist joints.
- **Supination**: the radius rotates about the ulna so that the palm faces upwards (like a soup bowl).

The wrist

The wrist is made up of the carpal bones (Table 14.3), which articulate with the distal ends of the radius and ulna in a **condyloid joint**, and with the metacarpals of the hand. Most force is transmitted between the large distal head of the radius and the eight carpal bones (Fig. 14.7):

- The **proximal** row: scaphoid, lunate, triquetral and pisiform

- The **distal** row: trapezium, trapezoid, capitate and hamate.

The hand

The bones in the hand are the metacarpals and phalanges. The five metacarpal bones articulate proximally with the carpal bones and distally with the proximal phalanges. There is one set of three phalanges (proximal, middle and distal) in each digit, apart from the thumb, which lacks a middle phalanx. There are also many small sesamoid bones to provide extra leverage and reduce pressure on the underlying tissue.

Movement of the hand relies on a complicated system of muscles and tendons. Muscles can be divided into the following:

- **Intrinsic muscles** are small muscles with their bodies in the hand; they allow fine movements. The intrinsic muscles include the thenar muscles (thumb), hypothenar muscles (fifth finger), interosseus muscles (between the metacarpals) and lumbricals.
- **Extrinsic muscles** reside in the forearm and are connected to the insertion by a long tendon, so that their bulky contractile part does not interfere with the functioning of the hand, while allowing the significant contraction needed for larger movements:
  - **flexors** are found in the **anterior compartment of the forearm**
  - **extensors** are found in the **posterior compartment**.

The palmar aponeurosis

The aponeurosis is a thickened layer of fascia on the palm. The aponeurosis protects the soft tissue and tendons of the hands and provides a tough surface to help gripping.

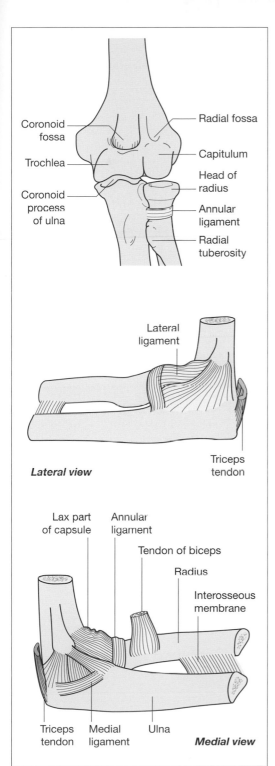

Lateral view

Medial view

 CLINICAL **Colles' fracture**

This is the most common wrist fracture. The distal part of the radius becomes displaced upwards, backwards and laterally, after a fall on an out-stretched hand. The ulna is not involved. Full correction must be achieved to enable full wrist movement in the future.

The arterial supply to the upper limb

The **brachial artery**, a continuation of the subclavian artery, supplies the arms. The subclavian artery becomes the axillary artery as it travels around the shoulder joint and, on entering the limb, it becomes the brachial artery, travelling on the anterior aspect of the arm, deep to many of the muscles (Fig. 14.8).

At the elbow the brachial artery divides into the cubital fossa to form the radial and ulnar arteries, which supply the forearm:

- The **radial artery** runs along the lateral (radial) side of the forearm supplying the **anterior compartment** of the forearm.
- The **ulnar artery** runs along the medial (medial) aspect of the forearm, supplying the **posterior compartment** of the forearm.

The radial and ulnar arteries continue into the hands where they give rise to the palmar arches:

- The deep palmar arch is primarily derived from the radial artery. It lies over the bases of the metacarpal bones.
- The superficial arch is derived primarily from the ulnar artery. It is located more distally than the deep arch.

Figure 14.6 The **elbow** is formed by the articulation of the humerus, ulna and radius. The humerus articulates with both the radial and the ulnar hinge joints, whereas the ulna and radius form a synovial plane joint. The annular ligament holds the radius to the ulna, allowing it to rotate around its axis. This allows pronation and supination of the forearm.

Table 14.3 The forearm joints, their muscles and movements

Joint	Structural and functional classification	Type and range of movements	Main muscle groups acting
Wrist	Synovial, ellipsoid	Flexion	Anterior compartment of forearm
		Extension	Posterior compartment of forearm
		Abduction/adduction	Combination of anterior and posterior compartments of forearm
		Circumduction/fixation	Flexors and extensors

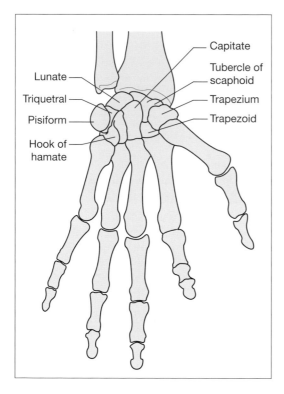

Typically, both arteries contribute to both palmar arches, although in some situations the palmar arches derive their blood supply from only one of the arteries.

> **Q CLINICAL Allen's test**
>
> Allen's test determines whether the palmar arterial arches of the hand receive contributions from both radial and ulnar arteries. This test is done before a procedure on the radial artery (such as an arterial blood gas sample) that could lead to obstruction of blood flow. Pressure is applied over both the radial and the ulnar arteries in the wrist, and blood in the hand is allowed to drain. One artery is then released and refilling of the hand noted. The same process is repeated for the other artery and it is noted whether both arteries result in rapid refilling (as noted by change in skin tone). Where a palmar arch is supplied by only one artery, there will be a marked difference in refilling between ulnar and palmar arteries.

Figure 14.7 Structure of the wrist and hand. The wrist is a condyloid synovial joint composed of eight small bones. Of these, the scaphoid, lunate and triquetral articulate with the distal radius and the fibrocartilage of the distal ulna, whereas remaining bones articulate with the metacarpals. The bones of the hand consist of the metacarpals and phalanges.

Figure 14.8 The arterial supply to the upper limb is derived from the axillary artery (which is a continuation of the subclavian artery). This becomes the brachial artery as it enters the arm, and gives off branches to the shoulder joint. As it travels along the humerus, the brachial artery gives off the profunda brachii branch, which supplies muscles in the posterior compartment. At the elbow the brachial artery divides into the radial and ulnar arteries, which travel with their respective bones. There are also posterior and interosseus branches from the arteries, which supply the muscles in the respective compartments of the forearm. The major pulse points are found at the elbow, where the brachial pulse can be felt, and at the wrist where both the ulnar and radial pulses can be detected.

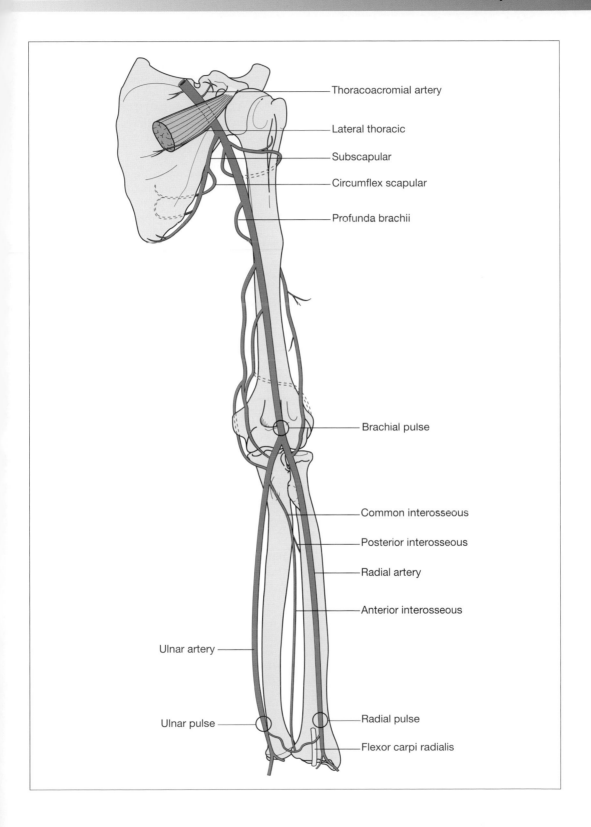

Thoracoacromial artery

Lateral thoracic

Subscapular

Circumflex scapular

Profunda brachii

Brachial pulse

Common interosseous

Posterior interosseous

Radial artery

Anterior interosseous

Ulnar artery

Ulnar pulse

Radial pulse

Flexor carpi radialis

The venous drainage of the upper limb

The superficial veins

The course of veins varies markedly between individuals. However, two major veins are commonly seen, both of which run superficially:

- The **basal vein** follows a course along the radial side of the arm.
- The **cephalic vein** follows a course along the ulnar side of the forearm.

The veins fuse near the proximal end of the upper limb to form the axillary vein, which drains into the subclavian vein.

 CLINICAL Venepuncture

A common site for sampling venous blood is the **antecubital fossa** at the front of the elbow, where the median cubital vein crosses. The median cubital vein runs relatively superficially at this point, connecting the basal and cephalic veins; it is not near other structures that are liable to be damaged.

The deep veins of the arm

The deep veins accompany the arteries and anastomose with them around the artery that they accompany. They consist of paired radial and medial veins that anastomose frequently, and feed into the paired brachial veins.

Lymphatic drainage of the upper limb

The lymphatic drainage of the upper limb consists of the following:

- **Superficial drainage** drains the hand and runs with the cephalic and basilar veins. Many of the vessels enter the cubital nodes at the elbow, and subsequently drain into the axillary lymph nodes.
- **Deep drainage** follows the course of the deep veins in the upper limb and also drains into the axillary lymph nodes.

Innervation of the upper limb

The brachial plexus

At the base of each upper limb the anterior primary rami of the spinal nerves form a plexus that organises the spinal roots of the nerves into the separate branches, which innervate distinct compartments of the limbs. The nerve roots from C5–T1 merge to form three trunks: **upper (C5–6)**, **middle (C7)** and **lower (C8)**. The cords then further divide into anterior and posterior fibres which recombine to form the three cords of the brachial plexus (Fig. 14.9):

- The **lateral cord** forms from the anterior divisions of the upper and middle trunks.
- The **posterior cord** forms from the posterior divisions of all three trunks.
- The **medial cord** is made up of the remainder of the lower trunk.

The cords are finally organised into branches that form the nerves of the upper limb. Although there are many different branches, there are four major nerves that innervate the skin and the major muscles in the upper limb (Fig. 14.10):

- The **radial nerve (C5–T1)**
- The **ulnar nerve (C8–T1)**
- The **median nerve (C5–T1)**
- The **musculocutaneous nerve (C5–7)**.

The radial nerve

The radial nerve arises from the posterior cord of the brachial plexus and contains roots from C5 to T1. It enters the arm behind the brachial artery, before travelling down the back of the arm on the medial side and entering the radial groove of the humerus, with the brachial artery. The radial nerve emerges on the lateral aspect of the humerus, and passes through the intermuscular septum into the anterior compartment of the forearm. At the distal end of the forearm it divides into two branches:

- The **motor branch** penetrates the supinator muscle and becomes known as the posterior interosseus nerve. It travels in the posterior compartment of the forearm and innervates the muscles in that compartment.
- The **sensory branch** remains relatively superficial as it passes through the forearm on the radial side. It then pierces the deep fascia to enter the hand on the posterior surface of the wrist. Sensory innervation is to the posterior surface of the hand and to the skin on the dorsal surface above the thumb and the next one-and-a-half fingers, up to the most distal phalangeal joint.

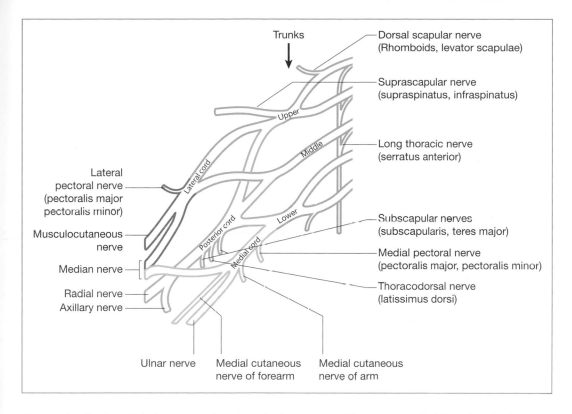

Figure 14.9 The **brachial plexus** organises the spinal nerves supplying the upper limb into the mixed nerves. Initially, the spinal nerves exit and form three trunks (upper, lower and middle). Further rearrangement leads to the generation of three cords (lateral, medial and posterior). The posterior cord forms the radial nerve, whereas the medial gives rise to the ulnar nerve and the lateral the musculocutaneous nerve. The median nerve is formed from divisions of the lateral and medial cords.

 CLINICAL Radial nerve palsy (saturday night palsy)

The radial nerve is at risk of injury in the upper arm at the site where it spirals around the humerus, when a patient spends an extensive period with an arm in a position with too much pressure on the radial nerve. This condition is known as '**Saturday night palsy**' because patients often present after falling asleep with an arm over the back of a chair when they have had too much alcohol to drink. However, another common presentation occurs with incorrect use of long crutches.

Damage leads to paralysis of the extensor muscles of the forearm and, therefore, a 'wrist drop' – the inability to flex the wrist upwards when the palm is faced down.

The ulnar nerve

The ulnar nerve is derived from the medial cord of the brachial plexus and travels down the posterior aspect of the arm on the medial side to reach the elbow. At the elbow it runs superficially to the medial epicondyle, where it is at risk of injury. It then passes into the forearm and travels alongside the ulnar, before entering the palm of the hand through the ulnar canal, superficial to **flexor retinaculum**.

The ulnar nerve carries both motor and sensory fibres:

- The **ulnar nerve** supplies many of the intrinsic muscles of the hand.
- **Sensory innervation** is to the medial side of the hand (both the dorsal and palmar aspects), and the medial side of the fourth digit, as well as the entire fifth finger.

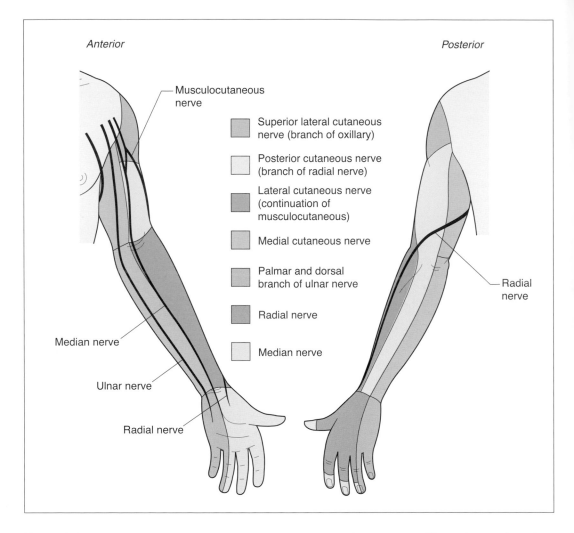

Figure 14.10 **The nervous distribution to the upper limb**: the brachial plexus gives off five major nerve branches, each of which courses into the lower limb to provide a mixture of sensory cutaneous and muscular innervation.

Median nerve

The median nerve is derived from the medial and lateral cords of the brachial plexus before passing down the arm's medial aspect. The nerve emerges in the cubital fossa to pass on the anterior side of the forearm to the wrist, where it passes through the **carpal tunnel** to enter the hand.

The median nerve has both motor and sensory components:

- The **motor** branches supply the flexors of the forearm (anterior compartment), the first and second lumbricals and the thenar eminence.
- The **sensory** component supplies the skin of the lateral part of the palm and the palmar side of the

thumb, the index and middle fingers, and half of the ring finger, as well as the most distal tips of those fingers on the dorsal side.

 DEFINITION The carpal tunnel

The carpal tunnel is a sheath formed by flexor retinaculum, a thick ligamentous layer that links the hook of the hamate with the scaphoid. The resulting 'tunnel' carries many tendons and the median nerve into the hand. Inflammation in this region can compress the median nerve, resulting in **carpal tunnel syndrome**.

CLINICAL **Carpal tunnel syndrome**

Carpal tunnel syndrome results from compression of the median nerve in the carpal tunnel. It is characterised by a tingling in the regions of the palm supplied by the median nerve. As it progresses the sensations become progressively more painful, particularly at night, when it can cause the patient to wake, and may make gripping and other movements difficult.

Carpal tunnel syndrome has become more prevalent in recent years with the increase in office jobs involving repetitive movements that increase stress on the wrist and may promote inflammation. Although painkillers may be prescribed, wrist splints are often effective to rest the wrist. In severe cases surgery may be performed to decompress the nerve.

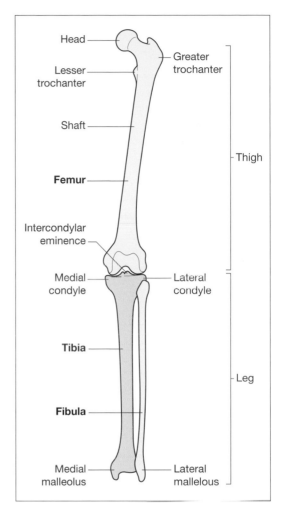

Figure 14.11 The **lower limb**. The major portion of the lower limb is made up of the femur, tibia and fibula, which articular at the knee joint. The bones of the lower limb are thicker than their counterparts in the upper limb, reflecting their adaptation for load bearing. This also results in a more limited degree of movement in the lower limb.

The musculocutaneous nerve

The **musculocutaneous nerve** arises from the lateral cord of the brachial plexus and travels through the arm on its lateral aspect to the forearm. It supplies the flexors (anterior compartment) of the arm and gives a sensory supply to the lateral aspect of the forearm.

The lower limb

The lower limb skeleton has evolved for locomotion and weight bearing; its bones are larger and thicker compared with the upper limb (Fig. 14.11). The lower limb skeleton is composed of the:

- pelvis and thigh: composed of the ilium, ischium and pubis, and the **femur**
- bones of the leg: **tibia** and **fibula**
- bones of the ankle: tibia, fibula and **talus**
- bones of the foot: **tarsal bones**, **metatarsals** and **phalanges**.

The pelvis

The pelvic girdle transmits force from the spine to the legs and forms a bony structure to protect the pelvic organs. The load-bearing role of the pelvis is reflected in its formation of a complete girdle that is less manoeuvrable, but more stable, than the shoulder girdle.

The pelvis is made up of three bones – the ischium, ilium and pubis – which are fused by **fibrous joints** and articulate with the femur at the **acetabulum**. The roof and the posterior wall are formed by the sacrum. The remainder of the pelvis is composed of the iliac bones which articulate with the sacrum via sacroiliac joints. In addition, the pelvic girdle is completed anteriorly by the pubic symphysis, a cartilaginous joint between the pubic bones in the midline (Fig. 14.12).

The ilium, ischium and pubis contribute to important anatomical landmarks:

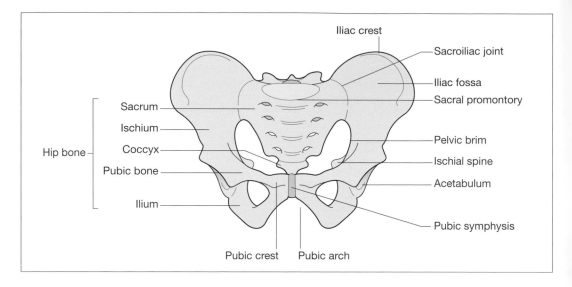

Figure 14.12 The pelvic girdle is a rigid structure made up of the fused bones of the ilium, ischium and pubis, which is connected to the axial skeleton through the fused sacrum, which forms the posterior aspect of the pelvic girdle. The two pelvic bones are connected anteriorly at the pelvic symphysis.

- The **acetabulum** has contributions from the ilium, ischium and pubis.
- **Obturator foramen** is bound by the pubis and ischium.
- The **greater sciatic notch** is bound by ischium and ilium and lies above ischial spine. The lesser sciatic notch lies below the ischial spine.

The pelvis is often thought of as a tube-like structure with two openings:

1 The 'inlet of the pelvis' runs from the most superior part of the sacrum to the superior part of the symphysis pubis.
2 The 'outlet of pelvis' runs from the inferior part of the pubic symphysis to the most distal part of the coccyx.

 CLINICAL Surface anatomy of the pelvis

The iliac crest can be traced from the coccyx to the anterior superior iliac spine (ASIS). The pelvic bone cannot be followed medially from the ASIS due to the presence of muscles. However, the pubic symphysis can be located in the midline and the pubic tubercle can be found on the upper part of the thigh. The inguinal ligament is located between the pubic tubercle and the anterior superior iliac spine.

The hip joint

The hip joint (Table 14.4) is the articulation of the head of the femur with the bones of the pelvis. The head of the femur sits in the **acetabular fossa**, which is a deep depression at the site of fusion of all three pelvic bones. Its deep nature reflects the load-bearing role of the pelvis, as movement at the joint is sacrificed to produce a more stable joint. The joint is further stabilised by several features, in particular:

- The acetabular fossa is surrounded by a ring of fibrocartilage, the **acetabular labrum**, which allows the joint to accommodate 50% of the head of the femur.
- The hip joint is further stabilised by a ring of ligaments surrounding the acetabular fossa.

The differences in the pelvis in the female and male

The structure of the pelvis differs between the sexes (Table 14.5). The shape of the female pelvis enables childbirth to be facilitated, whereas the male pelvis is adapted for greater strength and movement to enable primitive humans to hunt and gather.

Table 14.4 The pelvic girdle, its muscles and movements

Joint	Structural and functional classification	Type and range of movements	Main muscles acting
Pubic symphysis	Cartilaginous	Little movement	
Sacroiliac	Synovial	Little movement	
Hip	Synovial ball and socket	Flexion	Iliopsoas, Sartorius, Tensor fascia lata, Rectus femoris, Pectineus, Adductor muscles, Gracilis
		Extension	Hamstrings, adductor magnus, gluteus maximus
		Abduction	Gluteus medius and minimus, tensor of fascia lata
		Adduction	Adductor muscles, Gracilis, Pectineus, Obturator externus
		Medial rotation	Anterior parts of gluteus medius and minimus, tensor of fascia lata
		Lateral rotation	Obturator muscles, Gemelli, Quadratus femoris, Gluteus maximus

The knee

The knee joint is **complex joint** consisting of a synovial **condyloid joint** between the femur and tibia, and a synovial **plane joint** between the femur and patella. The patella lies on the patellar groove at the front of the femur (Fig. 14.13). The articulations in the knee joint are not very stable themselves; there are three features that contribute to the stability of the joint:

- The ligaments of the knee joint
- The menisci
- The muscles surrounding the knee joint.

The ligaments of the knee

The anterior and posterior cruciate ligaments are found inside the knee capsule and are crucial in stabilising the joint. Their names refer to the location of their attachment to the tibia.

Other ligaments are found outside the capsule:

- The **patellar ligament** connects the patella to the tuberosity of the tibia and gives the patella mechanical leverage.
- The **medial collateral ligament** stretches from the medial epicondyle of the femur to the medial tibial condyle, and helps the knee resist stresses to the lateral side of the knee.

Table 14.5 The differences between a male pelvis and a female pelvis, reflecting the adaptation of the female pelvis for childbirth

Pelvic characteristic	Male	Female
Pelvic inlet	Heart-shaped	Oval-shaped
Iliac fossa	Narrower and longer	Wider and shorter
Pubic arch – formed by the convergence of the ischium and pubis on either side	Narrower and less round	Broader and more rounded
The pubic bone	Smaller	Larger
Inferior pubic ramus	Everted and thickened by the attachment of ischiocavernosus	
Greater sciatic notch – created inferiorly by the ischial spine and superiorly by the sacrospinous ligament	Narrower	Wider

- The **lateral collateral ligament** extends from the lateral epicondyle of the femur to the head of the fibula, and protects the knee from stresses to the medial side of the knee.

Menisci

The condyles of the femur articulates with the tibia at two rounded prominences, each resting on a cartilage pad – known as a meniscus. The menisci act as shock absorbers and also deepen the knee joint, helping its stability.

Stabilising muscles of the knee

Although principally a synovial hinge joint, the muscles surrounding the knee joint can contract to stabilise it (Table 14.6). In particular, the knee can twist slightly, tightening the ligaments in an action known as 'locking' the knee. This generates a more stable but immobile structure, while the muscles can be temporarily relaxed. The knee can be unlocked through contraction of the popliteus muscle, which rotates the knee slightly.

 CLINICAL Ruptured cruciate ligament

Cruciate ligaments are two thick rounded cords, which lie centrally in the joint capsule but outside the synovial cavity; if the anterior cruciate is ruptured the tibia can be moved in front of the femur, and this is common in skiing accidents. When the posterior cruciate is damaged, the leg will noticeably droop if it is supported horizontally at the ankle; posterior cruciate ligament rupture may occur if someone lands on the tibial tuberosity with the knee flexed.

Small tears may be treated by stabilising the knee in a brace to allow the individual to continue to use the joint, while relieving strain on the ligament to help healing. Severe tears are treated surgically, and may require more than 6 months of rehabilitation for the individual to regain previous function.

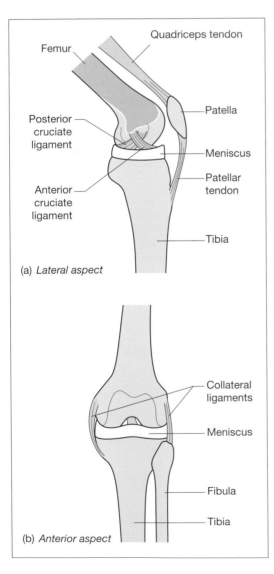

(a) *Lateral aspect*

(b) *Anterior aspect*

Figure 14.13 The knee joint: (a) the medial aspect of the right knee joint. The knee joint is made up of two synovial joints – a synovial hinge joint between the tibia and the femur and a plane joint between the femur and patella. The joint between the femur and the tibia results in the condyles of the femur articulating with the tibia. The interaction is cushioned by the cartilage on the femur, which articulates with the menisci (cartilaginous pads) found on the tibia. The joint is stabilised by the two cruciate ligaments, the posterior ligament being located more laterally. The patella is a large sesamoid bone, which acts as a pivot for the transference of the force of contraction of quadriceps to the leg. It is located in the patellar tendon, which is continuous superiorly with the quadriceps tendon. (b) The anterior aspect of the right knee joint of the right knee joint (patella not shown). The articulation between the femur and the tibia is stabilised by the collateral ligaments, which link the epicondyles of the femur with the condyles of the tibia, and via the muscles surrounding the knee can contribute stability to the joint.

Table 14.6 The knee's joints, muscles and movements

Joint	Structural and functional classification	Type and range of movements	Main muscle groups acting
Knee	Compound hinge, synovial joint	Flexion	Posterior compartment of thigh
		Extension	Anterior compartment of thigh
		Small active (lateral) and passive (medial) rotation movements	Medial and lateral compartments of thigh.

The ankle

The distal ends of the tibia and fibula are enlarged to form processes known as **malleoli**. The ankle is a synovial hinge joint between the malleoli of the tibia and fibula and the **talus** bone of the foot, which allows **dorsiflexion** and **plantarflexion**; in this the sole of the foot moves so that the toes point upwards and downwards, respectively (Fig. 14.14).

The foot is also capable of **inversion** and **eversion** where the foot tilts medially and laterally, respectively. These movements occur at the tarsal joint below the level of the ankle.

Stabilisation of the ankle joint

The deltoid ligament and two lateral ligaments support the ankle joint:

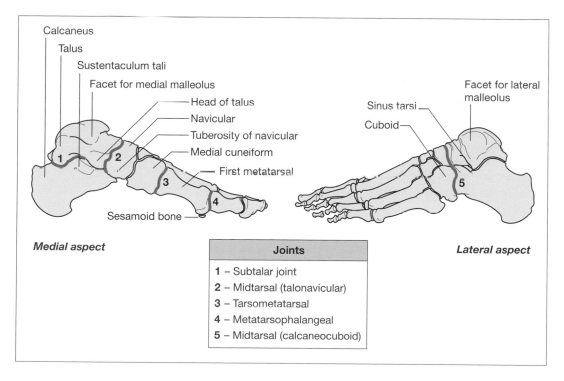

Calcaneus
Talus
Sustentaculum tali
Facet for medial malleolus
Head of talus
Navicular
Tuberosity of navicular
Medial cuneiform
First metatarsal
Sesamoid bone

Sinus tarsi
Cuboid
Facet for lateral malleolus

Medial aspect

Lateral aspect

Joints
1 – Subtalar joint
2 – Midtarsal (talonavicular)
3 – Tarsometatarsal
4 – Metatarsophalangeal
5 – Midtarsal (calcaneocuboid)

Figure 14.14 The foot is made up of the tarsal bones and the metatarsals. The talus articulates with the tibia and fibula to form the ankle joint and the calcaneus forms the heel of the foot. The remaining tarsals form a series of synovial plane joints in the foot. This arrangement allows the foot to absorb and transmit shock and impact between the ground and the body. The tarsals articulate anteriorly with the metatarsals, which extend to the phalanges that make up the toes.

- The **deltoid ligament** is a flat, triangular band stretching from the tarsal bones to the medial malleolus of the tibia; it has superficial and deep layers.
- The **lateral ligaments** connect the lateral malleolus to the tarsal bones.

The foot

The foot transmits body weight to the ground to enable standing and locomotion. It has a similar structure to the hand due to its evolutionary origin, although the structure is altered to reflect the different roles. The foot is composed of tarsals, metatarsals and phalanges. The tarsal bones correspond to the carpals of the wrist, the metatarsals to the metacarpals and the phalanges to those of the hand. The tarsal bones are composed of:

- the talus – interacts with the tibia and fibula to form the ankle joint
- the calcaneus – forms the heel of the foot
- the cuboid
- the navicular
- three cuneiform bones.

The metatarsal bones are the long bones of the foot. Each of the five metatarsal bones articulates with at least one of the tarsal bones proximally and one of the proximal phalanges distally. The number of phalanges in each toe corresponds with that in the fingers, i.e. three in each, apart from the toe in which there are only two.

The tarsal and metatarsal bones are arranged in a series of arches (medial and longitudinal), maintained by muscles and ligaments to enable shock absorption.

The muscles of the foot (Table 14.7) act in a similar way to those of the hand: there are intrinsic and extrinsic muscles. The intrinsic muscles act to maintain the arches. The bulk of the extrinsic muscles are situated in the lower leg and their tendons extend into the feet to enable gross movements of the foot.

The muscle compartments of the lower limb

There are three fascial compartments in the thigh:

- The **anterior compartment of the thigh** consists of quadriceps, which extends the leg at the knee joint. It also stabilises the hip and helps flexion of the thigh. The anterior compartment is innervated by the **femoral nerve**.
- The **medial compartment of the thigh** is responsible for the thigh's adduction, and also mediates rotation at the hip.
- The **posterior compartment of the thigh** extends the thigh, flexes the leg and contributes to rotation. The posterior compartment is innervated by the sciatic nerve.

There are three fascial compartments in the leg:

- The **anterior compartment of the leg** dorsiflexes the ankle and extends the toes. It is innervated by the deep peroneal nerve.
- The **lateral compartment of the leg** everts the foot and contributes to plantarflexion.
- The **posterior compartment of the leg** plantarflexes the ankle and inverts the foot.

The vasculature of the lower limb

The vasculature of the pelvis

The pelvic blood supply is derived from the branches of the abdominal aorta, and is discussed here briefly, but covered in more detail later:

Table 14.7 The joints, muscles and movements of the leg

Joint	Structural and functional classification	Type and range of movements	Main muscle groups acting
Tibiofibular	Plane, synovial	Fibula rotates slightly as the talus moves in the ankle joint	
Ankle	Synovial, hinge	Dorsiflexion	Anterior compartment of leg
		Plantarflexion	Posterior compartment of leg
		Inversion	Anterior compartment of leg
		Eversion	Posterior compartment of leg

- The **median sacral artery** supplies the fourth and fifth lumbar vertebrae, sacrum, coccyx and posterior surface of the rectum.
- The **common iliac arteries** bifurcate anterior to the sacroiliac joint. With few exceptions, the tissues of the pelvis are supplied by the internal iliac, and those of the leg are supplied by the external iliac:
  - each **external iliac** artery passes under the inguinal ligament to enter the thigh as the femoral artery
  - each **internal iliac** follows the sacroiliac joint and branches to supply: the pelvic viscera, gluteal region, perineum, lateral wall of the pelvis and medial aspect of the thigh (obturator artery), and skin and muscles of the posterior abdominal wall and lower back (iliolumbar and lateral sacral arteries).

Vasculature of the leg

The leg is supplied by the femoral artery (Fig. 14.15), a continuation of the external iliac artery. It travels from the inguinal ligament through the thigh, medial to the femur. At the popliteal fossa it becomes the popliteal artery, and divides into the anterior and posterior tibial arteries:

- The **anterior tibial artery** supplies the anterior compartment of the leg and the dorsal surface of the foot. It becomes dorsalis pedis as it crosses the anterior aspect of the ankle joint.
- The **posterior tibial artery** supplies the posterior compartment of the leg and the plantar surface of the foot. It gives rise to the **peroneal artery**.

Venous drainage of the pelvis

The pelvis is drained by veins that follow the same course as their respective arteries. They contribute to the common iliac veins, which unite to form the inferior vena cava. These veins have valve-less links to veins of the lumbar and sacral spine.

 CLINICAL Arterial pulse points

Arteries can be palpated at certain points to ensure that blood is flowing. This is essential if there is any query over blood supply being compromised to an area. In addition, the rate and rhythm of the heartbeat can be measured, often using the radial artery. The carotid artery in the neck can be palpated to assess the volume of the blood circulating in the body.

The venous drainage of the lower limb

The venous drainage of the lower limb can be divided into two distinct types of veins that are interconnected through communicating vessels. This allows flow of blood from the superficial vein to the deeper vessels:

- **Superficial veins** drain the skin and superficial fascia; examples include the short and long saphenous veins (Fig. 14.16). They give off communicating veins to allow flow of blood from the superficial to the deep venous system. Valves in the penetrating veins prevent blood flow from the deep to the superficial circulation.
- **Deep veins** accompany large arteries beneath the deep fascia. Venae comitantes are small paired veins, which drain the tissue supplied by smaller arteries. The blood from these veins drains into the deep veins.

The superficial part of the lateral side of the leg is drained by the **short saphenous vein**, which arises from the lateral part of the dorsal veins of the foot and passes behind the lateral malleolus. It runs posteriorly at the calf and drains into the popliteal vein (a deep vein), having passed through the deep fascia of the popliteal fossa. The popliteal vein empties into the femoral vein.

The remaining superficial parts of the leg are drained by the **long saphenous vein**, which arises from the medial end of the dorsal veins of the foot and runs anterior to the medial malleolus. It runs anterolaterally in the calf, passing behind the knee before running anteromedially in the thigh. The long saphenous vein passes through the fascia lata, 5 cm below the pubic tubercle on the medial aspect of the thigh. It then joins the femoral vein.

Venous pumps in the lower limb

Stasis of blood in the leg must be avoided, to ensure adequate return to the heart and to prevent the formation of thromboses. Two adaptations facilitate the return of blood from the lower limb, which is more difficult than from the arms due to the effects of gravity:

- **Valves** in the veins to prevent backflow of blood: the valves consist one to three folds of tissue that fill as the blood flows back, occluding the lumen. As the blood direction returns, the lumen is forced open and the valve pocket pushed to the side of the vessel.

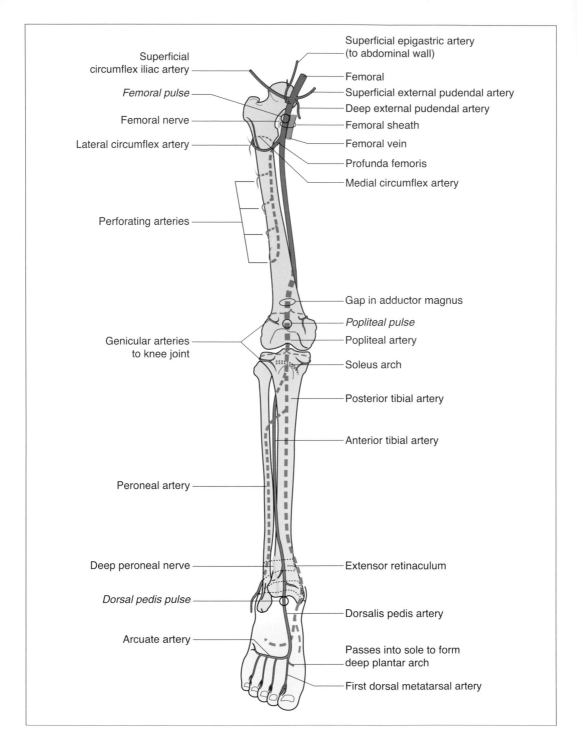

Figure 14.15 The arterial supply to the lower limb is derived from the femoral artery, which enters the leg on its anterior aspect and curves posteriorly as it becomes the popliteal artery, which runs posterior to the knee joint. In the leg, the popliteal artery splits to form three major branches: the fibular, and the anterior and posterior tibial branches. The anterior tibial branch becomes dorsalis pedis in the foot, whereas the posterior tibial artery gives rise to the lateral and medial plantar branches that supply the sole of the foot.

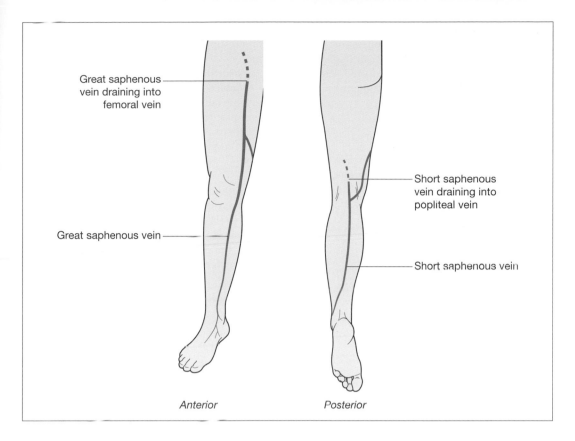

Figure 14.16 The saphenous veins provides the superficial venous drainage of the lower limb. The short saphenous vein is located on the posterior aspect of the leg and ascends to the popliteal fossa where it pierces the fascia and drains into the deep venous system. The great saphenous vein ascends the lateral aspect of the lower limb to the inguinal region, where it too pierces the fascia and drains into the deep femoral vein.

 CLINICAL **Varicose veins**

Varicose veins are dilated superficial veins. As a result, the valves of the veins become incompetent and the pooling of blood enlarges them further. Dilatation occurs for many reasons including genetics, pregnancy and obesity.

Varicose veins are painful, cosmetically ugly, compromise drainage of the skin and can cause severe ulceration. Conservative treatment includes compression stockings, leg elevation and exercise. Surgical management includes vein stripping when the affected vein is simply removed.

- **Muscle pump**: the veins run in fascial compartments among the muscles. During muscle relaxation, blood drains from the superficial veins to the deep veins through communicating veins, the valves of which open to accommodate this. During muscle contraction, the pressure in the fascial compartment rises and forces blood from the deep veins (including that which has drained from the superficial veins) towards the heart.

Lymphatic drainage of the lower limb

The lymphatic drainage is organised into superficial and deep vessels:

- The **superficial vessels** follow the course of the saphenous veins. Those travelling with the small saphenous vein drain into the popliteal lymph nodes in the popliteal fossa. The vessels accompanying the great saphenous vein drain into the external iliac nodes.

The **deep vessels** accompany the deep veins and drain into the popliteal lymph nodes. The lymph from the popliteal nodes travels through deep vessels with the femoral artery to the deep inguinal lymph nodes, and subsequently to the external iliac lymph nodes.

Innervation of the lower limb

The nerves supplying the pelvis and the lower limb are derived from the lumbosacral plexus, which receives spinal nerves T12–S4. The plexus can be divided into two separate, but linked, plexus (Fig. 14.17):

- The **lumbar plexus** is located in psoas major, a muscle in the lumbar region.
- The **sacral plexus** is found on the posterior surface of the pelvis between the piriformis muscle and pelvic fascia.

The lumbar plexus gives rise to several branches, the main ones being:

- The **femoral nerve** (posterior divisions of L2, -3, -4) supplies the anterior compartment of thigh.
- The **obturator nerve** (anterior divisions of L2, -3, -4) supplies the parietal peritoneum and medial thigh muscles. Four smaller branches supply the lower part of abdomen (T12, L1):
- The **genitofemoral nerve** (L1, -2) supplies skin overlying the femoral triangle and cremaster.

The major branches of the sacral plexus are:

- The **pudendal nerve** (S2, -3, -4) which supplies skin, anal canal, and reproductive and urinary tracts in the perineum
- **Combined S1, -2, -3, -4** which supply the muscles of the pelvic floor and the pelvic parasympathetic nerves of the pelvic viscera.

The sciatic nerve

The **sciatic nerve** is the longest single nerve, supplying all the skin of the leg, and the muscles of the

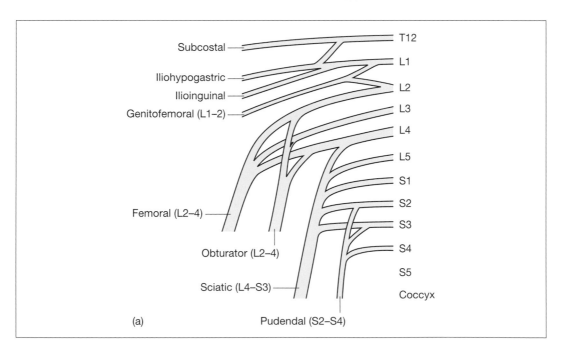

Subcostal

Iliohypogastric

Ilioinguinal

Genitofemoral (L1–2)

Femoral (L2–4)

Obturator (L2–4)

Sciatic (L4–S3)

T12
L1
L2
L3
L4
L5
S1
S2
S3
S4
S5
Coccyx

(a)

Pudendal (S2–S4)

Figure 14.17 Nervous supply to the lower limbs: (a) the nerves supplying the muscles of the lower body are derived from the lumbosacral plexus which organises the nerve roots emerging from T12–S5 into the mixed nerves that innervate the structures of the lower body. In particular, the major nerves supplying the leg are formed – the femoral, obturator and sciatic. (b) The sciatic nerve is responsible for the innervation of all the structures below the knee joint, as well as the hamstrings, in the thigh. The nerve forms two major branches that enter the different compartments of the leg – the tibial and common peroneal nerves.

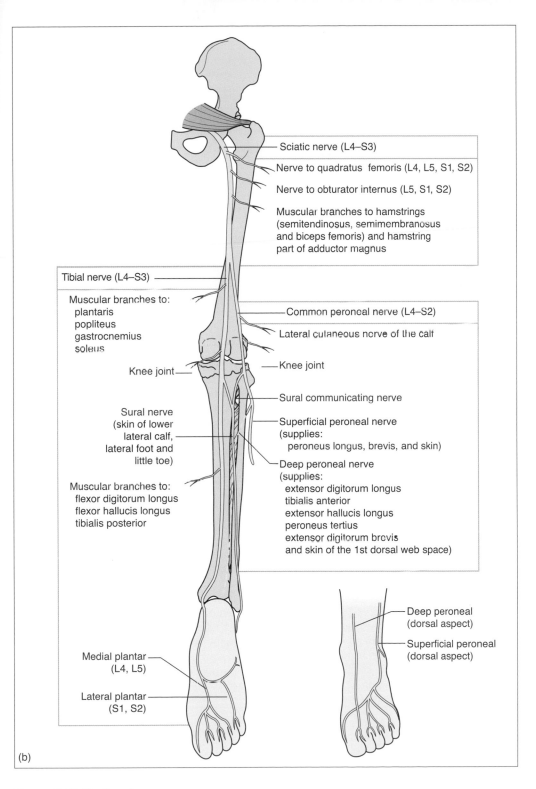

Sciatic nerve (L4–S3)

Nerve to quadratus femoris (L4, L5, S1, S2)

Nerve to obturator internus (L5, S1, S2)

Muscular branches to hamstrings (semitendinosus, semimembranosus and biceps femoris) and hamstring part of adductor magnus

Tibial nerve (L4–S3)

Muscular branches to:
  plantaris
  popliteus
  gastrocnemius
  soleus

Common peroneal nerve (L4–S2)

Lateral cutaneous nerve of the calf

Knee joint

Knee joint

Sural communicating nerve

Sural nerve
(skin of lower
lateral calf,
lateral foot and
little toe)

Superficial peroneal nerve
(supplies:
  peroneus longus, brevis, and skin)

Deep peroneal nerve
(supplies:
  extensor digitorum longus
  tibialis anterior
  extensor hallucis longus
  peroneus tertius
  extensor digitorum brevis
  and skin of the 1st dorsal web space)

Muscular branches to:
  flexor digitorum longus
  flexor hallucis longus
  tibialis posterior

Deep peroneal
(dorsal aspect)

Superficial peroneal
(dorsal aspect)

Medial plantar
(L4, L5)

Lateral plantar
(S1, S2)

(b)

Figure 14.17 (Continued)

posterior compartment of the thigh, and of the leg and foot. The sciatic nerve arises from L4–S3. It enters the lower limb through the greater sciatic foramen before descending the back of the thigh, which splits to form two branches in the lower third of the thigh:

- The **tibial nerve** supplies the muscles of the foot and muscles in the posterior compartment of the calf. It gives rise to two terminal branches – the lateral and medial plantar nerves.
- The **common peroneal nerve** winds around the neck of the fibula before dividing into superficial and deep branches.
- The **deep peroneal** nerve supplies the anterior compartment of the leg and foot, as well as the sensory supply to the area between the first and second toes.
- The **superficial peroneal nerve** supplies the muscles of the lateral compartment of the leg, the skin of the lateral lower two-thirds of the leg, and the whole of the dorsum of the foot excluding the region supplied by the deep nerve.

 CLINICAL Sciatica

Compression or irritation of the sciatic nerve causes severe pain in the distribution in the lower back, buttocks and various parts of the leg and foot. Although pain is the most obvious symptom, numbness and weakness may accompany it. The symptoms are usually unilateral and removed only when the cause of the irritation is resolved.

The skull

The head sits atop the neck and encloses the brain. Although this results in some vulnerability, it also allows the sensory organs in the head to move, allowing us to look around. The skull can be divided into two regions (Fig. 14.18):

- The **neurocranium** encloses the brain, having outlets only for the spinal cord, various nerves and veins, and inlets for only the arteries and nerves. The bones of the neurocranium are discussed in relation to the brain in Chapter 17, although their shape and contribution to the skull as a whole are discussed below.
- The **viscerocranium** makes up the face and contains the jaws, orbits and nasal cavity.

The neurocranium

The neurocranium is the dome-shaped superior part of the skull; it is made up of many bones fused by **fibrous joints**. The base of the cranium contributes to the roof of the nasal cavity, and the bones of the neurocranium make up part of the orbit. The internal aspects of the neurocranium have evolved to accommodate the brain, however, and are covered in Chapter 17. Some important aspects contribute to the external structure of the skull, where they form anatomical landmarks:

- The **frontal bone** makes up the forehead, articulating superiorly with the zygomatic and nasal bones of the viscerocranium, as well as bones of the neurocranium. The frontal bone develops as two halves that fuse in the midline early in life (in the first 5 years).
- Two **parietal bones** are found posterior to the frontal bone. These form much of the superior aspect of the head, articulating with the frontal bone at the **coronal suture**. The parietal bones also fuse with each other along the midline at the sagittal suture.
- The **temporal bones** lie on either side of the skull, immediately inferior to the parietal bones. The temporal bones contain the external acoustic meatus, and the styloid and mastoid processes, which are important muscle attachment points. The temporal bone also projects a zygomatic process laterally and anteriorly, which forms the **zygomatic arch** with the temporal bone.
- The **occipital bone** is a single bone at the posterior aspect of the skull, inferior to the parietal bones. It fuses with the temporal bones and

Figure 14.18 The skull is made up of several irregular bones and can be divided into those making up the neurocranium, which encloses the brain, and those making up the viscerocranium, which make up the face. The neurocranium itself forms a vault and base that surrounds the brain on all sides and the only points of access are the foramina, allowing vascular and nervous access to and from the brain. Most bones in the skull are joined by fibrous sutures that do not move; however, the mandible in the viscerocranium articulates with a synovial joint, as it forms the jaw and this allows chewing.

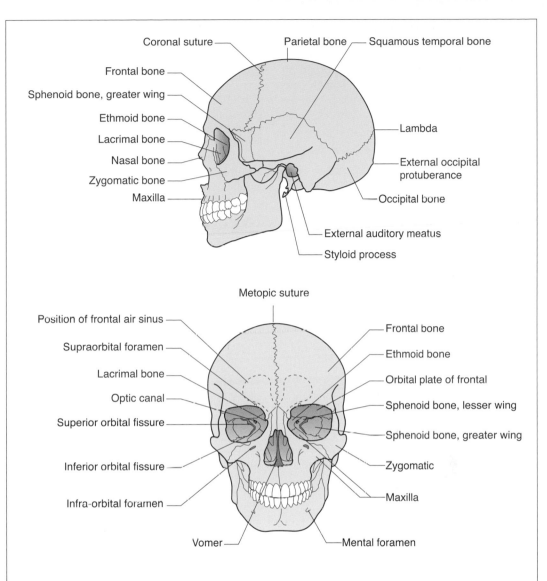

Coronal suture — Parietal bone — Squamous temporal bone

Frontal bone —

Sphenoid bone, greater wing —

Ethmoid bone —

Lacrimal bone —

Nasal bone —

Zygomatic bone —

Maxilla —

— Lambda

— External occipital protuberance

— Occipital bone

— External auditory meatus

— Styloid process

Metopic suture

Position of frontal air sinus —

Supraorbital foramen —

Lacrimal bone —

Optic canal —

Superior orbital fissure —

Inferior orbital fissure —

Infra-orbital foramen —

— Frontal bone

— Ethmoid bone

— Orbital plate of frontal

— Sphenoid bone, lesser wing

— Sphenoid bone, greater wing

— Zygomatic

— Maxilla

Vomer —

— Mental foramen

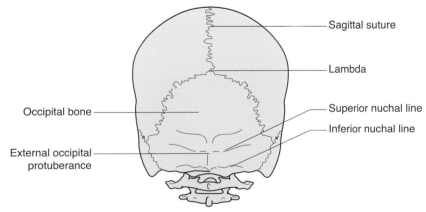

— Sagittal suture

— Lambda

Occipital bone —

— Superior nuchal line

— Inferior nuchal line

External occipital protuberance —

forms the posterior wall of the **foramen magnum**, which carries the spinal cord from the brain.

- The **sphenoid bone** makes up a large proportion of the floor of the cranial fossa, although contributes to small parts of the lateral aspect of the skull. It forms part of the lateral aspect of the skull, articulating with the frontal, zygomatic and parietal bones.

The viscerocranium

The viscerocranium forms the part of the skull that makes up the face. Our facial appearance is a result of structure of the bones and soft tissues that overlie it. The viscerocranium is made up of six pairs of bones and two unpaired bones, all of which are irregular in shape. The paired bones lie symmetrically about the midline of the face whereas the single bones lie directly on the midline itself:

- The **maxillae** form the skeleton of the upper jaw and serve as the points of insertion for the teeth of the upper jaw.
- The **zygomatic bones** make up the lower parts of the orbits and contribute to the cheek prominences. The zygomatic bones articulate with the maxillae, temporal, frontal and sphenoid bones. The temporal process of the zygomatic bone contributes to the zygomatic arch.
- The **nasal bones** form the bony part of the nose.
- The **lacrimal bones** contribute to the medial aspect of the orbit.
- The **palatine bones** are found in the roof of the mouth, making up the posterior part of the **hard palate**. They also contribute to the floor and lateral parts of the nasal cavities, and part of the base of the orbit.
- The **mandible** is a large single bone. It is U shaped and forms the jaw, providing attachment for the lower row of teeth.
- The **vomer** is a single bone lying in the midline of the face at the nasal cavity. It is extremely thin and forms the posterior bony part of the nasal septum.

The face

The face also contains many muscles responsible for facial expression, mastication and regulation of the opening of the orifices (Fig. 14.19), which connect the respiratory and gastrointestinal tracts to the external environment and provide openings for the special senses.

The muscles of facial expression

The muscles of facial expression develop from the second pharyngeal arch as a flat muscular sheet, which differentiates into functional groups of fibres surrounding the different orifices in the face. All the muscles associated with facial expression are innervated by the facial nerve (the seventh cranial nerve or CN VII).

The muscles around the orifices

The **eyelids** are controlled by the contraction of orbicularis oculi, which is attached to the palpebral ligament and the medial orbital margins, allowing its contraction to pull the eyelid shut.

The muscles around the **mouth** perform three functions: they convey facial expression, alter the shape of the lips to alter sound for speaking and singing, and close the mouth during eating.

The muscles of mastication

The muscles of the palate and those linking the mandible to the rest of the skull are responsible for allowing mastication (chewing). The muscles of mastication are derived from first pharyngeal arch, and are innervated by the mandibular branch of the trigeminal nerve (CN V_3, reflecting their common embryological origin. There are four muscles of mastication:

1 **Masseter** which is the largest of the muscles of mastication attaching from the maxilla and zygomatic arch to the angle of the mandible
2 **Temporalis**
3 **Lateral pterygoid**
4 **Medial pterygoid**.

 DEFINITION The zygomatic arch

The zygomatic arch is an arch of bone on the lateral aspect of the skull, which is made up of processes of the zygomatic and temporal bones. It is a point of attachment for muscles, including the masseter, and also forms a canal through which the temporalis muscle passes to its origin as a wide sheet on the lateral aspect of the skull.

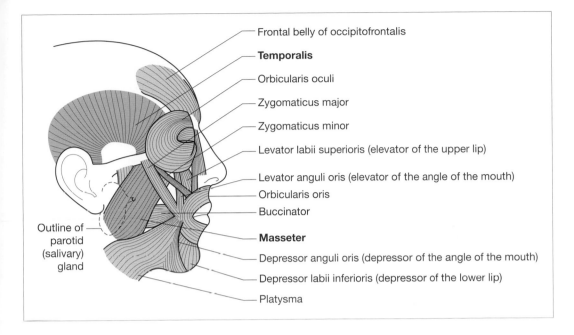

Figure 14.19 **The facial muscles**: the muscles in the face have a complex organisation. They can be predominantly organised into the muscles of facial expression. The orifices are surrounded by rings of muscle to control their opening. The eyes are surrounded by orbicularis oculi, whereas the mouth is surrounded by orbicularis oris. The masseter and temporalis muscles are the muscles of mastication, regulating the movement of the mandible relative to the skull.

Sensory innervation of the face

The major somatosensory nerve of the face is the sensory part of the three parts of the trigeminal nerve (CN V) (Fig. 14.20).

The ophthalmic nerve (CN V₁)

The ophthalmic nerve supplies structures in the orbit and the frontonasal cavity. This accounts for sensation in:

- the middle of the forehead, up to the hairline
- the conjunctiva
- the skin over the nose.

The maxillary nerve (CN V₂)

The maxillary nerve is purely sensory and supplies the skin and teeth around the maxilla, including sensation in:

- the zygomatic arch
- the cheek, and lateral sides of the nose
- the upper incisors and canines.

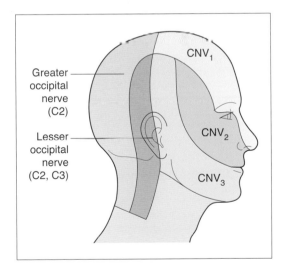

Figure 14.20 **Sensory innervation of the face**: The sensory innervation of the head is provided by the three branches of the trigeminal nerve (fifth cranial nerve or CN V), which between them supply the sensory innervation to the face. The innervation to the remainder of the head is supplied by the occipital nerves which are derived from the cervical nerves.

The mandibular nerve (CN V$_3$)

The mandibular nerve supplies sensory fibres to the skin around the mandible. It has three branches:

1 The **auriculotemporal branch** innervates the skin anterior to the ear and in the posterior temporal region. It also innervates much of the auricle and external acoustic meatus, and the tympanic membrane.
2 The **buccal branch** innervates the skin and mucosa of the cheek and much of the gums.
3 The **mental branch** innervates the skin in the chin and lower lip as well as the mucosa of the lower lip.

Vasculature of the face

The face is richly vascularised. Most of the arteries supplying the face are derived from the external carotid artery. In most cases, the arteries supplying the face are accompanied by their corresponding veins (Fig. 14.21):

• The **facial artery** is responsible for the blood supply to the face.
• The **occipital artery** runs to the back of the skull, where it supplies the scalp up to the vertex.
• The **posterior auricular artery** supplies the auricle and the region of scalp posterior to it.

• The **supraorbital** and **supratrochlear** arteries are unusual in that they are derived from the **internal carotid artery**. They supply the muscles and scalp around the forehead.

The oral cavity

The oral cavity (mouth) is the region through which food is ingested. It can be divided into two parts:

1 The **oral vestibule** is the thin potential space between the teeth and the cheeks.
2 The **oral cavity proper** is the space between the teeth. The superior surface of the cavity is formed by the palate.

The teeth

A major feature of the oral cavity is the teeth. These hard structures are set in the alveolar processes of the maxilla and mandible bones, forming the upper and lower sets, respectively. Their features and specialisation are discussed in Chapter 8 in relation to their function:

• The **upper set of teeth** is innervated by the superior alveolar nerve, a branch of the maxillary nerve (CN V$_2$), and receives blood from the

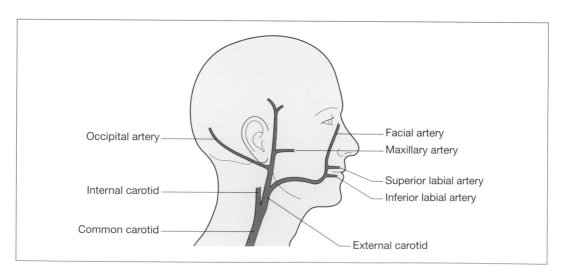

Figure 14.21 Vasculature of the face is supplied by branches of the external carotid artery. In particular the arterial supply to the face is supplied by branches of the facial artery. The head is also supplied by the occipital, auricular, supraorbital and supratrochlear branches, the branches of which anastomose and supply blood to the scalp.

superior alveolar artery, a branch of the maxillary artery.

- The **lower set of teeth** is innervated by the inferior alveolar nerve, a branch of the mandibular nerve (CN V$_3$), and receives blood from the inferior alveolar artery, a branch of the maxillary artery.

The venous drainage of the teeth follows a similar course to their arterial supply and the lymphatics from both sets of teeth drain to the submandibular lymph nodes.

The gingivae

The gingivae, or gums, are the fibrous tissue that surrounds the teeth and the surrounding bone. They are made up of two type of soft tissue:

1 **Gingiva proper** is the mucosa attached to the necks of the teeth and alveolar processes of the jaw. This tissue is strong, hard and keratinised.
2 The **alveolar mucosa** is a looser tissue surrounding the gingiva and is non-keratinised.

The palate

The palate separates the oropharynx from the nasopharynx. It is divided into two regions:

1 The **hard palate** is the bony portion formed from the palatine processes of the maxillae and the plates of the palatine bones. It accounts for the anterior two-thirds of the palate
2 The **soft palate** makes up the posterior third of the palate and is attached to the hard palate. The soft palate is made up of five muscles that help the formation of a bolus and swallowing. The soft palate tissue hangs inferiorly to form the uvula.

On its inferior surface the palate is covered in oral epithelium whereas on its superior surface the palate is covered by respiratory epithelium.

The tongue

The tongue forms the base of the oral cavity, and extends to the hyoid bone and mandible, where it is fixed to the rest of the body. It is important in both speech and eating and is both a muscular and a sensory structure, conveying the special sensation of taste. The detailed structure and function of the tongue is described in Chapter 8, whereas taste is discussed in Chapter 17.

The tongue receives many different sources of innervation:

- **All the muscles of the tongue** are supplied by the **hypoglossal nerve** (CN XII) *except* the **palatoglossus** muscle which is innervated the **accessory nerve** (CN IX).
- **General sensation** is carried by the lingual nerve (a branch of CN V$_3$) in the anterior two-thirds and the glossopharyngeal nerve (CN IX) in the posterior third.
- **Taste sensation** is carried by the chorda tympani nerve, a branch of the facial nerve (CN VII) in the anterior two-thirds, and the glossopharyngeal nerve (CN IX) in the posterior third.

Blood is supplied to the tongue by the lingual artery which is a branch of the external carotid artery. The venous drainage of the tongue is through the dorsal and deep lingual veins which drain into the internal jugular vein via the sublingual vein.

The nose and nasal cavity

The nose and nasal cavity allow the entry of air into the body. The nasal cavity also contains the olfactory receptors which sense smell.

The external structure of the nose

The nose projects from the face and is the entrance to the nasal cavity. It is made up of a fleshy tissue overlying a skeleton with bony and cartilaginous components. The nose is separated in the midline by the nasal septum, which contains a bony portion, made up of ethmoid bone and the vomer, and a cartilaginous portion; the two resulting passages to the nasal cavity through the nose are called the **chonae**. The nasal septum continues into the nasal cavity.

The nasal cavity

The nasal cavity lies posterior to the nose, is bounded by the bones of the skull and is lined with nasal epithelium. The cavity can be divided into two regions:

1 The **olfactory region** is found in the superior third of the nasal cavity and contains the olfactory receptors.
2 The **respiratory region** makes up the inferior two-thirds of the nasal cavity. It is richly vascularised to warm the air entering the respiratory tract.

The nasal cavity contains three pairs of **conchae** (Fig. 14.22). These are curved bony ridges that

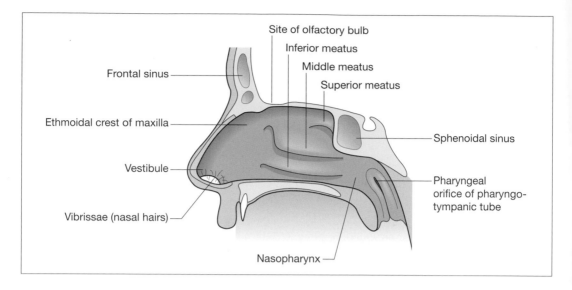

Figure 14.22 The lateral wall of the nasal cavity contains a series of processes that divide the cavity. The three conchae are highly vascularised and serve to warm and humidify the inspired air. The openings to the sinuses are also present in the lateral wall of the nasal cavity, as is the opening to the auditory tube.

increase the surface area and direct the flow of air through the nasal cavity.

Innervation and vasculature

The nasal cavity is highly vascularised, receiving branches from the labial, ethmoidal and palatine arteries, which anastomose around the nasal septum. The veins draining the nose also form a large plexus, which acts as a heat exchanger.

The superior part of the nasal cavity receives innervation from branches of the ophthalmic CN V_1 whereas the more posterior and inferior regions are innervated by branches of the maxillary nerve. The sense of smell is carried on the olfactory nerve (CN I).

The nasal sinuses

The nasal sinuses are a series of richly vascularised cavities in the bones of the face that are connected to the nasal cavity. These warm and humidify inspired air, helping gas exchange. There are four sinuses named after the bones in which they are located:

- The **frontal sinus** extends through much of the forehead. It drains into the nasal cavity in the space below the middle conchae.

- The **ethmoidal sinus** is a series of cavities in the ethmoid bone that drain directly into the nasal cavity.
- The **sphenoidal sinus** is derived from the cavities that form the ethmoidal sinus, and often has an uneven distribution. It opens directly into the superior part of the nasal cavity.
- The **maxillary sinus** is the largest of the sinuses occupying much of the maxillary bones, and opens into the nasal cavity at the same site as the frontal sinus.

The auricles

The auricles are the external parts of the ear. Although the internal structure of the ear is discussed in Chapter 17 in relation to its function, the anatomy of the external ear (the auricle) is discussed here.

The auricle is made up of fleshy tissue on a cartilage framework and forms a series of depressions, the largest being the **concha**, which is where the **external acoustic meatus** enters. The inferior part of the auricle lacks a cartilage skeleton and is known as the earlobe

The auricle is innervated by the **auriculotemporal nerve**, a branch of CN V_3, which supplies the skin superior to the external acoustic meatus. The rest of the auricle is innervated by the **great auricular** nerve, which is derived from the C2 and C3 spinal nerves.

The pharynx

The pharynx is the tract in the head and neck shared by the gastrointestinal (GI) and respiratory tracts. It conducts air to the lungs and food to the stomach, and runs to the inferior border of C6 and the cricoid cartilage. It can be divided into three distinct regions (Fig. 14.23):

- The nasopharynx
- The oropharynx
- The laryngopharynx.

The nasopharynx

The nasopharynx lies posterior to the nasal cavity. It extends backwards, so its posterior wall is made up of parts of the sphenoid. It is continuous inferiorly with the oropharynx. The nasopharynx warms and humidifies the air as it enters the respiratory tract. The nasopharynx also contains significant amounts of lymphoid tissue, arranged in a ring-like structure known as **Waldeyer's ring**, which is found in the superior part of the pharynx.

The oropharynx

The oropharynx is located directly behind the mouth. It is continuous superiorly with the nasopharynx and inferiorly with the laryngopharynx, running from the soft palate to the epiglottis. The oropharynx also contains the palatine tonsils, which are major accumulations of lymphoid tissue in the space between the palatine arches.

The other structures in the oropharynx are associated with swallowing and food and are discussed in more detail in Chapter 8.

The laryngopharynx

The laryngopharynx lies posterior to the larynx, starting at the epiglottis. The posterior and lateral aspects of the laryngopharynx are made up of the inferior and middle constrictor muscles which help swallowing.

Innervation of the pharynx

The pharyngeal plexus innervates the pharynx:

- The **motor innervation** is provided almost exclusively through the vagus nerve (CN X), exceptions being stylopharyngeus (CN IX) and tensor veli palatini (CN V$_3$).

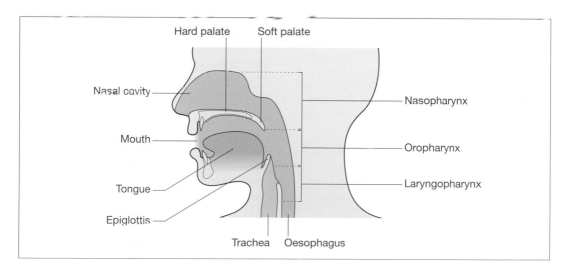

Figure 14.23 The pharynx is a tube that opens into the nasal cavity, mouth and larynx. It is effectively subdivided into three parts – the nasopharynx, oropharynx and laryngopharynx. The muscles in the larynx are important in the coordination of swallowing and are innervated by the pharyngeal branch of the vagus nerve. In addition, there is sensory innervation through the glossopharyngeal nerve.

- The **sensory innervation** of the pharynx is through the glossopharyngeal nerve (CN IX) which innervates all but the superior parts of the nasopharynx; these are innervated by the maxillary nerve (CN V_2).

The scalp

The scalp covers the surface of the skull. It is tightly apposed to the skull and continuous at the front with the skin of the face. The scalp consists of five layers:

1 The skin
2 Connective tissue that contains many of the vessels as well as the nerves
3 The aponeurosis
4 Connective tissue that is less attached than the preceding layers, allowing movement of the first three layers of the scalp
5 Pericranium – the periosteum of the skull.

Innervation of the scalp

The scalp is innervated by two main sets of nerves:

1 The branches of the **trigeminal nerve** supply the portion of the scalp anterior to the auricles.
2 The spinal cutaneous nerves (C2 and C3) supply the scalp posterior to the auricles.

The neck

The neck links the head to rest of the body. In doing so, it serves as a conduit for many vessels and nerves. The neck lacks much of the bony protection seen in the rest of the body because it must allow movement of the head. Many structures in the neck are derived from the pharyngeal arches.

The bones of the neck

There are two major bony structures in the neck:

1 The **cervical vertebrae** enclose the spinal cord and support the head.
2 The **hyoid bone** is a point of attachment for many of the anterior neck muscles.

The hyoid bone

The hyoid bone is a U-shaped bone that serves to keep the airway open. It is unusual in that it does not directly articulate with any other bones. It is suspended from the styloid process of the temporal bone by the stylohyoid ligament, and lies at the level of C3, between the angle of the mandible and the thyroid cartilage, to which is connected.

Fascial compartments of the neck

The neck can be subdivided into fascial compartments, which are important clinically in determining direction of potential spread of an infection. The neck is divided by the superficial fascia and the three layers of deep fascia.

The superficial fascia

The superficial fascia of the neck is found immediately below the skin and contains cutaneous nerves and vessels. On its anterolateral aspect, the superficial fascia of the neck contains the **platysma** muscle.

The deep fascia of the neck

The deep fasciae group in the neck structure allows smooth movement over each other and provides a protective covering (Fig. 14.24). Three layers of deep fascia are found in the neck:

- The **investing layer** surrounds the neck deep to the superficial fascia. Superiorly, it attaches to the inferior border of the mandible, and to the temporal and occipital bones. Inferiorly, it attaches to the pectoral girdle. The fascial layer splits around the sternocleidomastoid muscle and submandibular and parotid glands to develop fibrous capsules around them; it is continuous with the **nuchal ligament** posteriorly.
- The **pretracheal layer** runs in the anterior part of the neck from the hyoid bone and is continuous inferiorly with the fibrous pericardium. The pretracheal layer encloses the thyroid gland, oesophagus and trachea.
- The **prevertebral layer** surrounds the vertebral column and its associated muscles. The fascia runs from the base of the skull to T3. At the base of the neck the prevertebral layer surrounds the brachial plexus as the axillary sheath.

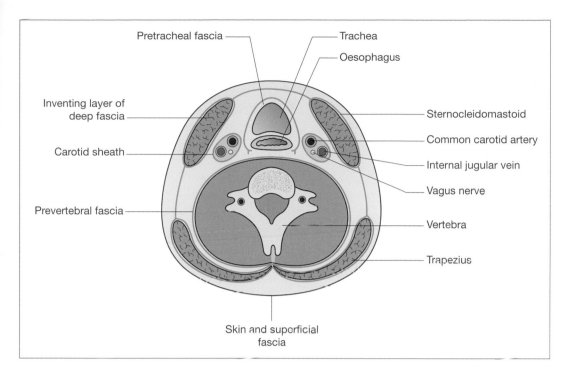

Figure 14.24 **The fascial layers of the neck**: the neck is surrounded by an investing layer of superficial fascia which is immediately deep to the skin in the neck. The deep fascia of the neck can be divided more readily into compartments. There is an investing layer of deep fascia that surrounds the entire neck and forms the floor of the cervical triangles. The pretracheal and prevertebral layers of deep fascia surround the trachea (and related structures) and the vertebrae, respectively. In addition there are fascial layers continuous with the investing layer that surround trapezius and sternocleidomastoid (SCM), whereas the carotid sheath is continuous with the investing and pretracheal layers of deep fascia.

The carotid sheath

The carotid sheath is a fascial structure continuous with the investing and pretracheal fascial layers and runs through the entire neck. The carotid sheath contains important structures:

- Common and internal carotid arteries
- The internal jugular vein
- The vagus nerve
- The deep cervical nerves
- Sympathetic nerve fibres.

Anatomical compartments of the neck

Many structures in the neck can be located by their relation to various muscles. In particular, the superficial muscles of the neck can divide it into two 'cervical triangles' which are used to describe the location of many organs and anatomical sites (Fig. 14.25).

The superficial muscles

There are three major superficial muscles in the neck:

- The **sternocleidomastoid (SCM)** muscle is responsible for turning the head. It also divides the neck into anterior and posterior triangles. Posteriorly, the muscle has two heads – one attaching to the manubrium of the sternum and one to the medial third of the clavicle. Superiorly, SCM attaches to the mastoid process of the temporal bone and occipital bone.
- The **platysma** muscle is a thin muscle in the anterior part of the neck. It is innervated by the fascial nerve, serving to tense the skin on the neck.
- The **trapezius** muscle is a large muscle found in the posterolateral part of the neck, extending on to the back. Trapezius attaches the pectoral girdle to the skull and vertebral column to support

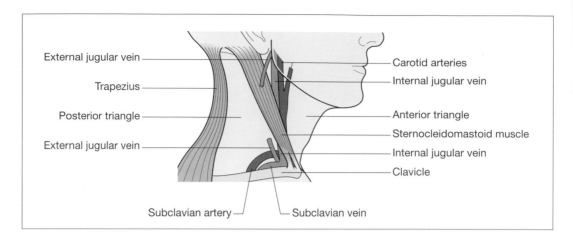

Figure 14.25 Cervical triangles: the more superficial structures of the neck have a course that can be described in relation to the two triangles of the neck. These are formed on the lateral aspects of the neck and are divided from each other by sternocleidomastoid. In particular, the course of the major vessels is described in this way, the carotid sheathe being a prominent feature that runs in the anterior triangle, whereas the subclavian artery and subclavian vein can be found in the base of the posterior triangle.

it. Motor innervation is from the spinal route of the accessory nerve, whereas the sensory innervation is from C3 and C4.

The posterior triangle of the neck

The posterior triangle is located between the investing and prevertebral layers of deep fascia. It has three borders made up of prominent muscular and bony landmarks:

- The **posterior border** is formed by the anterior border of trapezius.
- The **anterior border** is formed by the posterior border of SCM.
- The **inferior border** is made up of the middle third of the clavicle, between trapezius and SCM.

The posterior triangle contains many vessels supplying and draining the head:

- The **external jugular vein** is found in the anteroinferior aspect of the triangle. It drains blood from the side of the face and scalp. It terminates in the posterior triangle by forming the brachiocephalic vein with the subclavian.
- The **subclavian vein** passes anterior to the phrenic nerve and unites with the external jugular to form the **brachiocephalic vein** at the medial border of the anterior scalene muscle.
- Part of the **subclavian artery** runs through the posterior triangle. It lies in the inferior part of the posterior triangle, beneath the subclavian vein.

- The **accessory nerve** enters the posterior triangle posterior to SCM, running superficial to the investing layer of deep fascia.
- The **brachial plexus** starts in the posteroinferior part of the posterior triangle.
- The **phrenic nerve** passes briefly through the posterior triangle before descending into the thorax with the internal jugular.

The anterior cervical triangle

The anterior triangle is a more superficial structure than the posterior triangle, and has a roof made up of the subcutaneous tissue containing platysma and a floor formed by the thyroid, larynx and pharynx; its apex is located inferiorly:

- The **posterior border** is formed by the anterior boundary of SCM.
- The **anterior border** is formed by the median line of the neck.
- The **superior border** is made by the inferior border of the mandible.

Deep structures of the neck

The prevertebral muscles

These muscles lie in lateral to the vertebrae. Two groups of muscles can be identified:

1 The **anterior muscles** stabilise the head on the neck and allow flexion of the head and neck.

2 The **lateral muscles** are involved in the lateral flexion of the neck and may also elevate the ribs and scapulae.

The root of the neck

The root of the neck is the region connecting the neck to the thorax; it opens into the superior cervical aperture on the cervical side.

Arteries in the root of the neck

On the right side of the neck, the brachiocephalic trunk and the subclavian artery can be found.

Although the subclavian arteries supply the arms, they also give rise to the vertebral arteries, the internal thoracic and thyrocervical arteries, and the costocervical trunk.

On the left side, the left subclavian artery and left common carotid artery are present.

The veins in the root of the neck

Three pairs of veins in the root of the neck receive most of the blood from the arms and head. They unite to form the brachiocephalic veins:

- The **internal jugular vein** (IJV) drains the internal structures of the head; it travels through the neck in the carotid sheath and unites with the subclavian vein posterior to the medial end of the clavicle. The thoracic duct and the right lymphatic trunk drain into this site.
- The **external jugular vein** (EJV) receives blood mainly from the scalp and the face. It travels through the posterior triangle before passing through the investing deep fascia to unite with the IJV and the subclavian veins, to form the brachiocephalic veins.
- The **subclavian vein** is a continuation of the axillary vein and contributes to the formation of the brachiocephalic veins.

In addition to the paired veins in the root of the neck, an **anterior jugular vein** may arise superficially near the hyoid bone. There is variation in the course of the vein, although it runs in the midline and joins the termination of the EJV or subclavian vein in the neck.

Nerves in the root of the neck

Three major nervous structures are found in the neck (excluding the spinal cord, which is covered in Chapter 17).

The phrenic nerves

The phrenic nerves originate from C3–5 and are responsible for the motor innervation to their respective halves of the diaphragm. These pass through the neck between the subclavian vessels before entering the thorax.

The vagus nerve

The vagus nerve travels in the carotid sheath, between the IJV and the common carotid artery, and provides parasympathetic innervation to all the internal organs below the neck. In the inferior part of the neck, the vagus nerve gives off the recurrent laryngeal branches, which innervate the larynx and are responsible for controlling speech (Fig. 14.26):

- The **right recurrent laryngeal nerve** loops under the right subclavian artery before ascending to the larynx.
- The **left recurrent laryngeal nerve** loops under the arch of the aorta.

The vagus nerve also gives off branches in the neck that run along the arteries to the cardiac plexus.

Sympathetic ganglia

There are three sympathetic cervical ganglia, which are a continuation of the sympathetic chain and provide sympathetic innervation to the head and neck. They receive inputs that originate in the lower segments of the spinal column and have passed up the sympathetic chain. Branches from the cervical ganglia pass to the cervical spinal nerves or may leave as direct branches to the viscera. A lesion of the cervical trunk can cause a disturbance of the sympathetic innervation to the head – known as **Horner's syndrome**.

The viscera of the neck

The thyroid gland

The thyroid gland is responsible for the production of thyroid hormones and is found at the level of the second to fourth rings of cartilage in the larynx. It is made up of left and right lobes which are connected by a small midline region, the isthmus, and is enclosed in the pretracheal fascia which connects it to the larynx and the trachea (Fig. 14.27).

The thyroid gland receives a rich blood supply from three sets of arteries:

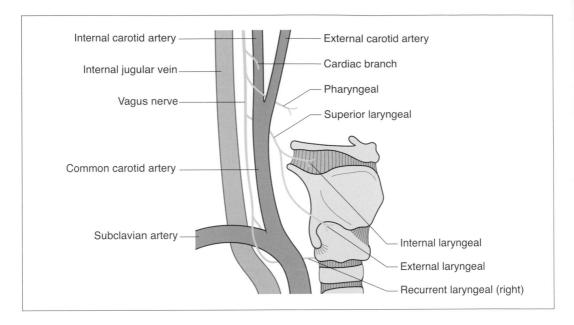

Internal carotid artery — External carotid artery

Internal jugular vein — Cardiac branch

— Pharyngeal

Vagus nerve — Superior laryngeal

Common carotid artery —

Subclavian artery — Internal laryngeal

External laryngeal

Recurrent laryngeal (right)

Figure 14.26 The **vagus nerve** arises from the medulla and provides much of the parasympathetic innervation to the viscera below the neck. It travels through the foramen magnum and passes through the neck in the carotid sheath. In the neck the vagus nerve gives off a pharyngeal branch, as well as superior, inferior and recurrent laryngeal branches. The recurrent laryngeal branch, in particular, takes an unusual course, looping under the subclavian artery on the right side, although on the left it arises lower and loops under the ligamentum arteriosum, before ascending to the larynx. The vagus nerve continues into the thorax and abdomen, giving off further branches to the viscera.

1 The **superior thyroid arteries** are derived from the external carotid arteries and enter the thyroid at the upper part of the left and right lobes. The external laryngeal nerve runs with this artery.

2 The **inferior thyroid arteries** are derived from the thyrocervical trunk and enter at the posterior surface of the gland. The inferior thyroid artery is accompanied by the recurrent laryngeal nerve.

3 The **thyroid ima artery** may be present. This is a small branch of the brachiocephalic trunk, of the arch of the aorta, and supplies the isthmus of the gland.

The thyroid gland is drained by three sets of veins:

- The **superior** and **middle thyroid veins** drain into the IJV.
- The **inferior thyroid veins** receive tributaries from the lower parts of the gland, and fuse to form a single vein that descends in front of the trachea and fuses with the left brachiocephalic vein.

The parathyroid glands

There are typically four parathyroid glands, two on each side. They are associated with the regulation of calcium through the production of parathyroid hormone (PTH). Each gland is enclosed in the fascia surrounding the thyroid gland:

- The **superior parathyroids** are located at the level of the middle of the thyroid gland.
- The **inferior parathyroids** lie at the level of the inferior poles of the lobes.

The parathyroids receive their blood supply from the superior and inferior thyroid arteries.

The trachea

The trachea is a muscular tube, reinforced by a series of cartilaginous rings that link the lungs and respiratory tree with the nasal and oral cavities. With the exception of the cricoid cartilage, all the rings are U-shaped so that the oesophagus, which sits immediately posterior to the trachea, can

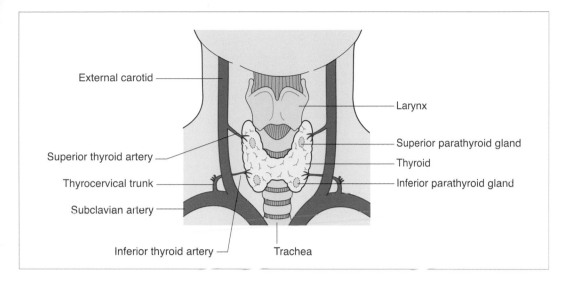

Figure 14.27 The thyroid and parathyroid glands: the thyroid gland is located in the neck anterior to, and just posterior to, the larynx. It consists of two lobes located either side of an isthmus. The thyroid is vascularised by the superior thyroid arteries which are branches of the external carotids, whereas the inferior thyroid arteries are derived from the thyrocervical trunk. The parathyroids are located posterior to the thyroid and consist of paired superior and inferior parathyroid glands. These receive their blood supply from branches of the superior and inferior thyroid arteries, respectively.

expand unimpeded to allow the passage of food into the stomach.

In the neck, the trachea is surrounded by many structures:

- The structures located **anteriorly** are the skin, fascia and isthmus of the thyroid.
- The major **posterior structures** are the vertebral column and oesophagus. The carotid sheaths are located **laterally** to the trachea.

Vasculature and innervation

The blood supply to the trachea is derived mainly from the inferior thyroid arteries, whereas the nerve supply is derived from the vagus nerve and the sympathetic trunks.

The oesophagus

The oesophagus is a muscular tube connecting the mouth with the stomach. The oesophagus begins at the level of the cricoid cartilage (located at the level of the C6 vertebra) anterior to the vertebral column, and descends initially in the midline, although as it descends into the thorax it moves to the left of the neck.

The vasculature and innervation

The blood supply to the oesophagus in the neck is provided by the inferior thyroid vessels. In the neck, the oesophagus is innervated by the recurrent laryngeal nerves.

The larynx

The larynx protects the airways from the entry of food and debris and allows the production of speech by passing air over the vocal folds to make them vibrate. The larynx is found between the trachea and the pharynx, and marks the point at which the airways separate from the GI tract. It consists of soft tissue supported on a cartilage frame (Fig. 14.28):

- The **cricoid cartilage** is a complete ring of cartilage located at the bottom of larynx. It holds the trachea open, and articulates with the thyroid cartilages.
- The two **thyroid cartilages** are located to the sides. They meet in the midline and in men are prominent on the surface of the neck, forming Adam's apple.
- The **arytenoid** cartilages are located to the back of the larynx at the upper border of the cricoid cartilage. They are attached to the vocal folds and the musculature that controls speech.

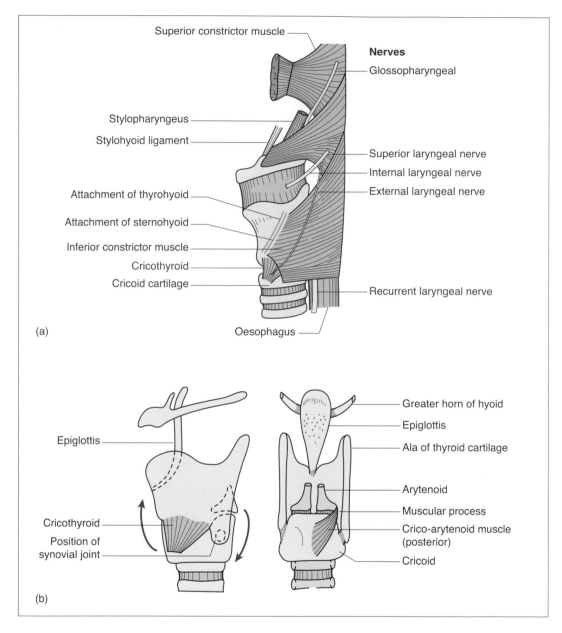

Figure 14.28 The larynx is made up of a cartilaginous frame, supported by a variety of ligaments and muscles. (a) It is supported by the attachment of the inferior constrictor muscle and of stylopharyngeus and the stylohyoid ligament, which anchor the larynx to the pharynx and hyoid bones, respectively. Here it is viewed the left lateral aspect is viewed. (b) The major cartilages in the larynx are the thyroid and cricoid cartilages. The thyroid cartilage contributes to Adam's apple and provides the points against which the vocal folds are attached. The cricoid cartilage is the opening to the trachea. From the posterior view of the larynx the arytenoid cartilages are visible. These are attached to the cricothyroid muscles and the vocal folds; the movement of these cartilages can alter the tension in the vocal folds, allowing alterations of pitch that contribute to voice.

- The smaller **cuneiform** and **corniculate** cartilages support the vocal folds.
- The **epiglottis** is a large flap of cartilage that is attached to the throat at its inferior border, although it is unattached at its superior border. The epiglottis is depressed during swallowing to close the entrance to the larynx and prevent food entering the respiratory airways, directing it towards the GI tract.

The cartilages of the larynx are linked by ligaments, which derive their names from the cartilages to which they are attached. Two are of particular importance:

- The **cricothyroid ligament** links the cricoid cartilage to the inferior border of the thyroid cartilage. The upper surface of the cricothyroid ligament is thickened on each side to produce the vocal ligaments.
- The **thyrohyoid membrane** connects the upper border of the thyroid cartilages to the hyoid bone.

The **vocal folds** are made up of tissue of the vocal ligament, which is stretched between the thyroid and arytenoid cartilages, at the back of the larynx. The **intrinsic muscles** of the larynx regulate the tension generated in the vocal folds. As air flows over the vocal folds it causes them to vibrate; alteration of the tension in the vocal folds can alter the pitch of the note.

The musculature of the larynx

The muscles of the larynx can be divided into two groups:

1 The **extrinsic muscles** move the larynx as a whole during swallowing and connect the larynx to other structures in the neck.
2 The **intrinsic muscles** control the vocal folds and inlet of the larynx. They are attached solely to structures in the larynx.

The movement of the larynx is also affected by movements of the hyoid bone, to which it is connected by a thyrohyoid membrane.

The extrinsic muscles of the larynx

The extrinsic muscles of the larynx consist of the elevators and depressors which move the larynx during swallowing.

The intrinsic muscles of the larynx

There are two tasks that the intrinsic muscles of the larynx perform:

- **Control of the sphincters in the larynx**: the sphincter at the larynx's inlet is closed during swallowing to prevent entry of food. In addition, there is a sphincter at the rima glottidis – the gap between the vocal folds. This can be used to close the airway and increase the pressure in the thorax, which occurs before coughing and sneezing. The sudden release of pressure helps to dislodge debris from the respiratory tract.
- **Voice production**: the release of air across the vocal folds can be used to generate noise, through vibration of the vocal folds. The pitch of the note produced is determined by the tension of the vocal folds, which relies on the action of the intrinsic muscles. The quality of the sound and normal speech is produced through altering the sound generated from the vocal folds in the mouth and pharynx.

Innervation and vasculature of the larynx

The innervation of the larynx is from three different branches of the vagus nerve:

- The **sensory supply** is through the internal laryngeal branch of the superior laryngeal branch of the vagus nerve.
- The **extrinsic muscles** of the larynx and the cricothyroid muscle are supplied by the external laryngeal branch of the superior laryngeal branch of the vagus nerve.
- The **intrinsic muscles** of the larynx are supplied by the recurrent laryngeal nerve, except for the cricothyroid muscle.

The upper structures of the larynx receive their blood supply from the superior laryngeal artery, a branch of the superior thyroid artery, whereas the lower structures of the larynx are supplied by the inferior laryngeal artery, a branch of the inferior thyroid artery.

The spine

The spine transmits the load of the body to the pelvis and consists of:

- 7 cervical vertebrae (C1–7)
- 12 thoracic vertebrae (T1–12)
- 5 lumbar vertebrae (L1–5)
- 5 sacral vertebrae (S1–5)
- the coccyx.

The common components of the vertebrae

A typical vertebra (Fig. 14.29) is contains the following components:

- The **vertebral bodies** form a strong column that transmits body weight to the pelvis. The vertebral bodies are separated and cushioned by the intervertebral discs.
- The **vertebral arch** is made from two pedicles and two laminae, and projects seven processes that either serve as articular surfaces or allow the attachment of muscles and ligaments:
  - the two **transverse processes** project laterally, on either side of the body
  - the single **spinous process** projects posteriorly from the body
  - the paired **superior** and **inferior articular facets** limit the range of movement at each region of the spine.

- The **vertebral foramina** are made up of the space surrounded by the vertebral arch. When the vertebrae are aligned, the vertebral foramina form a protective channel down the spinal column, which carries the spinal cord.
- The **intervertebral foramina** are the apertures between adjacent vertebrae. These allow lateral projection of the spinal nerves and vessels.

The cervical vertebrae

The seven cervical vertebrae are located in the neck. Although C1 and C2 are specialised, C3–7 demonstrate the common characteristics of cervical vertebrae; they have a transverse process pierced by a foramen to enable passage of vertebral vessels. The bifid spinous process (apart from C7) ('vertebra prominens') is the first palpable vertebra of the neck; it has a horizontal, non-bifid, spinous

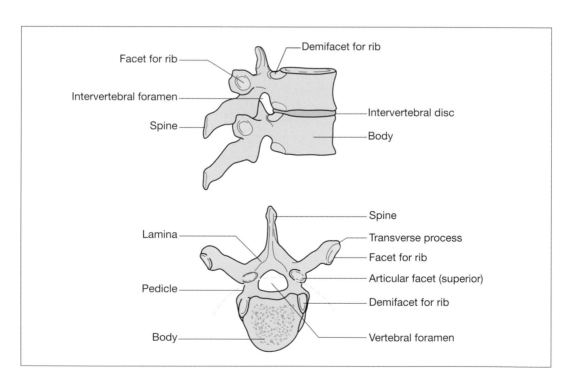

Figure 14.29 Typical **vertebrae** (a thoracic vertebra is shown – upper panel, right lateral aspect; lower panel, superior aspect) are composed of: a body, an arch – consisting, on either side, of a pedicle attached to the vertebral body and a broad lamina. The arch encloses the vertebral foramen in continuation with the vertebral body, a spine, which projects from the arch dorsally and medially, and two transverse processes; also paired superior and inferior articular facets – these project from the pedicles to enable the vertebral arch to articulate with the superior and inferior vertebrae.

process and the vertebral artery does not pass through its transverse process.

C1 – the atlas

The **C1 vertebra** (known as 'the atlas') forms the atlanto-occipital joint with the skull, a hinge joint that enables flexion and extension – nodding. It has no body, a prominent transverse process and several other specialised characteristics:

- A short **anterior arch**, which has an anterior tubercle for attachment of the cruciate ligament as well as an articular facet for the odontoid peg (dens). The cruciate ligament holds the odontoid peg in the arch whereas the ligament limits atlantoaxial joint movement to rotation only, and prevents the odontoid peg from slipping backwards and damaging the medulla and upper cervical spinal cord.
- The **posterior arch** is grooved superiorly by the vertebral artery and has a posterior tubercle replacing its spinous process.

The lateral masses of the atlas are each pierced by a foramen for the vertebral artery to pass through.

C2 – the axis

The **C2 vertebra** (known as 'the axis') articulates with the C1 vertebra and allows rotation of the skull. Its odontoid process (dens) has evolved from the body of the atlas. Its body has evident oval articular facets on which the atlas rotates.

The thoracic vertebrae

The thoracic vertebrae are specialised to allow articulation with the ribs and to accommodate lateral rotation of the spine. The thoracic vertebrae have several characteristic features related to their function:

- **'Heart-shaped' bodies** of increasing size which have upper and lower hemifacets for rib articulation
- A small vertebral foramen
- Thick, broad and overlapping laminae
- Long and posteriorly slanting spinous processes and substantial transverse processes, most of which have facets for articulation with the tubercles of the corresponding rib.

The lumbar vertebrae

The lumbar vertebrae are adapted to allow maximum weight bearing. They also allow flexion and extension. Consistent with their function, the lumbar vertebrae possess:

- **large**, **deep bodies**
- **interlocking articular processes** which allow flexion and extension of the lumbar spine but no rotation.

The sacrum

The sacrum is a large structure at the base of the spine. It is formed by the fusion of five vertebrae and contributes to the upper and posterior parts of the pelvic cavity. The pelvic surface of the sacrum has four anterior sacral foramina to allow spinal nerve passage and articular facets for articulation with the ilium.

The **sacrotuberous** and the **sacrospinous ligaments** reinforce the sacroiliac joint. The sacrospinous ligament converts the bony greater and lesser sciatic notch into the greater and lesser sciatic foramina. Important structures, such as the muscles that stabilise the joint between the acetabulum and the head of the femur, pass through these foramina.

The coccyx

The coccyx is non-weight bearing, but provides attachment for muscles; it has a limited shock-absorbing capacity when a person sits down. It is made up of three to five rudimentary fused vertebrae.

The joints of the spine

Intervertebral discs form fibrocartilaginous joints with adjacent vertebrae. Each disc has a fibrous outer ring and a more hydrated nucleus pulposus, which articulate with the vertebral bodies directly above and below it. The intervertebral disc allows some movement of the spine and maintains shock absorption.

Movements of the spine

The articular processes of flanking vertebrae are connected by plane synovial 'facet' joints which allow gliding movements. The orientation of these articular processes determines the movements that are allowed:

- The joint between the skull and the atlas allows **flexion** and **extension** of the head.

- The joint between the axis and atlas allows **rotation of the head** on the axial skeleton.
- Cervical and lumbar regions allow **flexion** and **extension**.
- The thoracic vertebrae allow **rotation** of the trunk.

> **CLINICAL 'Slipped' disc**
>
> A slipped disc occurs when the central nucleus pulposus herniates through a weakened annulus fibrosus. This often occurs in old age as the fibres of the annulus weaken, and usually follows excessive stress such as lifting a heavy object with poor posture.
>
> A slipped disc is most common in the lumbar region and typically herniates posteriorly; it can impinge on the spinal cord. Irritation of the cord causes sciatica.

The curvature of the spine

To improve balance and weight transmission, the vertebrae form a series of alternating curvatures of the spine. From anterior, the curve is concave at the neck and the lumbar region, but convex in the thorax and pelvis. Excessive curvature is pathological and can cause deterioration of health.

Organisation of the spinal nerves

Each segment of the spinal cord gives off one mixed spinal nerve composed of a series of rootlets within the spinal canal. There are 31 pairs of mixed spinal nerves:

- Eight **cervical** spinal nerves (C1–8)
- Twelve **thoracic** spinal nerves (T1–12)
- Five **lumbar** spinal nerves (L1–5)
- Five **sacral** spinal nerves (S1–5)
- One **coccygeal** spinal nerve (Co1).

The first seven nerves (C1–7) emerge above vertebrae C1–7. The eighth (C8) emerges below the vertebra C7. All other nerves emerge below the vertebrae of the same number.

> **CLINICAL Pathological curvatures of the spine**
>
> Excessive or abnormal curvatures of the spine can result in serious problems, through restrictive pathology that this is likely to result in the area affected. The effects and causes of such curvature depend on its location and orientation:
>
> - **Scoliosis** – the spine moves to the right or left of the midline vertical axis
> - **Kyphosis** – the spine has an excessive dorsal convexity
> - **Lordosis** – the spine has an excessive dorsal concavity for similar reasons to kyphosis.

The spinal ligaments

The spinal ligaments stabilise the vertebral column, to ensure that it maintains a strong, yet flexible structure:

- The **intrasegmental ligaments** link the vertebrae together in large groups. The intrasegmental system includes ligamentum flavum, and interspinous and intertransverse ligaments.
- The **intersegmental ligaments** connect individual vertebrae. The intersegmental system includes the anterior and posterior longitudinal ligaments, and the supraspinous ligaments.

The thorax

The chest contains the lungs and heart and their blood vessels. The borders of the chest are defined by the thoracic cage, which protects the contents of the chest. The thoracic cage is formed from the ribs and their cartilage, which articulate with the thoracic spinal column posteriorly and the sternum anteriorly.

The thorax is separated from the abdomen by the diaphragm. This is a domed fibromuscular sheet that is essential for breathing. It is attached anteriorly to the xiphisternum and posteriorly to the costal margins of each side and the upper lumbar vertebrae. As the diaphragm extends upwards, many of the upper abdominal organs are also protected by the thoracic skeletal framework. The diaphragm is supplied by the phrenic nerve and phrenic arteries, which are branches of the aorta.

The thorax can be divided into two regions:

1 The **lungs** take up most of the space in the thorax, projecting laterally.
2 The **mediastinum** is the central region of the thorax that is not occupied by the lungs.

The skeletal framework of the thorax

The skeletal framework of the thorax supports the thoracic viscera, to protect them and also enable the movements crucial for breathing (Fig. 14.30). The framework is composed of:

- the thoracic part of the **vertebral column**
- the **sternum**
- the **thoracic ribs** and their **costal cartilage**.

The sternum

The sternum is found anteriorly in the midline, and is connected (directly or indirectly) to the first 10 ribs, to create the ribcage. It is composed of three parts (superiorly to inferiorly):

1 **The manubrium** articulates laterally, with the medial part of each clavicle and the first/upper facet of second costal cartilages. Inferiorly, the

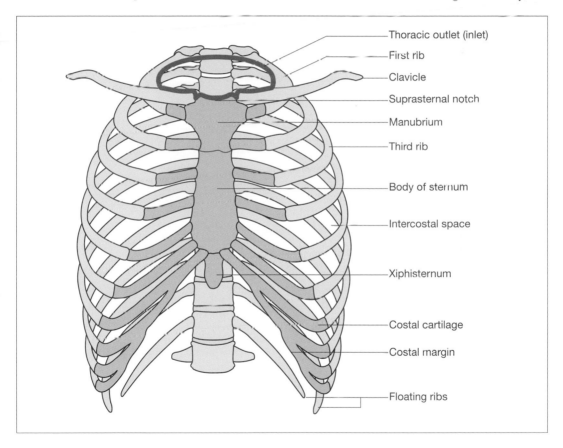

Figure 14.30 The thoracic cage consists of the vertebrae posteriorly and the sternum, anteriorly. These structures are linked by the ribs, which can be divided into three classes: the seven true ribs (first to seventh), which articulate directly with the sternum; the three false ribs (eighth, ninth and tenth), which articulate with the sternum via attachment to the costal cartilage of the ribs above and the two floating ribs (eleventh and twelfth). The sternum is made up of three components: the manubrium is the most superior part of the sternum, and articulates with the first costal cartilage and the upper part of the second costal cartilage. It is also the site of attachment of the clavicles. The manubrium attaches to the body of the sternum inferiorly at the angle of Louis. The body of the sternum provides attachment for the remainder of the costal cartilages. The xiphisternum is the most inferior part. It does not form a joint with any costal cartilages.

manubrium forms a fibrous joint with the body of the sternum. This joint can be palpated as the sternal angle (the angle of Louis).

2 **The body** articulates laterally with the second and seventh costal cartilages, and inferiorly with the xiphisternum.

3 **The xiphisternum** is the small rudimentary portion at the base of the sternum. It does not articulate with any ribs.

The ribs

The ribs have several common characteristics (Fig. 14.31a), including the following:

- A **head**: this has two hemifacets, one articulates of which with its corresponding vertebra and the other with the vertebra above; the area in between articulates with the intervertebral disc.
- A **neck**: this extends laterally from the head connecting it to the body.
- A **body**: the body of the rib is curved and contributes to the ribcage structure, protecting the internal organs. It stretches from the neck of the rib to the point where the rib articulates, directly or indirectly, with the sternum. At the inferior aspect of the rib lies the **costal groove** through which the intercostal nerves and vessels run.

> **Q CLINICAL Needle insertion into the thorax**
>
> A needle must be inserted into the chest immediately above a rib to avoid damaging the neurovascular bundle that lies in the costal groove directly beneath the rib (Fig. 14.31b).

The ribs can be divided into 'true' and 'false' ribs depending on their attachment to the sternum:

- The **'true' ribs** (1–7) articulate with the sternum.
- The **'false' ribs** (8–12) either are connected to the sternum via the costal cartilage of another rib or possess no connection with the sternum:
  - The costal cartilage of each of **ribs 8–10** does not articulate with the sternum; instead each is attached to the costal cartilage of the rib above.
  - **Ribs 11 and 12** (the 'floating' ribs) are not directly attached to the thoracic cage anteriorly.

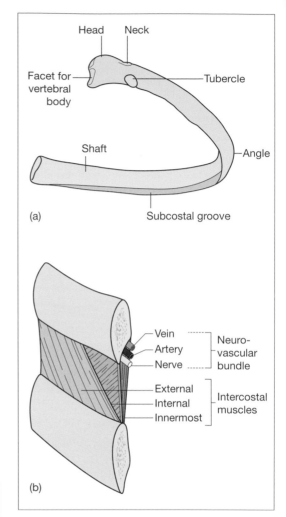

Figure 14.31 The structure of the ribs. (1) The **ribs** follow a **common structure**: the head articulates with the vertebral bodies. The smooth medial facet of the tubercle articulates with the transverse process of its corresponding vertebra. The subcostal groove allows room for the intercostal neurovascular bundle. (2) The **neurovascular bundle** is located beneath the rib. Clinically this arrangement is important because injections are made to the inferior aspect of the intercostal space, to avoid damaging the neurovascular bundle. The inner intercostal muscles contract during forced expiration, whereas the external intercostal muscles have a perpendicular organisation of fibres so that their contraction promotes the upward and outward movement of the ribs to help inspiration.

The intercostal muscles

The intercostal muscles occupy the spaces between the ribs. They are made up of three layers:

1 The **external intercostal muscles** run from the tubercle of the rib to the costochondral cartilage. The fibres in the muscles run inferolaterally, and contraction causes elevation of the ribs, as in **inspiration**.
2 The **internal intercostal muscles** run below the external muscles. Their fibres run at 90° to the fibres of the external intercostals, and on contraction cause depression of the ribcage, as in **expiration**.
3 The **innermost intercostal muscles** are the deepest layer of intercostal muscles. They perform a similar function to the internal intercostals and are separated from them by the intercostal vessels and nerves.

Breathing

Ventilation of the lungs occurs through expansion and contraction of the thoracic cavity. The muscles that enable ventilation of the lungs have different roles according to the extent of respiration required:

- The **diaphragm** is the main muscle used during **quiet ventilation**. Contraction of the diaphragm flattens it, increasing the volume of the thorax.
- The **intercostal muscles** are required to be more active when a greater degree of ventilation is necessary. During inspiration:
  - a **'water pump'** movement occurs in the upper ribs which move anteriorly and superiorly in a limited way, predominantly as a result of action of the external intercostals
  - the lower ribs glide upwards and outwards like lifting a **'bucket handle'**. It is the lower ribs that primarily affect the transverse diameter of the chest.
- On **forced respiration** accessory muscles may be used. These include the scalene muscles of the neck, sternocleidomastoids and limb muscles attached to the chest wall.

Morphology of the respiratory system

The lungs occupy most of the space in the thorax and allow gas exchange. They are connected to the environment by the airways.

The pleura and pleural cavities

The pleural cavities are lined on each side by a closed pleural sac, which reduces friction between the lungs and chest wall during ventilation. The pleurae are made up of two layers surrounding a potential space:

- The **parietal** pleural membrane which lines the chest wall, suprapleural membrane, diaphragm and mediastinum.
- The **visceral** pleural membrane
- The very narrow **pleural cavity** containing a thin film of pleural fluid.

 DEFINITION Mesothelium

Mesothelium forms the lining of many cavities: the thoracic cavity, heart sac and abdominal cavity. In the respective regions it is known as the pleura, pericardium and peritoneum. It is made up of two layers of specialised cells, each a single cell thick, which act to protect the organs by forming fluid between its layers; this has a lubricating action allowing easy movement of the layers over each other. The layer adjacent to the organs is known as the **visceral layer** and that covering the body walls is the **parietal layer**.

The lungs

The lungs are the site of gas exchange. They have a pyramidal shape and fill the lateral aspect of the thorax, leaving room for just the heart. The anterior surface of the left lung has an area where the pericardium is exposed – known as the **cardiac notch**.

Each lung is divided by the oblique fissure that passes from T3 to about the level of the sixth costal cartilage obliquely. Although this creates two lobes in the left lung, the right lung is additionally divided by the horizontal fissure, resulting in three lobes. The horizontal fissure runs from the oblique fissure in the midaxillary line to the fourth costal cartilage.

The airways

The nose and mouth are the entrance of the airways and both lead to the single trachea, which forms the start of the bronchial tree. This branching structure progresses into the lungs, generating many small vessels.

The nose and mouth contribute to the single airway that starts at the **larynx**, after its separation from the oesophagus, which marks the start of the GI tract. The **trachea** is continuous with the larynx and descends into the thorax, where it branches into the left and right main bronchi behind the sternal angle.

The main branches supplying the individual lungs are the **bronchi**. The left main bronchus separates into two branches to supply the upper and lower lobes of the left lung whereas the right main bronchus divides into three.

Quiet breathing occurs largely through the nose. As the nasal passages are enclosed in bone and have a limited diameter, the mouth is recruited when increased ventilation is required. Similarly, the laryngeal airway and trachea are limited by their cartilaginous casing. The C-shaped rings of cartilage of the trachea maintain the patency of the trachea while allowing it to accommodate large boluses of food moving down the oesophagus. The bronchi are supported by cartilaginous plates that are made up of smooth muscle to constrict effectively. At rest, the bronchi are usually tonically constricted to some extent – providing some capacity for an increase in diameter.

 CLINICAL Inhaling foreign objects

Inhaled objects may pass through the pharynx, down the trachea and into the lung. Objects are more commonly inhaled into the right lung, which is shorter, wider and more vertical than the left in the adult.

The respiratory tract is lined by the mucociliary escalator:

- **Mucus**, which is secreted onto the tract surface, traps foreign particles.
- The **cilia**, which line the surface of the respiratory epithelial cells, and the movement of the cilia, which moves the particle-laden mucus to the pharynx where it is swallowed.

The vasculature of the airways and lungs

The lungs have a dual blood supply:

- The **pulmonary arteries** supply deoxygenated blood to the lungs. Each pulmonary artery carries blood from the right ventricle. The pulmonary arteries branch to create a capillary network surrounding the alveoli to allow gas exchange. The **pulmonary veins** are formed from the alveolar capillaries and take the oxygenated blood away from the lungs to the left atrium.
- The **bronchial arteries** provide oxygenated blood to supply the bronchial tree. These arise from the aorta near the carina of the trachea, and lie behind each main bronchus. One bronchial artery supplies the right lung whereas two supply the left.

The bronchial arterioles anastomose with the pulmonary arterioles; together they supply the visceral pleura, which results in limited mixing of oxygenated and deoxygenated blood. Most of the blood supplied by the bronchial arteries is drained by the pulmonary veins and the remainder by the bronchial veins.

 CLINICAL Surface anatomy of the lungs

The lungs extend from the base of the neck to the diaphragm. When examining a patient it is important to be able to relate the signs elicited to specific areas of the lungs, and important to be aware of the various boundaries (Fig. 14.32).

In particular, the pleura extends to the level of the eighth rib anteriorly and the twelfth posteriorly, whereas the lungs extend only to the level of the sixth rib anteriorly.

The innervation of the airways and lungs

A plexus of nerves surrounds the bronchi:

- **Sympathetic fibres** derived from the ganglia of T1–5 supply the bronchial muscle, secretory glands and blood vessels. They induce opening of the airways to decrease airway resistance, helping ventilation and therefore a greater supply of oxygenated blood to the body.
- **Parasympathetic** fibres, derived from the vagus nerve, cause contraction of bronchial smooth muscle and secretion from mucus-producing glands.
- **Efferent** fibres in the bronchial tissue give sensory information back to the central nervous system. They respond to stretch and irritants, among other sensations.

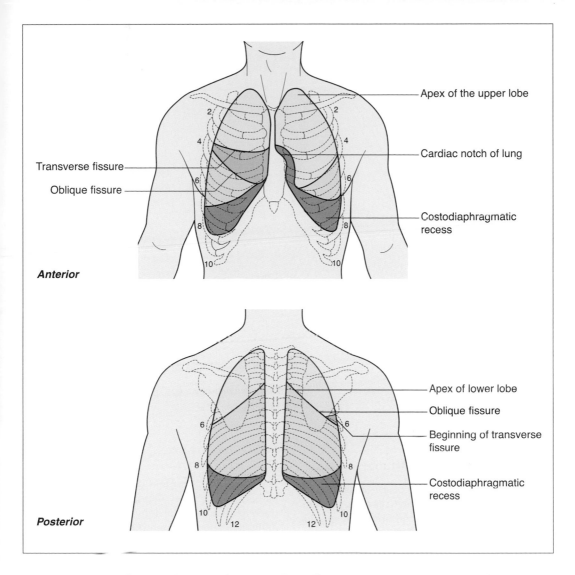

Figure 14.32 **The surface markings of the lungs and pleura**. The lungs and pleura make up much of the volume in the thoracic cavity. Although the pleurae extend down to the level of the twelfth rib posteriorly and the level of the tenth rib at the midaxillary line, they only reach the level of the eighth rib at the front. The lungs extend down to a level about two ribs above that of the pleura. As a result there is a gap – the costodiaphragmatic recess – not occupied by lung tissue. The lungs are divided into two lobes on the left and three on the right, and extend up superiorly to the level of the first rib posteriorly, with the cervical pleura projecting above the level of the clavicle.

The lymphatics of the airways and lungs

The lymph from the lungs drains to nodes found at the hila of the lung. In turn, the hilar nodes drain into nodes situated at the bifurcation of the trachea and then to mediastinal node trunks.

The mediastinum

The mediastinum refers to the structures found in the central part of the thorax. It is located between the lungs and stretches from the neck to the abdomen, consisting of four regions: superior, anterior, middle and posterior (Fig. 14.33).

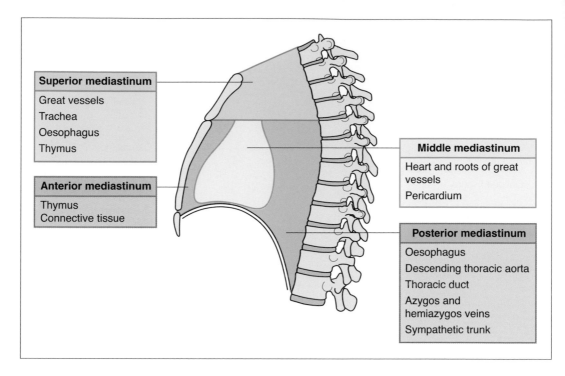

Superior mediastinum

Great vessels
Trachea
Oesophagus
Thymus

Anterior mediastinum

Thymus
Connective tissue

Middle mediastinum

Heart and roots of great vessels
Pericardium

Posterior mediastinum

Oesophagus
Descending thoracic aorta
Thoracic duct
Azygos and hemiazygos veins
Sympathetic trunk

Figure 14.33 The **mediastinum** is made up of the region of the thorax not occupied by the lungs and pleura. It can be divided into a series of distinct regions which, although part of a single anatomical compartment, are used to delineate structures clinically.

The superior mediastinum

The superior mediastinum consists of the medial section of the thorax, superior to the other sections. It is bordered inferiorly by an imaginary oblique plane that passes posteriorly from the sternomanubrial angle (angle of Louis) to the lower part of the body of the fourth thoracic vertebra. Laterally, it is bound by the pleurae. It contains many structures linking the head and neck to the rest of the body, as well as portions of the great vessels:

- The **trachea** which starts in the midline of the neck at C6 and lies anterior to the oesophagus; it divides into the main bronchi behind the sternal angle
- The **oesophagus**
- **Arch of the aorta**, **superior vena cava** and their major branches
- **Thoracic duct** and **bronchomediastinal lymph trunks** and their associated lymph nodes
- Upper parts of the **thymus**
- Parts of the **phrenic and vagus nerves** and the **sympathetic chain**.

The vagus nerve

The vagus nerve contains preganglionic parasympathetic and sensory neurons for the respiratory tract, heart and all the derivatives of the fore- and midgut in the abdomen. Branches of the vagus nerve are given off at the hila of the lungs. These supply the pulmonary plexus and the oesophageal plexus.

The phrenic nerve

The phrenic nerves supply the diaphragm and its coverings of pleura and peritoneum. They also supply sensory fibres to the pericardium and mediastinal pleura. They originate from spinal nerves C3–5 and enter the superior mediastinum between subclavian artery and vein.

The anterior mediastinum

The anterior mediastinum is narrow, located between the sternum and pericardium, and contains the internal thoracic vessels, internal thoracic lymphatics and most inferior part of the thymus, as well as a little fatty connective tissue. The parathyroid or thyroid glands are also located in the anterior mediastinum.

The middle mediastinum

The middle mediastinum contains the heart and great vessels. The middle mediastinum is bound and made up of the space between the pleura, between the diaphragm and the manubriosternal joint. It is bounded anteriorly and posteriorly by the pericardium.

The heart and great vessels

The heart is composed of two muscular pumps that work in series to pump blood through the great vessels:

- Deoxygenated blood is transported to the right side of the heart by two vessels (Fig. 14.34a):
  - the **superior vena cava** draining the upper limbs, head and thoracic walls; enters the upper extremity of the right atrium
  - the **inferior vena cava** draining the abdomen, pelvis and lower limbs; enters the right atrium directly after crossing the diaphragm.
- The **pulmonary trunk** carries deoxygenated blood away from the **right ventricle**. It bifurcates just beneath the arch of the aorta, forming the pulmonary arteries.
- The **pulmonary veins** carry oxygenated blood from the lungs to the left atrium
- The **aorta** carries oxygenated blood from the left ventricle and passes to the right of the pulmonary trunk. The arch of the aorta is a continuation of the ascending aorta, which passes backward and to the left, arching over the right pulmonary artery and left main bronchus. The aorta then descends at the left side of the fourth thoracic vertebra (Fig. 14.34b).

The heart is located in the middle mediastinum, positioned obliquely behind the sternum, one-third to the right of the midline and two-thirds to the left. It forms a broadly inverted pyramidal shape with the **apex** usually found behind the fifth intercostal space in the midclavicular line; the apex is the heart's most lateral and inferior part on the left.

The oblique position of the heart is better understood by considering which chambers of the heart create the surfaces (Fig. 14.35):

- The **left atrium** forms most of the base of the heart.

- The **right ventricle** forms most of the anterior surface of the heart and generates much of the inferior border of the heart.
- The right border is formed by the **right atrium**.
- The **left ventricle** forms most of the left border though the left atrium overlaps the most superior part.

Other blood vessels in the mediastinum

The aorta carries blood away from the left ventricle to the body. At the arch three important arteries arise:

1 The **brachiocephalic artery** bifurcates behind the right sternoclavicular joint to form the right subclavian and right common carotid arteries.
2 The **left common carotid** travels on the left of the trachea to supply the head.
3 The **left subclavian** supplies the left arm.

The inferior part of the aortic arch and the bifurcation of the pulmonary trunk are joined by the **ligamentum arteriosum**.

CLINICAL Aortic aneurysm

This is an abnormal dilatation of the aorta, due to a weakness in the wall, which may be one of the following:

- **Saccular**: a saccular aneurysm evolves when a weakness in the vessel wall allows the blood to force the intima and media to balloon out.
- **Dissecting**: dissection is a tear in the wall of the vessel that causes blood to stream between the layers of the aorta, forcing the layers apart.
- **Fusiform**: a fusiform aneurysm is spindle shaped, resulting from swelling around the circumference of the vessel with no protrusion of the inner layers.

Aneurysms can be further divided into two:

1 **True aneurysms** (such as saccular and dissecting aneurysms) involve an outpouching of all vessel layers and can be either congenital or acquired.
2 **False aneurysms** (such as dissecting aneurysms) occur when blood leaks out of the vessel but is confined by surrounding tissues. False aneurysms usually result from trauma and are a recognised complication of some arterial procedures.

Serious complications that can arise from an aneurysm include: rupture, thrombosis, embolism, pressure on other structures and infection.

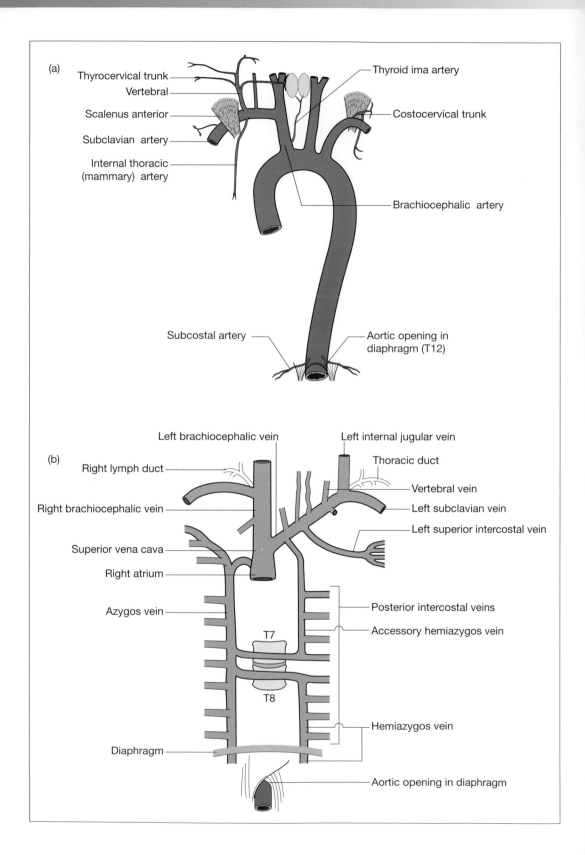

(a)

Thyrocervical trunk

Vertebral

Scalenus anterior

Subclavian artery

Internal thoracic
(mammary) artery

Thyroid ima artery

Costocervical trunk

Brachiocephalic artery

Subcostal artery

Aortic opening in
diaphragm (T12)

(b)

Left brachiocephalic vein

Right lymph duct

Right brachiocephalic vein

Superior vena cava

Right atrium

Azygos vein

Left internal jugular vein

Thoracic duct

Vertebral vein

Left subclavian vein

Left superior intercostal vein

Posterior intercostal veins

Accessory hemiazygos vein

T7

T8

Hemiazygos vein

Diaphragm

Aortic opening in diaphragm

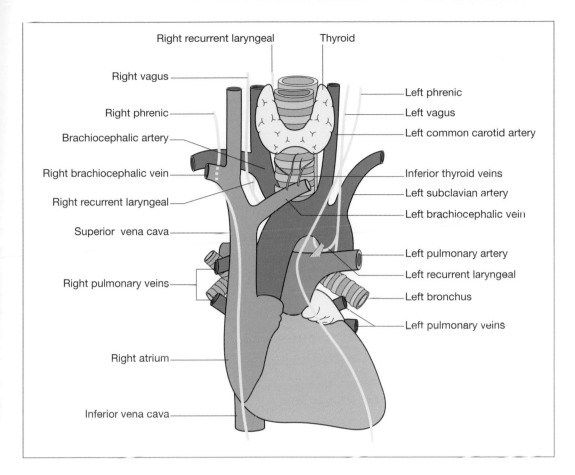

Figure 14.35 The anterior aspect of the heart and surrounding structures: the heart is located in the mediastinum, encased in pericardium, and most of its anterior aspect is made up of the walls of the left ventricle. Superiorly and laterally the great vessels enter the heart. The trachea and bronchi are also superior and posterior to the heart, whereas the left branch of the recurrent laryngeal nerve loops under the ligamentum arteriosum. The phrenic nerves also course along the surface of the pericardium, providing sensory innervation as they travel towards the diaphragm.

Figure 14.34 The thoracic aorta: (a) **The major branches of the thoracic aorta**. The thoracic aorta emerges from the left atrium where it ascends, arches and descends. It becomes the abdominal aorta at T12. (b) **The major venous drainage** occurs through the vena cavae. The inferior vena cava (not shown) is responsible for draining blood from the lower parts of the body, whereas the superior vena cava drains blood from the body above the heart. In addition the blood from the posterior wall of the thorax and abdomen can be drained through the azygos and hemiazygos veins. Although these originate from below the level of the heart, they drain into the superior vena cava.

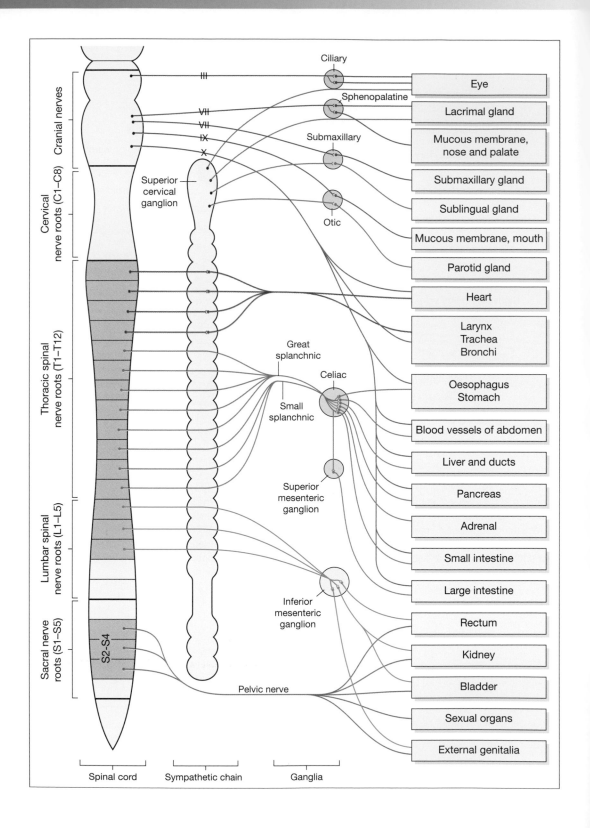

The posterior mediastinum

The posterior mediastinum lies posterior to the heart and great vessels. It is bordered anteriorly by the pericardium, inferiorly by the diaphragm, superiorly by the superior mediastinum, posteriorly by the thoracic vertebral column (T4–12) and laterally by the pleurae. It contains many structures and conduits travelling to or from the abdomen:

- The oesophagus
- The descending aorta and its branches
- The azygos vein and its tributaries
- The thoracic lymph duct and associated nodes
- The thoracic sympathetic chain and its branches.

The oesophagus

The oesophagus starts in the midline of the neck at C6, and lies slightly to the left of the midline as it descends behind the trachea. As it reaches the diaphragm, it travels to the left, crossing in front of the aorta and entering the abdomen at T10.

The descending aorta

The descending aorta extends from the aortic arch starting at the lower border of the fourth thoracic vertebra. It ends anterior to the lower border of the twelfth thoracic vertebra at the aortic hiatus in the diaphragm.

The azygos veins

Drainage of the posterior chest wall is achieved by the azygos veins, which travel to the right of the lower thoracic vertebral bodies and drain into the superior vena cava just before it enters the pericardium.

The thoracic duct

The thoracic duct originates from the **cisterna chyli**, a lymphatic sac, in the abdomen by the anterior surface of L1. Lymph from parts of the body below the diaphragm drains into the cisterna chyli. The thoracic duct arises from the abdomen behind the aorta. It ascends behind the oesophagus and anterior to the thoracic vertebrae, and drains into the junction of the left internal jugular and left subclavian veins. At the point of return to the venous system, the left lymphatic duct has acquired lymph from the left arm and left-hand side of the upper body.

The right lymphatic ducts empty here into the equivalent on the right side, and collect lymph from the right arm and right-hand side of the chest, neck and head.

The thoracic sympathetic chain

The sympathetic chain is a bundle of nerve fibres that travels vertically on the necks of the ribs on either side of the thoracic vertebral column from T5 to T12 (Fig. 14.36). The sympathetic chain extends further above T5 through three further ganglia, with their fibres inferior to them; these are responsible for supplying the sympathetic outflow to the head and neck.

The abdomen

The abdomen contains most of the alimentary canal and its supporting organs. It also contains other structures not directly related to GI function. The abdomen is clearly separated from the thorax by the diaphragm, although the division between the abdomen and pelvis is less clear.

 CLINICAL **Surface anatomy of the abdomen**

When the abdomen is examined it is divided into nine areas (Fig. 14.37). The left and right hypochondria are separated by the epigastric area, and are all found just below the ribs. The liver can be palpated in the right hypochondrium. Parts of the liver can be palpated in the epigastric area alongside the duodenum, pancreas and part of the stomach. The remaining part of the stomach can be palpated in the left epigastrium. The left and right lumbar regions are found directly below, separated by the umbilical region. In these areas, various parts of the bowel can be palpated as well as the kidneys. Below these are the left and right iliac areas, separated by the hypogastric region.

In the right iliac fossa, you can palpate the appendix and the caecum, whereas in the left you can feel the descending colon.

In women you may detect gynaecological pathology in those areas. In the hypogastric region, the bladder and uterus can be palpated.

Figure 14.36 The **autonomic outflow of the body** is divided into the sympathetic outflow which is through the sympathetic chain, derived from the thoracic region and the parasympathetic outflow that occurs from the cranial nerves (CN III, VII, IX, X and XI) and the sacral regions of the spinal cord (S2–4). Most organs in the body receive both sympathetic and parasympathetic innervations.

The anterior abdominal wall

The anterior abdominal wall secures the abdominal viscera. Its muscular layers allow increases in intra-abdominal pressure for functions such as bladder control.

The anterior abdominal wall is composed of a vertical muscle and three flat sheets of muscle that are encased by skin and superficial fascia.

- The **rectus abdominis** muscle is a vertical sheet that runs either side of the anterior wall of the abdomen and is divided in the midline by the linea alba, a band of connective tissue. The muscle runs from the xiphisternum and lower costal cartilages to the pubic symphysis.
- The **external oblique** muscle pulls the thorax downwards to compress the abdominal cavity and increase the pressure within it. The **internal oblique** muscle increases the abdominal pressure, encouraging the abdominal organs to push up into the diaphragm. This increases the pressure in the thorax to help expiration. The oblique muscles also help rotation and flexion of the trunk.
- **Transversus abdominis** provides core support to the trunk and is found deep to the internal oblique muscle.

The anterior abdominal muscles are supplied by the lower six intercostal nerves. The accompanying arteries, veins and lymphatics run between the internal oblique muscle and transversus abdominis.

The inguinal canal

The lower part of the abdominal wall covers the anterior part of the pelvis. In this region, it contains passages for the vessels of the gonads.

The **inguinal canal** stretches from the deep inguinal ring to the superficial inguinal ring. The deep inguinal ring transmits the spermatic cord in males and the round ligament in females; it is found at the midpoint between the anterosuperior iliac spine and pubic tubercle. The inferior epigastric branch of the external iliac artery lies medial to the deep ring. The superficial inguinal ring is located just above the pubic tubercle and is formed by separation of the fibres of the aponeurosis of the external oblique muscle. The boundaries of the canal are:

- superiorly, transversus abdominis and internal oblique
- inferiorly, the inguinal ligament
- anteriorly, the external oblique
- posteriorly, transversalis fascia.

 CLINICAL Hernias

A hernia is any structure that passes through the membrane or layer of muscle by which it should be contained, thus ending up in the incorrect place. It has three parts: the orifice, hernial sac and its contents. There are many types of hernia, the most prevalent related to the abdomen being:

- **Inguinal hernias** are the most common site of herniation in the male because they are at a point of weakness in the anterior abdominal wall; they can be:
  - **direct**: direct hernias protrude through the conjoint tendon, so direct hernias are more common in older men because the conjoint tendon is weaker
  - **indirect**: indirect hernias pass through the superficial ring and out through the direct ring.
- **Paraumbilical hernias** form when there is a weakness in the abdominal wall near to the umbilicus, causing an outpouching of the abdominal contents.

A **hiatus hernia** is a protrusion of the superior part of the stomach into the thorax through a weakness in the diaphragm, which causes the patient to experience a feeling like heartburn in some cases.

The posterior abdominal wall

The posterior abdominal wall provides support for many structures, particularly those not directly related to the GI tract, including the kidneys, adrenal glands, abdominal aorta and inferior vena cava, as well as important nerves and lymphatics.

The structure of the posterior abdominal wall

The posterior abdominal wall is composed of many structures and their vasculature:

- **Lumbar vertebrae** and their associated muscles and fascia

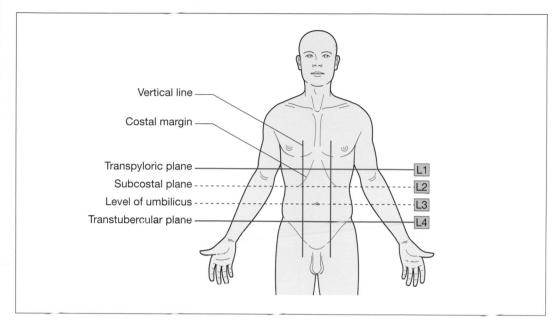

Figure 14.37 **The surface regions of the abdomen**: the abdomen is divided into nine surface clinical examination regions. These regions are delineated by the levels of L1–4 and a vertical line drawn from the point between the anterosuperior iliac spine and the pubic tubercle.

- The **diaphragm**, which is covered by peritoneum on its abdominal side
- **Psoas major**
- **Quadratus lumborus**
- **Iliacus**.

The blood vessels of the posterior and lateral abdominal walls

- The great vessels run on the posterior and lateral walls of the abdomen and pelvis.
- The **abdominal aorta** supplies the abdomen and lower limbs via its branches.
- The **inferiorvena cava** drains the veins of the posterior wall and returns blood to the right atrium.
- Lymphatics drain into the **cisterna chyli**.

  The **abdominal aorta** passes through the diaphragm as a continuation of the thoracic aorta. It then splits at L4 into the **two common iliac arteries**. Before its bifurcation, the abdominal aorta gives of several branches (Fig. 14.38):

- **Midline branches** carry blood to the gut and its associated structures. These include the coeliac artery, superior mesenteric artery and inferior mesenteric artery.
- **Lateral branches**, given off in pairs, supply organs that develop embryologically from the intermediate mesoderm – the adrenals, kidneys and gonads.
- **Paired branches to the anterior and posterior abdominal walls**
- The **median sacral artery** supplies the fourth and fifth lumbar vertebrae, sacrum, coccyx and posterior surface of the rectum.

The peritoneal cavity and the peritoneum

The peritoneum is the membrane that encases the peritoneal cavity, reducing friction between the viscera and abdominal walls. The peritoneum is located in the abdomen although it extends to enclose some organs in the pelvis and is made up of two layers. The parietal peritoneum lines the walls of the cavity. Visceral peritoneum covers many viscera partly or completely.

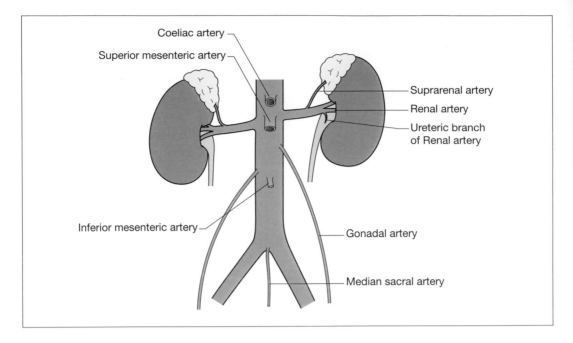

Coeliac artery

Superior mesenteric artery

Suprarenal artery

Renal artery

Ureteric branch
of Renal artery

Inferior mesenteric artery

Gonadal artery

Median sacral artery

Figure 14.38 **Abdominal aorta**: in the abdomen the major paired vessels coming from the aorta are those supplying the adrenal glands (the suprarenal arteries), the kidneys (the renal arteries) and the gonads (the gonadal arteries). In addition, single midline vessels that supply the gut arise, the coeliac artery, the superior mesenteric artery and the inferior mesenteric artery supplying the fore-, mid- and hindgut, respectively.

The organs covered by the peritoneum are suspended from the posterior abdominal wall by a double layer of peritoneum known as the **mesentery**, through which vessels and nerves run. The organs that are partially covered by peritoneum have 'bare areas' (uncovered areas). These are fused with other structures (Fig. 14.39).

The organs in the abdomen are described in relation to their covering of peritoneum:

- **Peritoneal organs** are those that are covered with visceral peritoneum (e.g. the stomach).
- **Retroperitoneal organs** are those that are partially (or not at all) covered with peritoneum. They can be further classed as:
  - **primarily retroperitoneal**, when the organs have not been covered in peritoneum at any point during development (e.g. the kidneys)
  - **secondarily retroperitoneal**, when the organs initially developed with a peritoneal covering, which was lost during development (e.g. the descending and ascending colon).

The omentum

The peritoneal membrane is also organised into two large folds – the omenta:

1 The **greater omentum** is a sheet of peritoneum that hangs down from the greater curvature of the stomach. The omentum folds back on itself and attaches to the anterior surface of the transverse colon.
2 The **lesser omentum** is a sheet of peritoneum that is attached to the lesser curvature of the stomach (forms the right border of the stomach beneath the entry of the oesophagus; it passes superiorly, backwards and laterally to the pylorus). It stretches up to the undersurface of the liver. It has a free edge on right-hand side which carries the common bile duct, hepatic artery and hepatic portal vein.

The gastrointestinal tract

The principle functions of the GI tract are digestion and excretion. The GI tract starts with the abdominal oesophagus. It then continues, in

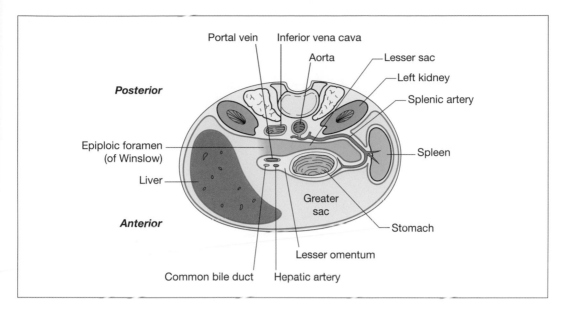

Figure 14.39 **Cross-section of the abdominal cavity**: the main portion of the abdomen is contained within the peritoneal cavity located at anteriorly to the abdomen. The great vessels, vertebrae and other retroperitoneal structures are located posteriorly. The omenta, which encases the stomach, divides the peritoneal cavity into the greater and lesser sacs, which meet at the epiploic foramen, the anterior edge of which is defined by the portal triad contained in the lesser omentum.

order, as: the stomach, small intestine, large intestine and rectum, and terminates at the anal canal (Fig. 14.40).

The oesophagus

The oesophagus is a muscular tube that carries food from the pharynx to the stomach. It passes through the neck and thorax before entering the abdomen anterior to T10, piercing the diaphragm to the left of the midline, before rapidly meeting the stomach.

The gastro-oesophageal junction is where it forms an acute angle with the fundus of the stomach to its left, creating the cardiac sphincter, which is a **physiological sphincter**. The sphincter prevents reflux of the gastric contents back into the oesophagus.

 DEFINITION **Physiological sphincters**

Physiological sphincters prevent the movement of a substance between two regions of a tube. However, such sphincters do not contain developed rings or thickening in the muscle.

The stomach

The stomach is the most dilated part of the GI tract with an adult capacity of 1.5 L. The stomach stores, sterilises, macerates and starts digestion of food before releasing it into the small intestine. The stomach has a curved shape – the small **lesser curvature** on the anterior aspect and the **greater curvature** along the posterior surface. The stomach is covered by peritoneum, the anterior surface of the stomach being covered by the peritoneum of the greater sac whereas the posterior surface is covered by peritoneum of the lesser sac. At the greater curvature the peritoneal sheets unite to form a double-layered sheet, which leaves the lower part of the greater curvature of the stomach as the **greater omentum**.

The stomach is divided into four regions, from proximal to distal (Fig. 14.41):

1 The **cardiac region**
2 The **fundus**
3 The **body**
4 The **pyloric region**.

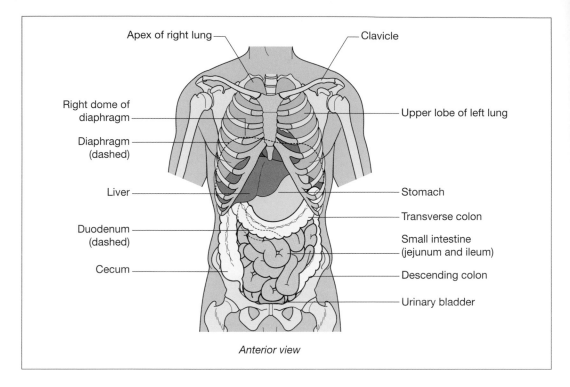

Apex of right lung

Clavicle

Right dome of
diaphragm

Upper lobe of left lung

Diaphragm
(dashed)

Liver

Stomach

Transverse colon

Duodenum
(dashed)

Small intestine
(jejunum and ileum)

Cecum

Descending colon

Urinary bladder

Anterior view

Figure 14.40 The abdominal organs are tightly packed. Much of the space in the peritoneal cavity is taken up by the small intestine, which descends into the pelvis. The spleen, liver and to a lesser extent the pancreas and stomach are packed closely to the diaphragm, and are protected in part by the lower part of the ribcage.

The mucosa in different regions of the stomach is specialised according to its function:

- The **cardiac region** contains mucus-secreting glands which protect the stomach epithelia from digesting itself.
- The **fundus** and **body** contains gastric glands. These secrete acid and pepsin, a digestive enzyme that breaks down proteins. The muscularis propria in the fundus and body contains an extra inner oblique layer of muscle, enabling folds to form in the mucosa.
- The **pyloric region** contains branched glands that produce mucus and gastrin. The mucus protects the gastroduodenal junction from acid and pepsin, and lubricates the passage of chyme.

Food enters the duodenum through the pylorus, which is situated just to the right of the midline, halfway between the suprasternal notch and the pubic symphysis. It crosses the tip of the ninth costal cartilage and the lower border of L1.

The small intestine

The small intestine completes digestion, neutralises acid and is the principal absorptive site of the GI tract. It stretches from the pyloric sphincter to the ileocaecal junction. In adults, the combined length of the small intestine is approximately 280 cm and it consists of three parts – the duodenum, jejunum and ileum – which differ subtly, reflecting their different specialisations.

The small intestines possess specialisations to increase the surface area available for absorption of the products of digestion:

- **Extended length**
- Mucosal/submucosal **folds**
- **Villi**, finger-like projections formed by the mucosa
- **Microvilli** found on the luminal surface of enterocytes, forming a brush border.

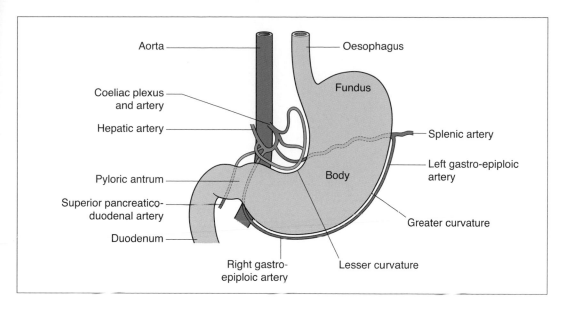

Figure 14.41 The stomach is a dilated portion of the gastrointestinal tract. It is located on the left side of abdomen, and has a curving course, resulting in the formation of the lesser and greater curvatures, along which the blood vessels lie – all of which are derived from the coeliac artery. The stomach can be divided into regions – the body and fundus make up the larger portion of the stomach, whereas food enters superiorly at the cardiac region through the oesophagus. The food is processed into chyme in the stomach and released through the pyloric sphincter into the small intestine.

The duodenum

The duodenum is the first part of the small intestine, receiving the chyme released from the pyloric sphincter. Initially, the duodenum is covered with peritoneum, but distal to the duodenal papilla it is retroperitoneal. The papilla is surrounded by the sphincter of Oddi where the hepatopancreatic ampulla enters the duodenum, which creates a C-shaped loop around the head of the pancreas and is divided into four parts (Fig. 14.42).

The jejunum

The jejunum is a continuation of the duodenum. It starts at the duodenojejunal flexure, where the suspensory ligament (of Trietz) connects the small intestine to the diaphragm. The jejunum and ileum are suspended from the posterior abdominal wall by small bowel **mesentery**. The mesentery is a folded layer of peritoneum which runs from the duodenojejunal flexure to the right iliac fossa, and contains all the vessels and nerves supplying the small bowel.

The ileum

The ileum is continuous with the jejunum. Differentiation relies on notable distinctions between the two (Table 14.8).

Table 14.8 Demonstration of the differences between the ileum and the jejunum

	Ileum	Jejunum
Diameter	Smaller	Larger
Mucosa	Thinner	Thicker
Circular folds	Less	More
Lymphoid tissue aggregates (Peyer's patches)	Yes, found at the antimesenteric border. Visible and palpable	No

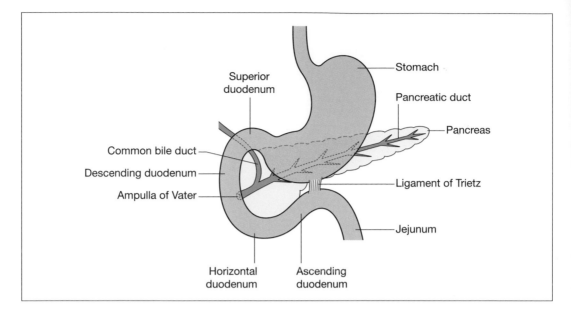

Figure 14.42 The **duodenum** connects the stomach with the rest of the small intestine. It is made up of four continuous parts, the first two being part of the foregut, and the last two part of the midgut. The division occurs at the ampulla of Vater where the enzymes from the pancreas and bile from the liver enter the gastrointestinal tract.

The large intestine

The large bowel stretches from the ileocaecal junction to the anorectal junction. Many of the specialisations of the large intestine are the result of its primary functions of reabsorbing water to produce faeces and moving faeces through the GI tract for expulsion:

- **A thick muscular wall** for powerful propulsion
- Predominance of **goblet cells** which secrete mucus for lubrication
- Many **crypts**, closely packed straight tubular glands, with a large surface area for absorption
- **Taeniae coli**: the longitudinal layer of muscle of muscularis propria forms three separate longitudinal bands, apart from in the rectum, which helps peristalsis.

The small and large intestines have characteristics essential to their function; these help their differentiation (Table 14.9).

The large intestine can be divided anatomically. Many of these regions have specific functions which are continuous, though blood supply and innervation differs in many cases. From proximal to distal, there are five parts of the large intestine (Fig. 14.43):

1. The **caecum**
2. The **appendix**
3. The **colon**
4. The **rectum**
5. The **anal canal**.

Table 14.9 The differences between the small and large intestine

	Small intestine	Large intestine
Calibre	Smaller	Larger
Villi	Yes	No
Taeniae coli	No	Yes
Haustrations	No	Yes
Appendices epiploicae	No	Yes, attached to the ascending, transverse, descending and sigmoid colon

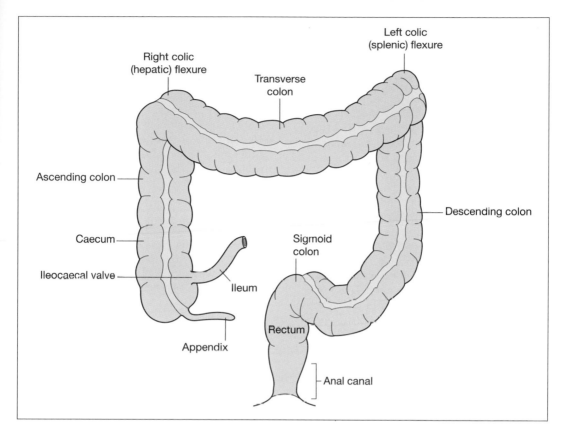

Figure 14.43 The **large intestine** is made up of five parts – the caecum is the site at which food enters from the small intestine, via the ileocaecal valve. This is continuous with the appendix – a dead-end tube, with no functional role in humans; it is also continuous with the ascending colon. Food travels along the ascending, transverse and descending colons, to reach the sigmoid colon, which is continuous with the rectum. It is in the rectum that faeces are stored until release through the anus. The transverse colon is the site where the midgut (supplied by the superior mesenteric artery) meets the hindgut (supplied by the inferior mesenteric artery), reflecting different embryonic origins.

 DEFINITION Haustrations

These are sacculations (outpouchings) of the wall of the large intestine. As each haustration fills it stimulates contraction, forcing the contents on to the next haustration.

 DEFINITION Appendices epiploicae

These are small tags of peritoneum filled with fat that do not appear to have a defined function. They are typically attached to the transverse and sigmoid colon, although they can also be found in the upper part of the rectum.

The caecum

The caecum is the first part of the large intestine. It is blind ended and dilated, starting at the ileocaecal junction. The ileum passes into the posteromedial wall of the caecum, entering as a horizontal slit surrounded by two folds of mucosa, which form a valve to prevent backflow.

The appendix

The appendix is a blind-ended tube that opens into the medial wall of the caecum. In humans, the appendix has no significant function, although it may become inflamed in **appendicitis**.

The colon

The colon forms the major length of the large intestine, taking a looping course around much of the anterior of the abdomen. It is divided into four parts:

1 The **ascending colon** travels from the right iliac fossa to the hepatic flexure which is located beneath the right lobe of the liver and is commonly attached to the posterior abdominal wall.
2 The **transverse colon** extends from the hepatic to the splenic flexure. The splenic flexure is the area of the colon in contact with the left kidney, tail of the pancreas, spleen and greater curvature of the stomach. The transverse colon has its own mesentery, the transverse mesocolon. Both the transverse colon and mesocolon are covered by the greater omentum.
3 The **descending colon** travels from the splenic flexure to the left iliac fossa. It is commonly retroperitoneal, i.e. attached to the posterior abdominal wall.
4 The **sigmoid colon** passes from the left iliac fossa to the rectum. The rectum usually begins at S3. It has its own mesentery, the sigmoid mesocolon.

The rectum

Faeces are temporarily stored in the rectum, before they are expelled through the anus. The rectum runs from the end of the sigmoid colon to the anorectal junction, where it passes through **levator ani**, a muscle responsible for supporting the pelvic organs. It is a midline structure that passes along the concave surface of the sacrum and coccyx.

Only the upper third of the rectum is covered in peritoneum. The peritoneum travels forwards from the middle third of the rectum, on to the bladder in males, and the vagina and uterus in females. This forms the rectovesical pouch or rectouterine pouch in males and females, respectively.

The anal canal

The anal canal is the passage through which faeces pass out of the body. It runs from the anorectal junction inferiorly and posteriorly to the anus.

The vasculature of the alimentary tract

The vessels that supply different parts of the alimentary tract in the abdomen relate to the embryological origins of the different areas:

- The **coeliac artery and its branches** supply the derivatives of the foregut: the foregut comprises the GI tract up to the duodenal papilla, i.e. predominantly the stomach and duodenum.
- The **superior mesenteric artery and its branches** supply the structures originating as the midgut: the midgut comprises the structures from the duodenal papilla to the splenic flexure.
- The **inferior mesenteric artery** supplies the structures originating as the hindgut: the hindgut stretches from the splenic flexure to the upper part of the anal canal.

The coeliac artery

This branch of the aorta originates at the level of T12 and supplies the foregut, including the liver, spleen and pancreas. It splits immediately to three major branches (Fig. 14.44):

- The **left gastric artery** ascends to supply the lower part of the oesophagus, before passing along the lesser curvature of the stomach, anastomosing with the right gastric artery – a branch of the hepatic artery.
- The **hepatic artery** directly supplies the pylorus of the stomach before giving rise to numerous branches. Its main branches are the right gastric artery and gastroduodenal artery, which arise near the pylorus. The **right gastric artery** anastomoses with the left gastric artery to supply to the lesser curvature of the stomach, whereas the gastroduodenal artery further divides into the right gastroepiploic artery and superior pancreaticoduodenal artery. The right gastroepiploic artery supplies the greater curvature of the stomach. The pancreaticoduodenal artery supplies both the pancreas and part of the duodenum before the duodenal papilla.
- The **splenic artery** directly supplies part of both the abdominal wall and the pancreas although its branches supply the stomach fundus and greater curvature of the stomach. The splenic artery passes along the posterior abdominal wall via the superior aspect of the pancreas. At the terminal point of the tail of the pancreas, it divides into the short gastric arteries and the left gastroepiploic artery. The short gastric arteries supply the stomach fundus. The left gastroepiploic artery anastomoses with the right gastroepiploic artery to supply the greater curvature of the stomach.

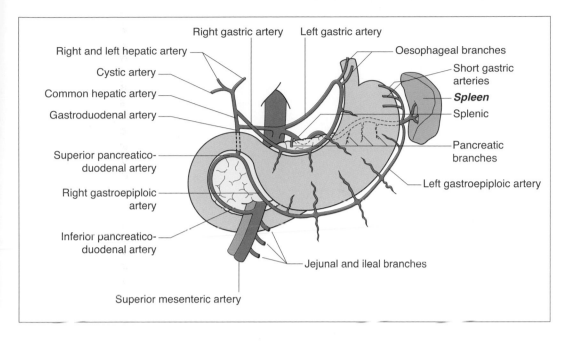

Figure 14.44 The coeliac trunk supplies the abdominal structures derived from the foregut. The coeliac trunk arises at the level of T12–L1 and provides three major branches: the splenic, hepatic and left gastric arteries.

The superior mesenteric artery

The superior mesenteric artery supplies the midgut-derived structures. It branches from the aorta anterior to L1, posterior to the neck of the pancreas, and crosses the third part of the duodenum to enter the small bowel mesentery. It forms many anastomosing branches (Fig. 14.45):

- The **inferior pancreaticoduodenal artery** is a single artery that branches off almost instantly and supplies the duodenum and head of the pancreas.
- Many **jejunal and ileal branches** enter the mesentery where they anastomose to form arcades. Terminal branches from these supply the wall of the bowel.
- The **ileocolic artery** travels to the right iliac fossa, supplying the terminal ileum and the caecum. The ileocolic artery gives off two main branches:
  - the **right colic artery** which crosses the posterior abdominal wall below the peritoneum to supply the ascending colon
  - the **middle colic artery** which enters the transverse mesocolon and supplies the remainder of the midgut.

The inferior mesenteric artery

The inferior mesenteric artery supplies the hindgut-derived bowel, which runs from the splenic flexure to the upper part of the anal canal. It originates from the aorta opposite L3 and travels downward and laterally to the left iliac fossa, and along its course it gives off anastomosing branches (Fig. 14.46):

- The **left colic artery** which supplies the splenic flexure and the descending colon.
- The **sigmoid arteries** which pass into the sigmoid mesocolon to supply the sigmoid colon.
- The **superior rectal artery**.

The arterial supply of the rectum and anal canal

The arterial supply differs along its length:

- The **upper two-thirds** of the rectal mucosa and muscle are supplied by the superior rectal artery.
- The **lower third** of the rectum is supplied by the middle rectal branch of the internal iliac artery.
- The **anal canal** is supplied by the inferior rectal arteries, which are derived from the internal pudendal branch of the internal iliac artery.

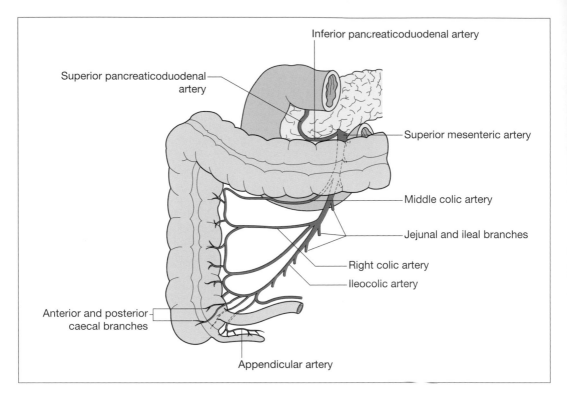

Inferior pancreaticoduodenal artery

Superior pancreaticoduodenal artery

Superior mesenteric artery

Middle colic artery

Jejunal and ileal branches

Right colic artery

Ileocolic artery

Anterior and posterior caecal branches

Appendicular artery

Figure 14.45 The superior mesenteric artery (SMA) supplies the abdominal structures derived from the midgut. It arises from the aorta at the level of L1 and passes behind the neck of the pancreas to the right iliac fossa, providing branches to the ileum and jejunum. The SMA gives rise to the right and middle colic arteries which supply parts of the colon.

The venous drainage of the GI tract

The veins draining the GI tract empty into the hepatic portal vein which is formed at the junction of the superior mesenteric and splenic veins, and then runs superiorly posterior to the first part of the duodenum and then to the liver (Fig. 14.47).

The venous drainage of the rectum

The rectum is drained partially by the inferior mesenteric vein and partly by the middle and inferior rectal veins. Due to the dual drainage by the portal and systemic circulations, an increase in pressure in the portal system will create anastomoses between the veins causing them to dilate (Fig. 14.48).

The lymphatic drainage of the GI tract

Lymphatic vessels follow a similar course to the arteries, although in the opposite direction,

emptying into the coeliac, superior mesenteric or inferior mesenteric preaortic nodes, which are found at the origin of the respective vessels.

In addition, lymph from parts of the anal canal drains into inguinal lymph nodes.

The autonomic innervation of the GI tract

Sympathetic innervation to the foregut derivatives arises from the coeliac plexus. The coeliac plexus is a group of ganglion cells formed from the preganglionic thoracic splanchnic nerves. Postganglionic fibres travel along the arteries to the stomach and duodenum. The superior and inferior mesenteric plexus innervate the midgut and hindgut in a similar manner.

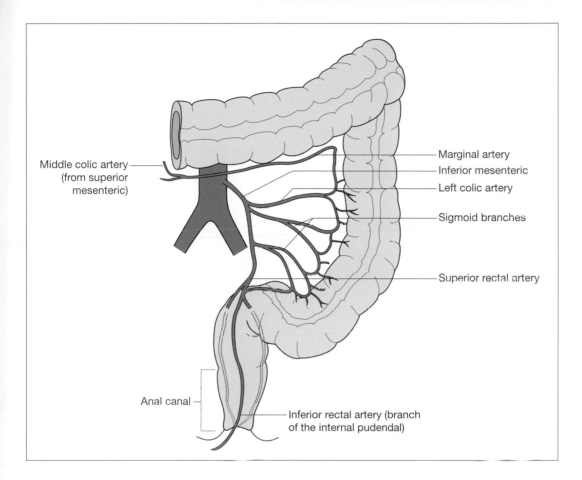

Middle colic artery
(from superior
mesenteric)

Marginal artery

Inferior mesenteric

Left colic artery

Sigmoid branches

Superior rectal artery

Anal canal

Inferior rectal artery (branch
of the internal pudendal)

Figure 14.46 The inferior mesenteric artery (IMA) supplies the abdominal structures derived from the hindgut. It arises from the aorta at the level of L3. The IMA has three major branches: the left colic artery which supplies the transverse and descending colon, the sigmoid branch, which supplies the sigmoid colon, and the superior rectal vessels, which supply the upper portion of the rectum. The inferior part of the rectum is supplied by the inferior rectal artery, which is a branch of the pudendal artery.

The innervation regulates blood flow to the tissues:

- The **sympathetic system** causes constriction of the blood vessels to reduce flow to the gut.
- The **parasympathetic** effect is dominant; during digestion, blood flow to the gut is maximised. The parasympathetic supply is mainly from the vagus nerve (CN X).

The histology of the GI tract

The GI tract is lined by mucous membrane which shows area-specific modifications corresponding to the particular region's function: ingestion,

fragmentation, digestion, absorption or elimination of waste products. The histological features of the GI tract and their adaptation to function are covered in Chapter 8.

The liver, biliary tract and pancreas

The liver

The liver is the largest solid organ in the body and has several vital functions in processing those nutrients received from the intestine,

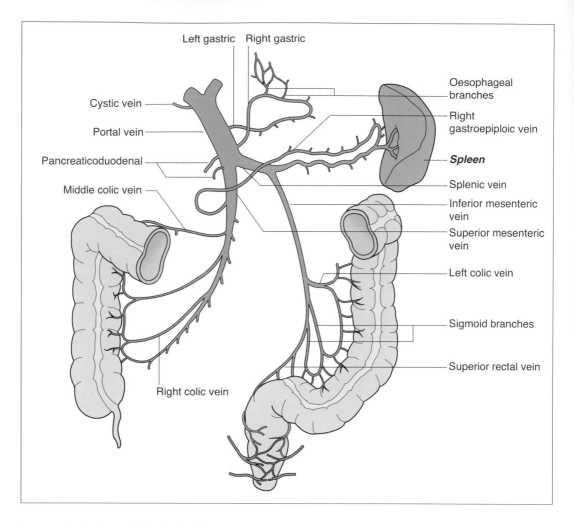

Figure 14.47 The portal circulation: the portal vessels drain the blood from the lower part of the oesophagus to the superior rectal veins of the large intestine. The blood drains into the portal vein, which carries it to the liver, where absorbed nutrients are processed. The portal circulation is distinct from the systemic venous system, although it forms anastomoses with the systemic circulation in the rectum and the oesophagus.

and in the production of various substances, both to aid digestion and to contribute to the blood:

- **Plasma protein production**
- **Mediator of carbohydrate/lipid/protein metabolism**
- **Removal of particulate matter from the blood** by macrophages (in this location they are known as Kupffer's cells)
- **Bile production**: bile is sent via the biliary tract to the duodenum.

 DEFINITION Porta hepatis

The porta hepatis is the entry point for the hepatic portal vein, hepatic artery, common hepatic duct, lymphatics and several nerves. It is also known as the transverse fissure of the liver and divides the caudate and the quadrate lobes. It is 5 cm long and extends across the inferior surface of the left side of the liver's right lobe. At the porta hepatis the vessels are organised to ensure efficient supply to the divisions of the liver.

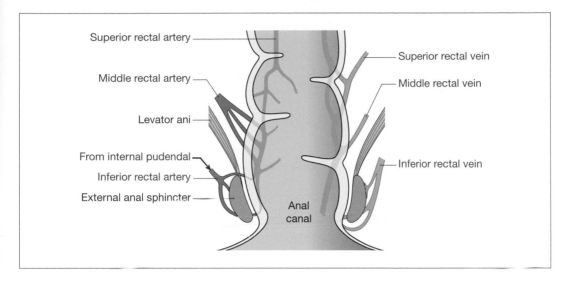

Figure 14.48 **Vasculature of the rectum**: the rectum is supplied by the superior, middle and inferior rectal arteries. The superior rectal artery is derived from the inferior mesenteric artery, the middle rectal artery from the internal inferior vesical and the inferior rectal artery from the internal pudendal artery; it supplies primarily the anal canal. Similarly the rectum is drained by the superior rectal veins, which drain into the portal system, whereas the middle and inferior rectal veins drain into the systemic circulation via the internal iliac and internal pudenal veins, respectively. In the rectum the venous systems are anastomosed which can cause the formation of varicosities if portal hypertension occurs. These can be a significant source of bleeding.

 CLINICAL Portal hypertension

Portal hypertension refers to high blood pressure in the portal system. Patients have portal hypertension most commonly as a result of liver cirrhosis, although many other conditions may be the cause, such as portal vein thrombosis, right heart failure and, in tropical countries, schistosomiasis.

Portal hypertension leads to dilated varices at the sites of portosystemic anastomoses, which are at risk of rupturing and bleeding. Common sites include:

- The **oesophagus** where the left gastric and oesophageal veins unite
- The **rectoanal junction** where the superior and middle rectal veins anastomose
- The **umbilicus** where small veins travelling with ligamentum teres join with the anterior abdominal wall veins
- The **attachment of the retroperitoneal bowel** where bowel veins unite with those of the posterior abdominal wall.

The position and structure of the liver

The liver lies beneath the right dome of the diaphragm and lower ribs. Its narrow apex extends leftwards to the fundus of the stomach, where it is protected by the right lower ribs. The liver occupies most of the right hypochondrium and part of the epigastrium and left hypochondrium (Fig. 14.49).

The liver has distinct anatomical and functional structures:

- **Anatomically** the liver is divided into four 'lobes'; these can be seen on the inferior surface of the liver as four distinct regions.
- **Functionally**, the liver can be divided into two halves – the left and right – which are not discernable anatomically. The right lobe is bigger than the left, with each lobe divided into four segments. Each segment has its own vasculature and biliary drainage.

Ligamentous attachments

The liver is secured by two major ligaments:

- The **falciform ligament** is a reflection of peritoneum on to the anterior abdominal wall above

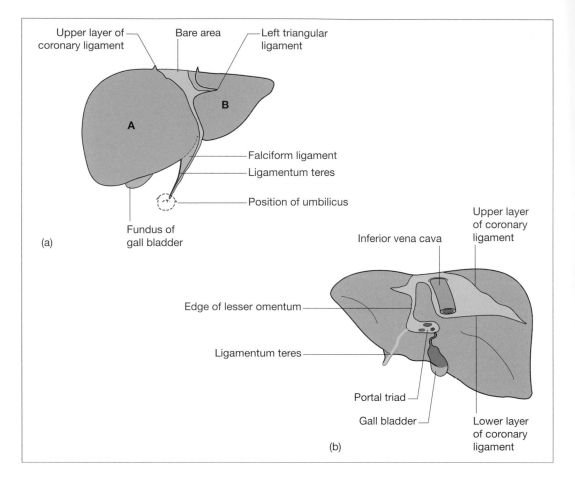

Upper layer of coronary ligament

Bare area

Left triangular ligament

B

A

Falciform ligament

Ligamentum teres

Position of umbilicus

Fundus of gall bladder

(a)

Inferior vena cava

Upper layer of coronary ligament

Edge of lesser omentum

Ligamentum teres

Portal triad

Gall bladder

Lower layer of coronary ligament

(b)

Figure 14.49 The liver: (a) the anterior aspect of the liver consists of a smooth surface that is closely apposed to the diaphragm. The bare area of the liver is the region directly in contact, whereas the peritoneum covers much of the rest of the anterior surface of the liver and forms the falciform ligament. (b) The posterior surface of the liver receives the portal triad, consisting of the portal vein, hepatic arteries and common bile duct. In addition the gallbladder is located on the posterior aspect of the liver. The coronary ligament is made up of the reflected layers of the mesentery and surrounds the inferior vena cava, which drains the blood from both the hepatic arteries and the portal circulation.

the umbilicus, which extends from the anterior surface of the liver. The falciform ligament divides the liver into the anatomical left and right lobes anteriorly.

- The **ligamentum teres** is the remnant of the left umbilical vein. It divides the left lobe of the liver in the lateral and medial parts.

The vessels of the liver

The liver receives oxygenated blood from the hepatic artery and nutrient-rich blood from the GI tract via the hepatic portal vein, both of which enter through the **porta hepatis**. The hepatic veins drain both blood supplies directly into the inferior vena cava.

The innervation of the liver

Sympathetic and parasympathetic fibres pass through the **porta hepatis** to innervate the liver. The function of these has not been determined.

The biliary tract and gallbladder

Bile is produced by the liver for emulsification of fats and excretion of some products. It can be secreted into the intestine at meal times, or stored and concentrated in the gallbladder, located on the undersurface of the liver.

Bile passes out of the liver through the hepatic duct. It then passes either straight into the common bile duct to enter the duodenum through the sphincter of Oddi or into the gallbladder for storage. Bile is released postprandially from the gallbladder, and then travels down the cystic duct to the common bile duct, which is formed when the cystic duct unites with the hepatic duct at the upper end of the lesser omentum (Fig. 14.50).

The pancreas

The pancreas has important exocrine and endocrine functions. The exocrine portion secretes its products into the GI tract to help digestion, whereas the endocrine portion secretes hormones directly into the bloodstream and is discussed in Chapters 8 and 10.

The morphology of the pancreas

The pancreas crosses from the concavity of the duodenum, anterior to the inferior vena cava, to the spleen across the posterior abdominal wall. The exocrine secretions are carried by the pancreatic duct which runs out of the head of the pancreas (Fig. 14.51). Anatomically, the pancreas is divided into five sections:

1 The **head** lies in the concavity of the duodenum anterior to the inferior vena cava. It is supplied by the superior and inferior pancreaticoduodenal arteries which are tributaries of the coeliac and superior mesenteric arteries, respectively.
2 The **uncinate** process extends to the neck, separated by the superior mesenteric vessels.

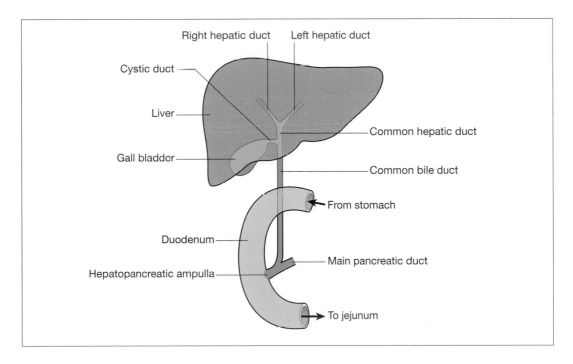

Figure 14.50 The biliary tree is responsible for the transport of bile. Bile is produced in the liver, and drains from the right and left hepatic ducts which are formed by the progressive union of biliary canaliculi. The hepatic ducts then unite to form the common hepatic duct. At most times the bile is diverted via the cystic duct where it is stored in the gallbladder, and concentrated until needed. The bile is drained into the gut via the common bile duct which enters the duodenum at the ampulla. The common bile duct merges with the pancreatic duct immediately before draining into the gut.

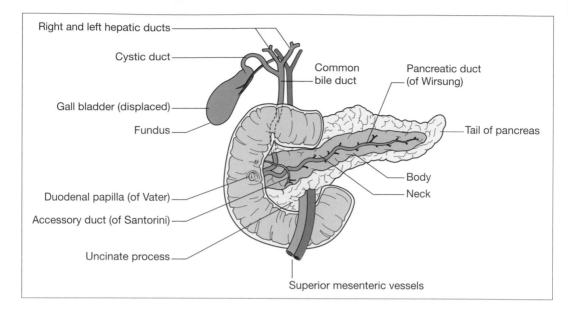

Right and left hepatic ducts

Cystic duct

Common bile duct

Pancreatic duct (of Wirsung)

Gall bladder (displaced)

Fundus

Tail of pancreas

Body

Neck

Duodenal papilla (of Vater)

Accessory duct (of Santorini)

Uncinate process

Superior mesenteric vessels

Figure 14.51 The pancreas is located in the abdomen surrounded by the duodenum. It is also closely related to the superior mesenteric artery.

3 The **neck** lies over the portal vein and the common bile duct.
4 The **body** crosses the aorta, the left adrenal gland and the left kidney.
5 The **tail** stretches to the spleen. The tail of the pancreas is supplied by the large splenic artery, a principal branch of the coeliac artery.

The pancreas is supplied by the splenic artery, superior mesenteric artery and gastroduodenal artery, and blood drains into the portal vein, which passes close behind the pancreas.

The spleen

The spleen is formed from highly vascular matter encapsulated by a fibrous casing and a layer of visceral peritoneum; although it does not contribute to the function of the GI tract, the spleen is discussed here, because it is located in the abdomen. The spleen is kidney shaped and found in the left hypochondrium below the ninth to eleventh ribs and is in contact with the diaphragm and most other neighbouring structures. The spleen contains two types of tissue – red and white pulp:

- The **red pulp** contains macrophages that remove old/damaged blood cells and particulate matter.

- The **white pulp** contains many leukocytes which are responsible for the production of immune responses to antigens in the blood.

The splenic artery, a branch of the coeliac artery, supplies the spleen, whereas it is drained by the splenic vein, which contributes to the portal system. Lymphatics follow the blood vessels and drain into nodes around the coeliac trunk, at the level of the T12 vertebral body.

The urinary system

The urinary system is responsible for the excretion of waste products and the conservation of water and essential ions. It is located predominantly in the pelvis and consists of two kidneys, two ureters, the bladder and the urethra (Fig. 14.52). The mechanisms by which the urinary system achieves these function are discussed in Chapter 9.

The kidneys

The kidneys balance the excretion of waste products with the conservation of water and vital ions.

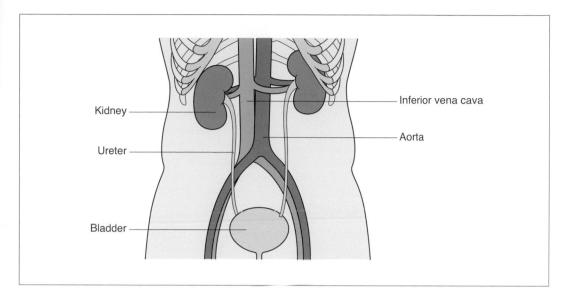

Figure 14.52 The urinary system is made up of three parts: the kidneys are located retroperitoneally on the posterior wall of the abdomen. They are supplied by the renal arteries which arise from the aorta at the level of L1. The renal arteries enter the kidney at the hilum, immediately posterior to the renal veins, which drain directly into the inferior vena cava. The ureters drain urine from the kidneys, and course through the abdomen to reach the bladder in the pelvis. Urine is stored in the bladder until it can be voided when it is released through the urethra. The bladder can easily expand to contain a large volume of urine and is located in the base of the pelvis on the anterior wall.

The kidneys receive a generous blood supply from the renal arteries, which allows it to sense the blood volume and composition and respond accordingly.

The position of the kidneys

The kidneys are retroperitoneal and lie on the posterior abdominal wall in the paravertebral gutters, either side of the vertebrae. The left kidney is higher than the right (due to the presence of the liver). The upper poles of the kidney are found at the level of the eleventh rib, on the left, and the twelfth rib, on the right. The kidneys are obliquely oriented, with their medial borders anterior to lateral borders.

The structure of the kidneys

Each kidney is enclosed in a thin capsule, with access occurring only at the hilum of each kidney. The hilum is found on the medial border of the kidney and carries (from anterior to posterior):

- The renal vein
- The renal artery with associated autonomic nerves and lymphatics
- The pelvis of the ureter.

If the kidney is cut vertically in cross-section three internal layers can be identified:

1 Outer pale **cortex**
2 Inner dark **medulla** containing triangular masses (known as pyramids), the apices of which appear striated
3 **Collecting tubules** draining to from 7–13 funnel-shaped **minor calyces**. These form two to three **major calyces** that drain into the **pelvis**.

The precise histology and function of each part of the kidneys are described in Chapter 13.

The vasculature of the kidneys

The **renal arteries** supply the kidney. The left artery is short and wide; the right artery is longer because it travels behind the inferior vena cava to arrive at the right kidney. Both arteries split into roughly five segmental branches before entering the hila of the kidneys. These, in turn, branch into progressively smaller vessels, leading to the production of many afferent arterioles, each one supplying a single glomerulus.

The venous drainage of the kidneys is through the **renal veins** which drain into the inferior vena cava:

- The right renal vein drains directly into the inferior vena cava.
- The left renal vein passes anterior to the aorta before entering the inferior vena cava.

The adrenal glands

The adrenal glands secrete several hormones into the bloodstream. One is located on each of the superior poles of the kidneys. The adrenal glands are composed of two distinct regions:

1 The **adrenal medulla** is the site of adrenaline and noradrenaline synthesis, as part of the sympathetic nervous response
2 The **adrenal cortex** produces the corticosteroid hormones:
   - **aldosterone** has a role in water and electrolyte concentration
   - **cortisol** is involved in the stress response
   - **androgen** has a role in sexual function.

The ureters

The ureters are the narrow muscular tubes that carry urine from the kidney to the bladder. The course of the ureters is long and they pass over many prominent structures. Each ureter travels downwards on psoas from the renal pelvis to the pelvic brim. At the sacroiliac joint, each ureter crosses the bifurcation of the common iliac artery to travel on the side wall of the pelvis. At the level of the ischial spine, each ureter passes forward and medially in the fascia of the pelvic floor to arrive at the lateral angle of the bladder.

Each ureter enters the bladder at an oblique angle. The ureters enter the bladder at the trigone, a region on the posteroinferior part of the bladder wall. The oblique entry acts as a valve to prevent reflux up the ureters when the pressure within the bladder is increased – as in voiding.

The structure and function of the bladder

The bladder is a hollow, muscular, distensible organ for short-term storage of urine. Its superior surface (fundus) reaches from the apex (which rests behind the pubic symphysis) to the ureters. The posterior surface (base) of the bladder continues from the two ureters downwards to the internal urethral orifice. Finally, the two

triangular side walls join in the midline from the apex to the internal urethral orifice. This structure is adapted to its function (Fig. 14.53):

- **Grossly**: the fundus has the capacity to expand upwards as the bladder fills. The peritoneum loosely covers it so that it can enlarge. Ligaments pass from the pubic symphysis to the bladder neck and facilitate urinary continence.
- **Internally**: the mucosa, lining the fundus, has multiple folds to enable expansion. The trigone is the exception because its mucosa is not thrown into folds and thus is unable to expand.
- **Orifices of the bladder**: the muscular wall of the bladder is adapted to expel urine through the internal urethral orifice effectively. It does this by increasing pressure in the bladder and also by altering its shape to form a funnel. In contrast, the ureteric orifices enter the

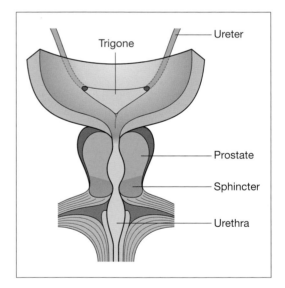

Figure 14.53 The bladder consists of various parts. In particular the **trigone** is located at the posterior wall of the bladder and is of a different embryological origin to the rest of the bladder. The main portion of the bladder constitutes the fundus, with the apex located inferiorly and the base located superiorly. The ureters enter the bladder at the superior corners of the trigone; they enter at an oblique angle to prevent the reflux of urine when the pressure is high inside the bladder. The urethra drains the bladder, and carries urine for voiding – the flow of urine from the bladder is regulated by the urinary sphincters.

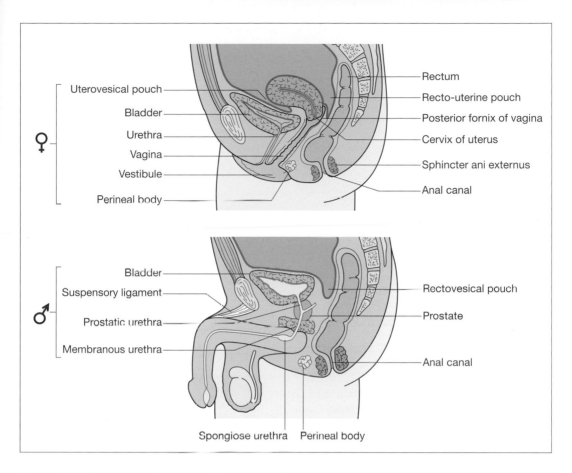

Uterovesical pouch
Bladder
Urethra
Vagina
Vestibule
Perineal body

Rectum
Recto-uterine pouch
Posterior fornix of vagina
Cervix of uterus
Sphincter ani externus
Anal canal

Bladder
Suspensory ligament
Prostatic urethra
Membranous urethra

Rectovesical pouch
Prostate

Anal canal

Spongiose urethra   Perineal body

Figure 14.54 The urethra: the course of the urethra differs considerable between the sexes, on account of the differing structures in the male and female pelvis. The female pelvis contains the uterus, located between the bladder and the rectum. The peritoneum forms two pouches between these structures – the uterovesical pouch and the rectouterine pouch. The female urethra is short, linking the bladder rapidly with the external environment. In the male pelvis the bladder and the rectum are separated by the rectouterine pouch, which is lined by the peritoneum. The male urethra is a much longer structure which passes through the prostate immediately on leaving the bladder, and then exits the body at the end of the penis.

bladder at an oblique angle, effectively preventing flow should the pressure in the bladder increase.

The reflex that empties the bladder (**micturition reflex**) relies on sensory nerves from the bladder which travel to the sacral spinal cord and parasympathetic innervation to the detrusor muscle.

The urethra

Urine leaves the bladder through the urethra. Due to the differences in pelvic anatomy, the urethra runs different courses in the different sexes (Fig. 14.54).

The female urethra

The female urethra is short and passes inferiorly and anteriorly from the bladder neck to the external urethral orifice. A voluntary external urethral sphincter encircles the urethra before it passes through the perineal membrane. The urethra is fixed to the anterior wall of the vagina and its external orifice appears anteroposteriorly superior to the vagina.

CLINICAL Cystitis

Cystitis is an infection of the bladder. It is extremely common; 2.5% of a GP practice population will consult with an infection every year.

Cystitis is more common in females than males due to the short length of the female urethra compared with the male one. Commonly, cystitis is due to infection with *Escherichia coli*. The common management is antibiotic treatment, such as nitrofurantoin or co-trimoxazole.

The male urethra

The male urethra is longer than the female one and extends from the bladder neck to the end of the penis. Anatomically, it can be broken down into four discrete parts:

1 The **preprostatic urethra** is continuous with the neck of the bladder and continues to the superior part of the prostate.
2 The **prostatic urethra** is the widest, most dilatable part or the urethra. It passes down through the prostate. The prostatic and ejaculatory ducts, which carry components of the seminal fluid, enter the urethra in the prostatic region.
3 The **membranous urethra** is the shortest, least dilatable part of the urethra. It starts at the lower end of the prostate, being continuous with the prostatic urethra. It is surrounded by the voluntary external urethral sphincter, and two bulbourethral glands lie on either side of it. The prostatic urethra travels through the pelvic floor and the perineal membrane before becoming the penile urethra.
4 The **penile urethra** starts below the perineal membrane and is surrounded by the corpus spongiosum. It is dilated in the region into which the ducts of the bulbourethral glands enter. The urethra passes through the glans penis to the external urethral orifice.

The lymph of the male urethra drains with the lymph of the tissues of the penis.

The vasculature of the urethra

The urethra receives an arterial supply from branches of the internal pudendal artery which is a terminal branch of the internal iliac. The pudendal artery leaves the pelvis via the greater sciatic foramen, entering the gluteal region. Next it curves around the sacrospinous ligament before passing through the lesser sciatic foramen to supply the perineum.

The pudendal vein runs with the pudendal artery and pudendal nerve in the pudendal canal, and empties into the internal iliac vein.

The reproductive system

The reproductive system is located in the pelvis. As the reproductive organs vary between the sexes, this is reflected in the structure of the pelvic bones, which are adapted for function.

The muscles and ligaments of the pelvis

The soft tissues of the pelvis are adapted not only for reproduction but also for weight transference. Therefore, ligaments, muscles and other soft-tissue structures complement the pelvic bones to form the walls of the pelvis.

Levator ani is the muscular septum that forms the floor of the pelvis; it is suspended from the walls of the pelvis. It is essential for control of both urinary and faecal continence.

The muscles of the pelvis insert into the fibrous **perineal body** which is found between the anal and urogenital openings in the **perineum**. The perineal body is the attachment site for the external anal sphincter, levator ani, the bulbospongiosus muscle and the superficial transverse perineal muscles, and it is crucial to maintain control of the pelvic floor.

Several structures support the internal structures of the pelvis:

- The **broad ligament** is a fold of peritoneum (not a ligament) that connects the uterus to the walls and floor of the pelvis.
- The **round ligament** maintains the uterus in an anteverted position.
- The **ovarian ligament** connects each ovary to the uterus at the uterotubal junction. It travels between the layers of the broad ligament.
- The **suspensory ligament** is a fold of peritoneum (not a ligament) that extends from each ovary to the wall of the pelvis and conveys the ovarian artery, ovarian vein and ovarian plexus.
- The **cardinal ligament** supports the cervix and the vault and lateral fornix of the vagina.

The perineum

The perineum is the superficial tissue found below the pelvic outlet, between the legs. It connects the outflow tracts of the urinary and faecal systems and is also the site of the external genitalia. The perineum is diamond shaped and stretches from the pubic symphysis to the coccyx. It is divided into two triangles by a line drawn transversely anterior to the two ischial tuberosities. The anterior part is sexually differentiated whereas the posterior part is the same in both sexes (Fig. 14.55).

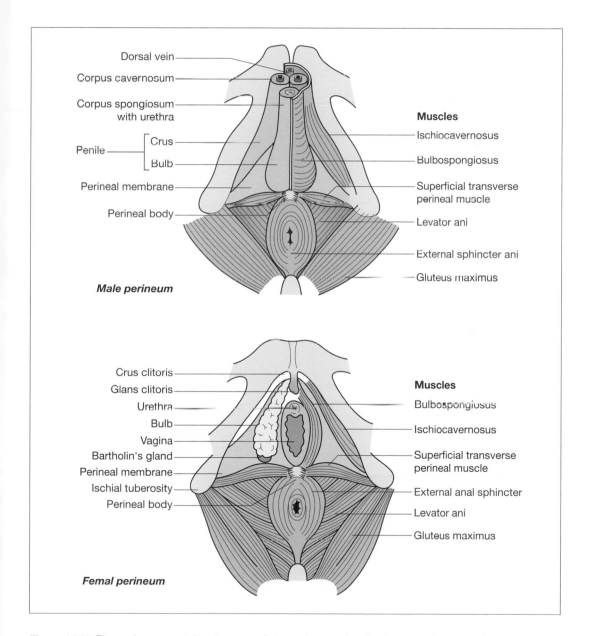

Figure 14.55 The perineum contains the urogenital openings and varies between the sexes. The perineum is divided by a line joining the ischial tuberosities. The anterior perineum contains the urogenital openings whilst the posterior perineum contains the anal region and has a similar structure between the two sexes.

The urogenital triangle

The urogenital triangle is bound by the pubic symphysis anteriorly and the two ischiopubic rami posteriorly. The urogenital triangle is divided into superficial and deep fascial compartments which are divided by the perineal membrane. The perineal membrane is composed of fibrous tissue and crosses from one ischiopubic ramus to the other. It is attached to levator ani, posteriorly, in the midline, at the perineal body. The perineal membrane is a less discrete layer in females than in males.

The male urogenital triangle

The **superficial perineal pouch** lies superficial to the perineal membrane and is derived from the membranous layer of superficial fascia of the anterior abdominal wall. The superficial pouch contains the root of the penis and its muscles, vessels, nerves, the testis, epididymis and vas (see Chapter 12). Branches of the pudendal artery supply the penis whereas the dorsal veins drain it. The penis is innervated by the pudendal nerve.

Deep to the perineal membrane is a potential space, unlike the superficial pouch, that is completely enclosed. Posteriorly, the deep perineal pouch is continuous with the ischiorectal fossa. Anteriorly, it is continuous with superficial perineal pouch a through slim opening between the perineal membrane and pubic symphysis. Its roof is formed from levator ani which passes laterally around the inferior aspect of the prostate to join the perineal body. The **membranous urethra** is found between the perineal membrane and the pelvic floor, surrounded by the external urethral sphincter. The bulbourethral glands are positioned either side of membranous urethra, their ducts piercing the bulb of the urethra.

The female urogenital triangle

The female urogenital triangle is where the urethra exits and the vagina enters, the vagina passing through the perineal membrane between the perineal body and the urethra:

- There is **no superficial perineal** pouch in the female.
- Deep to the perineal membrane, the urethra and external urethral sphincter are attached to the anterior wall of the vagina.

The urethra and the vagina pierce levator ani and the perineal membrane, and open directly on to skin of the anterior triangle.

The female urogenital triangle contains several structures:

- The **entrance of the urethra**
- The **vagina**
- The **labiaminora** which are two small cutaneous folds that form both the lateral and the anterior boundaries of the vestibule. They are attached, and surround, the clitoris, at the anterior border
- The **clitoris**: two masses of erectile tissue, the bulbs of the vestibule, unite; these are homologues of the male corpus spongiosum
- The **labia majora**, which are fat-filled cutaneous folds that run inferiorly and posteriorly away from the mons pubis. The mons pubis is the fatty eminence, directly above the pubic symphysis. The labia majora protect the vestibular glands (comparable to the bulbourethral glands of the male).

The blood vessels and nerves of the urogenital triangle

The urogenital triangle is supplied by the internal pudendal artery and pudendal nerve (S2, -3, -4) and drained by the pudendal vein. In the male, the deep and superficial dorsal veins drain the penis; these empty into the saphenous vein.

Most of the lymph passes with the pudendal artery to the internal iliac nodes. In the male, the lymph from the skin and fascia of the penis and scrotum drains to the superficial inguinal nodes.

The male genital system

The male genital system produces gametes and transfers them to the female. The scrotum encases the sperm-making apparatus: the testes, epididymis and vas deferens. The seminal vesicles and prostate produce chemicals to prime the sperm for delivery and the urethra provides a vehicle to transport them.

The scrotum

The scrotum is a pouch of skin that holds the testes and epididymis outside the body because the optimum conditions for sperm production is lower than the core body temperature.

The cremaster muscle, derived from the internal oblique muscle of the abdominal wall, is able to induce depression and elevation of the scrotum, to adjust its temperature. The cremaster is innervated by the genital branch of the genitofemoral nerve (L2).

The testes

The testes produce male gametes and sex hormones. Each testis is an oval body with a superior and inferior pole covered by derivatives of the serous, muscular and fibrous layers of the abdomen as a result of the journey that they make before birth. It is composed of numerous seminiferous tubules lined with spermatogenic epithelium. These tubules form the vasa efferentia from which sperm move to the vas deferens and then to the head of the epididymis (Fig. 14.56).

The testes are suspended in the scrotum by the **spermatic cord**, a cable-like structure that runs from the abdomen to each testicle. The spermatic cord is covered by layers of muscle derived from the abdominal wall: the internal spermatic fascia, cremaster and external spermatic fascia. Inside the inguinal canal, the spermatic cord travels alongside the ilioinguinal nerve and the genital branch of the genitofemoral nerve. The spermatic cord contains:

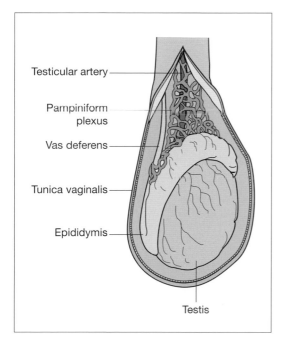

- the **vas deferens** with its arterial and lymphatic supply
- remnants of the **processus vaginalis**
- the **testicular vessels**, **lymphatics** and **sympathetic nerves**.

The testes release sperm into the **epididymis**, a series of coiled tubes that descend the testes. The epididymis continues inferiorly with the **vas deferens**, which conveys sperm to the ejaculatory ducts.

The testicular vessels

- The testicular artery supplies the testis and the epididymis. It arises from the aorta just below the level of the renal arteries at L2.
- The testicular veins form a network, the **pampiniform plexus**, which maintains temperature control of the testes to keep them at $1°$ below that of the rest of the body. It does this by surrounding the spermatic cord, thus cooling the incoming arterial blood. The right testicular vein drains directly into the inferior vena cava. The left, on the other hand, drains into the left renal vein.

The **lymphatic vessels** drain the epididymis. They follow the course of the testicular arteries and empty into the para-aortic nodes.

The **sympathetic nerves** accompany the testicular arteries and innervate **smooth muscle fibres** which enable the scrotal skin to wrinkle, and thus draw the testes closer to the body when the temperature is too low.

The accessory glands of the male reproductive system

The accessory glands secrete fluid into the urethra to provide the optimum atmosphere for sperm and lubrication to ease delivery. The glands are:

- the **seminal vesicles**
- the **prostate**
- the **bulbourethral glands**.

Seminal vesicles

The seminal vesicles are tubular glands that produce fructose and other substances for release in semen. The vesicles lie lateral to each vas deferens which they join to form the ejaculatory duct. The ejaculatory duct travels through the prostate and opens on the posterior wall of the prostatic urethra.

Figure 14.56 The testes are the site of sperm production. They are located outside the main body, in the scrotum which aids sperm production. The testes are encased in the tunica vaginalis, which also contains the testicular artery, supplying the testes and pampiniform plexus of veins that drains the testis and acts as a heat exchanger to maintain the cooler environment.

Labels in figure: Testicular artery, Pampiniform plexus, Vas deferens, Tunica vaginalis, Epididymis, Testis

The prostate

The prostate forms the acid phosphatase-rich part of the seminal fluid. The fluid drains into the urethra. This spherical gland with a firm muscular stroma encompasses the prostatic urethra. It lies on the pelvic floor, beneath the bladder, behind the pubic symphysis and in front of the rectum.

The penis

Semen is expelled through the urethra during emission and ejaculation. It is lengthened and encompassed in erectile tissue to form the penis; this allows semen to be deposited close to the uterus during sexual intercourse. The root of the penis joins the perineal membrane. The membranous urethra penetrates the perineal membrane anterior to its free posterior border. It then enlarges to form the bulb of the urethra. (Fig. 14.55)

Three masses of erectile tissue, the two corpora cavernosa and the corpus spongiosum, project from the root of the penis:

- The **corpora cavernosa** lies dorsally, attached at the midline.

- The **corpus spongiosum** lies ventrally and expands distally to form the glans penis, the most distal part of the penis.

The penis is supplied by branches of the internal pudendal arteries, whereas the penile skin is supplied by branches of the external pudendal arteries. The deep arteries of the penis supply the erectile tissue of the penis, and are involved in erection.

Lymph from the skin of the penis drains to the superficial inguinal nodes. However, lymph from the glans penis empties into a node in the femoral canal. The prostatic urethra is innervated, autonomically, from the pelvic plexus. Somatic sensory innervation is from branches of the pudendal nerve.

The female genital system

The female genital system encompasses the structures involved in the ripening and release of gametes and the support of the fetus during pregnancy. There are four major structures in the female reproductive system (Fig. 14.57):

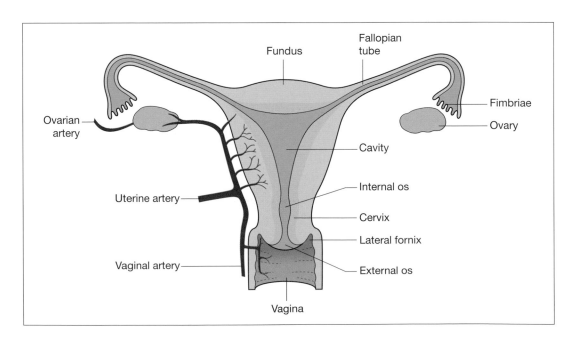

Figure 14.57 The female pelvic organs consist of the ovaries which mature and release ova; these are carried to the fallopian tubes where they are may be fertilised by sperm. If this is the case, the fertilised ovum implants in the uterus where it develops and grows during pregnancy. The ovarian and uterine arteries anastomose with each other, contributing to the supply of the pelvic organs.

1 The **ovaries** are the site of ovum release and oestrogen production.
2 The **fallopian tubes** carry the ovum to the uterus.
3 The **uterus** is the site where the fertilised ovum implants.
4 The **vagina** is the passage from the uterus to the external environment.

The ovaries

The ovaries are ovoid structures located in the **rectouterine pouch** alongside the distal ends of the fallopian tubes. The ovaries produce female gametes prenatally. Postnatally they are involved in female hormone production, egg maturation and release.

 DEFINITION The rectouterine pouch

The rectouterine pouch, also known as the pouch of Douglas, is formed by peritoneum. Peritoneum covers the upper third of the rectum anteriorly and laterally, but only the anterior surface of its middle third. The peritoneum is reflected forward from its middle third on to the posterior fornix of the vagina and uterus to form the rectouterine pouch.

The male equivalent is the rectovesical pouch in which the peritoneum is reflected on to the bladder.

The vasculature of the ovaries

The ovaries receive a rich blood supply from the ovarian arteries, which branch from the abdominal aorta beneath the renal arteries. Branches of the ovarian artery anastomose with the terminal branches of the uterine artery around the ovary.

Right and left ovarian veins empty into the inferior vena cava or the left renal vein, respectively. Lymph drains in the lymphatics which travel alongside the arteries in the opposite direction into the para-aortic nodes.

The fallopian tubes

Each fallopian tube lies in the broad ligament and links the ovaries to the superior part of the uterus, transporting an egg between these bodies. The end closest to the ovary is expanded to form the infundibulum which has numerous prolongations, known as **fimbriae**, to capture the ovum as it is released from the ovary.

The uterus

The uterus is the site of development of the fertilised ova. It is continuous with the cervix and positioned behind the bladder. The uterus is normally anteverted (tilting forwards) and anteflexed (flexed forwards); it is maintained in this position by the round ligaments. The uterus is mobile and its position changes during pregnancy; the round ligament has some oestrogen-dependent smooth muscle so its structure varies according to oestrogen production. The uterus can be divided into three major parts:

1 The **fundus** lies superior to the fallopian tube openings.
2 The **body** of the uterus makes up most of the organ.
3 The **cervix** is the neck of the uterus.

The vagina

The vagina is the muscular canal through which sperm enter the female reproductive tract and also the exit for menses, and the passage for birth of the fetus. The vagina stretches from the cervix to the opening on to the perineum and lies between the urethra and rectum.

The vasculature of the uterus and vagina

The vasculature of the female genital tract is derived from several vessels, the branches of which anastomose. The major supplying vessels are:

- the **uterine artery**, a branch of the internal iliac artery, which supplies the superior part of the vagina and the uterus
- the **ovarian artery** which contributes to supply the uterine tubes at the end of its courses, as well as supplying the ovaries.

The veins draining the uterus follow the course of the arteries and drain into the internal iliac vein and ovarian vein. Most of the lymph passes to the internal iliac nodes.

Medical imaging

A variety of techniques can be used to image the internal structure of the body. In general, images are generated in one of three planes, each of which is at 90° to the other:

- The **sagittal plane** is a vertical plane that lies in the anteroposterior plane. It is as if a knife has cut you between the eyes from front to back all the way down your body.
- The **coronal plane** is a vertical plane at right angles to this. It would be as if your body was cut from a line that stretched between your ears.
- The **transverse plane** is also known as the axial plane. It involves cutting the body into cross sections at different levels.

Five major techniques are commonly used to image the internal structures of the body:

- Plain radiographs
- Contrast media
- Computed tomography (CT)
- Magnetic resonance imaging (MRI)
- Ultrasonography.

Plain radiographs

Plain radiographs are obtained by passing X-rays through the patient on to photographic film. The degree of exposure that the film receives depends on the absorption of different tissues of the body. Air is radiolucent, bone and metal radio-opaque. The differences in radiodensity allow detection of breaks in the bones as well as the identification of other pathology if it has a different radiodensity to the surrounding tissue.

The chest radiograph

A plain radiograph is frequently taken to investigate thoracic pathology. Chest radiographs are commonly taken in a posteroanterior (PA) fashion – the patient faces the radiographic film and the X-rays are dispersed from back to front. The patient must have the shoulders protracted to give the best lung field exposure. The chest radiograph must also be taken when the patient is inspiring fully which generates large radiotranslucent fields, to improve the chance of detecting radio-opaque pathologies. This positioning enables the soft tissue structures to be seen most clearly (Fig. 14.58).

Computed tomography

CT is a type of three-dimensional radiography. X-rays are passed through the body and measured on emergence but, with CT, a narrow beam is used and an array of sensors used to receive the X-rays instead of film. The beam is rotated around the patient to enable measurements to be taken at many angles, allowing generation of three-dimensional images of the

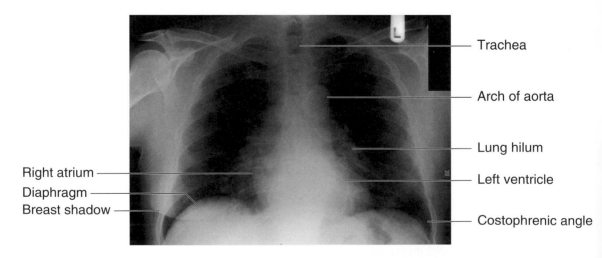

Figure 14.58 chest radiograph can allow identification of the major structures in the thorax. In particular, the borders of the right atrium and left ventricle can be seen either side of the spinal cord. Enlargement of these border may be seen in congestive heart failure, and other cardiomyopathies. The arch of the aorta and the ribs are also visible. The lungs are of low density and appear clear on the radiograph.

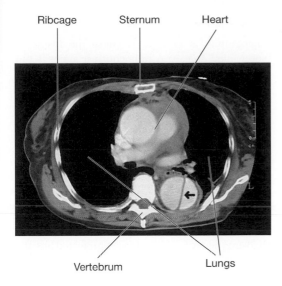

Ribcage   Sternum   Heart

Vertebrum   Lungs

Figure 14.59 Computed tomography allows the body to be viewed in three dimensions. The images are typically presented as axial slices viewed from the feet up. The slice shown here is from the thorax of a patient who has a dissection of the aorta. The intima can be clearly seen (arrow) and a false lumen has formed and filled with blood.

patient. CT scans are typically shown as a series of axial slices viewed from below (Fig. 14.59).

Magnetic resonance imaging

MR images are different to CT scans because they detect biochemical composition of the tissues rather than their density, which is detected by CT. In MRI patients are placed in a magnetic field and they are exposed to a sequence of magnetic pulses. This causes energy to be released from various molecules in the body, particularly water. The differences in energy released are shown on an image as changes in brightness. Depending on the type of MR scan, the characteristic intensity of signal varies. Similar to CT scans, MR images are viewed from the imaginary foot of the bed looking up towards the patient's head.

Two common methods used to differentiate tissue types further are T1- and T2-weighted images. These rely on slightly different manipulations of energy and are useful when looking for a particular pathology (Fig. 14.60):

- **T1-weighted images** cause fat to be white whereas fluid appears dark.

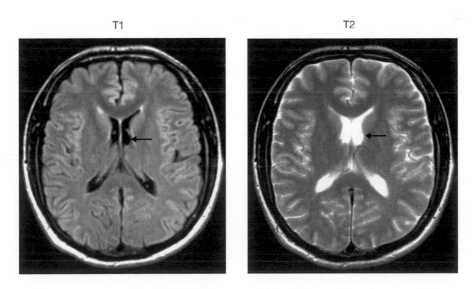

T1

T2

Figure 14.60 Magnetic resonance imaging can be performed with different weightings to the scan, allowing the highlighting of different tissue types and the identification of different pathologies. The two scans presented are of healthy brains. Both the T1- and the T2-weighted images highlight fatty tissue (white); however, in T2-weighted images the fluid (in this case, cerebrospinal fluid) is also highlighted. Similarly, fluid found in inflammation is illuminated in T2-weighted images.

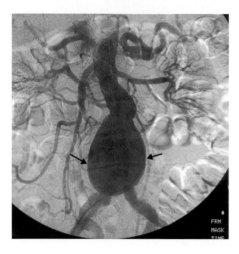

Figure 14.61 Angiography involves the placement of a catheter, allowing the release of a radio-opaque contrast medium into a blood vessel. This can then be imaged by a fluoroscope, which allows real-time X-ray imaging. In this figure, the aorta of the patient appears dark and a large aneurysm can be seen (arrows).

- In **T2-weighted images**, fat and fluid-filled tissues both appear bright, whereas those containing fat are darker, allowing identification of potential pathology (Fig. 14.60).

Angiography

Angiography is used to visualise the inside of blood-filled spaces. A radiocontrast agent is put into the bloodstream via a catheter into a peripheral artery. X-rays are then projected through the area of interest to visualise the inside of particular vessels or the heart (Fig. 14.61).

Ultrasonography

Ultrasonography is an imaging technique for visualising soft-tissue structures. It is commonly used to visualise the growing fetus, but has multiple other uses including visualisation of soft-tissue pathology of joints, the breast, abdomen, pelvis and heart. High-frequency sound waves are projected into the area of interest, and rebounding 'echoes' are captured as an image. Doppler can be combined with ultrasonography to picture moving images of blood flow through the heart and blood vessels.

→ RELATED CHAPTERS

15

Immunology

The human body must safeguard itself from constant attack by a variety of microorganisms, and from the development of cancerous cells. This is achieved by the immune system, a diverse group of cells and tissues. The immune system has two distinct parts: the innate immune system, which acts rapidly but recognises a limited set of antigens, and the adaptive immune system, which is slower in developing a response to a new antigen, yet able to respond specifically to an almost infinite variety of antigens – molecules derived from a pathogen. The adaptive immune system is able to 'remember' a previously encountered antigen and provide a more rapid and potent response if the antigen is re-encountered.

The rapidly acting innate system is able to promote the induction of the adaptive immune system and the adaptive immune system is able to recruit and modulate the behaviour of the innate immune system to help eliminate an infection.

The immune system may malfunction and an immune response can be directed against healthy tissue in the body, potentially resulting in severe autoimmune conditions.

Innate immunity

The innate immune system is evolutionarily very old, and is concerned not only with the protection of the individual from pathogens, but also with a variety of homoeostatic and repair functions.

The innate system is characterised by a number of features:

- **Germline-encoded receptors** recognise a variety of patterns that are conserved on a variety of pathogens. After recognition of a pathogen-associated molecular pattern (PAMP), a rapid response is triggered, e.g. **toll-like receptors**.

> **DEFINITION: Germ-line encode receptors**
>
> In the immune system most receptors are tran-scribed directly from the genome – the genetic code has not been modified. The receptors have a specific ligand or set of ligands. These receptors are referred to as **Germ-line encoded receptors** – and differ from receptors in the adaptive immune system which can be generated by **somatic recombination.**

> **DEFINITION: Toll-like receptors (TLRs)**
>
> Toll-like receptors are a series of germline-encoded receptors which recognise conserved patterns found in many pathogens. Unusually for a receptor, most TLRs are capable of recognising many different stimuli. For example, TLR4 recognises many molecules, including Lipopolysaccharide and heat schock proteins.
>
> The activation of a TLR results in the induction of cytokines, promoting an inflammatory response.

Biomedical Science Lecture Notes, First Edition. Ian Lyons.
© 2011 by Ian Lyons. Published 2011 by Blackwell Publishing Ltd.

- **Phagocytic cells** can engulf pathogens and mediate their destruction.
- **Rapid responses** to infection are possible because there is no need for the induction and expansion of cells.
- **Plasma protein cascades** result when an activated plasma protein acts as a proteolytic enzyme to activate the next protein in the cascade.

 DEFINITION: Pathogen-associated molecular pattern (PAMP)

PAMPs are molecules derived from a pathogen (e.g. LPS), or produced as a result of the damage and stress the body (e.g. The heat shock proteins) is placed under during infection. PAMPs can be recognised by several receptors in the immune system to stimulate and guide the immune response.

The innate immune system is critical to the function of the adaptive immune system, providing signals to induce and activate adaptive immunity. Innate immune cells are recruited by the adaptive immune cells to serve as an effector mechanism to promote the clearance of the infection.

Adaptive immunity

The adaptive immune system generates a very specific response to an antigen. The adaptive immune system centres on the B and T lymphocytes, which possess a huge diversity of antigen receptors specific to an almost limitless range of pathogens, although it is hindered by the length of time taken to induce a response. Adaptive immunity has a number of specific features:

- **Lymphocytes** are the key cell in the adaptive immune system; an individual lymphocyte is specific to a single antigen.
- **Diverse antigen receptors are** generated by somatic recombination.
- **Immunological memory** allows a more rapid response to a pathogen on a subsequent encounter, preventing a specific strain of pathogen repeatedly causing infection in the same individual.

Cells of the immune system

All the cells in the immune system are derived from lymphoid and myeloid progenitors which are themselves derived from the common haematopoietic stem cell (Fig. 15.1).

Myeloid cells

Myeloid cells are derived from the myeloid progenitor cell and make up most of the cells in the innate immune system. The two most prominent types are the **neutrophil**, the most common leukocyte in the blood and the first cell recruited to sites on inflammation, and the **monocyte**, which develops into many different cells, particularly the macrophage and dendritic cell.

Neutrophils

Neutrophils are the most common white blood cell, making up 40–70% of leukocytes found in peripheral blood. In tissue, their presence is an indicator of infection and is associated with **acute inflammation**.

Morphology and formation

Neutrophils develop from a myeloid progenitor cell in the bone marrow. These cells are typically 9–16 µm in diameter and possess a multilobed nucleus. The cytoplasm of neutrophils contains many granules containing degradative enzymes.

Role

Neutrophils have a relatively short lifespan, 2–3 days, and rapidly migrate to the site of infection; they are the first cells found in large numbers at a site of infection. Large numbers of neutrophils are also retained in a 'marginal pool', which can be mobilised during infection to increase the number of the cells able to respond. Neutrophils phagocytose pathogen and possess a large number of granules that can fuse with the phagosome to mediate killing. The neutrophil is a short-lived cell and, once its granules are exhausted, the cell dies and contributes to the formation of **pus**.

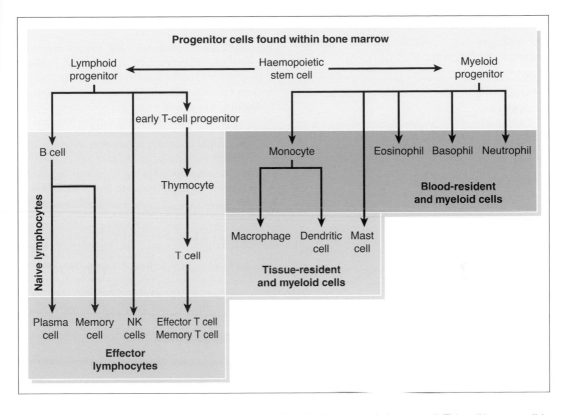

Figure 15.1 The cells of the immune system are derived from the haematopoietic stem cell. This cell is responsible for producing all the cells within the blood. Two progenitor cells derived from the haematopoietic cells give rise to the immune cells. The myeloid progenitor produces myeloid cells, which occupy compartments in the blood and tissues. The lymphoid progenitor gives rise to B cells, T cells and NK cells.

Macrophages and mononuclear cells

Macrophages are long-lived, tissue-resident cells that can detect pathogens in the tissue and produce mediators to initiate inflammation. Macrophages are one group of cell in the **mononuclear phagocyte system**, which is involved in many homoeostatic processes within the body.

Morphology and formation

Macrophages develop from circulating monocytes, which differentiate from the myeloid precursor. Monocytes make up around 5–6% of the circulating leukocytes, typically remaining in the circulation for 1–2 days before differentiating into macrophages on entering tissue. Macrophages are large cells, possessing many

cytotoxic granules, and have a single round nucleus.

 CLINICAL: The Mononuclear phagocyte cells

Macrophages are closely related to other cell groups in the body, which all have a role in tissue remodelling and homeostasis:

- **Kuppfer cells** and **splenic macrophages** remove senescent red blood cells from the circulation.
- **Osteoclasts** are involved in bone remodelling and calcium homeostasis, mediating the breakdown of the mineral deposits in bone.
- **Microglia** act as macrophages in the CNS. In embryonic development microglia are involved in phagocytosis of neurons that apoptose naturally as part of the development of the brain.

Role

Macrophages are involved in the immune response in many ways:

- Tissue-resident macrophages are the first cells to encounter a pathogen and **initiate an immune response**.
- Macrophages may **phagocytose** pathogens and induce a variety of killing mechanisms after their recruitment to the infection site.
- Macrophages are activated to **secrete cytokines,** which modulate the immune response.

Dendritic cells

Dendritic cells (DCs) provide a crucial link between the innate and adaptive immune systems. They are closely related to the mononuclear cells and may be derived from monocytes. There are many subtypes of DCs and their origin is poorly understood – both myeloid and lymphoid origins have been suggested for different subgroups.

DCs exist in an immature form in tissues, where they acquire antigen through **macropinocytosis** and **phagocytosis**. DCs may move to lymph nodes and present the acquired antigen to the adaptive immune system. In the resting state, this induces **self-tolerance**. However, in an inflammatory situation DCs can specifically activate the adaptive immune response to an antigen presents: DCs are the only cell type capable of activating naïve T cells.

 DEFINITION: Macropinocytosis and Phagocytosis

All cells are capable of taking up particles from their environment:

- In most cases small molecules are taken up through vesicles or through direct binding to a receptor.
- Specific types of cells (e.g. Macrophages and neutrophils) may be capable of taking up large (>1 µm) particles by **phagocytosis**.
- Dendritic cells have developed a mechanism of directly monitoring the external environment, sampling large amounts of fluid and particles by **macropinocytosis.**

Basophil

Basophils are blood-borne cells and are recruited to sites of inflammation, where they perform a similar function to **mast cells**. They are characterised by their alkaline granules which contain histamine. They have a number of features similar to mast cells – reflecting their similar function:

- **Cytoplasmic granules** containing inflammatory mediators including histamine
- The **IgE receptor** allowing basophils to release their granules in response to antigen binding to pre-bound IgE.

Eosinophils

Eosinophils respond to parasitic infection, through release of granules that contain molecules such as the eosinophil cationic protein and the major basic protein. Eosinophil granules stain red with the dye eosin.

Lymphoid cells

Three main groups of cells are derived from the lymphoid progenitor cell:

1. **T cells** which recognise protein antigen presented on major histocompatibility complex (MHC) molecules
2. **B cells** which produce antibodies that target extracellular antigens
3. **Natural killer (NK) cells** which can identify virally infected and cancerous cells.

T and B cells

T and B cells normally circulate through the blood and lymphatics in a dormant state or are found in the lymphoid tissues; they are small (approximately 7 µm) inactive cells that, on activation, swell to 9–15 µm in size. The antigen receptors of T and B cells are produced by genetic recombination; the receptor expressed on every T or B cell may be unique to that cell alone, resulting in a huge diversity of specificities in the whole population. T cells express a specific receptor which allows the detection of a unique protein antigen within a specific compartment of a host cell. B cells perform a similar task, detecting free-floating antigens through their immunoglobulin receptor.

T and B cells express a wide variety of additional molecules in their activated state which are involved in mediating effector functions:

- **Activated T cells** express co-stimulatory molecules to activate other parts of the immune system, or can release cytotoxic granules for killing pathogen-infected cells, although the composition of these granules is very different to that seen in myeloid cells.
- **Activated B cells** develop into plasma cells which are specialised for the secretion of antibody molecules.

Natural Killer (NK) cells

NK cells make up less than 5% of the circulating lymphocyte population. Unlike T and B cells, they express germline-encoded receptors that detect changes in the expression of a variety of molecules on the target cell's surface. These changes may indicate the presence of an infection, or a cancerous change. NK cells possess cytotoxic granules, allowing them to mediate killing of cells in which they detect pathology.

Non-cellular components of the immune system

Many proteins are initiators and/or effectors of an immune response. Some of these proteins may be produced directly by immune system cells (e.g. antibodies) whereas others are produced by the liver (e.g. complement).

Complement

The complement pathway consists of a cascade of blood-borne proteases which may be activated by some conserved elements of pathogens or some forms of antibody. Each activation pathway leads to the formation of a **C3 convertase**, which in turn leads to downstream functions promoting an effective immune response to clear the pathogen.

Production and nomenclature

Complement proteins are produced by the liver in an inactive form. They are activated as a result of proteolytic cleavage, which produces two fragments:

- The **uncleaved inactive form** of the protein is known by its number, e.g. C3.

- The small soluble fragment is designated 'a' (e.g. C3a) and can act as a mediator of inflammation.
- The larger 'b' fragment (e.g. C3b) binds to a membrane and can mediate the generation of other components in the complement cascade.

Activation of complement

There are three mechanisms by which the complement cascade may be activated (Fig. 15.2):

1 Classic pathway
2 Mannan-binding lectin pathway
3 Alternative pathway.

The **classic complement pathway** is initiated by the C1 complex, which binds to antibodies on the surface of pathogens. This molecule is made up of six 'heads' of C1q and two molecules each of C1s and C1r. The C1q molecules bind to a site on the constant region of antibodies and may also bind directly to the surface of some pathogens through the recognition of specific PAMPs. The binding of C1q activates C1s, a serine protease which recruits and cleaves C4, the next component on the complement cascade.

The cleavage of C4 into the membrane-bound C4b allows it to bind a C2 component, exposing it to the proteolytic activity of C1s, thus producing a C4bC2b molecule: an **active C3 convertase**.

The **mannan-binding lectin (MBL) pathway** is very similar to the classic complement pathway. However, it is initiated by MBL instead of C1. MBL has a similar structure to C1: six collectin 'heads' bind to common bacterial surface molecules, as opposed to the Fc regions of antibodies. Binding leads to the activation of **MASP-1** and **MASP-2**, which are serine proteases similar to C1s, and trigger cleavage of C4 and then C2, to produce the C4bC2b molecule.

The **alternative complement pathway** differs from the MBL and classic pathways because it is activated in the plasma, through the spontaneous hydrolysis of C3. This allows the binding of **plasma factor B**, which is then cleaved by another plasma-based factor, factor D. The resulting C3Bb complex is a fluid-phase **C3 convertase** and produces C3b, which binds to cell surfaces. The surface-bound C3b may recruit factor B to produce membrane-bound C3 convertase.

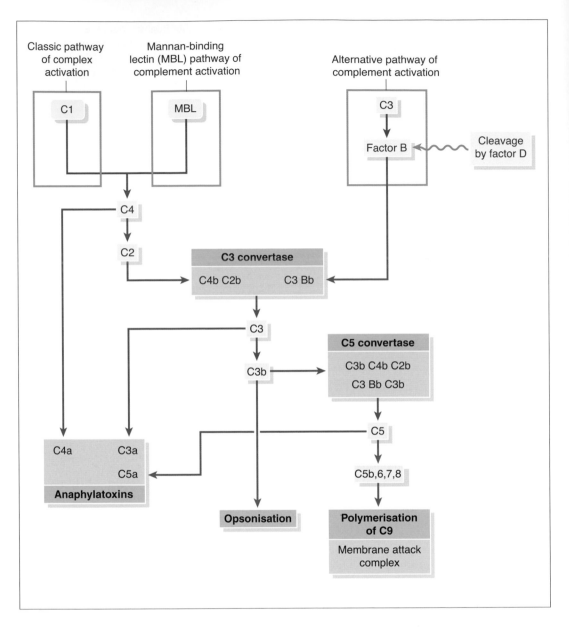

Figure 15.2 The complement cascade may be activated by three different methods, which converge of the formation of the C3 convertase. This contributes to the various effector mechanisms of complement: through the production of anaphylotoxins; the deposition of C3b; and the assembly of the membrane attack complex.

Host cells produce control proteins to prevent the build-up of C3 convertase on their surface; factors such as factor H and decay accelerating factor are able to displace the Bb molecule, inactivating the C3 convertase. The surface of a pathogen does not possess such inhibitory actions, and instead allows binding of **properdin (factor P)** which stabilises the C3 convertase, increasing its effectiveness.

Effector mechanisms

The C3 convertase forms the basis of the effector mechanisms in the complement pathway, which are classified into three main groups:

1 Opsonisation
2 Anaphylotoxins
3 Membrane attack complex.

Opsonisation

The C3 convertase produces membrane-bound C3b which is deposited on to the surface of pathogens. C3b can be recognised by many receptors on immune cells.

Anaphylatoxins

A series of small soluble fragments are produced by cleavage of the complement proteins: **C3a**, **C5a** and **C4a** (as part of the classic pathway). These molecules bind to receptors and mediate inflammatory changes. They have a variety of actions related to inflammation:

- Induce smooth muscle contraction
- Increase permeability of blood vessels
- Recruit leukocytes directly to sites of inflammation
- Trigger release of inflammatory molecules (e.g. histamine)
- Activate expression of adhesion molecules on the endothelium to recruit leukocytes.

The membrane–attack complex

The membrane–attack complex assembles a pore in the bacterial cell that disrupts the osmotic gradient into the bacterial cell, as well as allowing degradative enzymes into the pathogen. The production of **C5b** by **C5 convertase** (which is formed by the binding of C3b to a C3 convertase) is the first step in the production of a membrane–attack complex. **C5b** recruits **C7** and **C6** from the plasma, which bind to the pathogen surface and recruit **C8**, which inserts into the membrane. After this, **C9** is recruited and activated, when it can polymerise to form a pore in the bacterial cell membrane.

The membrane–attack complex is particularly important in the immune response to *Neisseria* species. This is highlighted in an increased susceptibility to infections by *Neisseria* spp. in those with deficiencies of the components.

Antibodies

Antibodies are produced by plasma cells, the differentiated form of B cells, and represent a major mechanism for specific recognition of pathogen. Varying classes of antibodies can be produced to recruit different parts of the immune response for an effective response to a specific pathogen (Fig. 15.3).

All antibodies share a conserved structure which is encoded by the imunoglobulin genes (Ig)

consisting of two heavy chains and two light chains. They are organised to form two main functional regions:

1 The **variable region** is made up of part of the heavy chain and part of the light chain. This has a highly variable structure and produces a highly specific binding site.
2 The **constant (Fc) region** varies between different classes of antigen and is made up of the heavy chain only. The Fc region can bind various receptors, determining the immune effector mechanisms recruited.

A **J chain** can bind to IgA and IgM, allowing them to form multimeric structures. This allows the antibody to bind at a lower affinity, through the presence of many more binding sites.

Cytokines

Cytokines are secreted molecules that allow signalling between cells and act on specific receptors. Three major cytokine groups have been identified in relation to their structure:

1 **Interleukins** (IL) are cytokines that are produced by and alter the behaviour and function of leukocytes. They often have a generalised function, such as the systemic response to inflammation (IL-1, IL-6).
2 **Interferon** can be subdivided into two groups:
   - **IFNα** and **IFNβ** are associated with the antiviral response to double-stranded RNA (dsRNA)
   - **IFNγ** is a crucial signal in the T-helper 1 (Th1) response, through its ability to activate macrophages.
3 **Tumour necrosis factor (TNF)-related molecules** are involved in a wide variety of process. Soluble examples such as TNFα may be involved in inflammation, whereas membrane-bound TNF-related proteins may undertake a variety of effector functions such as the Fas ligand in cytotoxic killing.

Inflammation and repair

A key feature of an early immune response is inflammation – the release of molecules that signal the presence of tissue damage, as well as of a pathogen. This process rapidly recruits neutrophils and other immune system components to the site to initiate an immune response.

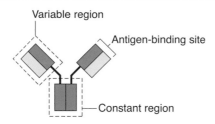

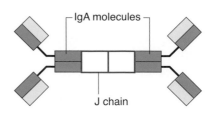

IgG

IgG is the most common form of antibody found in the plasma, playing a major role in post-infection immunity. It is found as a monomer; its small size allows it to enter tissue fluid which is not restricted to the bloodstream. There are many subclasses of IgG, with different Fc regions allowing different effector responses.

IgA

IgA is a higher affinity antibody produced later in the immune response. It is commonly found in the blood and secreted on to mucosa by means of a special transporter, where it mediates protection at the mucosal surface. In the mucosa it is found as a dimer linked by a J chain, and an additional secretory component that is involved in the transport of the molecule across the epithelial membrane. The secretory component mediates some protection against the proteolytic enzymes found in the gut.

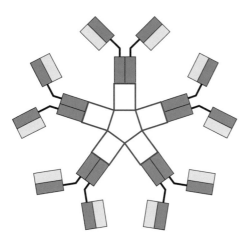

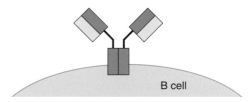

IgD

Expression of the IgD isoform is restricted to the surface of the B cells, where it is the major isoform expressed. IgD is not detectable in the plasma.

IgM

IgM is the first antibody isoform produced in a primary immune response. It may be found in a monomeric form on the surface of B cells where it acts as cellular receptor to activate them to differentiate and proliferate as an immune response. IgM antibodies have a relatively low binding affinity antibody, produced rapidly at the start of the adaptive immune response. They are found as a pentamer, producing a molecule with high avidity despite the low binding affinity of each Fab region. IgM recruits C1 of the complement pathway as an effector mechanism; IgM does not bind directly to a receptor.

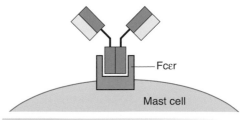

IgE

A high-affinity monomeric isoform that is capable of binding to its receptor on mast cells before binding to antigens. Upon binding antigen, it is able to mediate mast cell degranulation – important in tissue responses to pathogens, and also the basis of type I hypersensitivity.

The process of inflammation itself also damages tissues. As a result, repair is closely linked to inflammation.

Acute inflammation

Acute inflammation constitutes the rapid response to infection and injury, whereby the host attempts to limit damage and infection, and then promotes healing and recovery of function. Acute inflammation can be characterised by four cardinal features:

1 Heat
2 Redness
3 Swelling
4 Pain.

Histological changes

Acute inflammation is characterised by the influx of neutrophils which migrate into the tissue in large numbers from surrounding venules. The tissue layers become divided, as a result of the oedema, because of the increased vascularity of the vessels.

Pyogenic bacterial infections are controlled by phagocytosis, achieved primarily by neutrophils. This results in the formation of pus, which contains fluid, dead tissue, bacteria and other foreign bodies, as well as dead and living leukocytes. The whole structure becomes contained in an **abscess**. The influx of neutrophils is at its peak during the first 6 hours of inflammation. In later stages, macrophages are recruited.

 DEFINITION: Abscess

An abscess is a localised collection of pus contained in a cavity, preventing the escape of the bacteria into the system.

Leukocyte migration

To reach the site on infection, leukocytes must exit the circulation and migrate into the tissues. This process can be divided into four stages:

1 Leukocyte rolling
2 Adhesion to endothelium
3 Diapedesis
4 Leukocyte migration within the tissues (**chemotaxis**).

Leukocyte rolling

When leukocytes reach sites of inflammation they must first attach to the endothelium. Initially, this is by low-affinity interaction between **selectin** molecules and their carbohydrate ligands, both of which are constitutively expressed. This interaction causes 'leukocyte rolling' which is a normal physiological occurrence; 60–300% of circulating neutrophils are thought to exist in a marginal pool in this state which allows the leukocytes to sample cytokines and bind to other molecules expressed on the endothelial surface.

Adhesion to endothelium

In inflammation, cytokines and other inflammatory mediators causes the upregulation of adhesion molecules such as selectins and integrins on the endothelial cells. The cytokines also act on the leukocytes, where they trigger rapid changes in cell surface integrins. The conformational changes allow integrins on the leukocytes to bind with a high affinity to cell surface adhesion molecules (CAMs). The interaction between CAMs and integrins halts the leukocyte rolling, enabling a tight adherence.

Diapedesis

Leukocytes must cross the endothelium to reach the inflamed tissues. This process takes several minutes to occur and is tightly regulated by a variety of molecules, in particular by CD31 (PECAM-1 or platelet endothelial cell adhesion molecule 1), which is expressed by both leukocytes and endothelial cells. Leukocytes must also cross the basement membrane by producing various enzymes; neutrophils can express elastase and macrophages express collagenase. The release of the enzymes breaks down endothelial basement membrane to allow migration and contributes to the tissue damage that occurs during inflammation.

Figure 15.3 Antibodies can exist in many different classes. These are determined by the constant (Fc) regions of the antibody, which are made up solely from the heavy chains. The differences in Fc region allow antibodies to bind to different groups of receptors and other organising chains, which allows antibodies with the same specificity to perform different functions or form different multimeric structures.

Leukocyte chemotaxis

Once in the tissues, leukocytes migrate by following a chemokine gradient. Chemokines are produced at the site of inflammation and bind to the extracellular matrix. A major chemokine, IL-8, is produced by tissue-resident macrophages that first encounter pathogens and recruit neutrophils. Different chemokines can attract different cell types; later in inflammation, macrophages become the predominant migrating cell type and are recruited by chemokines such as macrophage chemotactic protein-1 (MCP-1).

Systemic response to acute inflammation

There is a systemic innate response to inflammation, which is triggered by macrophage-secreted cytokines, in particular IL-1, IL-6 and TNFα:

- **TNFα** increases the breakdown of the body's fat supplies to increase the available energy stores. Appetite is reduced causing weight loss during illness.
- Cytokines **act on the hypothalamus** to increase body temperature – with the aim to inhibit the replication of pathogens.
- **Synthesis of acute phase proteins** is triggered in the liver, including:
  - innate immune system molecules – complement components, etc.
  - clotting-related molecules, e.g. fibrinogen
  - regulatory molecules, e.g. α_1-antitrypsin.

Chronic inflammation

However, in some cases inflammation may persist – resulting in a chronic inflammation. Here there is T-cell involvement and the predominant cell becomes the macrophage, as opposed to the neutrophil. The precise nature of the inflammation varies with the cause – although the key difference to acute inflammation is that there is evidence of **repair**.

Histology

Chronic inflammation can be identified by its hard red swelling. It is typified by:

- A mononuclear cell infiltrate
- An absence of neutrophils
- Little oedema or pus
- Evidence of repair, in particular collagen deposition by recruited fibroblasts.

Pathogenesis

Both pathogens and foreign particles may cause forms of chronic inflammation. Non-toxic particles such as silica can be taken up by macrophages and trigger their activation. The secretion of toxic products such as H_2O_2 by macrophages, in an attempt to clear the silica, leads to tissue damage and chronic inflammation.

Formation of granulomatous inflammation

A specific form of chronic inflammation is granulomatous inflammation, which is characterised by the formation of discrete lesions, granulomas, that attempt to wall off the inflammation. A granuloma forms when the antigen triggering the inflammation cannot be removed by activated macrophages. Many macrophages (often activated) are found within the granuloma, as well as two other specialised cells, which are derived from them:

1. Multinucleated **giant cells**, formed by the fusion of many macrophages
2. Large **epithelioid cells** which appear to be specialised for a secretory function.

The presence of activated macrophages and the low oxygen contributes to cell death at the centre of the granuloma. This process is known as **caseous necrosis**, in which the necrotic tissues take on a 'cheesy' texture characteristic of a granuloma.

Surrounding the central granuloma are several different cell types, which contribute to the development of the typical structure:

- **Th1 cells** are thought to promote chronic inflammation through their release of IFNγ and other cytokines, which activate macrophages.
- **Th2 cells** are thought to be involved in the regulation of the inflammatory process, both to contain the infectious agent and to limit tissue damage.
- **Fibroblasts** limit the tissue damage and start repair. Their presence results in the laying down of collagen, which is seen in an established granuloma.

Treatment

Treatment of chronic inflammation has focused on two major methods: first, **elimination of the agent** triggers the inflammatory response, such as the use of isoniazid for *Mycobacterium tuberculosis* and, second, when the stimulus is not a pathogen, treatments have been tried that **reduce the immune response**. These treatments often focus on blocking macrophage activation, stopping the cell type responsible for the immune response.

Mediators of inflammation

Many protein cascades and pathways contribute to the development of an inflammatory response – five major mediators are discussed:

1 The coagulation cascade
2 The fibrinolytic cascade
3 The kinins
4 Arachidonic acid metabolites
5 Histamine.

Coagulation cascade

Clotting prevents the spread of microorganisms into the systemic circulation by producing a physical barrier of fibrin around the infection site. It may be activated by tissue damage, through the production of tissue factor or encountering a negatively charged surface.

Fibrinolytic cascade

Although the formation of a clot by the coagulation cascade limits the spread of infection, the clot must be cleared to allow wound repair and leukocyte access.

Activation of the fibrinolytic cascade produces plasmin from plasminogen which can break down the fibrin clots. Plasmin can also activate the classic complement pathway.

Kinins

The kinins are a group of proteins produced in direct response to tissue damage. Of particular importance is the peptide **bradykinin**, which is produced by the enzyme kallikrein. Bradykinin causes vascular muscle contraction which restricts blood flow to hinder spread of infection; it is also a major pain signal. In addition, kallikrein cleaves C5 into C5b and C5a, to trigger a complement-induced inflammatory response.

Arachidonic metabolites

Arachidonic acid is released from cell membranes by the action of the enzyme **phospholipase A$_2$** (PLA$_2$). The arachidonates promote increased blood flow and cell migration. They can be divided into two major families:

1 **Leukotrienes** are produced by lipoxgyenase enzymes. Leukotrienes, particularly, act in the lungs to mediate contraction of the bronchial smooth muscle and the coronary vessels. In other vessels, they are dilatory.
2 **Prostaglandins** are produced by the cyclooxygenase (COX) family of enzymes. The COX-2 isoform is upregulated in the inflammatory response, whereas COX-1 is a housekeeping enzyme. The action of the prostaglandins is typified by vasodilatation and the activation of endothelial cells. Prostaglandins increase the effect of other vasodilatory substances instead of directly causing vasodilatation themselves.

Histamine

Histamine is released from mast cell granules. The main actions of histamine are typified by:

- contraction of smooth muscle
- vasodilatation and increased vascular permeability
- increased heart rate and contraction.

When injected into the skin, the resulting response is similar to acute inflammation, **hyperalgesia** and oedema in the skin.

Regulation of inflammatory mediators

It is essential that inflammatory processes are restricted to the sites of infection, to prevent widespread tissue damage. Regulatory proteins are produced by the liver, to inhibit the inflammatory pathways, and are upregulated as part of the **acute phase response**.

α_1-**Antitrypsin** cleaves degradative enzymes such as elastinase, which is secreted by activated macrophages. This prevents proteinase enzymes from causing widespread tissue damage.

C1 inhibitor is important in controlling the complement pathway by inactivating spontaneously activated C1s. Deficiency of C1 inhibitor is associated with **hereditary spontaneous angioneurotic oedema**.

Anti-inflammatory therapies

Anti-inflammatory therapies reduce inflammation, through one or more methods:

- Preventing the synthesis of inflammatory mediators
- Inhibiting the binding of an inflammatory mediator to its receptor
- Modulating the behaviour of immune cells through modulation of their gene expression.

In each case, the result of giving an anti-inflammatory to a patient is diminished inflammation.

Aspirin and non-steroidal anti-inflammatories

Aspirin and non-steroidal anti-inflammatory drugs (NSAIDs) inhibit COX-2, which is responsible for producing prostaglandins from arachidonic acid. The inhibition of COX-2 is associated with three major therapeutic effects:

1 **Inhibition of inflammation**: the decrease of prostaglandin reduces vasodilatation, and therefore oedema, although the number of cells migrating to the site of inflammation does not appear to be greatly reduced.
2 **Analgesic effect**: prostaglandins contribute to an increased sensitivity in pain fibres to other pain signals, such as bradykinin.
3 **Antipyretic effect**: fever is decreased through the diminished prostaglandin levels, and indirectly through reduced IL-1.

Aspirin bonds irreversibly to COX-2, whereas other NSAIDs bond reversibly. This allows aspirin to inhibit COX-2 on platelets, which has a role in the treatment of cardiovascular disease.

Side effects

Side effects result from unwanted inhibition of COX-1, which is particularly important in the gut where it maintains mucus secretion.

NSAIDs are also associated with skin reactions, which may be severe. Renal insufficiency, liver disorders and bone marrow depression are rare complications.

Steroids

Glucocorticoids act on a wide range of cells to reduce the immune response:

- Glucocorticoids reduce leukocyte migration in response to acute inflammation, and limit the processes contributing to chronic inflammation.
- Reduced **clonal expansion** of T and B cells inhibits the adaptive immune response and reduces antibody production.

- Actions on the vasculature **reduce vasodilatation** and thus decrease oedema.
- **Decreased inflammation** results from decreased production of cytokines and arachidonate metabolites.
- **Inhibition of the acute phase response** in the liver reduces the level of complement components in the blood.

Side effects

Glucocorticoids cause widespread inhibition of the entire immune system. As a result of this, there is an increased susceptibility to infection and wound healing is impaired. Other side effects may be similar to the features of **Cushing's syndrome**.

Antihistamines

Antihistamines are H_1-receptor antagonists, although they also appear to act on other receptors in the central nervous system (CNS). The inhibition of H_1-receptors decreases vascular permeability, reduces oedema and inhibits bronchoconstriction.

Side effects

Side effects result from CNS effects. Antihistamines may promote sedation (e.g. promethazine) or they can have antiemetic effects (e.g. cinnarizine). Other side effects result from antimuscarinic actions, commonly resulting in a dry mouth and constipation.

Necrosis and apoptosis

There are two distinct forms of cell death that may occur:

- **Apoptosis** is programmed cell death that is important in development and tissue remodelling, as well as in immunity.
- **Necrosis** is a form of unplanned cell death, associated with injury that promotes an inflammatory reaction.

Necrosis

Necrosis occurs in cell injury from which the cell is unable to recover. It is associated with the release of a mediator signalling the cell's death and stimulating an immune response.

Mechanisms of cell injury

Many processes contribute to cell injury through:

- **loss of cell membrane integrity**
- **decreased ATP concentration**
- **reduced protein synthesis** and **damage to the genome**
- **generation of reactive oxidative species**
- **mitochondrial damage** and loss of calcium homoeostasis.

Many of the cell changes that occur may be reversible up to a point. Reversible cell injuries include general swelling, blebbing of the cell membrane, mitochondrial swelling and clumping of chromatin.

Irreversible forms of cell injury include the breakdown of the cell genome, loss of membrane function and large dense areas in the mitochondria.

Apoptosis

Apoptosis is a crucial process for development and tissue remodelling. Apoptosis is tightly regulated, and the cells play an active role in their death – it is effectively 'cell suicide'.

Apoptotic signals may be internal or external. Internally, signals include developmental programmes and irreparable damage to DNA, whereas extrinsic factors include those involved in cytoxic T-lymphocyte (CTL)-induced killing. It is the balance between proapoptotic and antiapoptotic signals that regulates the survival of the cells. There are two major mechanisms of apoptosis:

1 **Death domain proteins** – specific receptors possess intracellular domains that can recruit and activate death domain proteins which induce apoptosis.
2 **Changes in mitochondrial permeability** – specific mediators of apoptosis can be found in the mitochondria (e.g. the bcl-2 family of proteins). Release of these proteins into the cytoplasm can trigger apoptosis.

The apoptotic pathways activate **caspases**. Caspase activation results in a proteolytic cascade that is responsible for a variety of terminal changes:

- **Cross-linking of cell proteins**
- **Chromatin breakdown** – breakdown of DNA is mediated by caspase-activated DNAase
- **Breakdown of nuclear architecture** and DNA repair mechanisms.

Repair

Tissue damage must be repaired after resolution of inflammation and may be sufficient to restore function to the tissue. However, restoration of function is often not possible in the adult and scar tissue may result. In the fetus, full resolution of a wound is usually possible, and is likely to be due to the different healing processes within the fetus, in which there is no inflammation and differences in the signals regulate the repair process.

Compared with many animals, mammals have a relatively limited regenerative capacity although the scope for regeneration of different cell types varies widely, e.g. although epithelial cells can regenerate continuously, neurons are irreplaceable.

The process of repair

The repair process is discussed in relation to repair of an incision of the skin in five stages, which are continuous with one other.

Inflammation and clotting

An inflammatory response occurs and there is formation of a clot. The increased vascular permeability contributes to oedema and there is also leukocyte recruitment. The clotting results in the formation of a scab which protects the wound site while repair is occurring.

Fibrinolysis and would cleansing

After clotting, fibrinolysis occurs and macrophages take on a scavenger function, removing dead tissues from the wound site. Macrophages release plasminogen-activating factors to clear the clot, allowing the laying down of scar tissue.

Revascularisation

Underneath the scab, new capillary growth occurs, followed by the growth of lymphatic vessels, reducing oedema.

Tissue remodelling

Keratinocytes migrate rapidly over the wound to lay down a covering of skin, and fibroblasts migrate from surrounding tissue to lay down collagen, which is progressively remodelled to a stronger structure. Remodelling promotes wound contracture to produce a tight acellular scar.

Wound contraction

Where the wound is a clean incision, and the sides closely apposed, a small wound results and there is minimal production of scar tissue. Normally tissue damage is more extensive and debris must be removed from the site. Such wounds produce larger defects which, in turn, lead to the production of more scar tissue. Gradually, the scar tissue tightens to reduce the size of the wound site, resulting in scars that may be less than 20% of the size of the original wound.

Regulation of repair

Many cytokines and factors are involved in regulating the process of tissue repair. Particularly significant signals involved in wound repair include:

- **Platelet-derived growth factor** (PDGF) is produced by many cells at the wound site and increases the migration of macrophages and fibroblasts. PDGF stimulates proliferation of smooth muscle cells and fibroblasts and promotes production of the extracellular matrix.
- **Transforming growth factor-β** (TGFβ) regulates the production of extracellular matrix components.
- **Fibroblast growth factor** (FGF) production by macrophages induces the formation of new capillary vessels, allowing vascularisation of the wound.
- **Epidermal growth factor** (EGF) promotes epidermal repair by recruiting keratinocytes and fibroblasts to the wound site.

A variety of factors may prevent efficient wound healing:

- **Malnutrition** often hinders wound healing, although deficiency must be severe as wounds are give priority. **Vitamin C** is essential for the production of stable collagen fibres; furthermore, **zinc** has been implicated in helping wound healing.
- **Bacterial infection** and **foreign bodies** must be removed before proper healing can occur.
- **Immunosuppression** due to steroids and other drugs can reduce wound healing.
- **Genetic variation** is poorly understood, although errors in leukocyte migration and connective tissue are associated with a lack of wound healing.

Anatomy of the immune system

The different cell types in the immune system must be produced correctly and, where relevant, undergo selection. It is essential that the appropriate interactions occur between cells and pathogens to detect an infection, and then between different cell types to induce the correct response.

The lymphoid tissue is crucial to the generation of an immune response and can be divided into two types of tissue:

1 The production of immune cells is achieved by the **primary lymphoid organs**: the bone marrow and thymus.
2 The **secondary lymphoid tissue** is the site where antigen is presented to immune cells to generate an adaptive immune response.

Primary lymphoid tissue

Two organs are responsible for the production of immune cells:

1 **Bone marrow** is the site of the initial generation of all haematopoietic cells and where B cells develop.
2 The **thymus** is responsible for the development of naïve T cells (which migrate as immature cells from the bone marrow).

The bone marrow

Bone marrow is found in the hollow interior of the long bones. All lymphocytes are derived from a common lymphoid progenitor. Precursors of B cells mature in the bone marrow before entering the bloodstream to migrate to secondary lymphoid organs. Cells that are destined to become T cells develop in the thymus.

The thymus

The thymus is, a large gland located at the front of the chest in children. However, the gland atrophies in adults, although it is still responsible for producing T cells through an individual's life.

In the thymus, thymocytes (immature T cells) are nursed and selected to produce a variety of clones that can recognise foreign antigen, although those clones that recognise self-antigens are eliminated to reduce the potential for autoimmunity.

Secondary lymphoid tissue

Secondary lymphoid tissue is the site of initiation of an adaptive immune response. These consist of the lymph nodes, the mucosal lymphoid tissue and the spleen. T cells enter lymph nodes from the bloodstream and sample the contents. If they detect an antigen to which they are specific, they proliferate in the lymph node, starting an adaptive immune response.

Lymph nodes

Lymph nodes are located throughout the body and serve to 'trap' antigens from solid organs to increase the chance of detection by specific lymphocytes.

Lymph is derived from extracellular tissue fluid and flows to lymph nodes through afferent lymph vessels. The distinct structure (Fig. 15.4) allows the sampling of any antigen by adaptive immune cells in the fluid, be it free floating or carried in cells, by the adaptive immune cells. The specialised structure of the lymph node consists of the following:

- The **cortex** consists mainly of B cells that are grouped into primary and secondary follicles. Follicular DCs present antigen to the B cells.
- **Primary follicles** contain resting B cells.
- **Secondary follicles** are those in which rapid cell division is occurring. They are characterised by the presence of germinal centres, which are the sites of B-cell division and differentiation into plasma cells.
- The **paracortex** is made up of CD4$^+$ helper T cells. This region surrounds the cortex and regulates the different arms of the immune system to promote an effective response.
- The **medulla** of lymph node is made up of B cells, T cells and macrophages.

Naïve T cells constantly circulate through the lymph and bloodstream. They enter lymph nodes through **high endothelial venules** (HEVs) before finally leaving via efferent vessels to return to the bloodstream.

During an immune response, B and T cells in the node are activated and the subsequent accumulation of fluid and cells leads to swelling, causing the characteristic 'swollen glands'. The immune response is usually limited to the glands closest to the site of infection; generalised swollen lymph nodes may indicate a systemic infection.

After resolution of infection, nodes return to their normal size.

The spleen

The spleen regulates the immune response against blood-borne pathogens (see Fig. 15.4). It also removes opsonised microbes and red blood cells from the blood. These two functions occur in different areas of the spleen:

1 The **red pulp** makes the greater proportion of the spleen. It is made up primarily of macrophages which phagocytose senescent red blood cells and other opsonised cells.
2 The **white pulp** contains around 25% of the body's lymphocytes. The structure of splenic white pulp is different from that of lymph nodes. The T cells are located in periarteriolar lymphoid sheaths, which surround central arterioles.

B cells are found mostly in follicles and also in the marginal zone where T-independent responses are generated.

The mucosa-associated lymphoid tissue

Mucosa-associated lymphoid tissue (MALT) acquires antigens from mucosal surfaces and is made up mainly of lymph tissue in the gut and respiratory tract, consisting of the tonsils, adenoids, Peyer's patches and other small lymphoid structures. As the vast majority of pathogens infect their host through mucosal tissue, these tissues are crucial for induction of the adaptive immune response.

Peyer's patches are located in the gut and are a prototypical example of MALT, responsible for the acquisition of antigen from the gastrointestinal (GI) tract. They are the first point of contact between the host and many pathogens. Peyer's patches contain large numbers of B cells that secrete IgA across the epithelium. T cells are present that regulate the immune response. This structure is mirrored by other MALTs:

- **M cells** are located on mucosal surface above the MALT. These cells take up antigens by pinocytosis.
- **B cells** are located in follicles very close to the M cells.

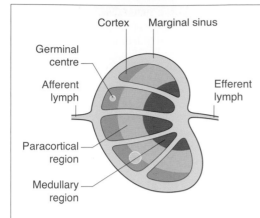

Lymph nodes

The lymph nodes receive a flow of lymph from the tissues through the afferent lymph. Antigens and cells present in the lymph flow through the various regions of the node, leaving the node through the efferent vessel, via the marginal sinus.

In the lymph node, the medullary regions contain T cells and macrophages. The cortical regions contain the follicles, which consist of B cells; these may be proliferating within germinal centres. The T cells are located primarily in the paracortical region. All lymph nodes receive a blood supply which allows the migration of naïve T cells into the node.

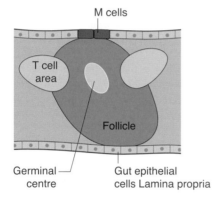

Peyer's patches

These lymphoid tissues collect antigen directly from the gut through specialised M (multi-fenestrated) cells. A follicle of B cells is located directly beneath the M cells, and is surrounded by small numbers of T cells. This arrangement ensures rapid presentation of gut-derived antigen to the immune system.

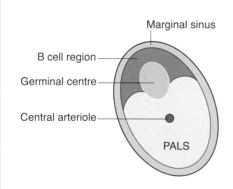

Spleen

The spleen is organised into red pulp, which is concerned with removal of senescent red blood cells, and white pulp, which is concerned with the immune response. The white pulp is organised around the central arteriole, which in turn is surrounded by a periarteriolar lymphoid sheath (PALS) of T cells. This is surrounded by a B-cell region which, when an active immune response occurs, will contain a germinal centre. The whole region is surrounded by a marginal zone of macrophages, which serve to capture antigen and present it to the T and B cells of the white pulp.

Figure 15.4 The secondary lymphoid tissue in the body is organised into specific structures. The most prominent of these are the Lymph nodes, Peyer's patches and white pulp of the spleen. Although the structure in each varies, they are organised to ensure that antigen is delivered effectively to both T and B cells and that an appropriate adaptive immune response can be developed.

Adaptive immunity

In response to a new pathogen, the adaptive immune system is far slower in its induction than the innate immune system. The almost limitless specificity of the antigen receptors that can be generated by the T and B cells allows them to respond to any antigen. Furthermore, T and B cells can develop into **memory cells**, allowing a second encounter with the same pathogen to be resolved much more rapidly.

Adaptive immunity is a double-edged sword, however; the huge diversity of receptors allows the generation of receptors specific to host proteins. These must be removed from the repertoire or autoimmune conditions may arise. This process, **tolerance**, occurs during maturation, after the generation of receptors by recombination or in the periphery.

Generation of diversity of antigen-binding sites

Both B and T cells generate a huge repertoire of receptors with different specificities through **genetic recombination**. The process by which this occurs in the two cell groups is very similar. The genes encoding the T-cell receptor (TCR) and immunoglobulin (Ig) are made up of a series of alternative regions. There are many copies of the variable (V), diversity (D) and joining (J) regions in the genes, which are recombined so that the final gene contains a single variant of each region to produce a unique gene product in each cell. The process of recombination in T and B cells is regulated by the recombination activity genes (RAGs). Further diversity is added by the potential for enzymatic removal or addition of nucleotides at the site of the joins between the various segments (Fig. 15.5).

It is important to ensure that each lymphocyte has a single specificity. This process requires **allelic exclusion**, to ensure that only one copy of the parental alleles is expressed in each cell. In B cells, both chains that contribute to the immunoglobulin molecules are regulated by allelic exclusion. However, in the TCR, only the β chain is subject to allelic exclusion; thus, a single T cell may express two different α chains, although it is not clear how this alters the specificity and function of an individual T cell.

T-cell development and clonal selection

As a result of recombination, some of the receptors produced will undoubtedly react to self-antigen. It is essential that the body remove or suppress these clones, because they provide a potential for autoimmunity.

Generation of the TCR

The TCR binds to a unique peptide antigen presented on an Major histocompatibility complex (MHC) molecule. The receptor is made up of two chains; in most T cells the α and β chains make up the TCR, although in about 5% of cells the TCR is made up of γ and δ chains. This section described generation of an αβ TCR, although generation of the γδ TCR occurs similarly.

The generation of a TCR is the result of recombination of various V, D and J regions within the α and the β chains, both of which contribute to binding. The TCR clones must be selected to ensure that they can recognise an antigen presented on the MHC and that they do not react to a self-antigen.

> **DEFINITION: γδ T cells**
>
> γδ T cells are found extensively in the mucosa and their role is not well known. They are derived separately from αβ T cells in the thymus and are thought to have a wide variety of roles, some of which may be regulatory.

Positive selection

Initially, thymocytes express both CD4 and CD8. With many different alleles of MHC, and a hugely diverse TCR repertoire, survival of a TCR clone depends on its ability to bind to either MHC Class I (MHC-I) or MHC Class II (MHC-II); if this occurs, the thymocyte becomes restricted to the appropriate co-receptor and enters **negative selection**.

If a thymocyte is incapable of binding MHC-I or MHC-II, it will undergo some TCR rearrangement using other copies of the TCR alleles; if that fails the lack of TCR signalling triggers its death. The large majority (around 90%) of thymocytes are eliminated in positive selection.

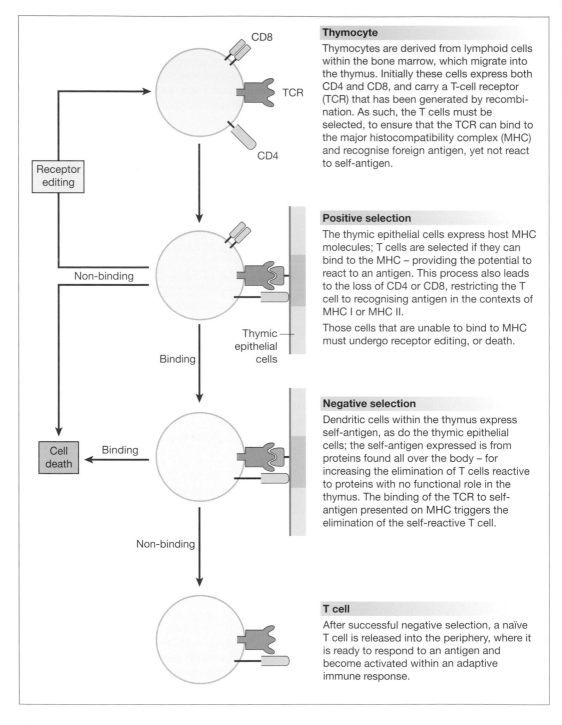

Thymocyte

Thymocytes are derived from lymphoid cells within the bone marrow, which migrate into the thymus. Initially these cells express both CD4 and CD8, and carry a T-cell receptor (TCR) that has been generated by recombination. As such, the T cells must be selected, to ensure that the TCR can bind to the major histocompatibility complex (MHC) and recognise foreign antigen, yet not react to self-antigen.

Positive selection

The thymic epithelial cells express host MHC molecules; T cells are selected if they can bind to the MHC – providing the potential to react to an antigen. This process also leads to the loss of CD4 or CD8, restricting the T cell to recognising antigen in the contexts of MHC I or MHC II.

Those cells that are unable to bind to MHC must undergo receptor editing, or death.

Negative selection

Dendritic cells within the thymus express self-antigen, as do the thymic epithelial cells; the self-antigen expressed is from proteins found all over the body – for increasing the elimination of T cells reactive to proteins with no functional role in the thymus. The binding of the TCR to self-antigen presented on MHC triggers the elimination of the self-reactive T cell.

T cell

After successful negative selection, a naïve T cell is released into the periphery, where it is ready to respond to an antigen and become activated within an adaptive immune response.

Figure 15.5 The thymocytes go through a carefully controlled developmental pathway in the thymus gland. Initially all cells express CD4, CD8 and the T-cell receptor and, after a series of selection, the expression of molecules is reduced and cells that react to self-antigen are removed from the repertoire or undergo cell death or T-cell receptor editing.

Negative selection

After positive selection, it is essential to ensure that TCR clones which react to self-antigens are removed. This achieved by the medullary thymic epithelial cells, which present a wide variety of self-antigen-derived peptides to the thymocytes. Recognition of self-peptide at this stage of thymocyte development triggers a variety of reactions based on the strength of the signal (Fig. 15.5):

- **No binding**: a small signal is required through the TCR to sustain the thymocytes. A complete absence of signal leads to cell death.
- **Weak interaction**: there is sufficient interaction to produce a small signal through the TCR. This results in the selection of the T-cell clone and its development into a naïve T cell.
- **Strong interaction**: a strong interaction through the binding of a TCR to a self-peptide present on the MHC by thymic epithelia would be harmful in the peripheral circulation. This premature activation triggers the cell to undergo receptor rearrangement. If receptor rearrangement fails, apoptosis occurs to prevent autoreactive T cells from entering the circulation.

The fate of self-reactive T cells

Should a thymocyte express a receptor specific to a self-antigen, this would trigger a reactivation of the *RAG* genes to create a new receptor through recombination of the second TCR allele. Failure to generate a suitable TCR results in death of the T-cell clone. In some cases a self-reactive T cell may develop into a regulatory T cell which can specifically suppress the immune response.

Generation of specificity in B cells

The process by which the B-cell receptor (BCR; immunoglobulin [Ig])) is generated is very similar to that of the TCR, although there are several key differences:

- The BCR genes are recombined, instead of the TCR genes.
- Development of the BCR occurs in the bone marrow.
- There is no positive selection, because the BCR recognises intact, unprocessed antigen.

Induction of the adaptive immune response

Induction of the adaptive immune response is tightly regulated through a series of specific receptor–ligand interactions to ensure that an appropriate response is mounted against a pathogen.

The T-cell surface molecules and T-cell activation

Many different surface molecules on the T cell have a role in their activation. These molecules can be divided into provision of three forms of information:

1. **Specificity for the antigen** is maintained by the TCR.
2. **Specific for the MHC molecule** presenting the antigen: the compartment from which the antigen is derived is therefore achieved by CD4 and CD8.
3. **Co-stimulation** is required to activate naïve T cells. It ensures that self- and non-harmful antigens do not induce an immune response. Many different surface molecules are involved in this, particularly CD40 and CD40 ligand (CD154), and CD28 and B7.

CD3

The CD3 complex allows the TCR into the interior of the cell – the TCR lacks a cytoplasmic signalling domain. A single TCR is associated with one each of CD3γ and CD3δ, two CD3ε chains and two CD3ζ chains. Signalling from CD3 occurs through motifs known as immunoreceptor tyrosine-based activation motifs (ITAMs):

- Binding of TCR allows phosphorylation of the ITAM by tyrosine kinase enzymes.
- Phosphorylation of ITAM allows binding of other tyrosine kinases (e.g. ZAP-70 which promotes T-cell activation.

Co-receptors: CD4 and CD8

TCRs are restricted to either MHC-I or -II as a result of their TCR specificity and are helped by CD8 or CD4. These co-receptors bind to MHC-I and MHC-II, respectively:

- **CD4** is found on helper T cells and binds to a conserved region of MHC-II. The cytoplasmic domain of CD4 is associated with Lck, a tyrosine kinase, which augments the signalling by CD3 and TCR.
- **CD8** is made up of a heterodimer of one CD8α and one CD8β chain; the CD8 molecule-conserved region on MHC-I augments the TCR signal (in a similar manner to CD4) and restricts the TCR to MHC-I.

MHC and antigen presentation

The major histocompatibility complex (MHC)

The MHC is located on chromosome 6 in humans and contains critical genes for antigen presentation, particularly the human leukocyte antigen (HLA). These are important in the presentation of antigens to T cells within the adaptive immune response.

Structure

The MHC is highly polymorphic. Specific alleles are numbered, e.g. HLA-B27, HLA-DR2. The MHC can be divided into three classes:

1 **MHC-I** encodes three genes – HLA-A, HLA-B and HLA-C – which are expressed ubiquitously on nucleated cells. The protein product of these genes combines with β_2-microglobulin. The complete MHC-I molecule presents peptides derived from the cytosolic compartment of the cells to CD8$^+$ cytotoxic T cells, allowing the detection of infection by intracellular pathogens.
2 **MHC-II** encodes genes for three major products – HLA-DP, HLA-DQ and HLA-DR. MHC-II molecules are made up of two chains, so both α and β chains are encoded for each molecule.
3 **MHC-III** refers to the other genes in the MHC, which are not highly polymorphic. Many of these genes are critical for normal immune function, including cytokines and complement components.

For a T cell to detect a pathogen, the epitope that it recognises must be processed and presented on the cell surface in a context that the T cell can recognise. The peptide epitope binds to a groove in the surface of the MHC molecule; it is the combination of peptide and MHC that is recognised by the TCR. To allow the presentation of a wide variety of peptides by an MHC molecule, the binding groove is in contact with the peptide at only a few residues, allowing a wide variation in the identity of those other residues.

The presence of MHC molecules allows the presentation of peptides derived from pathogens, and it is pathogens that are likely to have driven the polymorphic nature of the MHC. Were a pathogen able to evolve so that none of its peptides were capable of binding to an MHC molecule, it could evade the adaptive immune system in that host. By having such a variety of MHC, it would be unlikely that a pathogen would ever be able to evolve to escape every possible combination of MHC alleles found in the human population.

Presentation of peptides on MHC-I

MHC-I is recognised by CD8$^+$ cytotoxic T cells and presents peptides derived from the cytosol and nuclear compartments. This allows CTLs to detect infection by intracellular pathogens, such as viruses.

Structure of MHC-I and expression

The MHC-I molecule is made up of one 'heavy' chain consisting of three domains, which is encoded by HLA-A, -B or -C. It is associated with a β_2-microglobulin molecule, which is common to all alleles of MHC-I. The MHC heavy chain contains a peptide-binding groove that accommodates peptides, typically eight to nine amino acids in length.

As there is the potential for viruses and other intracellular pathogens to infect any cell in the body, MHC-I is expressed by all nucleated cells. However, some cell groups are irreplaceable and these express low levels of MHC-I, to reduce the potential for CTL-mediated killing, e.g. nerve cells.

Generation of peptides for MHC-I and antigen presentation

Large proportions (around 25%) of newly synthesised proteins are incorrectly folded and rapidly degraded by the **proteasome**, which generates peptide fragments by proteolytic cleavage. The peptide fragments are transported from the cytosol to the endoplasmic reticulum (ER) for loading on MHC-I molecules, through a specific peptide transporter – TAP. Peptides imported by TAP may be 'trimmed' by ER aminopeptidases to allow them to bind to the groove in MHC-I molecules, or may be of the appropriate length to bind directly. The binding of a peptide stabilises the MHC-I molecule and promotes its transport by the constitutive secretory pathway, to the cell surface.

Presentation of peptides by MHC-II molecules

MHC-II molecules present peptides derived from the endosomal compartment of the cell to CD4$^+$ Th cells. This permits the detection of infections and activation of the adaptive immune response to extracellular pathogens, which have been phagocytosed into the endosomal compartment by antigen-presenting cells (APCs).

The structure and expression of MHC-II

The MHC molecule is made up of two chains. The α and β chains both contain two domains and both contribute to the peptide-binding groove in the molecule. Unlike MHC-I, the peptide-binding groove is open ended, allowing a wide range of peptide sizes to be accommodated; MHC-II can typically accommodate peptides from 18 to 25 amino acids in length.

MHC-II has a more specialised role, and presents peptides derived, often, from extracellular sources. Its expression is restricted to specific cell groups – particularly those cells capable of phagocytosis:

- **Macrophages and dendritic cells**
- **B cells**
- Some **epithelial** and **endothelial** cell groups.

The synthesis of MHC-II and formation and transport of the MHC-II–peptide complex

MHC-II must present peptides from the endosomal compartment, yet it is synthesised in the ER. The loading of peptide in the ER onto an 'empty MHC-II' molecule must be prevented.

- MHC-II is synthesised in the ER, complete with an 'invariant chain' (Ii) that is bound across the MHC-II peptide-binding groove, preventing ER-derived peptides binding.
- The 'empty' MHC-II complexed with Ii is transported to the endosomal compartment.
- In the endosome, pathogen-derived proteins are broken down as a result of acidification and enzymatic activities.
- Acidification and the enzymatic activities promote the cleavage and dissociation of Ii from

MHC-II, allowing binding of a suitable pathogen-derived peptide.
- Binding of a pathogen-derived peptide to the groove stabilises the MHC molecule and promotes its transport to the surface for presentation to a TCR.

T-cell activation

There are two main subgroups of T cells, via their signals through their TCR, although other signals involved in the process differ:

- **CD8$^+$ cytotoxic T cells** detect intracellular pathogens, which present peptides on MHC-I.
- **CD4$^+$ Th cells** detect peptides derived from pathogens in the endosomal compartment, presenting peptides on MHC-II.

The crucial stage of activation of T cells is binding of the TCR, which signals to the interior of the cell through CD3. This can happen in two ways:

1 Through **binding of the TCR to an MHC molecule presenting the relevant peptide**: the specific allele of the MHC and the peptide structure are both crucial to the binding of the TCR, leading to activation. In addition, the co-receptor of CD4 or CD8 ensures that the binding is to the correct form of MHC, either MHC-I or MHC-II.

Superantigens are capable of binding to a TCR expressing a specific form of β chain; this can represent a large proportion of the T-cell population, resulting in an excessive immune response.

To activate a naïve T cell, it is not sufficient for a specific TCR to recognise the correct peptide–MHC combination. As there is a potential for the T cell to react to a host-derived peptide, additional co-stimulatory signals must be presented to activate the naïve T cell. These are provided by **DCs**, which are the only cells known to be capable of activating a naïve T cell. There are many signals in the innate immune response that can detect the presence of a pathogen:

- **Tissue damage**: necrotic damage is a hallmark of infection or wounding, which provides a potential for infection.
- **PAMPs**.

PAMPs, combined with an inflammatory response, activate DCs to 'mature' and migrate to lymph nodes to present the acquired antigenic

T cell

Three signals are required for the activation of a CD4+ T-helper cell and the polarisation of the helper T-cell response:

1. The specificity of the interaction is ensured by the requirement of the TCR to bind to the peptide–MHC complex; CD4 also binds to MHC II to ensure that the interaction is with the correct class of MHC molecule.

2. Co-stimulatory molecules such as CD40 and CD28 are expressed by the antigen-presenting cell (APC), to signal the need for the induction of adaptive immunity. These molecules bind to ligands on the T cell – CD40 ligand and B7, respectively.

3. The release of cytokines by the APC and other cells in the local environment can influence the polarisation of a T-helper (TH) response, towards TH1 or TH2.

Phagocytosis

An exogenous antigen may be taken up through phagocytosis or, in dendritic cells, through macropinocytosis. The antigen begins to be broken down in the phagosome.

CD4   CD3   Cytokine receptor

Co-stimulatory molecules

TCR

Cytokine release

Antigen-presenting cell

MHC-II loading

The presence of degradative enzymes, combined with the low pH, promotes the digestion and loss of the invariant chain, and allows peptides derived from the antigen to bind to the MHC-II molecule, stabilising it ready for presentation.

MHC-II presentation

MHC II is transported to the cell surface, for presentation to T cells. Under inflammatory conditions, the appropriate co-stimulatory signals are supplied to trigger the activation of specific T cells.

MHC synthesis

Major histocompatibility complex (MHC) II is produced in the endoplasmic reticulum (ER), where it is transported to the phagosome with an invariant chain that prevents binding of ER-derived peptides.

MHC-II

Endoplasmic reticulum

peptides. The maturation of a DC increases the presentation of MHC and promotes expression of high levels of co-stimulatory molecules.

The T cell needs the presentation of TCR signal and co-stimulatory signals to the T cell by a single APC. The binding of antigen to the TCR without co-stimulation leads to an anergic state in the T cell, hindering its activation even if it is later presented with co-stimulatory signals.

CD4$^+$ T cells

CD4$^+$ cells are activated to form Th cells, which direct and drive the immune response through the production of a variety of cytokines. These can act to activate or inhibit other cell types to coordinate an appropriate response; certainly the response required and the cell types involved in clearing an intracellular pathogen such as *M. tuberculosis* differ from the response to clear a helminth infection.

Initial activation by DCs can polarise cells to one of two main responses. The polarisation of a Th cell response can be determined by three signals (Fig. 15.6):

1 The **TCR (signal 1)**: the TCR binding to peptide–MHC is an essential signal, ensuring the activation of specific T-cell clones in response to infection.
2 **Co-stimulatory molecules (signal 2)**: co-stimulatory molecules such as CD40 and B7, presented by the DC, promotes the activation of a naïve cell, ensuring that any T-cell response is not due to the presentation of a self-peptide.
3 **Polarisation signal (signal 3)**: the various cytokines and inflammatory stimuli are thought to be integrated by the DC to lead to the expression of a pattern of cytokines and surface molecules that promote the polarisation of the T-cell response. The cytokine milieu in the lymph node itself is likely to contribute to this response, e.g. IL-12 is associated with the development of a Th1 response, whereas IL-4 and IL-10 are associated with the formation of a Th2 response.

The Th1 response (cell mediated)

A Th1 response is associated with macrophage activation. The prototypic infection in which such a response is seen is tuberculosis, where the bacterium is able to withstand the acidification and formation of phagolysosomes and thus withstand killing. A variety of molecules is associated with the Th1 response:

- **IFNγ**: this is the critical cytokine in the response that activates macrophages.
- **Fas ligand**: this surface molecule is important in killing chronically infected cells, allowing the release of any surviving pathogens, so that they may be cleared by fresh macrophages.
- **IL-2** promotes proliferation of T cells, increasing the number of T cells of the reactive clones.
- **TNFα**: upregulate the general innate immune response, in particular acting on endothelial cells to allow additional migration of macrophages towards sites of infection.

Th2 response (humorally mediated)

The Th2 response is seen in response to helminth infections and promotes the formation of high-affinity IgE antibodies. The Th2 response is closely associated with the activation of B cells, and with a polarising signal of **IL-4** and **IL-5** – cytokines associated with B-cell activation.

Other forms of Th cells

There are other subtypes of CD4$^+$ T cells that have been identified. Further subtypes of Th cells are continually being identified:

- **Regulatory T cells** respond to self-antigen and are able to specifically suppress the immune response.
- **Th17 cells** cause acute inflammation and are typified by the secretion of IL-17.

CD8$^+$ cytotoxic T cells

After activation, CTLs can migrate and detect viral infection through binding to cells expressing the relevant peptide–MHC specificity. On detecting an infected cell, an activated CTL will produce a cytotoxic response, inducing apoptosis of the target cell before the pathogen can replicate and escape the cell. The action of CTLs is tightly

Figure 15.6 Antigen-presenting cells are able to take up antigens through phagocytosis. Through a series of steps the antigen-presenting cells are able process the antigen and present it in the context of MHC-II molecules to allow it to bind to and stimulate CD4$^+$ helper T cells. Antigen-presenting cells are also capable of cytokine release, which may help direct the activation (or not) of the T cell.

regulated by the need to bind the TCR to a specific peptide–MHC-I combination.

The activation of CTLs requires a similar signal 1 and signal 2, from a DC:

- The specificity of the reaction is maintained by the **recognition of a peptide antigen bound to MHC-I**, by the TCR. MHC-I also binds to CD8, expressed by CTLs.
- The interaction of the various **co-stimulatory molecules** ensures that the antigen presented needs the development of an immune response.

On the binding of the TCR to the MHC molecule, many other molecules bind to form a tight 'immunological synapse' between the two cells. Cytotoxic molecules are expressed on the synapse or released from cytotoxic granules across this junction, limiting the cytotoxic effect solely to the cell in question.

CTLs possess a variety of mechanisms by which they can mediate their cytotoxic killing, three of which are particularly prominent:

1 **Perforin** inserts into the target cell membrane and polymerises to form pores, similar to the **membrane–attack complex** produced by complement. Perforin disrupts the integrity of the cell membrane, which contributes to killing, although its primary action is to permit entry of **granzymes** into the target cell.
2 **Granzymes** are released from the cytotoxic granules and enter the target cell through perforin pores. These proteases trigger **apoptosis** by activating **caspases**.
3 **Fas ligand** binds to Fas, which is expressed on the surface of the target cells. Binding of Fas ligand to Fas triggers the activation of caspases in the target cell, leading to apoptosis. Fas ligand-mediated killing is a perforin-independent process.

The cytotoxic granules possessed by CTLs have a variety of other enzymes and molecules that contribute to the induction of cell death in the target cell. CTLs may alter the function of other cells through the release of cytokines, in particular TNFα and IFNγ.

B cells: activation and T-cell help

The activation of most B cells requires the assistance of T cells, which are also involved in regulating **class switching** and **somatic hypermutation**, the process by which higher-affinity antibodies are generated. There are other groups of B cells that can generate antibodies without the assistance of T cells; however, these are unable to undergo class switching and somatic hypermutation.

B-cell subgroups

There are two groups of B cells in the body. The B-2 cells, the conventional B-cell group, are responsible for the antibodies produced in an adaptive immune response. There is a second smaller group of B cells – the B-1 cells – that produce the so-called 'natural antibodies'.

B-1 B cell

These B cells are found in large numbers at birth although the proportion of the B-cell population that they account for gradually diminishes. These B cells possess receptors that are effectively germline encoded and not generated by the same recombinatory process as B-2 cells. Often the antigens that the B cells recognises are self-antigens; anti-DNA antibodies and anti-blood groups antibodies are produced by B-1 cells. B-1 cells secrete IgM constitutively and do not undergo **class switching**.

B-2 B cells

These cells are the conventional B cells that are found located in the circulation and lymphoid tissue. B-2 cells require the binding of their specific antigen to activate them. B-cell activation can be classified into two groups, based on whether T-cell assistance is required for activation of the B cells: most antigens are T-dependent, although a few are T-independent.

T-independent (T-I) antigens

Some rare B-cell antigens are made up of long repeating units, promoting the cross-linking of the many receptors on the B-cell surface that are enough to allow activation of the B cell. Although this allows a more rapid induction of the B-cell response, T cells are crucial for **somatic hypermutation** and **class switching**, which produces higher-affinity antibodies with a greater degree of effector functions. Instead, T-I antigens result, almost exclusively, in the production of IgM antibodies.

Thymus-dependent (T-D) antigens

On the binding of an antigen to its specific immunoglobulin, the B cell internalises the receptor, complete with its bound antigen. Peptides derived from the internalised antigen are processed and presented on MHC-II molecules on the B cell. The T cells that possess a TCR specific to the antigen-derived peptides can now initiate the activation of the B cell.

B-cell activation triggers migration to germinal centres of the lymphoid tissue, where the division and differentiation of B cells into secreting plasma cells. Plasma cells have large amounts of rough ER and are specialised for secretion to produce high levels of antibody. Plasma cells are often found in the bone marrow – they do not need to remain in the lymph node to perform their function.

Class switching

One B-cell clone is capable of generating antibodies specific to a single epitope. However, depending on the stage of the immune response, and the type of pathogen against which it is directed, there may be a need for the antibody to employ different effector functions. Different classes of antibody possess differing constant (Fc) regions that mediate different effector functions. Class switching is the result of **alternative splicing** of the heavy chain mRNA. The final mRNA product of the alternative splicing expresses only a single constant region sequence, leading to the production of an antibody of that class.

The process of class switching is controlled by various immune signals, in particular cytokines.

- **Th2 response**: the Th2 cytokines, IL-4 and IL-5, promote the production of the IgE isoform which contributes to a Th2 response in the clearance of helminth pathogens.
- **The Th1 response** is more focused on cell-mediated immunity although there is a significant role for antibodies, particularly in protection from further infection. Although Th1 cytokines do not have a major role in promoting antibody production, they influence the classes that are produced. In particular, IgG2a and IgG3 help clear infection, through the binding of phagocytic receptor.

Development of high-affinity antibodies

In the germinal centre of a lymphoid follicle, B cells may undergo two processes: affinity maturation and somatic hypermutation. These processes act together to produce antibodies with a higher specificity.

Somatic hypermutation occurs during rapid division of B cells. Specific enzymes are expressed that generate point mutations in the immunoglobulin (Ig) gene. The resulting daughter B cells will have subtly differing specificities. Although many of the specificities produced are poorer than those of the parent cell, a few may be of higher affinity, leading to the production of a more effective antibody.

Affinity maturation ensures that any antibodies produced are of the highest specificity. As the survival of developing B cells depends on receiving sufficient signals through their B-cell receptor, higher-affinity B cells are able to bind antigen more effectively, which promotes the expansion of that clone, outcompeting other B-cell clones of weaker specificity.

Immunological memory

A key feature of the adaptive immune system is that an infection by a previously encountered pathogen is quickly dealt with through the rapid production of high-affinity antibodies and cell-mediated responses. This 'immunological memory' prevents the same pathogen causing severe disease twice in the same individual.

Immunological memory is mediated by the development of memory cells after resolution of the immune response. Memory cells do not require co-stimulation for their reactivation. They are produced after infection and migrate to the lymph nodes in small populations. There, they rapidly detect the presence of their antigen and mediate an immune response to it, without the need for the induction and expansion that is seen in a primary immune response.

B-cell memory

During the differentiation of B cells to plasma cells, a few develop by a different route to become **memory cells**. In a subsequent infection, these cells can be rapidly induced to proliferate and differentiate into antibody-secreting plasma cells. Thus, in a primary and secondary immune response, the production of IgG has a very different kinetics. Conversely, IgM is produced by naïve B cells in both cases, and has a similar response in both primary and secondary responses.

T-cell memory

Memory T cells are thought to develop directly from functional effector cells at the end of the immune response. These cells become dormant, but are reactivated rapidly in response to their antigen stimulus.

Effector mechanisms of the immune system

Once the body has identified a potential pathogen, it must activate suitable effector mechanisms to eliminate it. A variety of different mechanisms may be recruited based on the nature of the target. Broadly, they focus on the induction of apoptosis in pathogen-infected cells, the promotion of pathogen phagocytosis and the release of toxic.

Natural killer (NK) cells

NK cells express germline-encoded receptors; they do not express a receptor generated by recombination. They are important in the detection and killing of virally infected cells, and also in stimulating the adaptive immune response. They do not need to be activated in the same way as other lymphocytes, allowing a rapid response to a pathogen.

Activation and effector mechanisms

NK cells are activated rapidly in response to cytokines – in particular **IFNγ** and **IL-12**. This allows NK cells to be activated by either the innate or the adaptive immune systems. NK cells detect viral infection in cells through their surface receptors, some inhibitory and others stimulatory.

Natural killer receptors

NK receptors may be inhibitory or activating, relying on a balance between activating and inhibitory signals to activate the killing mechanisms:

- **Inhibitory receptors**: the best understood group of inhibitory receptors on NK cells acts through binding to the α chain of MHC-I molecules. These molecules are often downregulated during viral infections, in an attempt by the virus to evade detection by CTLs. Such downregulation reduces the ability of CTLs to detect infected cells, but increases the likelihood of NK cell-mediated killing, due to the absence of an inhibitory signal. NK cells have an important role during pregnancy in protection of the uterus and fetus. Unlike T and B cells, there is no potential for NK cells to attack fetal tissue as 'non-self'.
- **Activating receptors**: in response to a viral infection, the expression of many molecules is upregulated and they are detected by the varied activating receptors expressed by NK cells, stimulating killing.

Antibody-dependent cytotoxicity

NK cells may induce killing in response to detection of bound antibody. The FcγRIII receptor on NK cells recognises IgG-bound viral antigen on the surface of infected cells, triggering the NK cell to induce apoptosis in the infected cell.

Killing mechanisms

NK cells possess similar cytotoxic effector mechanisms to CTLs, using cytotoxic granules containing **perforin and granzyme**. The surface molecule Fas ligand, which can induce apoptosis, is also expressed. NK cells are a major source of IFNγ which stimulates macrophages and Th1 cells.

Macrophages and neutrophils

Macrophages and neutrophils can phagocytose pathogens and other particles, and then kill them through a variety of mechanisms; this is crucial for clearance of many infections. The phagocytic function of macrophages is also essential in tissue remodelling and wound repair.

Phagocytosis

A pathogen is internalised through binding of phagocytic receptors on the macrophage surface. These receptors recognise specific patterns on the pathogen surface, or **opsonins** – molecules such as antibodies or complement proteins coating the surface of pathogens. Ligation of phagocytic receptors triggers remodelling of the cell surface membrane, so that the pathogen can be engulfed.

Killing mechanisms

As some pathogens exploit phagocytosis as a method of entry into a cell, it is essential to ensure that pathogens do not survive in the macrophage. As macrophages must operate in both high and low oxygen conditions they possess a variety of killing mechanisms:

- **Phagosome acidification** occurs rapidly after phagocytosis, and creates a corrosive environment within the phagosome which, as well as being directly harmful to the engulfed pathogen, promotes the activation of many degradative enzymes, such as those released after lysosomal fusion. This creates an inhospitable environment to inhibit the growth of the pathogen and to destroy it.
- **Fusion of lysosomes** results in exposure of the pathogen to many degradative enzymes, allowing destruction of the pathogen. These enzymes are not oxygen dependent, allowing efficient killing to occur anaerobically.
- The **respiratory burst** results in the production of toxic oxygen species within the phagosome. These may act directly on the pathogen, or combine with nitrogen or chlorine species to produce other toxic molecules.

The production of $O_2{}^-$ is crucial in the respiratory burst – NADPH oxidase is the crucial enzyme in this process and its deficiency leads to serious immunodeficiency.

Inducible nitric oxide synthase (iNOS) is also expressed during the respiratory burst. This mediates the production of NO, which is directly toxic, or may combine with oxygen radicals to provide more reactive species such as peroxynitrite (ONOO$^-$).

Activation of macrophages

Activation of macrophages in response to IFNγ is a hallmark of the Th1 response. Activation results in a number of changes that stimulate macrophages to become efficient killers and inducers of the immune response:

- **MHC-II expression** increases, allowing macrophages to function as APCs.
- **Induction of killing mechanisms** such as the respiratory burst promote more efficient killing. Although this upregulation allows the clearance of very resistant infections, associated tissue damage is common as a result of the leakage of some of the toxic metabolites.
- Activated macrophages are potent **cytokine** producers and produce IL-12. This promotes the polarisation of newly activated T cells towards a Th1 phenotype.

Mast cells and basophils

Basophils and mast cells mediate early responses to infections, in particular to parasites and helminths. Mast cells reside in body tissues, whereas basophils are found in the circulating blood and are recruited to sites of inflammation.

Mediators of inflammation

Mast cells possess granules that contain inflammatory mediators:

- **Histamine** induces smooth muscle contraction in most tissues, except blood vessels. It also increases T-cell migration by increasing the permeability of blood vessels.
- **Cytokines** are produced that promote a Th2 response, triggering the production of eosinophils and preventing the formation of a Th1 response.
- **Enzymes**: a number of proteolytic enzymes are released from mast cell granules. The products of the enzymatic reactions promote mucus secretion and smooth muscle contraction, as well as activating the complement pathways and kinin pathways.

Other mediators of inflammation can be rapidly synthesised by mast cells following activation. PLA$_2$ liberates arachidonic acid which results in the production of **leukotrienes** (by the enzyme **lipoxygenase**) and **prostaglandins** (by the **cyclooxygenase** enzymes).

Hypersensitivity, immune regulation and immune defects

The regulation of the immune system requires a fine balance; if the system is too active, dangerous immune responses may be harmless antigens or such responses to self-antigens may occur. If the system is too weak it is insufficient to clear infection. There is also a need for the regulation of the immune system in transplantation. In this situation, immune responses against the transplanted organ must be suppressed to allow the graft in question to function and not be rejected.

Types and mechanisms of hypersensitivity

The immune response can produce inappropriate reaction against a stimulus. Such a reaction may be very damaging to the body and is known as a **hypersensitivity reaction**. This reaction may be caused by:

- **infectious agents** (e.g. tuberculosis)
- **self-antigens** (e.g. thyroid antigens in autoimmune thyroiditis)
- **environmental antigens** (e.g. peanut allergy).

There are four main forms of hypersensitivity reaction (types I–IV), classified by the immune mechanisms that cause them.

Type I hypersensitivity reaction: anaphylaxis and allergy

Type I hypersensitivity is commonly seen in allergies. Sensitisation to an antigen leads to the production of high-affinity IgE antibodies which associate with mast cells. On subsequent encounter with an antigen, binding to IgE triggers mast cell degranulation and inflammation, which may be severe. The severity of the reaction varies, and may be limited to a skin rash, or runny nose and irritation. In serious cases, **anaphylaxis** may result.

Chronic reaction

In many allergic reactions, such as those due to ingested food antigens, there is only an acute component. However, with some environmental antigens (e.g. house dust), prolonged exposure occurs, which produces a chronic condition, due to the presence of activated Th2 cells.

Type II hypersensitivity: antibody-mediated cytotoxic reaction

Type II hypersensitivity reactions result from the production of reactive antibodies that directly attack the body. This hypersensitivity reaction is responsible for some autoimmune diseases.

Type II hypersensitivity reactions can also occur as a result of antibodies produced against a pathogen that cross-reacts with self-antigens. Rheumatic fever occurs in this manner as antibodies produced against streptococcal antigens, which appear to cross-react with self-proteins).

Antibodies involved in type II hypersensitivity reactions usually result in loss of function, e.g.

autoimmune thyroiditis. Occasionally, the autoantibodies produced are activating: Graves' disease is caused by an overactive thyroid in response to autoantibodies that bind to and activate the thyroid-stimulating hormone receptor on thyroid follicular cells. This activating response is referred to as a **type V** hypersensitivity reaction.

Type III hypersensitivity: immune-complex mediated

Type III hypersensitivity is also antibody-mediated, although damage results from activation of complement by antigen–antibody (Ag/Ab) complexes. Type III hypersensitivity reactions may occur in a localised or systemic fashion depending on the antigen:

- **Localised antigen** leads to the formation of complexes at the site of antigen exposure (e.g. the lungs in response to inflamed antigens).
- **Systemic antigen** may lead to the deposition of immune complexes in many locations throughout the body. This is particularly important in joints in which inflammation may contribute to arthritis and in the glomerulus of the kidneys, which can cause glomerulitis, as is seen in systemic lupus erythematosus.

Type IV hypersensitivity: delayed-type hypersensitivity

Type IV hypersensitivity differs from the other hypersensitivity reactions in that it is **T-cell mediated**; there is no role for antibodies. This delayed-type hypersensitivity causes chronic inflammation; as a result of a persistent stimulus, chronic inflammation and tissue damage occur. *M. tuberculosis* infection is an example of a type IV hypersensitivity reaction.

This delayed-type hypersensitivity often takes days to develop, because it needs the activation of large numbers of T cells, which must accumulate before they can mediate an inflammatory response.

Transplantation and rejection

An organ may become damaged, to the point that it is irreparable, even with medical intervention. At this point, transplantation of the diseased organ is required. Although there are mechanical replacements for some organs, these are unable to reproduce the same function and lead to a lower standard of life, e.g. dialysis is currently used to treat kidney failure and involves repeated visits to the hospital.

Transplants between individuals are hindered because genetic information may be different, resulting in the production of different proteins – and thus a different set of peptides presented on the MHC. Moreover, the MHC of the donor and recipient usually differ. These differences contribute to the activation of T cells that target an immune response against the graft. For the graft to survive, it must be tolerated, and the immune response against it stopped, or at least strongly ameliorated.

Forms of rejection

The mechanisms by which rejection occurs can be classified into three classes based on the timeframe and the mechanisms involved:

1 **Hyperacute rejection** requires the existence of preformed antibodies that react to allograft antigens (alloantigens), e.g. ABO blood group mismatch results in hyperacute rejection due to preformed antibodies produced by B-1 cells.
2 **Acute rejection** results from the recognition of alloantigens by the T cells, mediating an immune result targeted directly at the allograft. This process is mediated predominantly by mismatch within the MHC genes; T cells react strongly to foreign MHC – so that as much as **10% may be activated by a foreign MHC haplotype**. Acute rejection occurs over days to weeks. It is this process that current transplant protocols aim to impede to promote allograft survival. The acute phase of rejection is similar to **type IV hypersensitivity**.
3 **Chronic rejection** is a complex and relatively poorly understood process that leads to gradual narrowing of lumen of vessels in the graft. This process leads to a loss of graft function and occurs over months or years.

Tolerance

There is the potential for newly produced TCRs to react to peptides derived from self-proteins, or for host B cells to react to self-molecules. There are many processes in place to ensure that this does not occur:

- **Central tolerance** is the result of **negative selection** of T and B cells.
- **Peripheral tolerance** allows for the removal of any self-reactive clones that have escaped central tolerance.
- **Suppression by regulatory T cells** in the thymus, some self-reactive T cells are not deleted, but develop into regulatory T cells that can specifically inhibit the adaptive immune response. Regulatory T cells shut down and limit the immune response to a self-antigen, thus contributing to peripheral tolerance.

Immunodeficiency

Immunodeficiency may be acquired or inherited. Typically deficiencies can be identified by an abnormal susceptibility to infection – the type of infection is often highly indicative of the immune deficiency. Inherited immune deficiencies are typically recessive. Hence, X-linked diseases tend to be the most common of such defects.

Inherited defects

Inherited defects often manifest rapidly after birth, and may be associated with other congenital defects. The susceptibility of the affected individual to infections depends on the nature of the defect:

- **T-cell deficiencies** lead to an increased tendency to develop infections by intracellular pathogens. A typical inherited T-cell deficiency is **DiGeorge syndrome**.
- **B-cell deficiencies** are linked to a lack of antibody production, resulting in susceptibility to repeated viral infection and to infection by extracellular bacteria. **Bruton's agammaglobulinaemia** is a common inherited B-cell deficiency, which results from a defect in signalling of the B cells.
- **Cellular defects of the innate immune system** typically focus on defective migration of cells or defective killing mechanisms.

Acquired defects

An individual born with a competent immune system may develop an immunodeficiency, typically through the depletion or loss of a component of the immune system. The most clinically significant condition is Acquired immunodeficiency syndrome (AIDS), which results from the loss of CD4$^+$ T cells during infection by Human immunodeficiency virus (HIV).

Autoimmunity

Autoimmunity is a hypersensitivity reaction to a self-antigen. Once activated, autoimmune syndromes may last for days or the remainder of the person's life, due to the ever-present nature of the antigen driving the reaction. Although not fully understood, many factors are implicated in the development of autoimmunity:

- **Breakdown of central tolerance**
- **Breakdown of peripheral tolerance**
- **Molecular mimicry**: an antibody or TCR that reacts with a pathogen may cross-react with a self-peptide; clearance of the infection resolves the autoimmune condition
- Tissue APCs may **present self-antigen during infection:** professional APCs are recruited to sites of infection. Although tolerance provides a good safeguard, self-peptides may be acquired and presented under inflammatory stimuli. If there are reactive T cells present, an immune response against a harmless self-antigen may develop
- **Cryptic antigens**: some antigens are kept physically separate from the immune system (e.g. sperm antigens). The exposure of cryptic antigens to the immune system later in life can lead to an immune response, if there is no central tolerance to that antigen (e.g. post-vasectomy).

Genetics of autoimmunity

There is a strong genetic association in many autoimmune diseases, which has been identified through studies of twins. The MHC haplotype is often the strongest predetermining factor; this is best illustrated by **ankylosing spondylitis**, in

which the presence of the **HLA-B27** allele is seen in about 90% of cases.

 CLINICAL: Ankylosing Spondylitis

Ankylosing Spondylitis is an autoimmune disease, very much more common in men. Initial symptoms are pain in the lower back and thighs. Sclerosis of the spinal joints occurs, leading to restrictions in movement of the spine in all planes. In the spine, the vertebrae become linked through 'bony bridging' and calcification of the ligaments.

Whilst most cases of Ankylosing Spondylitis express the HLA-B27 allele, the vast majority of individuals expressing HLA-B27 are not afflicted by Ankylosing Spondylitis.

One of the best-studied autoimmune conditions is type 1 diabetes. Genetic analysis has suggested that the HLA-DR3 and DR4 alleles are linked with susceptibility to type 1 diabetes. It is thought that these MHC alleles reduce the body's ability to generate tolerance against a self-antigen associated with the condition – in this case, insulin has been implicated.

There is a strong environmental component to all autoimmune diseases – studies of identical twins have shown that there is only about a 30–50% **concordance**, suggesting that at least half of the factors contributing to the generation of type 1 diabetes in an individual are the result of environmental stimuli, such as an infection.

 RELATED CHAPTERS

16

Microbiology

Microorganisms that cause disease are termed 'pathogens'. The source of these organisms may be external to the body or another location in the body (e.g. the gut).

In many cases, disease is a by-product of the infection and provides no advantage to the pathogen in terms of helping its replication and transmission. In others, the symptoms of disease specifically aid the survival and replication of the pathogen.

Infectious diseases are still a major cause of illness and death, even in the developed world. With the increasing emergence of drug-resistant strains of pathogen, an understanding of the lifecycle of a pathogen is becoming evermore important: both to identify new potential drug targets, and to develop methods to prevent transmission.

Microorganisms that cause infectious disease can be grouped into four broad categories, based on their structure: acellular pathogens, bacteria, fungi and parasites. In each group, different strains of pathogen cause a huge variety of different disease, and have evolved mechanisms of replication and immune evasion. To illustrate this, examples of common pathogens are discussed in detail.

Basic concepts

The body may be colonised by a variety of microorganisms. Some of these comprise the commensal organisms that occur naturally on the skin and at other sites. In their *usual* site commensal organisms do not cause disease. In the case of other microorganisms, their presence always results in disease.

The relationship between a microbe and its host can be described in one of three ways:

1 **Mutualism** – both organisms benefit from the relationship
2 **Commensalism** – one organism benefits, although the other neither is harmed nor benefits from the relationship
3 **Parasitism** – one organism benefits while causing damage to its host.

When a microorganism causes disease it is termed a pathogen, but it may be further classified as a **professional** or a **non-professional** pathogen:

- **Professional pathogens** cause the symptoms of disease to promote their survival and replication, e.g. enterobacteria tend to cause diarrhoea which promotes transmission by the faeco-oral route.
- **Non-professional pathogens** cause symptoms of disease incidentally and derive little (if any) benefit from it. *Neisseria meningitidis* causes meningitis, which is likely to be fatal if untreated and therefore does not help transmission of the disease to another host.

In the terms of microbiology, a **disease** can be considered as infection by microorganisms that have pathology.

Koch's postulates

To establish that an organism causes a specific disease it must fulfil **Koch's postulates**:

Biomedical Science Lecture Notes, First Edition. Ian Lyons.
© 2011 by Ian Lyons. Published 2011 by Blackwell Publishing Ltd.

- The organism can be isolated from each case of the disease.
- The organism can be grown in culture.
- Injecting the organism into a suitable recipient will reproduce the symptoms of the disease and the organism can be re-isolated from the recipient.

Koch's postulates can only be fulfilled if the microorganism is indeed the cause of infection. In practice, it may be difficult for the postulate to be fulfilled for a number of reasons:

- There may not be a suitable culture system for the pathogen.
- There is no suitable recipient model.
- The disease may have a latent stage, making it difficult to isolate or detect.

Routes and transmission of infection

Infectious diseases must be transmitted to new hosts so that the causative organism can survive and replicate. Many routes of transmission have been identified that vary with the pathogen and its source including:

- **Airborne** (e.g. influenza virus) in fluid droplets
- **Faeco-oral** (e.g. poliovirus)
- **Mucosal** (e.g. HIV)
- **Vector borne** (e.g. malaria – caused by *Plasmodium* spp. transmitted by a bite from a mosquito)
- **Blood** (e.g. hepatitis B virus [HBV])
- **Animal bite** (e.g. rabies)
- **Neonatal** – transmission from mother to child across the placenta, or at or around birth (e.g. group B streptococci).

Neonatal transmission typically leads to chronic infections, as a result of the baby's developing immune system. Transmission may occur in three situations:

1 Virus crossing the placenta into the neonatal circulation
2 At childbirth, as a result of exposure to pathogens present in the birth canal
3 Virus present in infected milk.

Prevention of infection

The potential for a disease to occur can be reduced by preventing the spread of the organism to the individual. The potential for infection can be abrogated by eliminating or reducing the number of potential pathogens at possible sites of contamination.

Sterilisation and disinfection

Physical methods of destroying microbes rely on heat, which kills or denatures the infectious agent, or on chemical disruption of microbes by disinfectants.

Heat treatment may be used either to kill all microbes or to remove those that are potentially harmful (e.g. pasteurisation of milk). Depending on the nature of the materials to be sterilised, either wet or dry heat is used:

- **Wet heat** is generally preferred as it works more quickly, reducing the amount of time that a high temperature must be maintained. **Autoclaving** is the standard method of sterilisation, which maintains steam at high pressure for 20 min, ensuring the killing of all microorganisms, including spores.
- **Dry heat** is used to sterilise materials that cannot be exposed to moisture. In contrast to the relatively short periods of heating required in autoclaving, dry heat sterilisation requires several hours, usually at 160 °C or more to ensure killing.

Pasteurisation is often used in industry to kill milk-borne pathogens through heating to 72 °C for about 30 seconds. This kills many, but not all, pathogens; it reduces the risk of developing illness from milk-borne pathogens, and lengthens the storage life of milk.

Chemical agents can be used to kill microorganisms through:

- disruption of lipid membrane, e.g. detergents
- modification of proteins, e.g. hypochlorite in bleach is an oxidising agent
- modification of DNA.

 CLINICAL Nosocomial infections

Hospitals are a source of pathogens; the specific pathogens and strains differ from those found in the community. Furthermore, hospitalised patients are likely to have depressed immune systems, increasing the likelihood of infection. Many pathogen strains common in hospitals have acquired resistance to antibiotics (e.g. meticillin-resistant *Staphylococcus aureus* or MRSA), making them difficult to treat.

Gamma irradiation can be used to sterilise items by inducing fatal mutation in the microorganisms exposed to it. The gamma rays break down the bacterial DNA preventing the replication of the bacteria.

Vaccination (active immunisation)

Vaccines are used to protect against infection by inducing active immunity. Vaccines act by inducing immunological memory through the production of antibodies and memory T cells. Vaccines can be 'live' or may be 'killed' when a dead version or non-infectious components of the pathogen are used:

Live vaccines

Live vaccines contain an attenuated (weakened) form of the pathogen or closely related organism. A common example is the BCG vaccine, used to protect against tuberculosis (TB):

- **Advantages**: live vaccines stimulate production of immunoglobulin IgA and IgG antibody immunity, as well as cell-mediated immunity. Such vaccines provide long-lasting protection because the replicating, but attenuated pathogen (or a closely related organism) mimics a natural infection. As a live culture can be maintained, live vaccines are inexpensive to manufacture.
- **Disadvantages**: a 'live' vaccine may spontaneously revert to its wild form (e.g. polio vaccine) and be spread into environment. If such a vaccine is administered to an immunocompromised patient, it may cause life-threatening infection. In terms of transportation, live vaccines are difficult because they are unstable at room temperature and require storage in refrigerated vessels.

Killed (inactivated vaccines)

Dead or inactivated vaccines are incapable of infectivity or toxicity because they contain no component that can replicate. Common examples are the tetanus toxoid (formalin-inactivated tetanus toxin) and the influenza vaccine (formalin-treated virus particles):

- **Advantages**: Inactivated vaccines are safer than live vaccines because they cannot cause or transmit disease. They are far more stable than live vaccines, helping their transport and storage.
- **Disadvantages**: as the vaccine does not replicate, it generates a shorter-lasting immunity than live

vaccines and it is not focused on the normal life-cycle of the pathogen. The response is restricted primarily to antibody production; little cell-mediated immunity is elicited. In terms of cost, inactivated vaccines are relatively expensive.

Passive immunisation

Passive immunisation is achieved by the transference of antibodies to an individual. The protection that this provides is only temporary because the circulating antibodies are gradually cleared and not replaced.

Passive immunisation occurs from a mother to her child through IgG, which crosses the placenta to the fetus from the maternal circulation. Moreover, a mother's breast milk is rich in IgA, which protects the neonate's mucosal surfaces from pathogen entry.

In a clinical setting, passive immunisation has been exploited to treat a number of conditions. In particular, rabies can be treated by the injection of sera containing antibodies against the rabies virus into the wound site. Similar treatments can be used to treat tetanus and snake bites. The serum used in passive immunisation is often produced from horses and can lead to an immune reaction to the foreign proteins within the serum, known as 'serum sickness'.

Other methods of prevention

Although vaccination is a commonly used method of prophylaxis, other, less 'hi-tech' approaches are often just as effective including:

- **Physical methods**, such as quarantine, can be very effective in preventing the transmission of disease. The principle behind quarantine is to isolate the individual to allow any infection, if present, to manifest itself. This procedure is very expensive and inconvenient to the patient. Other methods of prevention include barriers. In the hospital, gloves are commonly used to prevent the potential spread of infection to and from patients.
- **Control of vectors and reservoirs** of a pathogen can prevent transmission of infection. This form of prevention has been effective in combating malaria through the use of insecticides to kill malaria-carrying mosquitoes.
- **Good hygienic practice** is important in the preparation of food to prevent transmission of enteric bacteria. Practices such as hand washing

between examining patients are essential to reduce spread of nosocomial infections.
- **Education**: teaching on how infectious diseases spread and how they can be prevented is important in their control.

Epidemiology

Epidemiology is the study of the effects of health and disease in populations. A variety of factors must be considered when studying a disease and its effects on the population

- **Demographic factors**, e.g. age, ethnic group, gender
- **Biological and genetic,** e.g. blood groups, MHC (major histocompatibility compex) haplotype
- **Socioeconomic**, e.g. occupation, income
- **Personal habits**, e.g. smoking, alcohol consumption, drug use.

The **basic reproductive rate** of an infection (R_0), is a key value to consider. It is defined as the number of cases that would result directly from the introduction of a single infectious individual into a susceptible population. It can be influenced by a number of factors, including:

- The duration of the infectious period
- The ease of transmission
- The density of the host population.

An R_0 of 1 means that a single infectious case is likely to cause one new case in a population; prevention mechanisms aim to reduce R_0.

- **For an infection to spread $R_0 > 1$**.
- If $R_0 < 1$, the infection is **shrinking**.

With any microbial infection there must be a careful balance between the severity of the ensuing disease and allowing its host to survive without extensive morbidity:

- If infection relies on **high motility of host**, infection must not cause high morbidity, e.g. HIV has a long asymptomatic period which promotes sexual transmission of the virus to many sexual partners.
- If an infection is **highly virulent** there is little need for host motility, e.g. arthropod-borne diseases in which the vector is able to move rapidly and the host effectively acts as a reservoir for infection.
- There are some pathogens that are capable of surviving outside their host. The pathogen may

 DEFINITION Herd immunity

Vaccination/immunisation aims to reduce the density of individuals who are susceptible to an infection. An immunised individual cannot become infectious, and thus cannot transmit the infection. If there are enough individuals within a population who are immune to infection, this will hinder the transmission of the infection between susceptible individuals and is known as **herd immunity**. There is a critical level for eradication of an infection, p_c, where $p_c = 1 - (1/R_0)$. R_0 is the basic reproductive rate. If the immunised proportion exceeds p_c, the proportion of non-susceptible individuals is high enough to break the transmission cycle between susceptible individuals.

In the case of measles, R_0 is estimated to be around 10, so the critical level for heard immunity would be:

$$p_c = 1 - \left(\frac{1}{10}\right) = \frac{9}{10}.$$

This suggests that, for herd immunity to be maintained, at least 90% of the population must be immunised.

seek to kill its host rapidly, because it provides a large source of dead tissue in which it can survive.

If an infection is too virulent it is likely to limit the life of its host, and reduce the potential for the spread of infection to new hosts. The transmission rate of the disease determines the virulence of an infection.

Some zoonoses, infections that have evolved to infect a specific animal host, are fatal in humans which are not their normal host. Humans may be 'dead-end' hosts, from whom further transmission of the pathogen will not occur, e.g. rabies is almost always fatal in humans, if untreated. In bats, the usual host, the disease takes a more chronic form.

Acellular pathogens: viruses and prions

Viruses and prions are acellular pathogens that use host proteins for their replication. They are unable to replicate outside live cells:

- Viruses are a few hundred nanometres at most.
- Prions are aggregates of a misfolded host protein.

Classification of viruses and related particles

The term 'virus' refers to the assembly of proteins, lipids and nucleic acids that replicates in cells. In addition to the typical virus particles, other particles exhibit many of the features that have also been described in viruses, some of which are produced aberrantly during a viral infection:

- **Virion** refers to a normal, infectious viral particle which is capable of attaching and entering a new cell and replicating within it to produce further virions.
- **Defective viruses** contain viral proteins and a genome, although they lack some components essential for replication due to mutation or deletion of part of the viral genome. Defective viruses can only replicate in cells that are also infected with a fully functional 'helper' virus (e.g. hepatitis δ requires cells to be infected with hepatitis B virus for it to replicate).
- **Pseudovirions** possess a fragment of host DNA instead of the viral genome. They may form when the host DNA becomes fragmented in infected cells.
- **Viroids** consist solely of a circular molecule of RNA without associated protein or envelope. They can cause disease in plants, but no human disease has yet been described.

Viral components

Virions are minute (20–300 nm), too small to be seen by a light microscope. The following are common components of a virion (Fig 16.1):

- The **genome** encodes the proteins necessary for the assembly and replication of new virions. A viral genome may be made up of RNA or DNA, either double or single stranded.
- The **capsid** is made up of repeated protein subunits which form a stable structure containing the viral genome. The capsid subunits determine the shape of the virus. In non-enveloped viruses, the capsid also contains the viral-binding site.
- **Viral proteins** perform a variety of functions. Some bind to host cell protein to allow entry into the cell, whereas others have a structural

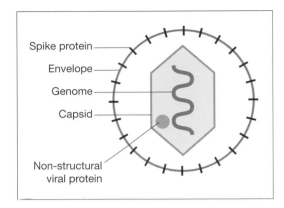

Figure 16.1 Components of a virion.

role, e.g. capsid proteins. Internal proteins, such as RNA polymerase, aid the replication and assembly of progeny virions. Accessory proteins help viral survival by potentiating their evasion of the immune response. Viral proteins provide the targets by which both antibodies and T cells recognise the pathogen.
- The **envelope** is a lipid bilayer that encloses the capsid. It is found in many viruses and derived from the host membrane. The formation of an envelope requires the expression of a matrix protein to mediate interactions between capsid and envelope. Viral 'spike' glycoproteins are inserted into the envelope, forming binding sites to allow virus entry into the host cell. Due to the presence of this additional structure, enveloped viruses tend to be less stable than non-enveloped viruses.

Types of virus

Viruses are classified according to the type of nucleic acids that make up the genome and the transcriptase enzyme involved in the replication of the viral genome, both of which determine the nature of the viral replication cycle.

Viruses can be classified into seven distinct groups – the Baltimore classification:

1 Single-stranded **positive polarity** RNA virus (e.g. poliovirus)
2 Single-stranded **negative polarity** RNA virus (e.g. influenza virus)
3 Double-stranded RNA virus (e.g. rotavirus)
4 Single-stranded DNA virus (e.g. parvovirus)

5 Double-stranded DNA virus (e.g. herpesvirus)
6 Retrovirus (e.g. human immunodeficiency virus)
7 Hepadnavirus (e.g. hepatitis B virus).

The viral life cycle

Viruses must enter a host cell and hijack its internal machinery in order to replicate. Viral proteins must be synthesised, to regulate replication of the genome and produce new virions, and the viral genome must be copied. After this, many progeny virions are assembled and released from the host cell. The life cycle consists of five distinct stages (Fig. 16.2):

1 Attachment to the target cell
2 Entry into the cytoplasm (and, if necessary, nucleus) of the cell
3 Replication of viral genome and proteins
4 Assembly of progeny virions
5 Release of progeny from cell.

Attachment and entry into cells

Proteins on the virion surface bind to specific receptors on the cell surface; the specificity of this interaction determines which species and cell types the virus can infect.

For **enveloped viruses**, fusion of the envelope with the cell membrane is required for entry of the viral genome and associated proteins into the cell. This may occur at the cell surface, or after endocytosis into an endosome. Viral proteins (e.g. gp120 and gp41 in HIV) are able to trigger the fusion of the cell membrane with the viral envelope.

Interactions of cell proteins directly with the capsid of **non-enveloped** viruses lead to conformational changes which release the capsid contents into the cell cytoplasm.

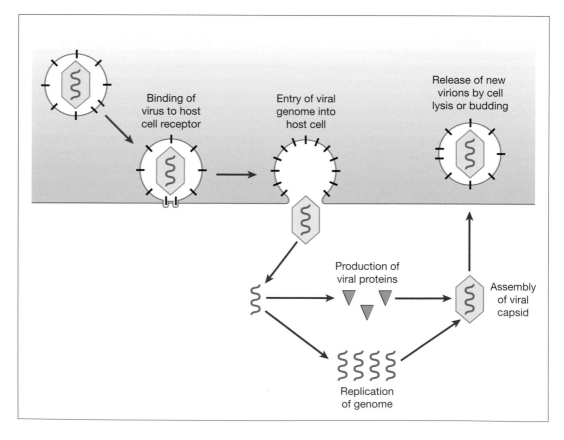

Figure 16.2 The viral lifecycle.

Replication

On entering a host cell, viruses must synthesise the proteins necessary to allow genome replication, as well as those that form new virions. The path by which this process occurs is determined by the nature of the viral genome.

DNA viruses replicate in the nucleus. Host cell polymerases produce mRNA and copy the viral genome. Poxviruses are unusual in that they replicate in the cytoplasm, because they carry a viral DNA polymerase.

RNA virus replication is restricted to the cytoplasm in almost all cases. The major exceptions are the influenza virus and retroviruses. RNA viruses are divided into four major groups with different strategies for replication:

1 **Single-stranded positive-polarity RNA viruses** can use host machinery to produce viral proteins, including an RNA polymerase, directly from the viral genome. This RNA polymerase is used to produce a negative-polarity copy of the viral genome which acts as a template for the synthesis of further genome copies.
2 **Single-stranded negative-polarity RNA viruses** carry their own RNA polymerase for mRNA production, as well as to synthesise a template for new viral genomes.
3 **Double-stranded RNA viruses** must carry their own polymerase, similar to single-stranded negative-polarity RNA viruses.
4 **Retroviruses** possess a single-stranded RNA genome which is transcribed into DNA by the viral enzyme, reverse transcriptase, for integration into host cell DNA. Retroviruses are unusual in that they carry two copies of the genome in each particle.

Viral mRNA is translated into protein by the host cell ribosomes.

In some viruses, mRNA is translated into precursor polypeptides (e.g. poliovirus), and then cleaved into functional proteins by viral protease. In other viruses, individual mRNAs are translated directly into proteins, e.g. influenza virus.

Assembly and release

The viral genome and internal proteins must be packaged in the capsid. After packaging, the virus particles are then released from the cell:

- Non-enveloped viruses are typically released by **cell lysis**, resulting in cell death.

- Enveloped viruses **bud** through the cell membrane to form an envelope, although in the case of the herpesvirus the envelope is derived from the nuclear membrane. Budding does not directly cause cell death.

Effects of viral infection on the host

The precise effects of infection depend on the nature of the virus, the cell that it infects and the state of the host.

There are four main outcomes of infection of a cell by a virus:

1 Death, as a direct effect of the virus or through the host immune response
2 Fusion of infected cells to form syncytia
3 Malignant transformation (e.g. Epstein–Barr virus, papillomavirus)
4 No apparent change (as a result of latency), or a cell may produce virus with no apparent ill effects.

Spread of virus within the host

Local spread of virus occurs after a short incubation through transmission of virus to other cells at the initial site of infection. The virus may also spread to local lymph nodes, as free virus or within phagocytes.

Viraemia allows systemic infection, against which it is more difficult to mount an effective immune response because the infection is no longer restricted to a single site.

Symptoms of viral disease

Most viral diseases have similar general symptoms – fever, myalgia, malaise – reflecting a general antiviral response as a result of the release of cytokines and other mediators of inflammation. Viruses cause specific symptoms due to the cell types that they infect, e.g. paralysis occurs in poliomyelitis from infection of motor neurons.

Viral titre during infection

The course of a viral infection can be charted by the viral titre and broadly classified as acute or chronic. It can be also be defined by the eventual outcome of the disease in the host: resolution of infection, chronic carrier state or death of the host.

Immediately after virus enters the host, a **viral eclipse phase** ensues, in which no free virus particles are detectable because they have entered host cells for replication. The viral level increases as progeny virus are produced:

In an **acute infection**, a successful immune response eradicates the virus. In a **chronic infection**, a steady state is set up in which virus production offsets destruction due to cell-mediated killing of infected cells. The symptoms of disease may be the result of repeated damage due to an incomplete cell-mediated immune response (e.g. in hepatitis B infection) as well as any direct effects of the virus itself.

Immune response to viral infection

The immune system is equipped to combat viral infection. The precise response is specific to an individual virus, but the basic mechanisms and pathways are similar for all viruses.

Interferon

Most viruses produce double-stranded RNA (dsRNA) during their lifecycle, a nucleic acid structure not produced by host cells. The interferon (IFN) pathway is triggered by the presence of dsRNA within a cell. Two types of interferon, IFNα and IFNβ, are produced as part of the innate antiviral responses. IFNα and IFNβ are secreted by infected cells on both the infected cell and its uninfected neighbours, binding to a common surface receptor. The interferon receptor signals through JAK/STAT tyrosine kinases and induces expression of genes that inhibit viral replication.

IFNα and IFNβ induce expression of antiviral proteins including:

- **RNAase L** – an endoribonuclease that degrades both host and viral RNA
- **2′,5′-oligoadenylate synthase** which polymerases ATP to prevent its use as an energy source.

IFNα and IFNβ upregulate the adaptive immune response and activate **natural killer (NK) cells**. They also promote expression of major histocompatibility complex class I (MHC-I) molecules, thereby increasing presentation of viral peptides to cytotoxic lymphocytes.

Clearance of virus-infected cells

Much of the viral lifecycle occurs in host cells, protected from the antibody response. Moreover,

in HIV and some other infections, the viral genome can become integrated into the host cell genome; the infected cells must be killed to remove the virus:

- **Cytotoxic T cells** recognise viral peptides, presented on MHC-I molecules through their unique T-cell receptor, and may mediate killing.
- **NK cells** are capable of clearing virus-infected cells and are not specific to an antigen (they recognise broad changes associated with infection or malignancy), allowing a rapid response as part of the innate immune system.

Antibodies in the antiviral immune response

Antibodies neutralise viruses by either blocking viral binding to surface receptors or disrupting the structure of the virus. Viruses may also be cross-linked by antibodies to form complexes, which can recruit proteins in the **complement pathway** to help their clearance. Although antibodies often play a limited role in recovery from a primary infection, due to the largely intracellular lifecycle of viruses, they have an important role in the prevention of reinfection. The presence of IgG in serum and IgA on mucosal surfaces plays a particularly important role in protection.

Evasion of the immune system

Viruses have developed methods to avoid the host immune response, attempting to prolong the period during which the host is infectious, so as to promote transmission to other hosts.

Mutation and recombination

Viral polymerases are rather inaccurate during their replication of the viral genome. The resulting mutations can change antigenic epitopes on the viral proteins. The influenza virus is also able to recombine segments of genome, resulting in a major change in the antigenicity of the virus; this process is known as antigenic shift.

Speed

The adaptive immune response requires about 1 week to develop. Some small RNA viruses may reproduce rapidly and overwhelm the host before a strong immune response is generated.

Subversion

Viruses may express proteins to alter or modify the immune response so that it is less effective. This approach is typically employed by large DNA viruses, e.g. HIV encodes proteins to downregulate MHC-I expression.

Location

Viruses may infect specific cell types to help their immune evasion. This is particularly evident in the herpes simplex virus which infects nerve cells. Nerve cells express low levels of MHC-I, reducing the likelihood of cell-mediated killing.

Latency

Cellular latency occurs in viruses that are able to shut down production of new viruses while the viral genomes remain in the infected cell, reducing targets of the immune response. The virus may be reactivated at a later stage – possibly when the immune system is weakened.

> **DEFINITION Cellular and clinical latency**
>
> **Cellular latency** occurs when there is no new virus production in a cell, despite the cell being infected. **Clinical latency** is a transient asymptomatic period during viral infection: this may be the result of cellular latency or other factors such as an active immune response.

Laboratory diagnosis of viral infection

Viruses cannot be seen under a light microscope and require specific cell cultures in order to be grown in a lab. Identification of viruses typically relies on serological tests and other mechanisms of detecting antigens or antibodies to viral proteins from samples isolated from the patient.

The methods of detecting viral infection can be divided into direct and indirect:

- **Direct methods** of identification aim to detect some feature of the virus itself – either detecting presence of the viral genome by polymerase chain reaction (PCR), or detecting viral antigens using a test such as the enzyme-linked immunosorbent assay (ELISA).

- **Indirect methods** look for changes that result directly from the viral infection, such as the development and increased titre of antibodies specific to viral antigens.

Identification of virus using cell culture

Inoculation

Inoculation of a cell culture with a clinical sample can provide evidence of viral infection because the virus may produce characteristic cytopathic effects, allowing a presumptive diagnosis based on time to appear and the cell types used in the culture.

Microscopic identification

Virus may be detected by direct examination of clinical samples. Light microscopy may show characteristic morphological changes of host cells, such as inclusion bodies and formation of giant cells. Under electron microscopy, individual virus particles can be visualised, allowing identification of the virus based on size and morphology.

Serological methods

A rise in the antibody titre in a patient must be detected to distinguish between current infection and antibodies generated from a previous infection. Serological diagnosis is often retrospective because the patient is usually recovering before results are obtained. In some cases, levels of IgM antibody may be used to diagnose current infection.

Detection of viral proteins or nucleic acids

Detection of **viral proteins** is achieved using an antibody to a known viral antigen (e.g. for HIV and hepatitis B virus), most commonly through an ELISA test.

The method for detection of **nucleic acids** uses PCR to amplify sequences specific to a virus, allowing detection even with low levels of virus in the sample. An assay in which the level of viral nucleic acid is assessed can be used to monitor the course of a chronic infection (e.g. in HIV).

DEFINITION Enzyme-linked immunosorbent assay (ELISA)

The ELISA is a standard laboratory test that can be used to identify a virus and determine its titre. Antigen from a clinical sample is bound to the surface of plastic wells and antibodies of a known specificity are added. These can bind to the antigen and excess unbound antibody is washed away. The antibody may be linked to an enzyme, or a secondary antibody can be added that is specific to the first antibody and conjugated to an enzyme. The enzyme catalyses a colour change in a soluble substrate. A photometer can then be used to estimate viral titre based on the intensity of colour.

 CLINICAL Influenza

After a short incubation period (24–48 hours) sore throat, fever, myalgia and headache can develop. The sore throat and cough are a local symptom caused by necrosis of respiratory epithelium. Systemic symptoms are caused by the cytokine response to viral infection. Resolution usually occurs in 4–7 days, although pneumonia may develop (bacterial or viral). Influenza has a significant mortality, particularly in elderly and young people. Those individuals most at risk are immunised annually. Diagnosis of influenza is usually made on clinical grounds.

Treatments of viral infection

Drug therapies rely on targeting proteins that are unique to the pathogen. As viruses exploit the host cellular machinery, such targets are limited. Research is ongoing to develop inhibitors of proteins unique to viruses. Current examples of such drugs are reverse transcriptase inhibitors and protease inhibitors. Antiviral drugs are often ineffective in acute infections because they often need to be given early before many patients have even seen a doctor.

Other treatments have focused on enhancing the immune response to the infection, e.g. IFNβ therapy for hepatitis B infection.

Protection can be achieved by an antibody response – IgA and IgG – neutralising the virus in the blood or at sites of entry. Protective antibodies can be raised by immunisation or temporarily by administration of specific antiviral antibodies, as in post-exposure prophylaxis for rabies.

Influenza virus

The influenza virus, an orthomyxovirus, has been responsible for a huge number of deaths throughout history. Major outbreaks of influenza have occurred as a result of the widespread antigenic variation that the virus can undergo, particularly through recombination of its genome with that of influenza from another animal species.

Morphology and structure

Influenza virus is an enveloped virus around 100 nm in size, containing a segmented, single-stranded, negative-sense RNA genome. The eight genome segments are associated with viral proteins, including RNA polymerase, to form ribonucleoprotein.

The viral envelope has two types of viral spike:

1 **Haemagglutinin** binds to the cell surface receptor, sialic acid, mediating entry into host cells.
2 **Neuraminidase** can cleave sialic (neuraminic) acid on host cells to allow release of progeny.

These spikes are the major antigenic targets on the virion – changes in antigenicity of haemagglutinin and neuraminidase are important in establishing epidemics. Influenza strains are identified by the types of haemagglutinin and neuraminidase that they contain, e.g. H5N1: avian influenza.

Phylogeny and transmission

Three types of influenza virus can infect humans:

1 Influenza A is found in many different species of animal and can lead to pandemics.
2 Influenza B is a milder form and infects only humans.
3 Influenza C causes only mild respiratory infections and not full-blown influenza.

Transmission of Influenza virus is by respiratory aerosol. This infection is limited to the upper respiratory tract because it expresses specific enzymes that are necessary for the function of haemagglutinin in host cells. Viraemia is very rare.

Replication cycle and pathogenesis of disease

Attachment and entry

Haemagglutinin binding to sialic acid triggers endocytosis. Subsequent entry into the cytoplasm depends on acidification of the endosome. This induces a structural change in haemagglutinin, which allows it to fuse with the envelope of the endosome.

Replication

Unusually for an RNA virus, replication of the genome occurs in the nucleus where the virion RNA polymerase transcribes the eight viral genome segments into mRNA; each segment encodes a different protein. The genome is replicated from positive-polarity templates and associates with viral protein to form ribonucleoprotein.

Release

The capsid is assembled around ribonucleoproteins and progeny virions are released through budding. Influenza virus is cytopathic as a result of the damage that is caused to the internal machinery of the cell during replication.

Immune evasion

The influenza A virus has developed two mechanisms of mutating to evade immune responses:

1 **Antigenic shift** occurs through reassortment of genome segments between species and results from a cell being infected with two different strains of influenza. This may occur in pigs, which can be infected with both human and avian influenza A. This recombination results in a major shift in the antigenic epitopes of the virus and may lead to pandemic because existing antibodies are unlikely to offer protective immunity. Antigenic shift occurs only with influenza A, because it is found in a variety of animal species.
2 **Antigenic drift** occurs through mutations introduced by error-prone transcription. Existing protective antibodies are likely to exhibit some cross-reactivity due to the less drastic change in the antigenic epitopes of the virus.

Immune response

Infection is primarily controlled by the interferon response to dsRNA and cytotoxic T lymphocytes (CTLs) specific for influenza-derived epitopes. Protective immunity results from the generation of IgA antibodies which are secreted into the respiratory mucosa, although these are strain specific.

Treatment

Treatment of influenza includes **amantadine**, which prevents viral entry from endosome to cytoplasm by inhibiting the viral M2 protein that is involved in endosome acidification. Amantadine is effective only against influenza A and resistant strains have been identified.

Zanamivir inhibits neuraminidase, to prevent release of virus from the host cell. It is effective against influenza A and influenza B viruses.

The usefulness of both therapies is limited by the fact that they must be given early on in the infection, often before an accurate diagnosis can be made.

Prevention

Immunisation to prevent infection is preferred to treatment. The vaccine is grown in chicken eggs, purified and inactivated. Consequently, the strains of influenza to be included in the vaccine must be decided 6–9 months in advance, to allow sufficient time for vaccine production. Protection lasts for around 6 months because the inactivated virus triggers rather poor IgA and IgG production.

Hepatitis B virus

Hepatitis B virus (HBV), the causative agent of hepatitis B, is a hepadnavirus that is thought to chronically infect over 300 million people. HBV is a severe global health problem because it is highly transmissible and infection results in many chronic carriers, who show few clinical symptoms.

Morphology and structure

HBV is an enveloped virus with an icosahedral nucleocapsid that contains a partly double-stranded circular DNA genome. The viral envelope contains surface antigen protein (HBsAg) which is produced in excess during infection. Tubes of HBsAg in the blood of an infected individual are visible under the electron microscope and are an important diagnostic marker.

Transmission and phylogeny

Humans are the natural host for HBV. There are three main routes of transmission:

1 Via infected blood, e.g. drug abuse
2 During sexual intercourse
3 From mother to child during childbirth.

After transmission to a new host, the virus enters the blood and infects hepatocytes through a specific cell receptor found on the hepatocyte surface. Replication is restricted to hepatocytes through the need for a specific transcription factor within the cells.

The surface antigen of HBV is sufficiently conserved for protection from all strains to be conferred by a single vaccine. From epidemiological studies four distinct strains can be identified.

> ### CLINICAL **Symptoms of hepatitis B**
>
> Many HBV infections are asymptomatic and can be detected only by antibody to HBsAg. Clinical symptoms include fever, anorexia and vomiting. Impaired liver function leads to jaundice, dark urine, pale faeces and high levels of transaminases. Most chronic carriers are asymptomatic, although some may have active chronic hepatitis, which can lead to cirrhosis and ultimately death.

Replication and pathogenesis of disease

Attachment and entry

HBV binds the sialoglycoprotein receptor which is thought to mediate uptake into the cells via endosomes.

Replication

After entering the cell, the virion DNA polymerase synthesises the missing portion of DNA to form a complete circular DNA genome, from which mRNA is synthesised by cellular RNA polymerase. A template of the viral genome is also synthesised.

Assembly and release

New viral DNA genomes are produced in the new virus particle from the positive-polarity RNA template using the reverse transcriptase activity of viral DNA polymerase. Progeny HBV with an HBsAg envelope are released by budding through the cell membrane in a non-cytopathic process.

Pathogenesis of disease

Viral infection is controlled by cytotoxic T cells that mediate the killing of infected hepatocytes. The symptoms of disease result from cell-mediated immune injury. HBV has a particularly long

incubation period before symptoms manifest – typically 4–20 weeks.

Chronic HBV infection occurs in about 10% and is associated with hepatocellular carcinoma. This is due to the repeated damage sustained by the liver from the immune system, leading to a necessary constant regeneration and therefore a high potential for cancer-inducing mutation.

A variety of factors promote a chronic state:

- **CTL escape mutants**
- **MHC alleles**
- **Virus strain variation**
- **Clonal exhaustion** due to high antigen load.

The weaker immune system found in newborns makes them likely to become chronic carriers.

> ### DEFINITION **Hepatitis viruses**
>
> There are many different hepatitis viruses that are found worldwide. These are capable of causing hepatitis, often chronic:
>
> - **Hepatitis A**: this picornavirus is transmitted by the faeco-oral route. It usually causes a mild infection and is now less common due to an effective vaccine.
> - **Hepatitis C**: a flavivirus found throughout the world. It is transmitted by blood and, although an acute infection is mild, chronic infection often occurs.
> - **Hepatitis δ**: incomplete (dependovirus) virus – contains circular single-stranded RNA genome. It can replicate only within cells also infected with HBV. Hepatitis δ virus increases the symptoms of HBV infection.
>
> Specific symptoms of viral hepatitis are similar as because reflect a decrease in liver function leading to jaundice, dark urine, pale stools, etc.

Immune response

The immune response to HBV results in the proliferation of cytotoxic T cells. Antibodies are generated against the HBsAg which provide lifelong immunity after recovery.

Treatment

IFNα is used to treat chronic hepatitis B infections. Reverse transcriptase inhibitors are also useful.

Prevention

A vaccine containing recombinant HBsAg produced by genetically modified yeast cells has been developed. The HBV vaccine is administered to those at high risk of exposure, e.g. healthcare workers.

Immunoglobulin pooled from patients who have recovered from HBV can be used to provide passive immunity in those exposed to HBV-contaminated blood (e.g. after a needle-stick injury).

 CLINICAL Needle-stick injury

HBV is very easily transmitted by infected blood, and needle-stick injuries carry a significant risk of passing on HBV infection. There is as much as a 30% chance that a needle-stick injury from a patient infected with HBV infects the recipient, hence the need immunise healthcare workers. In contrast, there is about a 3% chance of developing HCV from a needle-stick injury from contaminated blood and, for HIV, about a 0.3% chance of infection.

Poliovirus

Poliovirus is the causative agent of poliomyelitis. This severe paralytic disease has been almost eradicated due to the development of an effective vaccine, and the fact that humans are its only natural host.

Structure and morphology

The poliovirus is a small (20–30 nm) member of the picornavirus family. These are non-enveloped viruses with icosahedral nucleocapsids and a single-stranded, positive-polarity, linear RNA genome.

Transmission and phylogeny

Poliovirus is transmitted by the faeco-oral route, initially infecting gut epithelial cells. The poliovirus exists in three distinct antigenic types.

Replication cycle and pathogenesis of disease

Attachment and entry

Entry is mediated through binding of the viral capsid to the poliovirus receptor (PVR) on the host cell surface. This binding induces a conformational shift in the viral capsid, allowing the viral genome to enter the host cell.

Replication

The poliovirus genome functions as mRNA – it is translated into one large polypeptide and cleaved by a protease encoded within the polypeptide itself. A complementary negative strand of RNA is also synthesised, which acts as a template for new copies of the genome.

Assembly and release

Progeny virion particles are assembled in the cytoplasm and released by cell lysis.

Pathogenesis

Most poliovirus infections are minor and restricted to the gut. In most cases the infection is asymptomatic, although a mild febrile illness may ensue. Severe infections can result from the spread of poliovirus to the central nervous system (CNS) where it infects motor neuron cells. Bulbar poliomyelitis results from infection of the respiratory neurons in the brain stem, contributing to respiratory paralysis.

 CLINICAL Symptoms of poliomyelitis

Most poliovirus infections are asymptomatic. Rarely, severe forms of poliomyelitis are associated with viral infection of motor neurons in the spinal cord or brain stem, leading to flaccid paralysis of the muscles. The motor damage is permanent due to lysis of the neurons, although some recovery of motor function is possible after recovery from infection. In the most severe forms of poliomyelitis, infection of the brain stem occurs, leading to paralysis of muscles involved in breathing.

Treatment

Treatment is by relief of symptoms, buying time for the body's immune response to counteract the virus through supporting essential functions, in particular breathing.

Prevention

Immunisation is possible due to the virus' antigenic stability. Two vaccines are in clinical use:

1 **Salk vaccine**, containing formalin-inactivated virus
2 **Sabin vaccine**, containing 'live' attenuated virus. This type of vaccine produces more effective, longer-lasting immunity, although it is potentially infectious and there is a risk of causing disease in immunocompromised individuals.

As there are effective vaccines, and as humans are the only hosts, the World Health Organization aims to eradicate poliovirus in the next few years. As a result, the Salk (formalin-inactivated) vaccine is now used, because the number of cases of polio resulting from the 'live' vaccine was exceeding those occurring from the wild-type disease.

Epstein–Barr virus

The Epstein–Barr virus (EBV) is the causative agent of infectious mononucleosis ('glandular fever') and has been implicated in the development of some tumours. EBV is common throughout the world and, by adulthood, the vast majority of people possess protective antibodies.

Structure and morphology

EBV is a large virus (120–200 nm) consisting of a icosahedral capsid surrounded by a lipid envelope, which contains a linear, dsDNA genome. EBV is a member of the herpesvirus family.

Transmission and phylogeny

Humans are the natural hosts for EBV. Transmission occurs mainly through exchange of saliva. Infection in early years of life is asymptomatic, whereas clinically apparent infectious mononucleosis is more common in adults.

Replication cycle and pathogenesis of disease

Attachment and entry

Infection occurs in the oropharynx, spreading to the blood and primarily infecting B cells. Entry is mediated by the glycoprotein, gp340, which binds the CR3 complement receptor on B cells. The viral particle is taken up in an endocytic vesicle and the viral genome enters the cell after fusion of the viral envelope with the membrane of the endocytic vesicle.

Replication

EBV sets up a latent infection in B cells. The viral genome may integrate into the host cell genome, although most copies of the genome are found in the cytoplasm. The linear viral genome becomes circular when it enters the cell and replication relies on the transcription of the DNA genome to mRNA by host-cell RNA polymerase. The EBV genome contains many 'accessory proteins' which are involved in subversion of the immune response, a hallmark of herpesvirus infections.

Assembly and release

EBV is unusual in that it has two replication strategies. The **latent stage** of infection results in the low expression of viral proteins. EBV may also switch to a **lytic mode** of replication, in which there is release of large amounts of virus from infected cells. The mechanism triggering switching from one mode of replication to the other is not fully understood.

 CLINICAL Infectious mononucleosis

Characterised by fever, sore throat, lymphadenopathy, anorexia and tiredness. Recovery usually occurs within 2–3 weeks, although infection may often recur.

In immunocompromised patients, more serious conditions can result from EBV infection; a severe progressive form of infectious mononucleosis can be seen in children with X-linked immunosuppressive syndrome and EBV has been linked with various cancers.

 CLINICAL EBV and cancer

EBV has been associated with cancers that have a lymphoid origin – it predisposes individuals to cancer, although other co-factors are required. It is linked with Burkitt's lymphoma in African children, nasopharyngeal cancer in Chinese populations and thymus cancer in the USA.

Immune response

The immune response to the primary infection focuses on the generation of cytotoxic T cells to kill infected B cells. Antibodies are produced against the viral capsid antigen.

Treatment and prevention

No effective therapy is available for EBV infection, although in serious cases aciclovir, a thymidine kinase inhibitor, may be used because it has a small amount of activity.

No vaccine currently exists for EBV.

HIV

The human immunodeficiency virus was first identified in the 1980s, following the identification of acquired immune deficiency syndrome (AIDS), for which it is the causative agent. Since then the disease has spread across the world. It is estimated that over 40 million people have been infected in this pandemic, many of whom live in sub-Saharan Africa.

Properties and structure of the HIV virion

HIV is a lentivirus, a form of retrovirus that causes slow, chronic infections. Two species exist:

1 **HIV-1**, found throughout the world
2 **HIV-2**, found predominantly in West Africa.

An HIV virion contains two copies of the viral genome, and reverse transcriptase, protease and integrase proteins contained within a bar-shaped capsid and envelope (Fig. 16.3). The viral envelope contains the glycoproteins, gp120 and gp41, which mediate cell entry.

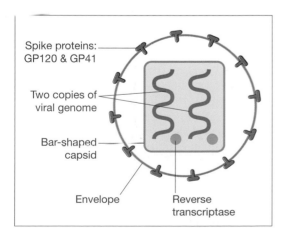

Figure 16.3 The HIV virion.

The glycoprotein gp120 initiates entry of HIV into host cells through binding to CD4 found on CD4$^+$ T cells, and also macrophages and dendritic cells. The binding of gp120 to CD4 induces a conformational shift in gp120, which enables it to bind to cellular co-receptors, causing the viral gp41 fusion protein to mediate viral uncoating and entry of the genome and internal viral proteins into the cell.

The HIV genome contains nine genes:

- **Gag** encodes the internal core proteins
- **Pol** encodes reverse transcriptase, an integrase and a protease
- **Env** encodes the protein gp160, which is cleaved to form gp120 and gp41
- Two additional genes for replication are encoded – **tat** and **rev**
- Four accessory genes are encoded – **nef**, **vpu**, **vpr** and **vif**.

Immune evasion

The glycoprotein gp120 possesses many 'hypervariable' regions that mutate particularly rapidly, preventing block antibodies from binding to conserved binding sites. This allows a site to be conserved to mediate entry to host cells through binding the target receptors, while allowing huge variation in antibody-binding epitopes.

The high mutation rate which occurs in the HIV genome is the result of two steps of replication by an RNA transcriptase, generating large numbers of mutations.

Transmission and epidemiology

The main route of transmission is by sexual contact. Transfer by infected blood (e.g. in intravenous drug use) and perinatal transmission are other significant routes of infection. The transmission of HIV by blood transfusion has been effectively eliminated after the introduction of screening. Humans are the only natural hosts of HIV

After the first cases of AIDS in the 1980s, infection has spread widely, resulting in a pandemic. In the 1980s in Europe and the USA, HIV infection occurred predominantly in homosexual men and intravenous drug users or people with haemophilia (as a result of infected pooled clotting factors). In recent years, however, heterosexual transmission has become a more common route of transmission.

The infectious dose required to cause HIV infection is relatively high. Consequently, even repeated prolonged exposure and needle-stick injuries rarely lead to infection in healthcare workers.

Replication cycle

After fusion of viral envelope, the viral genome and proteins enter the nucleus; viral reverse transcriptase then transcribes the RNA genome into dsDNA which is integrated into the host cell DNA. Integration, mediated by the integrase enzyme, can occur at many sites in the host genome. Integrated viral DNA is transcribed by host RNA polymerase. The genome is assembled with the capsid and internal proteins into a virion particle in the cytoplasm and budding occurs by cleavage of envelope polypeptides at the cell membrane.

Pathogenesis of HIV and the immune response

Infection initially targets dendritic cells and macrophages in the genital tract. These cells migrate to the lymph nodes, where infection of $CD4^+$ T cells subsequently occurs. Viraemia happens about a week after infection. After an initial viraemia the virus level drops, which may reflect control of infection by the adaptive immune response. HIV causes persistent infection of T cells. A patient infected with HIV is considered to be infected for life.

The main immune response to HIV is through the activation of specific CTLs. Their failure to control HIV infection leads to an increase in viral titre associated with the decline in the $CD4^+$ T-cell count that typifies AIDS. CTLs lose their effectiveness because they no longer receive cytokine signals to sustain activation due to lack of $CD4^+$ T cells.

The virus genome mutates at a high rate; 'escape mutants' may develop to which the CTLs are incapable of responding. Antibodies produced in response to HIV infection are poorly neutralising and so have little effect on disease progression.

HIV has developed three main mechanisms to aid immune evasion:

1. The **integration of viral DNA** into host cell DNA causing persistent infection
2. The high rate of **mutation** of genome resulting in rapid changes to antigens
3. Production of **tat** and **nef** proteins which act to **downregulate MHC-I**, preventing recognition of infected cells by CTLs.

 CLINICAL AIDS

AIDS is defined by a number of criteria, which may include the presence of an 'AIDS-defining pathology' (such as Kaposi's sarcoma or *Pneumocystis* pneumonia) or a $CD4^+$ cell count <200 cells/μL of blood.

AIDS results from the low $CD4^+$ count caused by severe HIV infection. The weakened immune system allows opportunistic infections. Additional effects of chronic HIV infection include dementia, as a result of infection of microglia in the brain, and the development of tumours, often as a result of infection by a tumour-causing virus.

After an initial viraemia, a set point occurs where the viral titre is maintained at a low level by cell-mediated immune response. This is typified by a low or absent level of virus in the blood and a long period of clinical latency, although virus levels remain high in the lymph nodes.

Towards the end of the latent phase, AIDS-related complex, characterised by fever, fatigue and weight loss, may occur. AIDS-related complex usually advances rapidly to AIDS.

Treatment of HIV infection

The standard therapy for HIV infection is HAART (highly active antiretroviral therapy), consisting of two reverse transcriptase inhibitors and a protease inhibitor. Use of more than one drug acting on different targets reduces the ability of the virus to mutate to escape the action of all the drugs.

Reverse transcriptase inhibitors

These may be **nucleoside analogues** (e.g. zidovudine) that reverse transcriptase incorporates into transcripts, causing chain termination. These nucleoside analogues are not used by host cell polymerase so there is no effect on host cell nucleic acid polymerisation. The **non-nucleoside reverse transcriptase inhibitors** (e.g. nevirapine) act directly on the reverse transcriptase enzyme, at a different site. Reverse transcriptase inhibitors are also used to treat retroviral infections and HBV.

Protease inhibitors (e.g. saquinivir)

Many viruses encode a protease to produce viral proteins, the inhibition of which prevents formation of functional viral proteins, thus preventing formation of progeny virions. The protease structure is distinct from host cell proteases, allowing the development of specific drugs.

HAART cannot cure HIV infection, although it is effective in prolonging life. It improves health and quality of life and allows an increase in CD4$^+$ T cells.

Prevention of HIV

There is currently no vaccine available. Prevention of transmission is the best way of avoiding infection. Methods of prevention include promotion of condom use and (in drug addicts) avoidance of needle sharing.

Steps taken to reduce the likelihood of transmission from mother to child include:

- giving antiretroviral drugs to mother and child around the time of birth
- avoidance of breastfeeding to prevent passing on the virus in milk
- caesarean section to lower the risk of HIV transmission during birth.

Prions

Prions are a misfolded version of a normal host cellular protein, prion-related peptide (PrP), which are thought to be induced to misfold as a result of interactions with the prion.

Variant Creutzfeldt–Jakob disease (vCJD) is the most well-known prion disease; it is believed to result from the ingestion of meat derived from cattle with bovine spongiform encephalopathy (BSE or 'mad cow disease').

Prion diseases are characterised by:

- spongiform degeneration of nerve cells
- formation of amyloid plaques – aggregates of prion protein
- loss of nerve cells.

 CLINICAL Symptoms of vCJD

Variant CJD is a neurodegenerative disease, characterised by dementia and gradual loss of cognitive function; it is accompanied by movement problems such as an abnormal gait and myoclonus.

Presumptive diagnosis is based on clinical symptoms. Definitive diagnosis requires a brain biopsy during life or histological examination of postmortem tissues.

There is currently no known treatment or vaccine for prion diseases. Little is known about the precise mechanisms by which ingestion of prions leads to prion diseases.

Bacteria

Bacteria are prokaryotes that can colonise a huge variety of niches in the environment and in a host, both inside and outside host cells. Bacteria are capable of independent replication, and many have adapted to cause disease to aid their replication. With some bacteria disease is 'accidental' – it does not help replication or survival of the bacterial colony.

Bacterial structure and morphology

Bacteria are much smaller than eukaryotic cells, typically around 1 μm in length. Some organelles are possessed by all bacteria, but there is a wide variety in morphology and other features.

Morphology

Bacteria are classified by their shape. Three common morphologies are:

1 **bacilli** – rod shaped (e.g. *Clostridium tetani*)
2 **cocci** – round (e.g. *Staphylococcus aureus*)
3 **spirochaetes** – spiral shaped (e.g. *Treponema pallidum*).

Bacteria can be further identified by their characteristic arrangement as individuals, in clusters, chains or pairs.

Structures

Bacteria do not have membrane-bound organelles, although four essential structures can be identified (Fig. 16.4):

- The **nucleoid** is a single circular chromosome around 10^6–10^7 base-pairs in length. It is free floating in the cytoplasm.
- The **cytoplasm** contains ribosomes and the nucleoid. Bacterial ribosomes are smaller (70S) than eukaryotic ribosomes (80S). In addition, the cytoplasm contains a bacterial cytoskeleton.

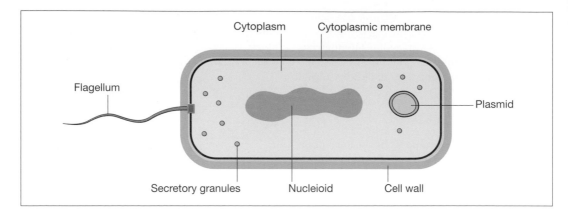

Figure 16.4 Structure of a bacterium.

- The **cytoplasmic membrane** encloses the bacteria. This lipid bilayer has a number of functions:
  - regulation of transport of molecules into and out of the cell
  - permeability barrier to maintain osmotic pressure
  - maintenance of gradient for energy generation.
- The **mesosome** is an invagination in the cytoplasmic membrane that is crucial in cell division.
- **The cell wall** maintains cell shape and provides protection.

  Bacteria may also possess other structures:

- **Pili and fimbriae** – short projections that are involved in movement or conjugation. Pili may express adhesin proteins which mediate attachment to surfaces.
- **Flagella** – a whip-like tail structure associated with motility. Bacteria may be multiflagellated, possess a single flagellum or have no flagella.

- **Photosynthetic material,**
- **Storage granules,**
- **Capsule** – this provides additional protection from phagocytosis by immune cells, and from drying out in the external environment.
- **Plasmids** are small accessory chromosomes, usually circular and around 2–1000 kilobasepairs in size, which can replicate independently of the nucleoid and provide accessory functions. Plasmids may be transmitted between bacteria through **conjugation**.

The bacterial cell wall

The classic method of identifying bacteria in a clinical sample is by means of a Gram stain (Fig. 16.5):

- A **Gram-positive** cell wall contains a thick layer of peptidoglycan containing fibres of lipoteichoic acid that protrude out of the cell wall.

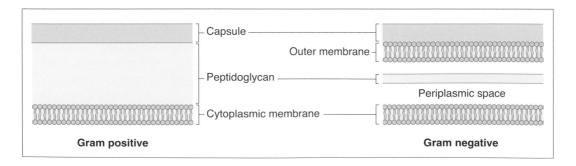

Figure 16.5 Structure of the bacterial cell wall.

- The **Gram-negative** cell wall has a more complex structure, possessing an outer membrane and a periplasmic space containing a thin layer of peptidoglycan. Gram-negative cell walls contain the endotoxin **lipopolysaccharide** (LPS).

A few bacteria cannot be classified using the Gram stain. The most clinically significant bacteria in these groups are the mycobacteria, which possess **acid-fast** cells walls. These cell walls are not decoloured by acid alcohol after staining by carbolfuchsin, due to the high concentrations of mycolic acids.

 DEFINITION Gram stain

The Gram stain is performed by smearing bacteria on to a slide and then staining with crystal violet. Iodine is added, colouring all the cells blue due to the iodine–violet complex that results. An organic solvent is used to wash away the violet stain from the Gram-negative bacteria only:

- Gram-positive bacteria retain the **blue** stain due to the high levels of peptidoglycan.
- Safranin is used to counterstain Gram-negative bacteria a **pink** colour.

 DEFINITION Peptidoglycan

Peptidoglycan is an essential component of the bacterial cell wall. It is a network of carbohydrate strands cross-linked by short peptides made up of both D- and L-amino acid molecules. D-Amino acids are not used by the human body because it is these that are targeted by the penicillin family of antibiotics, allowing selective toxic action on bacteria.

Bacterial cell growth

Bacteria reproduce by binary fission, one parent dividing into two daughter cells, although the rate at which this occurs – the doubling time – varies between species. *Escherichia coli* may divide every 20 min, whereas mycobacteria divide only every 24 hours.

Bacterial growth can be divided into four phases (Fig. 16.6.), the standard growth curve:

1 **Lag phase** – vigorous metabolic activity occurs, although little growth, as the bacteria acclimatise to their new conditions.
2 **Log phase** – during this phase there is rapid growth and cell division, because environmental conditions are optimal for the bacteria.

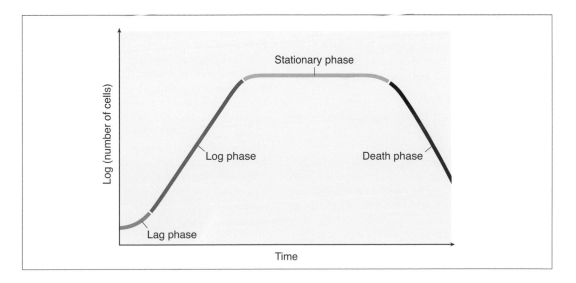

Figure 16.6 The phases of bacterial cell growth.

3 **Stationary phase** – new cells resulting from replication match the number of dying cells, reaching a steady state. The stationary phase may be caused by nutrient depletion, the presence of toxins, or a combination of these and other factors.

4 **Death phase** – the rate of death in the culture exceeds the rate at which the cells are being replaced by the generation of new cells.

Bacterial pathogenesis

Bacterial infections must establish themselves as a colony before causing disease. This is achieved in a series of continuous steps:

- **Entry into body** – or in the case of commensals, this may be by moving from one site in the body to another.
- **Evasion of primary defences**, such as stomach acid and mucus secretions.
- **Adherence to and colonisation of host** – many bacteria have specialised structures to aid adherence (e.g. pili of *E. coli* mediate attachment to urinary tract epithelium). Foreign bodies help infection because host phagocytes are unable to adhere well due to a lack of binding proteins.
- **Evasion of host immune response**.

Local effects and secretions in bacterial infection

Bacteria secrete compounds to help their colonisation of the local environment. Many are enzymes that digest and dissolve the local surroundings, allowing uptake of nutrients by passive diffusion. Other toxins, such as **leukocidins**, protect the bacteria through killing host leukocytes. Bacteria may also secrete toxins to aid their replication and survival.

Systemic effects of bacterial infection

Systemic effects result from bacteria within the blood, **bacteraemia**, or the release of a bacterial toxin into the blood. **Septic shock** may result from severe bacterial infection and can be caused by a variety of toxins.

LPS is the most well-established cause of septic shock. This endotoxin is an integral part of Gram-negative cell walls and is not secreted. The toxic portion of LPS is lipid A which is made up of disaccharides with several fatty acids attached.

 CLINICAL Septic shock

Septic shock is characterised by high fever and hypotension. It results from excessive release of cytokines in response to bacterial toxins such as LPS and toxic shock syndrome toxin. Cytokine release triggers mass vasodilatation and may activate many immune cells, such as macrophages and T cells, triggering further cytokine production. There is a high risk of mortality (as much as 70%) due to the occurrence of **disseminated intravascular coagulation**. The decreased movement of blood stimulates the onset of clotting in the capillaries of organs throughout the body, triggering multiple organ failure.

Types of toxin

The toxins produced by bacteria can be divided into two classes:

1 **Exotoxins** are actively secreted by bacteria, usually to help the organism survive. Some exotoxins break down tissues to provide nutrients and others prevent an effective immune response.

2 **Endotoxins** are not secreted; they are an integral part of the bacteria and are released on the death of the organism.

Immune evasion

Evasion of the immune system is essential if bacteria are to colonise tissues and survive. Bacteria, similar to viruses, have developed a variety of different mechanisms to achieve this:

- **Host mimicry** – antigenic targets on bacteria (e.g. capsule antigens) may mimic the structure of a host molecule, preventing the immune response from developing effective antibodies to the pathogen, e.g. *Neisseria meningitidis* group B, in which the capsule polysaccharide is identical to a host molecule, NCAM-1
- **Absence of tissue damage** – the lack of 'danger signals' due to tissue damage slows the immune response. Many of the mediators that recruit leukocytes to a site of infection are not produced, hindering such a response.
- **Antigenic variation** – varying the antigen molecules that a pathogen presents will impede the immune response, because each effective response is rapidly made obsolete, through the bacteria presenting new antigenic epitopes and losing the old, e.g. *N. gonorrhoeae*.

- **Intracellular phase** – bacteria that are situated in cells are protected from antibodies and phagocytosis, e.g. *Mycobacterium tuberculosis*.
- **Antibody inactivation/proteolysis** – some bacteria possess IgA protease (e.g. streptococci) which can hydrolyse IgA found in mucus secretions. Other bacteria use antibodies in other ways to evade the immune response, e.g. staphylococci present **protein A** in cell walls that binds to the Fc portion of IgG. This prevents activation of complement and restricts opsonisation of bacteria.
- **Cytotoxins** – some bacteria secrete exotoxins that kill host (particularly immune) cells, e.g. leukocidins kill both neutrophils and macrophages.

Gene motility in bacteria

Some bacteria possess mechanisms for transferring genetic information between strains, or even between species. Such mobile genetic elements include genes that encode virulence determinants, such as toxins, and genes aiding antibiotic resistance.

Vectors by which genes may be transferred

Bacteriophages

Viruses that infect bacteria may, in some cases, produce virus particles that transport a section of bacterial DNA instead of the viral genome, allowing transfer of genetic information to another bacterium

Plasmids

Plasmids are small additional molecules dsDNA external to the nucleoid and capable of replication independent of the nucleoid. They are usually **circular**, although they may be linear. An individual bacterium may contain several plasmids. Plasmids may carry genes with medical importance (e.g. toxins or antibiotic resistance genes).

Transposons

These mobile segments of DNA may move between bacteria or between DNA of bacteria, plasmids and bacteriophages. In addition to the genes regulating excision from genetic material and integration at a new site, transposons can also contain genes for drug resistance enzymes or toxins. Unlike plasmids, transposons are not capable of independent replication, and replicate with the recipient DNA.

Mechanisms of gene transfer

Horizontal transfer of genes between bacteria is particularly significant when the transferred genes encode toxins or antibiotic resistance proteins. **Three methods** for horizontal gene transfer have been identified:

1. **Conjugation** is the mating of two bacteria, where DNA is transferred from donor to recipient cell. This process is controlled by genes within the plasmid by which the plasmid is transferred to the recipient cell through a sex pilus. Newly acquired genes can recombine into the recipient genome
2. **Transduction** is transfer of DNA via a bacteriophage virus. During viral assembly in the infected cell, bacterial DNA may be incorporated into a viral particle and carried to a recipient cell. This process may result in the recipient cell becoming pathogenic, e.g. cholera toxin gene is acquired through transduction.
3. **Transformation** occurs when there is transfer of DNA between cells. This occurs in nature when dying cells release their DNA, which may be taken up by living cells. Transformation is frequently used in research to genetically alter bacteria, although it is not clear if it has a role in disease.

The transfer of genes between sites in a bacterium is achieved by transposons. This process can be exploited in antigenic variation, as is the case in *Borrelia* species. Rearrangement results in movement of genes from silent storage sites to an active site where transcription and translation of the gene can occur, resulting in the expression of a different antigenic protein.

Many virulence factors are often clustered together in 'pathogenicity islands' and may represent large regions of genome inherited as a single block. This is a common feature in many Gram-negative rods, e.g. *E. coli*, *Salmonella* spp.

Commensal bacteria

The human body naturally has a microflora of many different strains of bacteria, which colonise the skin and mucosa; the presence of bacteria on these surfaces is not an indication of disease. The internal organs and blood are usually sterile; the presence of bacteria at these sites is an indication of disease.

The normal flora in the body varies with site, owing to the different microenvironments present.

Commensal bacteria can be advantageous to the host in preventing colonisation of the site by pathogenic strains and may also produce compounds that are of benefit to the host. Normal flora may be made up of bacteria and fungi, never viruses and parasites.

Normal flora of the skin

Staphylococcus epidermis is a bacterium normally prevalent on the skin. It is non-pathogenic in this locale, but may cause disease at other sites, e.g. on prosthetic heart valves. Most commensals live on the skin surface, although some reside in hair follicles. The yeast *Candida albicans* is also part of the normal skin flora.

Normal flora of the respiratory tract

The upper respiratory tract is colonised by a wide variety of organisms, whereas the lower respiratory tract is sterile. In the nose, staphylococci and streptococci are prevalent. *Staphylococcus aureus* may reside here as a commensal, and can be a source of infection in other loci. In the throat, *Streptococcus viridans* and staphylococci predominate, and prevent the growth of pathogenic species on the pharyngeal mucosa. Anaerobic bacteria may be found in crevices in the gums.

Normal flora of the gastrointestinal tract

The stomach is essentially sterile due to the harsh, low pH environment, although the small intestine is usually colonised by streptococci, lactobacilli and yeasts. There are large numbers of bacteria in the colon, including many anaerobic strains. Intestinal bacteria can produce small amounts of vitamin B and vitamin K and may be an important source of these vitamins in malnourished individuals.

Commensals in the gastrointestinal (GI) tract help prevent the growth of pathogenic strains. The use of antibiotics can, however, suppress the growth of normal flora and so lead to the growth of pathogenic strains. Due to the high number of bacteria, the GI tract may be a source of infection in other parts of the body. In particular *E. coli* is a major cause of urinary tract infection.

Normal flora of the Genitourinary (GU) tract

The vaginal mucosa is primarily colonised by lactobacilli, inhibiting colonisation by pathogens such as *C. albicans*. Bacteria found in the vaginal canal may cause infection during childbirth. Urine in the bladder and ureters is sterile in a normal individual.

Laboratory identification of bacteria

To start effective treatment of a bacterial infection, it is necessary to identify the strain of bacteria through a variety of tests. The presence of bacteria in the skin and mucosa is normal and is not sufficient to indicate disease. In contrast, presence of bacteria in the blood or the cerebrospinal fluid (CSF) is always an indicator of disease.

Initial identification of bacteria involves the Gram stain to determine cell wall structure. In addition, the morphology of individual bacteria and the general structure of bacterial colonies may help identification. The clinical features of an illness, the bacterial morphology and the Gram stain are often sufficient for presumptive diagnosis. Selective media can be used to aid isolation and identification of bacteria:

- **Blood agar** is the medium used to grow most bacteria.
- **Chocolate agar** is used primarily in the culture of *Neisseria* spp. It is made up of blood agar that has been heated to inactivate complement proteins.
- **MacConkey's agar** allows the culture of enteric bacteria and contains bile salts to restrict the growth of non-enteric species. The medium also contains lactose and an indicator, allowing the distinction of lactose-fermenting bacteria.
- **Löwenstein-Jensen medium** contains a complex mix of substances, including egg proteins. It allows the culture of mycobacteria, while preventing the growth of many other species that would normally outcompete mycobacterial growth.

After the use of selective media, bacterial morphology and clinical symptoms, more detailed identification of bacteria may include specific tests to identify the presence of specific enzymes and the detection of specific antigenic markers. A limited number of laboratory tests can be used to identify many clinically important bacteria (Fig. 16.7).

Treatment of bacterial infection

The main method of treatment for most bacterial infections is antibiotics – drugs that act specifically to kill bacteria. Physical methods of removing bacteria can be used to aid healing.

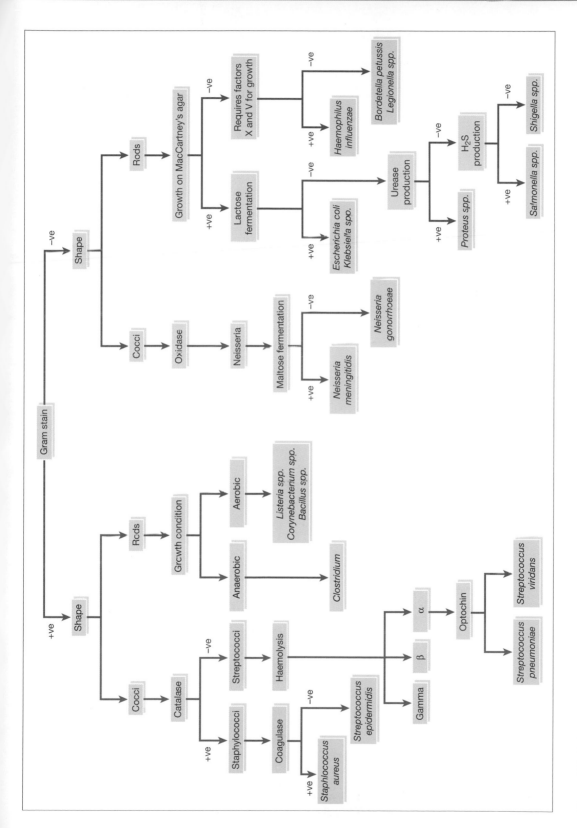

Figure 16.7 Laboratory tests used to identify common bacterial pathogens.

Physical methods of treatment

Debridement is the cleaning of an open wound, which allows removal of foreign bodies and dead tissue to help healing. **Surgical drainage** can be used to remove pus and bacteria from an abscess, although the wound resulting from drainage may become a source of infection itself.

Antibiotics

Antibiotics inhibit the growth of the microorganism while causing minimal damage to the human host. They work on the principle of **selective toxicity**, targeting an aspect of the microorganism's physiology that differs from that of a human. Antibiotics can be classified as bactericidal or bacteriostatic, and can be narrow spectrum or broad spectrum. Often more than one antibiotic is given at the same time, because drug resistance is prevalent. Using a second (or even a third or fourth) drug in combination reduces the risk of drug resistance developing.

> **DEFINITION Bactericidal and bacteriostatic antibiotics**
>
> Bactericidal antibiotics kill bacteria, whereas bacteriostatic antibiotics inhibit their replication – the host immune defence systems are required for elimination of bacteria.

> **DEFINITION Narrow- and broad-spectrum antibiotics**
>
> Broad-spectrum antibiotics are effective against a wide range of organisms.
> In contrast, narrow-spectrum antibiotics are effective against one, or very few types of, organisms.

Inhibition of bacterial cell wall synthesis (e.g. penicillins, cephalosporins)

Inhibition of bacterial wall synthesis occurs through inhibition of transpeptidases, the enzymes that catalyse the cross-linking of **peptidoglycan**.

The β-**lactam ring** structure of these antibiotics mimics that of the terminal dipeptide in the peptidoglycan chain – D-alanyl-D-alanine – competitively inhibiting the transpeptidase enzyme's active site.

Penicillins and cephalosporins are only bactericidal during the bacterial growth period when new peptidoglycan is being synthesised.

Vancomycin blocks transpeptidation through a different mechanism. It binds directly to D-alanyl-D-alanine, preventing recognition by the enzyme's active site.

Inhibition of protein synthesis

Drugs that target the smaller ribosomal subunit The selectivity of these ribosomal inhibitors is based on increased uptake into bacterial cells compared with human cells. They are capable of inhibiting the ribosomal target in both humans and bacteria.

- **Tetracyclines** (e.g. doxycycline) bind the smaller ribosomal subunit preventing tRNA from binding to an acceptor site on the ribosome.
- **Aminoglycosides** inhibit initiation of translation and cause misreading of mRNA such that incorrect amino acids are inserted. This leads to membrane damage and bacterial death.

Drugs that target the larger ribosomal subunit

- **Chloramphenicol** inhibits peptidyltransferase, preventing formation of new peptide bonds. Some bone marrow toxicity may occur due to incomplete selectivity for bacteria over the human host.
- **Macrolides** (e.g. erythromycin) prevent release of uncharged transfer RNA (tRNA) from the donor site after the peptide bond has been formed.

Inhibition of nucleic acid synthesis

- **Sulphonamides** inhibit synthesis of tetrahydrofolic acid, required as a methyl donor in the synthesis of nucleotides.
- **Trimethoprim** also inhibits synthesis of tetrahydrofolic acid, but by inhibiting a different enzyme target to sulphonamides. This enzyme is present in both humans and bacteria, although trimethoprim has a higher affinity for the bacterial form of the enzyme.
- **Quinolones** (e.g. ciprofloxacin) inhibit bacterial DNA gyrase.
- **Rifampicin** inhibits bacterial RNA polymerase.

Inhibitors of mycolic acid synthesis

These inhibitors (e.g. isoniazid) are used to treat mycobacterial infections.

Specificity for anaerobic environment

Metronidazole acts as an electron sink, preventing metabolic reduction. On acquiring electrons, the drug ring is cleaved to a toxic intermediate that damages DNA.

Use of antibiotics in combination

Combinations of antibiotics may be used to treat serious infections. The acquisition of resistance to multiple antibiotics is much less likely than resistance to a single antibiotic.

Antibiotics may work **synergistically** (e.g. trimethoprim and sulphonamides, which act on the same metabolic pathway) to produce a greater effect than either agent individually. Other combinations of antibiotics may be less effective together, e.g. using penicillins (which act on growing cells) with another antibiotic that inhibits cell growth.

Antibiotic resistance

Innate resistance

Some bacteria have an innate resistance to certain antibiotics as a result of their metabolism and structure, e.g. *Mycoplasma* spp. lack cell walls, so penicillin has no effect.

Acquired resistance

Acquired resistance can occur as a result of a genetic change:

- **Mutation** may occur in the gene encoding the target molecule, or the transport mechanism by which the drug is taken up.
- **Acquisition of a resistance gene** on a plasmid or transposon. A variety of different mechanisms are employed by resistance genes:
  - the gene product may **inactivate** the drug, e.g. penicillin resistance by β-lactamase
  - resistance genes may encode an enzyme that **alters the drug target site**, e.g. erythromycin-resistant protein methylates a 50-S ribosomal subunit, preventing binding of drug
  - a resistance gene may encode proteins that can **actively remove the drug** from cells, e.g. sulphonamide resistance results from a specific transport protein.

Antibiotic resistance is an increasing problem due to:

- inappropriate prescription by doctors
- use of antibiotics in farming
- failure by patients to complete their course of treatment.

> **CLINICAL Testing for antibiotic resistance**
>
> Efficacy of an antibiotic against a specific organism can be tested. Antibiotic-impregnated discs are placed on agar inoculated with target bacteria. The diameter of the zone of growth inhibition of the microorganism around the disc is compared with standards to determine sensitivity of the bacterium to the antibiotic.

Probiotics

Live non-pathogenic strains of bacteria (probiotics) may be used to treat or prevent disease; *Lactobacillus* sp. has been used to reduce occurrence of childhood diarrhoea. These probiotics are thought to act in a number of ways: they may colonise a niche preventing a pathogenic strain from causing infection, or they may promote an immune response that is effective against the pathogen.

Pyogenic Gram-positive bacteria

Pyogenic, 'pus-forming' bacteria are a common source of infections. Typically, infection with pyogenic bacteria results in **abscesses**, although more serious infections can also occur. Two clinically important pyogenic bacteria are *Strep. pyogenes* and *Staph. aureus*.

Streptococcus pyogenes

Strep. pyogenes is the leading bacterial cause of pharyngitis and cellulitis, and is found as a commensal on the skin and in the oropharynx of many individuals; it can cause infection on entering the tissues or blood.

Structure and morphology

Streptococci are Gram-positive cocci, typically arranged in chains or pairs. They can be distinguished from staphylococci that are catalase positive. Streptococci can cause a wide range of diseases due to pyogenic inflammation, exotoxins and immunological cross-reaction.

Characterisation of streptococci

Different species can be identified by the type of haemolysis around colonies grown on blood agar:

- **α-Haemolysis**: incomplete lysis of red blood cells in agar produces a green-coloured zone around colonies.
- **β-Haemolysis**: complete lysis of red blood cells in agar leads to a clear zone around colonies. Further grouping of β-haemolytic streptococci is based on characterisation of the C-carbohydrate antigen in the cell wall using the Lancefield test.
- **γ-Haemolytic**: no lysis of red blood cells

 CLINICAL Lancefield groups

β-Haemolytic streptococci can be classified based on antigenic differences in the C carbohydrate, which can be detected by specific antibodies. The Lancefield groups are classified A–U; group A includes *Strep. pyogenes*, whereas group D includes enteric strains of streptococci. Groups A, B and D streptococci are particularly associated with causing disease in humans.

Transmission and phylogeny

Strep. pyogenes is typically present on the surface of the skin in small numbers. For disease to result bacteria must infect the tissues or the blood.

Strep. pyogenes is a group A, β-haemolytic strain of streptococci, and can be further classified based on its C carbohydrate, allowing the identification of antigenically distinct substrains.

Pathogenesis of disease

Mechanisms of causing disease

Strep. pyogenes is capable of causing disease by three mechanisms:

1 **Pyogenic inflammation** induced locally
2 **Toxin production** causing systemic symptoms throughout body

3 **Immunological cross-reaction** whereby antibodies against the streptococci cross-react with normal tissue.

 CLINICAL The range of streptococcal diseases

Strep. pyogenes is the most common bacterial cause of sore throat. Pharyngitis is associated with inflammation, exudate, fever and tender cervical lymph nodes. Spontaneous recovery usually occurs within 10 days if untreated. However, the infection may spread, leading to otitis media, sinusitis, mastoiditis or even meningitis.

If the bacterium produces the appropriate toxin, scarlet fever or toxic shock syndrome may occur.

If *Strep. pyogenes* gains access to the skin through skin defects, it can produce cellulites, necrotising fasciitis or pyoderma (impetigo) – a superficial skin infection, which is communicable among small children.

Pyogenic inflammation occurs as a result of the body's acute inflammatory response. *Strep. pyogenes* produces inflammation-related enzymes:

- **Hyaluronidase** breaks down hyaluronic acids, a major component of the extracellular matrix.
- **Streptokinase** facilitates blood clot break down through activation of plasmin.
- **DNAase**.

Various toxins may be produced with local or systemic effects:

- **Streptolysins** cause β-haemolysis.
- **Exotoxin B** is a protease that rapidly degrades tissue. It is produced in large amounts by strains that cause necrotising fasciitis.
- **Erythrogenic toxin** has a similar mode of action to toxic shock syndrome toxin produced by *Staph. aureus* and causes the rash in scarlet fever.
- **Pyogenic exotoxin A** is the superantigen responsible for streptococcal toxic shock syndrome.

After infection, poststreptococcal diseases may occur due to the cross-reactivity of anti-streptococcal antibodies with human tissues.

Immune response

The immune response mainly involves phagocytic cells of the innate immune system, although these may be activated by T cells. Protection from future infection is mediated by the generation of antibodies to the bacteria. These antibodies may be cross-reactive with self-antigen and can result in the development of **poststreptococcal conditions**.

 CLINICAL Poststreptococcal diseases

Local infection by group A strepococci is sometimes followed later by inflammation in a non-infected organ. Antibodies produced against the streptococcal M protein in the capsule may cross-react with host tissue. These conditions typically occur around 2–3 weeks after local infection. Occurrence of these diseases can be reduced by prompt treatment of the initial infection.

Acute glomerulonephritis (AGN) occasionally occurs, usually after skin infection. AGN is characterised by hypertension, oedema of the face and ankles, and 'smoky' urine (due to red blood cells in the urine). This is the result of antibody–antigen complexes in the glomerular basement membrane.

Rheumatic fever may occur after streptococcal pharyngitis. Symptoms are a fever, polyarthritis and carditis, as a result of antibodies that cross-react with the heart and joint tissue. Carditis may damage both myocardial and endocardial tissue, typically leading to mitral and aortic valve damage.

Treatment

Strep. pyogenes infection can be treated with **penicillin**.

Prevention

Although it has no effect on rheumatic fever or acute glomerulonephritis, penicillin can be used prophylactically in those who have had rheumatic fever to protect from reinfection by streptococci, which may reactivate the rheumatic fever.

Staphylococcus aureus

Staph. aureus is responsible for causing many forms of pyogenic infection, food poisoning and toxic shock syndrome. Drug-resistant strains are a significant problem in hospitals where it is a common cause of pneumonia, septicaemia and surgical wound infections.

Morphology and structure

Staphylococci are spherical, Gram-positive cocci that form irregular clusters. Distinction of staphylococci from streptococci can be achieved by examining for organisation of clusters and also by catalase production. *Staph. aureus* can be distinguished from other staphylococci by its coagulase production, as well as the typical formation of golden colonies that are β-haemolytic.

Transmission and phylogeny

Staph. aureus is salt resistant and can be found on the skin. It can be isolated from nasal swabs of a small proportion of people, particularly health-care workers, who are at a high risk of exposure due to the prevalence of drug-resistant strains of *Staph. aureus* in hospitals. *Staph. aureus* is a commensal in these people and does not cause disease.

A variety of different strains of *Staph. aureus* exist, which possess different toxins and virulence factors, or may possess different antibiotic resistance cassettes. Different serotypes of *Staph. aureus* can be identified based on antigenic differences in the capsule of the bacteria.

Disease pathogenesis

There are many ways in which *Staph. aureus* can cause disease; several clinically important toxins can be produced by *Staph. aureus*:

- **Enterotoxin** acts as a superantigen in the gut, stimulating massive cytokine release which can trigger vomiting on ingestion. Food poisoning by enterotoxin does not require ingestion of live bacteria; the enterotoxin alone is sufficient.
- **Toxic shock syndrome toxin** causes toxic shock syndrome through the mass activation of T cells.
- **Exfoliatin** cleaves proteins within the epidermis and causes scalded skin syndrome in children.
- **Leukocidins** are capable of killing host cells, in particular the immune system cells responding to the infection.
- **Coagulase** creates a barrier through the induction of clotting, which prevents leukocytes reaching the site of infection.

The diseases caused by *S. aureus* can be divided into:

- **inflammatory diseases**, e.g. skin infections
- **toxin-mediated diseases**, e.g. toxic shock syndrome, food poisoning.

CLINICAL Toxin-mediated diseases

Food poisoning, toxic shock syndrome and scalded skin syndrome are all toxin-mediated staphylococcal diseases. Food poisoning is caused by ingestion of enterotoxin, which is preformed in contaminated food.

- **Staphylococcal food poisoning** occurs after a rapid incubation period (1–8 hours) and is characterised by more prominent vomiting than diarrhoea.
- **Toxic shock syndrome** follows the course characteristic of septic shock, and can involve many organs, including the liver, kidneys, muscles and CNS.
- **Scalded skin syndrome** predominantly occurs in young children and is characterised by a rash and fever, and the sloughing off of large areas of skin. Hair and nails may be lost and there is a risk of ion imbalance and fluid loss. Recovery is usually within 10 days.

Treatment

Treatment of *Staph. aureus* infection is difficult due to the high proportion of bacteria that have developed drug resistance. Most strains of *Staph. aureus* possess β-lactamase but, about 20% of strains are resistant to penicillins that are not broken down by β-lactamase. These methicillin-resistant *Staph. aureus* (MRSA) strains cause a significant problem in hospital-acquired infections. Treatment of such strains requires vancomycin; worryingly, a few strains have been isolated with vancomycin resistance.

Treatment of toxic shock syndrome also involves treatment of the symptoms.

 CLINICAL Inflammatory diseases caused by *Staph. aureus*

The typical inflammatory diseases caused by *Staph. aureus* are pyogenic skin infections, such as impetigo, or a surgical wound infection. Spread of bacteria to the lungs can lead to a staphylococcal pneumonia, which is a particularly common hospital-acquired infection. Trauma can lead to infection of the joints or bones – arthritis or osteomyelitis may occur. In addition, septicaemia, spreading from a localised infection may be a complication.

Prevention

There is no effective vaccine to *S. aureus* or its toxins. Good hygienic practice can limit spread of infection in hospitals.

Clostridium tetani

Clostridium tetani is an anaerobic bacillus, which causes tetanus. The spores of *C. tetani* are common in the soil and enter the body through a wound site.

Structure and morphology

C. tetani is a Gram-positive rod-shaped bacillus. Its spores require anaerobic tissue to germinate.

Transmission and phylogeny

C. tetani spores enter the body through a wound site and germinate in the anaerobic conditions of the wound. Neonatal tetanus is a problem in developing countries because the organism enters through a contaminated umbilicus or circumcision wound.

Tetanus toxin, which is responsible for the symptoms of tetanus infection, is found in a single antigenic type.

Replication and pathogenesis of disease

C. tetani is restricted to the wound site due to its obligate anaerobic nature. Tetanus toxin is produced by *C. tetani* in the wound site, following germination. This toxin is a zinc-dependent protease that inhibits vesicle release from inhibitory nerves in the spine. The toxin is carried by retrograde axonal transport to the CNS, so it is highly toxic in even minute amounts.

Treatment

Tetanus immunoglobulin, which neutralises the toxin, is given after an injury that is likely to have resulted in *C. tetani* spores entering the body. Penicillin may be useful to kill bacteria. Treatment also focuses on alleviating the symptoms; the airway must be maintained and respiratory support given. Muscle spasms can be reduced by benzodiazepines.

Prevention

Immunisation is by administration of tetanus toxoid (formaldehyde-treated toxin). This is given during childhood, and every 10 years thereafter. After trauma, tetanus toxoid should be administered and the wound debrided. Tetanus immunoglobulin should also be given, but at a different site to prevent neutralisation of the vaccine.

Enteric bacteria

Three clinically important strains of enteric bacteria are *E. coli*, and *Salmonella* and *Shigella* spp. Enterobacteria commonly cause diarrhoea which, in turn, promote transmission of the pathogen by the faeco-oral route.

Morphology and identification

All three clinically important enteric bacteria mentioned above are Gram-negative rods and can be grown and isolated on MacConkey's agar. *E. coli* can be distinguished from *Shigella* and *Salmonella* spp. by its ability to ferment lactose and its production of indole from tryptophan, which also allows it to be distinguished from other lactose-fermenting bacteria.

Salmonella and *Shigella* spp. can be distinguished from each other by H_2S production –*Shigella* sp. does not produce H_2S, whereas *Salmonella* sp. does.

E. coli, and *Salmonella* and *Shigella* spp. all exist as many different serotypes. Thus infection can occur repeatedly as the antibody response to one serotype does not protect against other serotypes.

Enteric bacterial infection of the gut is usually through the ingestion of contaminated food. Prevention of infection by enteric bacteria requires good hygiene practices to break the route of transmission. There are four main methods of transmission of enteric bacteria to cause infection: food, flies, fingers and faeces

Escherichia coli

Most strains of *E. coli* are harmless commensals in the gut. Some strains, however, can cause a variety of infections inside and outside the GI tract, including urinary tract infections, travellers' diarrhoea and neonatal meningitis.

Transmission and phylogeny

E. coli is transmitted in undercooked food and can also be present in contaminated water, although this is rare due to chlorination.

Different strains of *E. coli* can be distinguished by the presence of a number of different antigens associated with the cell wall (O antigen), flagella (H antigen) and capsule (K antigen). More than 1000 distinct serotypes have been identified based on their O, K and H antigens. Specific serotypes are associated with distinct diseases.

Disease pathogenesis

Intestinal tract infection occurs after adherence of pathogenic strains to cells in the small intestine. Bacteria synthesise enterotoxin which causes watery, non-bloody diarrhoea associated with inflammation. Such an infection usually resolves within 3 days.

E. coli strains that invade the epithelium of the large intestine cause bloody diarrhoea and inflammation. Infection with the O157:H7 strain can be complicated by haemolytic uraemic syndrome.

 CLINICAL O157:H7 and haemolytic uraemic syndrome

The O157:H7 serotype of *E. coli* produces verotoxin, similar to the toxins produced by *Shigella* spp. This results in bloody diarrhoea, fever and abdominal pains with little inflammation.

Haemolytic uraemic syndrome is a life-threatening complication. It is an acute renal failure associated with haemolytic anaemia and thrombocytopenia.

Systemic infection by *E. coli* can lead to septic shock mediated by LPS found in the bacterial cell wall.

Urinary tract infection is caused by serotypes in which the bacterial pili contain adhesins for specific proteins on urinary epithelium, allowing the organism to ascend the urinary tract to the bladder and kidneys.

E. coli is the most common cause of hospital-acquired urinary tract infections (UTIs):

- **Neonatal meningitis** is often caused by *E. coli* exposure during child birth.
- **Pathogenic features**: *E. coli* has several features that contribute to its pathogenic nature.
- **Pili** allow attachment to epithelial cells for colonisation of the GI and urinary tracts.
- **Capsules** can prevent phagocytosis.
- **Enterotoxins** may be produced in intestinal tract infection. There are two distinct toxins:
  - a high-molecular-weight toxin, similar to cholera toxin, that stimulates adenylyl cyclase, triggering loss of K^+, Cl^- and fluid
  - the low-molecular-weight toxin acts through stimulation of guanylyl cyclase.
- **Endotoxin** – Lipopolysaccharide.

Treatment

The treatment of *E. coli* infection varies with the site of infection:

- Lower UTIs are often treated with **penicillin** or **trimethoprim**
- Neonatal meningitis is treated with **ampicillin** and **cefotaxime**
- Treatment is not normally required in diarrhoea, though **rehydration** may be needed

Prevention

E. coli infection can be prevented by reducing the risk of exposure to bacteria:

- Ensure that food is properly prepared and thoroughly cooked.
- Travellers' diarrhoea can be prevented by prophylactic antibiotics.

Salmonella spp.

Salmonella spp. are associated with enterocolitis and enteric fevers such as typhoid fever. It can also cause infections in other parts of the body, such as osteomyelitis and septicaemia.

Phylogeny and transmission

Three antigens are important in identification of strains: the O (cell wall) antigen, H (flagellar) antigen and Vi (capsular) antigen.

A distinction is made between those species that cause typhoid fever and those that do not: *S. typhi* and *S. paratyphi* can cause typhoid fever; *S. enteriditis* is not typhoidal.

Salmonella spp. can be transmitted by ingestion of contaminated food. Most species of *Salmonella* have animal reservoirs, although *S. typhi* infects only humans and may be transmitted by the faeco-oral route. Salmonella infection is frequently contracted from uncooked poultry or eggs.

Disease pathogenesis

Three different types of infection may be caused by *Salmonella* spp.:

1 **Enterocolitis** results from invasion of gut tissue. Infection is limited to the gut and lymph nodes.
2 **Typhoid and other enteric fevers** are caused by initial infection in the small intestine. Bacteria enter phagocytes in the gut and spread to the lymph tissue, spleen, liver and gallbladder. In particular, invasion of the gallbladder is associated with the individual becoming a chronic carrier
3 **Septicaemia** can lead to seeding of bacteria in other organs, which can result in meningitis, osteomyelitis and pneumonia.

 CLINICAL Symptoms of salmonella infection

Enterocolitis occurs after a short incubation period (12–48 hours). It is characterised by symptoms of nausea, vomiting, diarrhoea and abdominal pain, and is normally self-limiting.

Typhoid fever is caused by *S. typhi*, and enteric fever by *S. paratyphi*. Initially, infection causes fever and constipation. Septicaemia leads to a high fever, delirium and painful abdomen. A rash on the abdomen may occur. There is a small risk of patients becoming chronic carriers.

Treatment

Many infections will resolve without antibiotics. However drug-resistant strains of *Salmonella* spp. are common, making testing of resistance essential if they are to be used. Fluid and ion replacement may be required to treat dehydration.

Prevention

Salmonella infection can be prevented by good hygiene. Vaccines against *S. typhi* are available but confer limited protection (about 65–75%).

Shigella

Shigella sp. is a highly infectious bacterium that causes dysentery. It is estimated that fewer than 100 organisms are sufficient to cause disease.

Structure and morphology

Shigella sp. is a non-lactose-fermenting, Gram-negative rod. It can be distinguished from *Salmonella* spp. because it does not produce H_2S.

Phylogeny, transmission and disease pathogenesis

The cell wall antigen is used to group the bacteria into four groups – A–D.

Shigella sp. infects only humans, commonly through food, invading the GI tract and causing bloody diarrhoea. Some strains also produce a toxin – shiga toxin.

 CLINICAL Shigellosis

Incubation of infection takes approximately 1–4 days, and is followed by abdominal cramps and bloody diarrhoea. Disease may vary in severity – young children and elderly people may be particularly badly affected. Infection usually resolves within a few days, although in severe cases antibiotics may be needed to help recovery.

Treatment

In severe cases, antibiotics may be used, e.g. fluoroquinone, although drug resistance is a common problem. Usually only rehydration and ion replacement are needed.

Prevention

Shigella infection is prevented by breaking the faeco-oral route of transmission. No vaccine is currently available.

Neisseria spp

Neisseria spp. are Gram-negative cocci of which two species are clinically important – *N. gonorrhoeae* and *N. meningitidis*. The bacteria are closely related, but nevertheless show marked differences. *N. gonorrhoeae* is a professional pathogen and causes disease to help its transmission and survival. In contrast, *N. meningitidis* gains little advantage through causing meningitis because it precipitates death.

Morphology and identification

Neisseria spp. are oxidase-expressing bacteria that grow on chocolate agar. Microscopically, they are found in pairs (diplococci), resembling paired kidney beans. *N. meningitidis* can be distinguished from *N. gonorrhoeae* by its ability to ferment maltose.

Neisseria meningitidis

N. meningitidis causes meningitis, and is the leading cause of death from infection in children in the USA. Identification is carried out on blood and CSF samples. The presence of Gram-negative cocci in spinal fluid is sufficient for a presumptive diagnosis of meningococcal meningitis.

Transmission and phylogeny

Humans are the only known hosts for meningococci. About 10% of the population are asymptomatic carriers, with the nasopharynx being the most common site of colonisation. Infection occurs in less than 0.01% of population, resulting from bacteria spreading to other regions of the body. Transmission between individuals is by respiratory aerosol.

Pathogenesis

N. meningitidis has three main virulence factors:

1 **Capsule** – inhibits phagocytosis
2 **Endotoxin** – LPS
3 **IgA protease**.

Neisseria spp. also possess pili that project through the capsule. These pili help attachment and can be extended to help motility. To help adhesion, *N. meningitidis* also possess Opa (opacity-associated) proteins, which are a family of proteins that determine tropism of bacteria.

Resistance to disease is due to protective antibodies to the capsule, mediating group-specific immunity. Complement also plays a role in defence against *N. meningitidis*; individuals with deficiencies of late complement components are susceptible to neisseria infection

---

 CLINICAL Meningitis and meningococcaemia

As a result of bacteraemia, *N. meningitidis* can spread to distant organs and may seed in the meninges. The resulting meningitis results in the characteristic symptoms – fever, stiff neck, sensitivity to bright light.

The most severe manifestation of *N. meningitidis* infection is meningococcaemia. The resultant septic shock leads to high fever, widespread rash and disseminated intravascular coagulation.

Treatment

N. meningitidis infection can be managed by penicillin, although more severe forms of infection also require management of symptoms.

Individuals who have come into close contact with meningitis sufferers are given prophylactic antibiotic treatment – typically rifampicin.

Prevention

Vaccines have been developed against the poly-saccharide capsule of some serogroups. However, this is not possible for serogroup B, in which the capsule antigen is identical to the host molecule, NCAM-1.

Neisseria gonorrhoeae

N. gonorrhoeae is the causative agent of gonor-rhoea, a sexually transmitted infection. It can also cause pelvic inflammatory disease and neonatal conjunctivitis.

Transmission

N. gonorrhoeae infects only humans and is usually transmitted sexually, although it can be transmit-ted from mother to newborn during birth. The genital tract is the most common source of the bacteria, although they can also be found in the pharynx and rectum.

Pathogenesis

N. gonorrhoeae is a professional pathogen, almost always causing disease in the host. Although usually symptomatic in males, gonococcal infection is often asymptomatic in females, helping transmission.

Diagnosis in men can be made by detection of Gram-negative diplococci within neutrophils in urethral discharge. In women, cultures are nor-mally required for diagnosis.

N. gonorrhoeae has several important virulence factors:

- **Pili** mediate attachment of bacteria to cell sur-faces. The pili are retractable, limiting presenta-tion of an antigen to the period when the pilus is performing an essential function.
- **Cell walls** contain lipo-oligosaccharide (LOS), a mild endotoxin causing less severe endotoxic shock than LPS.
- **IgA protease**.

Immune response

The main host defence against *N. gonorrhoeae* is production of antibodies (IgG and IgA), but com-plement and neutrophils also have a role. Repeated gonococcal infection may occur due to antigenic variation – **phase switching**.

 DEFINITION Phase switching

Phase variation is a process whereby some genes in the genome are reversibly switched on or off. In *Neisseria* spp. this leads to antigenic variation, be-cause the genes that are turned on and off are enzymes associated with the production of antigenic polysaccharides.

The genes contain tracts of repeated nucleotides within their coding region. During replication, the tracts may be lengthened or shortened as a result of inaccurate copying by the bacterial polymerases; the resulting frame shift produces a non-functional product.

Treatment

Ceftriaxone and penicillins can be used to treat *N. gonorrhoeae* infection, although penicillin-resistant isolates have been identified.

Prevention

No vaccine currently exists. Prevention focuses on condom use and prompt treatment of infected individuals and their contacts.

 CLINICAL Symptoms of gonococcal diseases

Gonorrhoea is the most common disease caused by *N. gonorrhoeae*. In men, it is characterised by purulent discharge and pain on urination. In women, infection occurs in the endometrium, causing discharge and intermenstrual bleeding. A common complication is spread of infection up the fallopian tubes, which can result in sterility or ectopic pregnancy as a result of scarring in the fallopian tubes. Disseminated infection can lead to arthritis and tenosynovitis.

Newborn babies may acquire *N. gonorrhoeae* from an infected mother during childbirth, resulting in neonatal conjunctivitis. This condition can be pre-vented by prophylactic erythromycin eye ointment.

Mycobacterium tuberculosis

M. tuberculosis causes more deaths than any other bacterial infection – it is estimated that approxi-mately a third of the world population may be infected. Tuberculosis as a world health issue has been compounded by the spread of AIDS, because severe TB can occur in immunosup-pressed patients.

Structure and morphology

M. tuberculosis is an acid-fast bacillus. It must also be grown on special medium (e.g. Löwenstein-Jensen) to help its growth while inhibiting the culture of faster-growing bacteria.

M. tuberculosis can be distinguished form other mycobacteria by the production of niacin. It is an obligate aerobe, normally infecting highly oxygenated tissue, e.g. lungs.

The cell wall is rich in lipids due to the mycolic acids (long-chain fatty acids), which contribute to its acid-fast nature, and phosphatides, which play a role in caseous necrosis. In addition, *M. tuberculosis* is relatively resistant to NaOH, which is used to isolate bacteria from clinical specimens. It is also resistant to dehydration, which may help respiratory transmission because it can survive in dried sputum.

Transmission and pathogenesis

Transmission is by respiratory aerosol. The initial site of infection is within the lungs where *M. tuberculosis* is taken up and can survive within alveolar macrophages. Disseminated disease occurs in only a small proportion of infected individuals.

M. tuberculosis survives and multiplies within the phagosome. It is capable of inhibiting lysosomal fusion with the phagosome. Survival of *M. tuberculosis* within the macrophage leads to formation of granulomas with the bacteria.

A typical granuloma is made up of a central area of multinucleate giant cells containing bacilli, surrounded by epithelioid cells, lymphocytes and fibroblasts. The last result in a repair process that is ongoing. Many granulomas in TB contain a central region of necrotic caseous ('cheesy') tissue. *M. tuberculosis* can reside within granulomas for many years, isolated from the rest of the host. The walled-off granuloma is known as a tubercle and may calcify over time, although it is still likely to contain live *M. tuberculosis*.

 DEFINITION Giant and epithelioid lesions

Giant and epithelioid cells within a granuloma appear to be specialised forms of macrophages. Giant cells are multinucleated cells, thought to result from the fusion of infected macrophages. Epithelioid cells appear to be specialised for secretion, showing aspects of morphology similar to epithelial cells.

Immune response

M. tuberculosis does not directly damage the host. The damage is the result of the cell-mediated immune response to the bacteria. Antibodies are formed, but play no significant protective role.

Patients with weakened cell-mediated immune response are unable to contain the bacteria, leading to disseminated infection (e.g. in AIDS). The strength of the host immune response appears to be an important determinant of disease state.

 CLINICAL Disseminated TB infection

A tubercle may rupture into a bronchus and bacteria may spread to other areas of the lungs or enter the blood, from where bacilli may infect distant sites. Many organs may become involved in disseminated infection, leading to generalised symptoms of fever, tiredness and weight loss. Pulmonary TB is associated with a severe cough and haemoptysis (blood in sputum). Common disseminated forms include miliary TB (characterised by small millet-seed-like lesions throughout the body and lungs), tuberculous meningitis and tuberculous osteomyelitis, in particular, Pott's disease (vertebral osteomyelitis).

Treatment

Treatment of TB is difficult because many drug-resistant strains have developed. Consequently, drug resistance tests are essential for management of the disease. **Isoniazid** is the main therapeutic agent used in combination with other drugs such as rifampicin and ethambutol. A long period of treatment (9–12 months) with multiple drugs is required due to:

- **intracellular location** of the organism
- **caseous material** blocking penetration by drug
- **slow growth of the organism**
- **metabolic inactivity** – a portion of bacteria do not take up drugs, and thus are not killed.

Problems are exacerbated due to lack of patient compliance over a long period.

Immunisation

Prior infection can be detected by a positive tuberculin skin test. However, previous immunisation will also yield a positive response.

BCG (Bacillus Camille–Guérin) vaccine is used to protect against TB. The BCG bacterium is an attenuated strain of *M. bovis*, a related bacterium, and results in only partial protection. BCG cannot be given to immunocompromised patients because it is a **live vaccine**.

Fungi

Fungi are eukaryotic organisms and cause some important clinical diseases. With the exception of *Candida albicans* (a skin commensal), fungi naturally reside in the environment.

Structure and morphology

Fungal cell walls differ from those of other organisms because they consist primarily of chitin. Fungal cell walls contain ergosterol instead of **cholesterol**. As human cells do not synthesise or use ergosterol, this difference is exploited by the selective action of azole antifungal drugs. Fungi can be found in two states:

1 **Yeasts** grow as single cells.
2 **Moulds** grow as hyphae (long filaments).

Many fungi can grow in both states – they are dimorphic. Most medically important fungi replicate asexually.

Common fungal conditions

Two common fungal infections are candidiasis caused by *Candida albicans* and tinea pedis caused by *Trichophyton* spp.

C. albicans is the causative agent of **thrush**. It is commonly found as a skin commensal, although it can cause infection at other sites. In immunocompromised individuals, *Candida* spp. may cause disseminated infection. Treatment is by azole drugs which inhibit the synthesis of ergosterol, found in fungal cell walls.

Athlete's foot is caused by tinea pedis. Other fungal infections are rare, opportunistic fungal infections associated with a compromised immune system (particularly pneumocystis pneumonia in AIDS).

Parasites

Parasites occur in two distinct forms – single-celled **protozoa** and multicellular **helminths**. These organisms are a serious cause of illness in the developing world. Parasites tend to have a complex lifecycle with stages in humans and other animals. All parasites are eukaryotic.

Protozoal parasites

Protozoal parasites are typically vector borne and affect many millions of people each year. The lifecycle of these parasites is complex, with different stages for the host and the vector, and they may employ both sexual and asexual reproduction in their lifecycle.

Malaria

Around 300 million people each year are affected by malaria, with more than 1 million people a year dying from the disease. Malaria is mainly confined to Africa, southern Asia and Latin America. Treatment has become more challenging due to the emergence of drug-resistant strains.

Malaria is caused by the parasites of the genus *Plasmodium*, of which four species may cause malaria in humans:

- *Plasmodium falciparum* – the most virulent
- *Plasmodium vivax*
- *Plasmodium ovale*
- *Plasmodium malariae.*

 CLINICAL Symptoms of malaria

Clinical symptoms are often non-specific: fever, headache, chills, vomiting, diarrhoea. More specific symptoms include splenomegaly, anaemia, hypoglycaemia, and pulmonary or renal dysfunction. Clinical manifestations of malaria are associated with the synchronous rupture of infected red blood cells.

Falciparum malaria can rapidly progress to a more severe form which may be fatal. This results from attachment of infected cells to small blood vessels, which may cause CNS involvement (cerebral malaria), as well as acute renal failure and respiratory distress.

Splenomegaly and occasionally splenic rupture are known complications of *P. vivax* infection. Infection with *P. malariae* may be complicated by nephrotic syndrome.

Transmission and lifecycle

Malaria is transmitted by the bite of an infected female *Anopheles* mosquito (Fig. 16.8). *Plasmodium* develops in the gut of the mosquito and sporozoites are passed on in the saliva of the insect. When an infected mosquito bites, the parasites enter the victim's bloodstream and migrate to the liver where they multiply.

Over the next 2 weeks, *Plasmodium* undergoes rapid asexual reproduction to produce thousand of merozoites in each liver cell, which are released when the hepatocyte ruptures. These merozoites infect red blood cells and undergo further asexual reproduction to produce a schizont, containing around 15 merozoites. Some merozoites may differentiate into sexual forms – gametocytes. The male and female gametocytes are taken up by a female anopheline mosquito on biting an infected human. Sexual reproduction occurs in the midgut of the mosquito.

P. vivax and *P. ovale* can produce a recurrent infection because they may also exist in the liver in a dormant stage. They may form hypnozoites that can persist for several years and lead to relapses.

Immune response and evasion

Plasmodium parasites are specialised for entry into hepatocytes and red blood cells, where they live within a vacuole. The parasite is able to remodel the red blood cell surface – *P. falciparum* causes the expression of PfEMP-1 (*P. falciparum* erythrocyte membrane protein 1) on the red blood cell surface, which mediates attachment to the surface of small blood vessels, preventing clearance of the infected red blood cell in the spleen. There are many antigenically distinct variants of PfEMP-1, impairing formation of an effective antibody response.

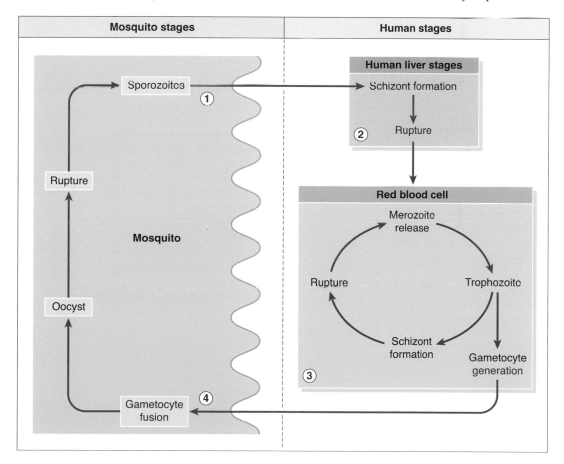

Figure 16.8 **Lifecycle of malaria**. (1) Sporozoites are injected into a host when it is bitten by an infected mosquito. (2) The sporozoites infect hepatocytes were they divide rapidly and form a schizont. The schizont then ruptures releasing merozoites into the blood stream. (3) Merozoites infected red blood cells and these infect the cells and may develop into further merozoites, or undergo and alternative development to form gametocytes. (4) The gametocytes may be taken up by a mosquito when it infects an infected human. They undergo sexual reproduction in the gut of the mosquito, and subsequently divide into sporozoites.

P. falciparum is capable of antigenic variation at various stages of its lifecycle, impeding the production of an effective immune response against any form of the parasite. Nevertheless partial immunity can be built up due to the development of antibodies that provide some protection and act against the merozoites.

The hepatocyte stage of the parasite lifecycle can result in the development of CTLs that are specific for *Plasmodium*-derived epitopes. Given the lack of MHC-I molecules on red blood cells, the CTLs play little part in the removal of merozoites.

Treatment

Many drug-resistant strains of *Plasmodium* have emerged; there is a desperate need for the development of new drug regimens and therapies. Three major drugs are currently used whereas antibiotics such as tetracycline can be used to treat acute episodes:

1 **Chloroquine** acts to kill the merozoite stage of all four species of *Plasmodium*. They prevent the digestion of haemoglobin, which is toxic to the parasite) and its conversion to haemozoin, which is non-toxic. Resistance to chloroquine is common, particularly in *P. falciparum*.
2 **Pyrimethamine** inhibits the formation of tetrahydrofolate in the parasite, which is crucial for DNA synthesis. Pyrimethamine has a higher affinity for the parasitic enzyme than its human equivalent. Some strains have developed resistance to pyrimethamine, although these are less common than chloroquine-resistant strains.
3 **Artemesinin** kills schizonts during acute malaria. The mechanism is not clear, although it is thought it may act through promoting the generation of free radicals which damage the parasite, as well as potentially inhibiting the protozoal Ca^{2+} ATPase.

Prevention

Chloroquine is typically used as prophylactic and must be taken for about 2 weeks before arrival in a malaria-endemic area and for about 6 weeks after departure. However, drug-resistant strains have emerged. Other drugs may also be used prophylactically, often doxycycline or larium, each with varying efficacy and side effects.

Mosquito nets are frequently used to reduce access of the vector to host and management of malaria has also been attempted through removal of the vector. The drainage of stagnant water near communities reduces the mosquito population and insecticides have been tried, although mosquitoes have developed resistance to some of these.

Currently, no vaccine is available although many are in development, targeting different stages of the lifecycle.

Helminths

Multicellular parasites – helminths – are a serious cause of mortality and morbidity in the developing world. Many millions of people are affected, particularly by schistosomiasis and onchocerciasis (river blindness).

Classification

Helminths can be divided into two main groups:

1 **Nematodes** (roundworms) possess a cylindrical body and are covered in a protective cuticle. Nematodes have separate sexes – the female is usually larger than the male.
2 **Platyminths** (flatworms) can be further divided into **trematodes** and **cestodes**:
   – **trematodes** (flukes) have a leaf-shaped body, although this takes on very different morphologies at different points in the lifecycle; they often have a complex lifecycle, with stages in a human host and a snail intermediate, and they are usually hermaphrodites
   – **cestodes** (tapeworms) vary in length from 2–3 mm (typically three to four proglottids) to 7–10 m long (several thousand proglottids). They have a segmented body made up of a scolex (head) and a chain of **proglottids** and are hermaphrodites.

The severity of helminthic infection is often directly related to the number of parasites infecting the host. Infection with a single parasite will be asymptomatic, whereas infection with several thousand parasites is likely to cause severe pathology. Low numbers of parasites may cause a severe illness if infection occurs in a critical location (e.g. the brain).

⊙ RELATED CHAPTERS

17

Neuroscience

Neuroscience is the study of neuroanatomy, the spatial arrangement of structures in the nervous system, and of neurophysiology, the functioning of the nervous system.

The nervous system is divided into the central nervous system (CNS) – the brain and spinal cord – and the peripheral nervous system (PNS), which comprises all nervous matter outside of these structures.

 DEFINITION Grey and white matter in the CNS

The tissue in the CNS is broadly divided into grey and white matter, which have different roles and features:

- **Grey matter**: darker coloured tissues of the CNS, rich in neuron cell bodies, branching dendrites and supporting cells, glia.
- **White matter**: paler coloured tissues of the CNS, rich in the insulating material, myelin, which surrounds nerve fibres.

The nervous system comprises not only neurons but also other cells that support neuronal function. The bony structures of the skull and vertebral column, the tissue meninges investing the CNS, the cerebrospinal fluid (CSF) and blood vessels have a supportive role, and are covered in this chapter.

The functioning of the nervous system can be broadly categorised into:

- **motor systems**, which control both voluntary and involuntary muscle contraction and relaxation
- **sensory systems** which detect touch, pain and limb position (proprioception)
- **special senses** including sight, hearing, smell, taste and balance
- **higher cortical functions**, including memory, sleep and consciousness.

The skull

The skull is the bony structure of the head that encases the brain and also contributes to the face. The skull can be broken up into two regions with distinct roles (Fig. 17.1):

1 The **neurocranium** is the region of the skull that encases and protects the brain.
2 The facial skeleton (**viscerocranium**) makes up the remainder of the skull and is covered in Chapter 14.

The bones of the neurocranium are mainly flat or irregular in shape and are joined by fibrous joints, forming a thick, tight structure. In children, the bones are linked by hyaline cartilage. This

---

Biomedical Science Lecture Notes, First Edition. Ian Lyons.
© 2011 by Ian Lyons. Published 2011 by Blackwell Publishing Ltd.

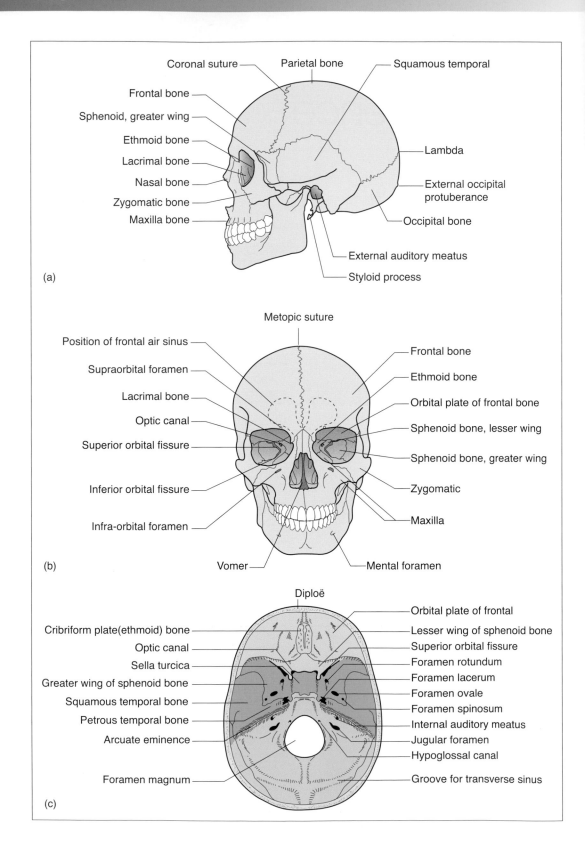

(a)

Coronal suture — Parietal bone — Squamous temporal

Frontal bone —
Sphenoid, greater wing —
Ethmoid bone —
Lacrimal bone —
Nasal bone —
Zygomatic bone —
Maxilla bone —

— Lambda
— External occipital protuberance
— Occipital bone
— External auditory meatus
— Styloid process

(b)

Metopic suture

Position of frontal air sinus —
Supraorbital foramen —
Lacrimal bone —
Optic canal —
Superior orbital fissure —
Inferior orbital fissure —
Infra-orbital foramen —

— Frontal bone
— Ethmoid bone
— Orbital plate of frontal bone
— Sphenoid bone, lesser wing
— Sphenoid bone, greater wing
— Zygomatic
— Maxilla

Vomer — — Mental foramen

(c)

Diploë

Cribriform plate(ethmoid) bone —
Optic canal —
Sella turcica —
Greater wing of sphenoid bone —
Squamous temporal bone —
Petrous temporal bone —
Arcuate eminence —
Foramen magnum —

— Orbital plate of frontal
— Lesser wing of sphenoid bone
— Superior orbital fissure
— Foramen rotundum
— Foramen lacerum
— Foramen ovale
— Foramen spinosum
— Internal auditory meatus
— Jugular foramen
— Hypoglossal canal
— Groove for transverse sinus

increases the flexibility of the skull, facilitating birth. Eight bones make up the neurocranium:

- Frontal bone
- Occipital bone
- Sphenoid bone
- Ethmoid bone
- Two parietal bones
- Two temporal bones.

The cranial cavity

The brain is housed in the cranial cavity. Three depressions (fossae), on which the brain sits, can be identified:

1 The **anterior cranial fossa** is the shallowest of the fossae and contains the frontal lobes of the brain. The fossa is made up of the frontal bone, and is located immediately posterior to the frontal sinuses. In the middle of this fossa is the **cribriform plate**, which possesses a series of small holes to allow entry of the olfactory nerve fibres.
2 The **middle cranial fossa** consists of two deep depressions on each side of a small prominence, the sella turcica – a formation in the middle of the sphenoid bone that contains a slight depression in the middle, in which the pituitary gland sits. The middle cranial fossa is formed by the sphenoid and temporal bones.
3 The **posterior cranial fossa** is the deepest of the fossae, accommodating the cerebellum, pons and medulla; it contains the foramen magnum in its base. It is made up mainly by occipital bone.

Foramina of the skull

There must be points of entry and exit in the neurocranium to allow communication between the brain and the body. Four types of tracts or conduits link the brain and the rest of the body (see Fig. 17.1):

1 The **arterial supply** of the brain and structures internal to the skull is derived almost exclusively from the internal carotid and vertebral arteries. The only exception is the middle meningeal artery, which is a branch of the external carotid artery.

2 The **venous drainage** of the brain is through the internal jugular veins.
3 The **cranial nerves** must exit the skull to innervate structures in the face and in body.
4 The **spinal cord** is a continuation of the CNS.

Foramina in the anterior cranial fossa

There are two major foramina in the anterior cranial fossa that serve the nose and eyes:

1 The **cribriform plate** is located in the midline in the ethmoid bone. It contains many small perforations that allow the olfactory nerve to enter the nose.
2 The **optic canal** carries the optic nerve and the ophthalmic artery to the eye.

Foramina in the middle cranial fossa

The middle cranial fossa contains many foramina for the cranial nerves innervating the muscles and skin of the face, as well as carrying much of the vasculature:

- The **superior orbital fissure** is located at the anterior aspect of the middle cranial fossa and carries branches of the trigeminal nerve and ophthalmic veins. In addition it carries the cranial nerves (CN) responsible for eye movements (CN III, IV and VI)
- The **foramen rotundum** carries the maxillary branch of the trigeminal nerve.
- The **foramen ovale** carries the mandibular branch of the trigeminal nerve.
- The **foramen spinosum** carries the middle meningeal artery.
- The **foramen lacerum** carries the internal carotid artery.

The foramina of the posterior cranial fossa

The foramina in the posterior cranial fossa carry many of the connections between the brain and the rest of the body:

- The **foramen magnum** carries the lower part of the medulla, which connects inferiorly with the

Figure 17.1 The skull is made up of a series of irregular bones. In the bones of the skull there is a series of foramina to allow the communication of the brain with the rest of the body. The most prominent is the foramen magnum which takes the spinal cord as well as some other nerves and vessels. The other major foramina are the carotid canal and the foramina rotundum, ovale and spinosum. The foramen lacerum is seen in skulls, although it is not a true foramen – nothing passes through it, and in humans it is covered by a layer of cartilage.

spinal cord. It also carries the vertebral arteries and the spinal accessory nerve.

- The **internal auditory meatus** in the petrous temporal bone carries the facial and vestibulo-cochlear nerves.
- The **jugular foramen** carries the internal jugular vein and CN IX, X and XI.
- The **hypoglossal canal** allows exit of the hypoglossal nerve from the skull.

The meninges

The brain is supported by three tissue layers known as the meninges:

1 The **pia mater** is the innermost layer. It consists of a very rich network of fibres containing many vessels and a rich lymphoid system.
2 The **arachnoid mater** is made up of many irregular connecting fibres and contains a layer of CSF so that the entire brain tissue is bathed in the fluid.
3 The **dura mater** is the outermost layer. It is a tough fibrous covering of tissue encasing the CNS.

The meninges are richly innervated and vascularised. Due to their large blood supply, the meninges may rupture and bleed, which is a clinical emergency. A haemorrhage can be classified based on its location in relation to the meninges:

- **Subarachnoid** haemorrhage
- **Subdural** haemorrhage
- **Extradural** haemorrhage.

The signs and symptoms of the different forms of bleeds differ, although in each case the condition is serious, because the pressure caused by the pooling of blood is likely to press on the brain tissue and cause damage.

 CLINICAL Subarachnoid haemorrhage

A subarachnoid haemorrhage results in blood entering the subarachnoid space. This usually results from the rupture of an aneurysm, often in the circle of Willis. The bleeding causes meningeal irritation and a severe headache with loss of consciousness. Neurological symptoms are often not seen. Subarachnoid haemorrhages are particularly severe and those resulting from the rupture of an aneurysm have about a 50% mortality rate pre-admission.

 CLINICAL Subdural haemorrhage

Subdural haemorrhages result from leakage of venous blood into the potential space between the dura and arachnoid, as a result of trauma. Similar to an extradural haemorrhage, the symptoms result from accumulation of pressure on the brain. The onset of symptoms is usually prolonged due to the low pressure of venous blood and may take up to 2 weeks to develop. The symptoms include altered consciousness, headaches, disorientation and amnesia, slurred speech, ataxia and altered breathing patterns.

 CLINICAL Extradural haemorrhage

In an extradural haemorrhage, blood collects between the skull and the external part of the dura. This usually occurs due to a blow to the head and is typically characterised by a sequence of brief concussion, followed by a period in which the patient appears lucid, followed later by drowsiness and coma. The symptoms are caused by the build-up of pressure on the brain due to the accumulating volume of blood after tearing of the arteries.

Cell types in the brain

The brain is made up mainly of two cell groups: neurons and glia (supporting cells).

Neurons

The structure of a neuron

Neurons are highly specialised cells involved in the initiation and conduction of action potentials allowing the processing and transmission of information. There are a number of subtypes, although they share a variety of features reflecting their common purpose in receiving and integrating signals from other cells and conducting action potentials:

- The **dendrites** are small projections arising from the cell body. They typically form the site of synapses with other neurons.

- The **axon** is the section of the nerve cell specialised for the conduction of an action potential. It is often myelinated, contains many voltage-gated channels and can be long.

Classification of neurons

Neurons can be classed by:

- shape (Table 17.1)
- neurotransmitter, which may be inhibitory or excitatory
- function: according to either the neuronal system in which that neuron plays a part or whether the neuron is excitatory or inhibitory; it can be both at different synapses.

Neurons are classed as inhibitory or excitatory according to their effect on the membrane potential of the postsynaptic cell:

- **Excitatory neurons** induce depolarisation of the postsynaptic membranes, potentially leading to the generation of an action potential
- **Inhibitory neurons** typically hyperpolarise the postsynaptic membranes, inhibiting the generation of an action potential (reducing the excitability of the postsynaptic cell).

In the brain the main excitatory neurotransmitter is glutamate, although in the spinal cord acetylcholine is the major excitatory neurotransmitter. Conversely, in the brain γ-aminobutyric acid (GABA) is the predominant inhibitory neurotransmitter, whereas in the spinal cord glycine is the major inhibitory neurotransmitter.

The input and output cells of different regions of the brain can be considered predominantly as either inhibitory or excitatory; however, the actual behaviour of cells is extremely complex and not fully understood, e.g. the input and output from the cortex are mainly excitatory, whereas the output from the cerebellum is predominantly inhibitory

Functional classification of nerve fibres

In the sensory and motor nervous systems, different receptors are innervated by specific fibre types, with different conducting velocities (Tables 17.2 and 17.3).

Neural repair and regeneration

The ability of nerves to regenerate differs in the PNS and CNS. As many cells have long axons, cutting an axon results in death of the portion of the cell not connected to the cell body, although the rest of the nerve may be able to regenerate.

In both the PNS and CNS, the stump of the damaged axon will rapidly develop new sprouts. A series of processes following injury must occur for the nerve cell to regrow along its original pathway (Fig. 17.2):

- Degeneration of the damaged axon
- Regrowth and elongation of the axonal sprout
- Remyelination of the nerve fibre.

Degeneration

When a nerve is cut, a characteristic process occurs, known as **wallerian degeneration**. After cutting, the axon region distal to the cut rapidly dies and the axon and synaptic endings rapidly disintegrate. If the axon were myelinated, the myelin sheath should also disintegrate, although the cells

---

Table 17.1 Classification of neurons according to morphological characteristics

Number of axons	Unipolar (one neurite)	Bipolar (two neurites)	Multipolar (three or more neurites)
Shape of cell body	Pyramidal		
Pattern of dendritic tree	Stellate cells: star like arrangement	Purkinje cells: two-dimensional array	Single long axon, many dendrites receiving impulses
Length of axon	Projection neurons: long axons	Interneurons: short axons	
		Sensory neurons: long axons	

Table 17.2 Sensory nerve fibre types

Class	Conduction velocity	Diameter	Myelinated?	Sensory receptors
Ia	80–120 m/s	13–20 μm	Yes	Muscle spindle
Ib	80–120 m/s	13–20 μm	Yes	Golgi tendon organs
Aβ (II)	~50 m/s	6–12 μm	Yes	Touch, vibration and pressure sensors in the skin
Aδ	5–30 m/s	2–5 μm	Yes	Free nerve endings sensing touch and pressure. Cold thermoreceptors. Nociceptors, typically responding to mechanical stimuli
C	0.5–2 m/s	0.2–1.5 μm	No	Nociceptors. Typically responding to noxious stimuli. Warmth thermoreceptors

themselves would remain viable. The dying axon and myelin are removed by macrophages in phagocytosis. If the axon were the sole source of input to the cell downstream, the postsynaptic cell could also degenerate – this is seen in muscle cells in which atrophy occurs after neuronal damage.

Regrowth and axonal sprouting

After degeneration, the viable axon sprouts and attempts to regrow, guided by the various growth factors that may be present. In the PNS regrowth is guided by the Schwann cells, allowing the axons to reach their target tissue. Nerve cells may be more than 1 metre long and growth rate is limited by axonal transport. This regrowth rarely exceeds 1 mm/day.

Regrowth of axons in the CNS does not occur for three main reasons:

- The oligodendrocytes myelinate many cells, and do not provide the guide path for regrowth provided by Schwann cells in the PNS.
- Astrocytes in the CNS rapidly form scar tissue and obstruct the path of axonal growth.
- The growth factors found centrally may differ from those in the periphery, and may alter the potential for regrowth.

Remyelination

After regrowth of the axon in the periphery, Schwann cells regenerate a myelin coating around the nerve cell. In this process the membrane of the Schwann cell progressively wraps around the axon. The membrane contains many insulating products such as myelin, which promote saltatory conduction between the nodes of the exposed axon.

Neuroglia

The neuroglia are the cells that support the function of the neurons. In fact, they outnumber the neurons by approximately 10:1. Three types of neuroglia can be identified:

1 Astrocytes
2 Microglia
3 Myelinating glia.

Astrocytes

Astrocytes are the most numerous glial cells. They act as interstitial cells, filling much of the space not containing blood vessels or neurons, and may be involved in regulating the precise space that a neuron can occupy.

Table 17.3 Lower motor neuron fibre types

Class	Conduction velocity	Diameter	Myelinated?	Target
α	70–120 m/s	12–20 μm	Yes	Muscle fibres
γ	4–25 m/s	3–6 μm	Yes	Motor innervation of muscle spindles

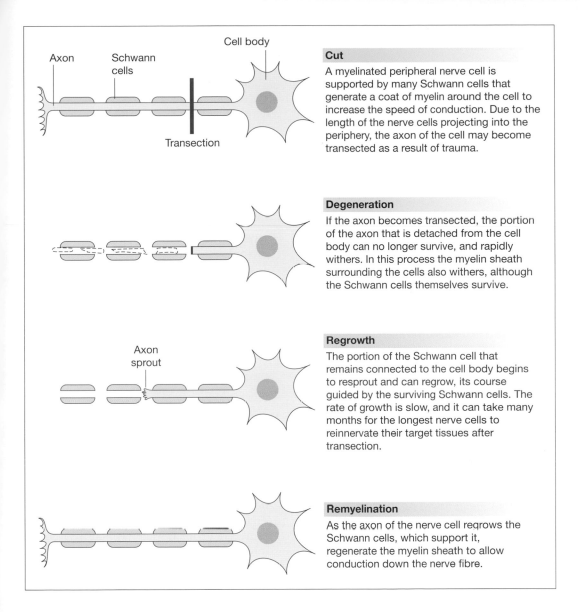

Cut

A myelinated peripheral nerve cell is supported by many Schwann cells that generate a coat of myelin around the cell to increase the speed of conduction. Due to the length of the nerve cells projecting into the periphery, the axon of the cell may become transected as a result of trauma.

Degeneration

If the axon becomes transected, the portion of the axon that is detached from the cell body can no longer survive, and rapidly withers. In this process the myelin sheath surrounding the cells also withers, although the Schwann cells themselves survive.

Regrowth

The portion of the Schwann cell that remains connected to the cell body begins to resprout and can regrow, its course guided by the surviving Schwann cells. The rate of growth is slow, and it can take many months for the longest nerve cells to reinnervate their target tissues after transection.

Remyelination

As the axon of the nerve cell regrows the Schwann cells, which support it, regenerate the myelin sheath to allow conduction down the nerve fibre.

Figure 17.2 Nerve cells may be exceptionally long; if the axon is cut, the portion attached to the cell body may regrow. In the periphery, the existence of Schwann cells to guide this axonal growth can allow it to reinnervate its original target organ, to return some innervation that may have been lost by the initial transection.

Astrocytes regulate the concentration of ions in the extracellular space, particularly those that affect neuronal function. They also contain stores of glycogen, which can be broken down into glucose during the sympathetic response to boost neuronal function and energy. Astrocytes are tightly packed around synapses and may regulate the contents of the synapse, preventing the leak of neurotransmitters. In addition, astrocytes have high affinity uptake systems for neurotransmitters such as serotonin (5-hydroxytryptamine or 5-HT) to aid removal of neurotransmitters from the synapse.

Microglia

Microglia are the smallest glial cells. They can differentiate into macrophages in response to damage and inflammation, allowing an immune response within the CNS.

Myelinating glial cells

Some glial cells provide the neurons with layers of myelin to insulate the nervous cell and promote saltatory conduction to speed up action potential conduction. In the PNS myelination is achieved by Schwann cells, which myelinate a single neural cell. In the CNS, the arrangement is more complex because a single oligodendrocyte can myelinate many neurons.

In the PNS and the CNS not all axons are myelinated; these typically have a slow conduction speed due to their small diameter, as well as their lack of myelin.

Oligodendrocytes and Schwann cells also help the axonal growth of nerve cells by directing their growth pathway. In the cerebellum, the Bergmann glia are a specialised set of cells found during development that direct the migration of granule cells toward their correct locations.

The ventricular system and the blood–brain barrier

The brain is a metabolically active organ. Although it makes up about 2% of the total body weight, it requires around 15% of the resting cardiac output, and accounts for about 20% of total body oxygen consumption. The brain is very sensitive to changes in its environment, which is tightly regulated and somewhat different in its make-up to blood. The brain and the body are separated by the **blood–brain barrier**, which is made up of a continuous endothelial layer with a particularly dense basement membrane, allowing transport of substances in an almost entirely selective manner.

There are a few sites where the barrier is not present are normally associated with secretion of substances from the CNS into the blood:

- Pituitary gland
- Pineal gland
- Epithelium of the choroid plexus
- Preoptic recess
- Paraphysis.

Structure of the blood–brain barrier

The endothelial cells in blood vessels in the brain are continuous, containing no fenestrations. They possess tight junctions, which prevent the movement even of ions. The endothelial cells are surrounded by a layer of pericyte-like cells to regulate blood flow, and the basolateral surface of the endothelial cells is covered by processes from astroglial cells, which cover over 95% of the endothelial surface.

Transport across the blood–brain barrier

Given the restrictive nature of the blood–brain barrier, transport of substances into, or out of, the brain requires selective transport by protein transporters. This is reflected in the high levels of mitochondria present in the endothelial cells. The large amount of transport accounts for a proportion of the brain's high energy requirement. Entry of substances into the CSF is achieved in three distinct ways:

1 Lipid-soluble substances are capable of **direct diffusion** across the endothelial cell membranes, although if they are too lipid soluble they are unlikely to be present in the blood in sufficient concentrations; they may also bind serum albumin, which is likely to reduce their delivery.
2 Transport by **facilitated diffusion** allows the transport of many water-soluble substances into the CSF. In particular, glucose, which is almost the exclusive food of the brain, is transported by this method through the GLUT1 transporter.
3 Many small amino acids are produced in the brain and must be removed by **active transport**. In particular, glycine which is used as an inhibitory neurotransmitter must be removed against its concentration gradient.

Transport of drugs across the blood–brain barrier

The transport of drugs into the brain presents a difficult problem, first due to the nature of the regulated transport by the blood–brain barrier. The endothelial cells express the multidrug resistance (MDR) transporter. This transporter has a physiological role in transporting steroid molecules out of the brain, although it can also act to transport many drugs out.

The metabolic blood–brain barrier

Endothelial cells in the blood–brain barrier express enzymes that can metabolise solutes before they are transported into the brain. These systems may also influence the delivery of drugs, e.g. L-dopa. L-Dopa is readily transported into endothelial cells, although it is then degraded by the enzymes monoamine oxygenase and dopa decarboxylase. To ensure effective treatment for parkinsonism, L-dopa requires administration with a dopa decarboxylase inhibitor.

 CLINICAL Breakdown of the blood–brain barrier

Some diseases (e.g. bacterial meningitis) can cause increased permeability of the blood–brain barrier. This may allow drugs access to the CNS, which is not usually possible.

Cerebrospinal fluid

The cells of the brain are bathed in CSF, maintaining a constant environment for them. CSF is produced by the choroid plexus in the ventricular system and circulates through to the subarachnoid spaces, before draining into the **venous sinuses** of the brain. This drainage system allows the removal of many metabolites from the brain that are potentially toxic. The CSF performs several functions:

- Serves as a mechanical cushion for the brain
- Provides nutrients for the cells for the CNS
- Acts as a conduit for some hormones secreted by the hypothalamus, which act on remote sites of the brain
- Allows sensing of pH changes to regulate cerebral blood flow and pulmonary ventilation
- Removes metabolites from cells
- Acts as a lymphatic system for the brain.

The ventricular system

The CSF circulates through the ventricular system, bathing the brain cells. The ventricular system is made up of four ventricles which are connected by a series of conduits, all of which develop from the cavity of the neural tube. The chambers in the ventricular system are filled with CSF and lined with ependymal cells. There are four ventricles (Fig. 17.3):

- Two lateral ventricles – one in each cerebral hemisphere
- The third ventricle
- The fourth ventricle.

The lateral ventricle

The lateral ventricle is C shaped and contained within the parietal lobe of the cerebrum. The ventricle has three horns – anterior, posterior and inferior – which project into the frontal, occipital and temporal lobes, respectively. On the medial aspect of each ventricle is an interventricular foramen, which communicates with the third ventricle and lies between the anterior fornix and the anterior aspect of the thalamus. The choroid plexus lies on the medial aspect of the lateral ventricles between the body of the fornix and the superior surface of the thalamus.

The third ventricle

The third ventricle is a slit-like chamber in the midline, between the two thalami. It is connected to the lateral ventricles through the interventricular foramina, and with the fourth ventricle through the cerebral aqueduct. The third ventricle is bounded anteriorly by the anterior commissure, posteriorly by the cerebral aqueduct and (more superiorly) by the posterior commissure. The roof of the ventricle is also lined with choroid plexus and has a blood supply from the internal carotid and basilar arteries.

The cerebral aqueduct

This short (<2.5 cm) channel connects the third and fourth ventricles, allowing a flow of CSF from the third to the fourth ventricle. The aqueduct contains no choroid plexus and is surrounded by a region of grey matter – the **periaqueductal grey** – which is important in the response to pain.

The fourth ventricle

The fourth ventricle is located between the cerebellum and pons and is continuous with the cerebral aqueduct, which links it to the third ventricle. The fourth ventricle is continuous inferiorly

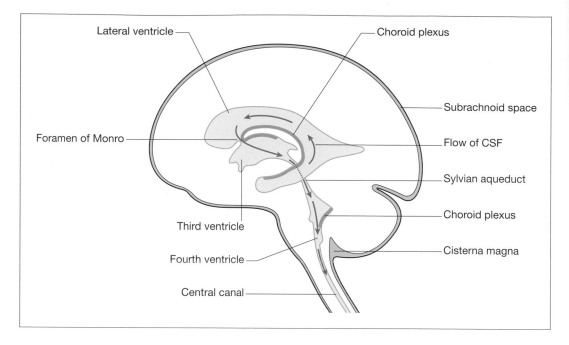

Figure 17.3 The ventricular system of the central nervous system allows flow of cerebrospinal fluid (CSF), which bathes the cells of the central nervous system. CSF is produced by the choroid plexus, which is located in the lateral, third and fourth ventricles. The flow of CSF is from the lateral ventricles, which are located in the cerebral hemispheres, to the third ventricle, which is located deep in the brain, and surrounded by the thalamus. From there CSF flows to the very thin fourth ventricle and onwards to the central canal of the spinal cord. The fourth ventricle is also connected by other foramina to the cisternae, which are collections of CSF. The CSF collects in cisternae and subsequently flows to the subarachnoid space, where it is reabsorbed into the venous blood through arachnoid granulations.

with the central canal of the medulla and spinal cord, and is bounded laterally by the inferior cerebellar peduncles. The choroid plexus of the fourth ventricle is suspended from its roof and is supplied by the posteroinferior cerebella arteries.

Central canal of the spinal cord and medulla oblongata

The central canal is located inferior to the fourth ventricle, extending down through the lower part of the medulla, to the bottom of the spinal cord. At the bottom-most point, there is an expanded chamber – the conus medullaris. The central canal is closed at its lower end and lined with ependymal cells, although no choroid plexus is present.

The cisterns and subarachnoid space

The subarachnoid space is filled with CSF and completely surrounds the brain, extending along the olfactory nerves towards the nose. In most regions this is a small space, because the meninges

follow the surface of the brain closely; however, in regions at the base of the brain, the subarachnoid space becomes expanded into a cistern.

The subarachnoid space extends to surround the spinal cord, and invests the cauda equina, to the level of S2–3. The subarachnoid space also surrounds the cranial and spinal nerves to the point at which they leave the skull and the spinal cord. The meninges then fuse with the perineurium of the nerve.

Ependymal cells

Ependymal cells line the ventricular system of the brain and spinal cord. They are ciliated and assemble as a single layer of cells, directing the flow of CSF through the ventricular system. Ependymal cells can be classified as follows:

- **Ependymocytes** line the ventricles and the central canal of the spinal cord. The cells are connected by gap junctions which allow CSF through, to communicate with the cells of the CNS.

- **Tanycytes** are specialised ependymal cells lining the floor of the third ventricle over the median eminence of the hypothalamus. These have long processes that protrude between the median eminence cells, coming into direct contact with the capillaries.

The ependymal cells in the choroid plexus are joined by tight junctions to prevent CSF flowing between them and leaking into the underlying tissues.

Reabsorption of CSF

CSF is reabsorbed through the arachnoid granulations. These are sites at which the arachnoid tissue protrudes through the dura and into the venous sinuses as villi. These villi act as one-way valves to allow the flow of CSF into the venous sinuses. The villi contain fine vessels through which the CSF flows. An increase in pressure closes these vessels and prevents the flow of blood through the villi into the CSF.

 CLINICAL Lumbar puncture

Access beyond the blood–brain barrier may be required to administer drugs to the CNS or to acquire a sample of CSF. Access is obtained through a lumbar puncture. Although the spinal cord ends at around the level of L1 in the adult, the subarachnoid space continues until S2. By introducing a needle at the level of the iliac crests (L4–5) a sample of CSF can be obtained without damage to the CNS.

To reach the vertebral canal several layers of structure must be passed:

- Skin
- Fascia
- Supraspinous ligament
- Interspinous ligament
- Ligamentum flavum
- Connective tissue
- Dura mater
- Arachnoid mater.

 CLINICAL Hydrocephalus

If the production or removal of CSF is not correctly regulated, the volume of fluid in the skull may increase, resulting in hydrocephalus. This condition may be *congenital* or *acquired* later in life.

Congenital hydrocephalus is often caused by stenosis of the cerebral aqueduct – through the overgrowth of neuroglial cells – or the replacement of the aqueduct with a series of minute channels, which do not provide sufficient drainage. Hydrocephalus can be diagnosed on ultrasonography. It causes enlargement of the fetal head and can contribute to a difficult labour.

In the adult, raised intracranial pressure due to hydrocephalus causes headaches, unsteadiness and mental impairment:

- **Obstructive hydrocephalus** is likely to develop due to the growth of a tumour blocking the ventricular system.
- **Communicating hydrocephalus** is caused by a blockage in the drainage of the arachnoid granulations – it can occur due to adhesion of the meninges subsequent to trauma or meningitis.

Hydrocephalus, regardless of its cause, is treated by insertion of a shunt, normally into the jugular vein, to allow adequate drainage of fluid.

The vasculature of the brain

Arterial supply

The brain receives a large blood supply through four major vessels – the paired internal carotid arteries and the paired vertebral arteries. The main blood supply to the meninges is the middle meningeal artery which is a branch of the external carotid artery:

- The **circle of Willis** receives blood from the four major arteries supplying the brain, forming a circle that sends off branches to supply the cerebral cortex and many subcortical structures (Fig. 17.4). This arterial arrangement has a survival advantage, because, if there is a stenosis of one vessel, the others may be able to compensate to ensure that sufficient blood continues to reach the brain.
- The **internal carotid arteries** are direct continuations of the common carotids. They contribute to the circle of Willis and the anterior circulation of the brain. Unlike the external carotid arteries, the internal carotids have no branches in the neck and enter the skull through the carotid

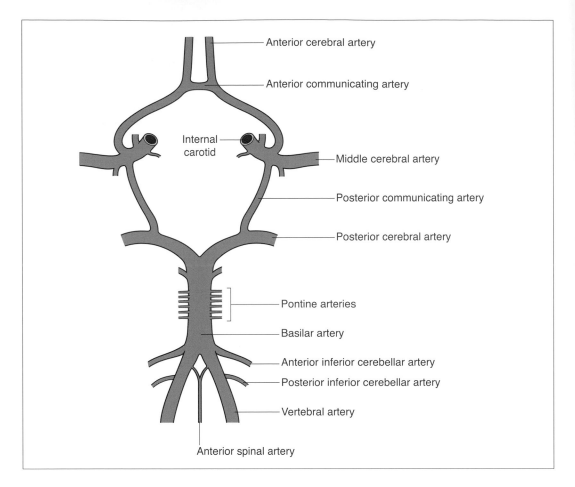

Figure 17.4 The major blood vessels supplying the brain anastomose in the **circle of Willis**, which gives of the anterior, middle and posterior cerebral arteries – the vessels supplying the cerebral hemispheres. The circle of Willis is supplied by the internal carotid arteries and the basilar artery. The basilar artery is itself formed by the fusion of the two vertebral arteries and gives many branches off to other regions of the branch as is ascends through the foramen magnum before joining the circle.

canal located in the temporal bones. In the skull, the internal carotid arteries pass through the cavernous sinus. The internal carotids arise in the neck at the level of the thyroid cartilage, at the bifurcation of the common carotid artery into the internal and external branches. The carotid bodies are located at the site of bifurcation and have an important role in the regulation of the blood composition. The **vertebral arteries** supply the posterior circulation of the brain, and are the first branches of subclavian arteries. They travel through the transverse foramina of the vertebra and are usually of unequal size, with the left typically being larger. The arteries travel in the subarachnoid space and enter the neurocranium through the **foramen magnum**.

At the inferior border of the pons, the vertebral arteries unite to form a single basilar artery which travels up the anterior aspect of the posterior fossa. The basilar artery gives off many branches before branching into two terminal branches, the posterior communicating arteries of the circle of Willis.

The basilar artery

The **basilar artery** results from fusion of the vertebral arteries and is responsible for supplying the brain stem, cerebellum and posterior parts of the cerebrum. It gives off many significant branches to supply structures close to its path.

The posterior inferior cerebellar artery

The posterior inferior cerebellar artery (PICA) is the largest branch of the basilar artery and follows a course between the medulla and cerebellum. It sends off branches that supply the posterior part of the cerebellum, the inferior vermis and central nuclei of the cerebellum, and the choroid plexus of the fourth ventricle.

 CLINICAL Wallenberg's syndrome

Wallenberg's, or lateral medullary, syndrome results from an occlusion of the PICA. The symptoms reflect the damage caused through infarction of the lateral medulla:

- Loss of pain and temperature sensation on the contralateral side of the body due to disruption of the spinothalamic tract
- Loss of pain sensation on the ipsilateral side of the face due to disruption of the trigeminal nucleus
- Vestibular dysfunction (dizziness, vertigo and nystagmus) as a result of disruption of the cerebellum
- Ipsilateral Horner's syndrome due to the disruption of the descending sympathetic fibres
- Ataxia, due to damage to the cerebellum or the inferior cerebellar peduncle.

Vasculature of the hypothalamus

The hypothalamus and the surrounding **median eminence** structures do not possess a conventional blood–brain barrier, as is reflected in their ability to secrete hormones. They are supplied by two hypophyseal arteries, both derived from the internal carotids:

1 The **inferior hypophyseal artery** supplies only the posterior pituitary gland.
2 The **superior hypophyseal artery** supplies the hypothalamus.

Venous drainage of the brain

The brain is drained by a series of venous sinuses that coalesce to drain into the internal jugular veins, returning blood to the systemic circulation. Venous sinuses are composed of cavities in the dura, lined by endothelial cells. There are some prominent sinuses that drain blood from large regions of the brain:

- The **superior sagittal sinus** runs along the superior aspect of the brain on the line of the great longitudinal fissure. It runs at the site of attachment of the falx cerebri to the skull.
- The **inferior sagittal fissure** runs along the inferior aspect of the **falx cerebri** above the corpus callosum.
- The **transverse sagittal sinus** is a major sinus that winds along the occipital bone and the parietal and temporal bones at the back of the skull. It receives blood from the **superior** and **inferior** sagittal sinuses and transports it to the jugular foramen, where it drains into the jugular vein via the sigmoid sinus.
- The **cavernous sinus** is found between the sphenoid and temporal bones lateral to the sella turcica. It carries many nerves and vessels within it. In particular, the internal carotids and the nerves associated with eye movement (CN III, IV and VI), and the ophthalmic and maxillary branches of the trigeminal nerve, pass through the carotid sinus.
- The **sigmoidal sinus** is found in the temporal bone and drains into the internal jugular vein.

 DEFINITION Falx cerebri and tentorium cerebelli

Two prominent folds of dura divide the gross structures of the brain:

1 **Falx cerebri**: a sickle-shaped fold of dura mater that dips down from the frontal bone and separates the cerebral hemispheres
2 **Tentorium cerebelli**: a tent-like infolding of the dura mater that separates the cerebellum below from the occipital lobes of the cerebral hemispheres above.

The gross structure of the brain

Developmentally, the brain is made up of three regions – forebrain, midbrain and hindbrain – of which the forebrain makes up the largest volume.

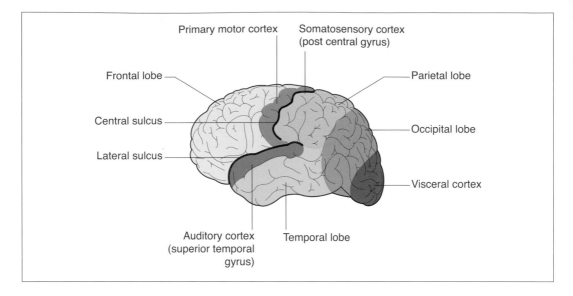

Figure 17.5 The lateral aspect of the cerebral hemispheres. The cortex is divided into four major regions, the four lobes – each of which is broadly associated with a specific range of functions. Although the functional regions of the cortex are not accurately delineated on the cortex, most functional regions can be localised approximately to specific anatomical parts of the cortex. In particular, the somatosensory and primary motor cortices can be found posterior and anterior, respectively, to the central sulcus. Similarly, the auditory cortex can be found on the superior temporal gyrus.

Neuroanatomical divisions do not always correspond to functional divisions. Instead, they are based on structural distinctions (Fig. 17.5).

The forebrain

The forebrain is the largest part of the brain and is divided into two **cerebral hemispheres** separated by the **great transverse fissure** which runs sagittally in the midline. The cerebral cortex of each hemisphere can be divided into four major lobes, which are named in relation to the neighbouring bones:

1 The **frontal lobe** is the anterior part of the brain, sitting in the anterior cranial fossa. It contains regions associated with higher cognitive functions and some aspects of movement. The frontal lobe is separated from the parietal cortex by the central sulcus, which runs out from the great transverse fissure to the lateral cerebral fissure.
2 The **parietal lobe** lies posterior to the frontal lobe and sits in the middle cranial fossa. The anterior region of the parietal lobe is concerned with somatosensory inputs, whereas the posterior aspect contains the association cortex, which interprets sensory information and contributes to higher functions such as language and recognition.

3 The **temporal lobe** is located inferiorly to the parietal and frontal lobes, and separated from them by the **lateral fissure**. The temporal lobe contains the primary auditory complex, which processes sound information, and also the auditory association cortex, including **Wernicke's area** which is responsible for understanding speech. The inferomedial part of the temporal cortex contains the **hippocampus** and the **amygdala**.
4 The **occipital lobe** is the most posterior of the lobes, and is separated from the parietal lobe by the parieto-occipital sulcus. At the most posterior regions the occipital lobe contains the primary visual cortex which processes information from the eyes. This region is marked by the **calcarine sulcus**.

The structure of the cerebral cortex

The cerebral cortex covers the surface of the brain and is folded to increase the available area. The cortex is made up of several layers of unmyelinated neurons which are connected in complex manners, allowing the processing of neural inputs. In the cortex, regions are organised into different areas with different functions:

- **Primary sensory cortices** receive direct inputs from the various senses of the body and process this information so that it can be used by other regions of the brain.
- **Association and secondary sensory cortices** receive inputs from the primary cortex and are involved in processing information from the primary cortex. Regions of secondary and association cortex are involved in speech and language comprehension (Wernicke's area).
- The **prefrontal and association cortices** are involved in decision-making and higher cognitive functions. These cortices receive inputs from the sensory cortices as well as from other subcortical structures – particularly the limbic system.
- The **primary motor cortex** receives inputs from the sensory structures, allowing feedback on movement. It also receives inputs from secondary and association motor cortices and the prefrontal cortex to instruct the muscles. The primary motor cortex sends signals down a variety of spinal tracts by which it communicates with the muscles in the body.

The structure of the cortex varies based on its function, although two main types can be identified with very distinct structures:

1 **Neocortex** makes up about 95% of the cortex, and consists of a structure of six layers of heavily interlinked neurons.
2 **Archicortex** is evolutionarily older and consists of only three layers of neurons. Although it makes up a small proportion of the cortex, it has many important functions, e.g. the hippocampus.

Organisation of the cortex

The neocortex is arranged into six layers, which are arranged from the outside to the inside:

- **Layers 1** and **2** consist of scattered neurons and pyramidal cells.
- **Layer 3** is made up of many pyramidal cells and is the site of many cortical–cortical connections.
- **Layer 4** contains many different cell types. It receives connections from other regions of the cortex, and also from the thalamus.
- **Layer 5** contains many large pyramidal cells and forms many subcortical connections.
- **Layer 6** sends connections to the thalamus.

Gyri in the cerebrum

The gyri are raised areas in the cerebral hemispheres, many of which have significant functions. The gyri are separated by numerous grooves in the cortex, known as sulci:

- The **calcarine gyri** are located at either side of the calcarine sulcus on the occipital lobe and contain the primary visual cortex.
- The **superior temporal gyri** run parallel to the lateral fissure and contain the primary auditory cortex on their superior side.
- The **precentral gyrus** is found anterior to the central sulcus and contains the primary motor region controlling the contralateral half of the body.
- The **postcentral gyrus** contains the primary somatosensory cortex and is found posterior to the central sulcus, on the parietal lobe. The somatosensory cortex receives input from the contralateral half of the body.
- The **insula** is an area of cortex located deep in the lateral sulcus and cannot be seen without moving the lips of the sulcus. It is associated with the processing of taste.
- The **uncus** is the medial protrusion of the parahippocampal gyrus and makes up the cortical part of the amygdala. The uncus contains the primary olfactory cortex.

Internal structures of the cerebral hemispheres

Beneath the cortex are many white matter structures of the hemispheres. These myelinated tracts of fibres link different cortical regions and may link the two cerebral hemispheres. Three different types of fibres can be found in the white matter of the cerebral hemispheres:

- **Association fibres** connect different cortical sites in the *same* hemispheres, often connecting primary cortices to their related association areas.
- **Commissural fibres** form connections *between* the hemispheres. The most prominent of these structures is the **corpus callosum**.
- **Projection fibres** link parts of the cerebral cortex with subcortical regions. Most projection fibres are contained in the corona radiata of the internal capsule.

The corpus callosum

The corpus callosum is a huge network of myelinated fibres linking the two cerebral hemispheres. It can be seen at the base of the great transverse fissure and links the corresponding regions in each hemisphere. Although it links all the structures, the corpus callosum is shorter than the hemispheres, which leads to bowing of the fibres at both the anterior and posterior edges of the structure.

The internal capsule

Most of the fibres that link the cerebral cortex with subcortical structures are contained in a large sheet, the internal capsule. The capsule starts close to the cortex as a wide radial sheet – the corona radiata – and converges as it travels between the thalamus and the caudate nucleus, towards the brain stem. The internal capsule can be divided into regions that have different connections:

- The **anterior limb** of the internal capsule connects the prefrontal cortex to the mediodorsal nucleus of the thalamus and to the pontine.
- The **genu** of the internal capsule is a flexion between the anterior and posterior limbs.
- The **posteriorlimb** of the internal capsule contains the corticobulbar fibres, which connect the cortex to the medulla. It contains fibres of the corticospinal motor tract and the fibres linking the ventroposterior nucleus of the thalamus to the primary somatosensory cortex, and the ventrolateral nuclei with the motor regions of the frontal lobe.
- The **retrolenticular part** of the internal capsule is the most posterior region and contains fibres from the lateral and medial geniculate nuclei of the thalamus, which pass to the auditory and visual cortices, respectively.

The fornix

The fornix is the major outflow tract from the hippocampus. This bundle of fibres passes in a large loop to connect to the mamillary bodies of the hypothalamus. The outflow of the hippocampus starts at its posterior aspect and forms the posterior columns of the fornix, which fuse together in the midline to allow communication between the two hippocampi and follow a course anteriorly, over the thalamus, and immediately inferior to the corpus callosum. The fornix then divides into two anterior columns, each connecting to its respective hypothalamus.

Basal ganglia

The basal ganglia are a series of subcortical nuclei that are involved in the initiation of movement. The role of these structures is discussed later in relation to movement, although there anatomy is briefly outlined here. Two main regions can be identified:

1 The caudate nucleus
2 The lentiform nucleus, made up of the globus pallidus and the putamen.

The caudate nucleus

The caudate nucleus is a large region of grey matter close to the lateral ventricle, which lies lateral to the thalamus. The large round body of the caudate nucleus forms the lateral wall of the anterior horn of the lateral ventricle and is continuous inferiorly with the putamen of the lentiform nucleus. Posterior to the body of the caudate nucleus is a long slender tail that follows the lateral ventricle and terminates posteriorly in the amygdala.

The lentiform nucleus

The lentiform nucleus is made up of two sections: the putamen and globus pallidus.

The putamen is continuous inferiorly with the head of the caudate nucleus and consists of a wedge of grey matter located between the internal and external capsules. The globus pallidus is the lighter portion of the lentiform nucleus, due to its high proportion of white matter. It is separated from the medial aspect of the putamen by a thin sheet of white matter.

The diencephalon

The diencephalon contains structures concerned with regulation of body function, and serves as a relay for fibres projecting to and from the cortex. It is a paired forebrain structure continuous with the midbrain, and is almost entirely surrounded by the cerebral hemispheres. It consists of four structures:

- The **thalamus** – the largest part of the diencephalon

- The **hypothalamus** – crucial for regulation of the neuroendocrine system.
- The **epithalamus** – containing the melatonin-secreting pineal gland
- The **subthalamus** – part of the basal ganglia.

The thalamus

The thalamus (fig. 17.6) is a relay to process information being transmitted to the cortex and has a large number of reciprocal connections with the cortex; this allows it to moderate transmission of information to the cortex. The thalamus can regulate the rate and quantity of information reaching specific regions of the cortex.

Location and structure

The thalamus is roughly ovoid in shape and makes up part of the lateral wall of the third ventricle. The internal capsule lies lateral to it, with the caudate nucleus being located anterolaterally. The paired thalami are connected through the interthalamic adhesion, which joins them across the ventricle.

Organisation of the thalamus

The thalamus is made up of nuclei that receive a distinct tract of neurons and relay them to the cortex via the internal capsule. There are two types of nuclei found in the thalamus:

1 **Relay nuclei** are made up of specific groups of cells and closely associated with a particular cortical region.
2 **Diffuse nuclei** are located in the midline of the thalamus or the internal medullary lamina of the thalamus.

The nuclei project to many structures, both in the cortex and deep to it. The internal medullary lamina serves to split the thalamus into three regions that contain relay nuclei. The thalamic relay nuclei are arranged into four groups:

- The **anterior nucleus** is involved in memory and emotion, receiving inputs from the mamillary bodies of the hypothalamus and the hippocampus. It projects to the cingulate and frontal cortices.
- The **medial nuclei** are implicated in memory. The major nucleus in this group is the mediodorsal nucleus which receives inputs from the basal ganglia, amygdala and midbrain, and projects to the frontal cortex.
- The **ventral nuclei** are responsible for relaying sensory and motor information to the cortex. The major motor nuclei are the ventral anterior and ventral lateral nuclei. The ventral posterior lateral nucleus is particularly important in relaying somatosensation.

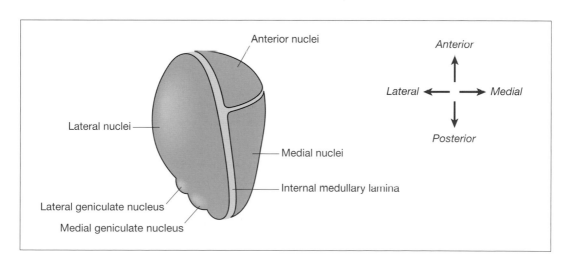

Figure 17.6 The thalamus (there, the right thalamus, viewed superiorly) is split by the internal medullary lamina, which splits the thalamus into anterior, lateral and medial nuclei. At the posterior region of the lateral nuclei are two regions, the lateral and medial geniculate nuclei. Furthermore, the thalamus is surrounded by a capsule of fibres on the lateral aspect – the reticular nucleus.

- The **posterior nuclei** are responsible for relaying auditory and visual signals and integrating them. In particular, the lateral and medial geniculate nuclei receive visual and auditory information, respectively, and relay them to their respective cortical areas.

The reticular nucleus

The outermost sheet of neurons in the thalamus forms a diffuse network that receives collateral fibres from other thalamic nuclei. The reticular nucleus receives inputs from the brain stem's reticular formation, enabling it to moderate cortical transmission according to arousal levels. Unlike the other neurons in the thalamus, the predominant neurotransmitter is the inhibitory neurotransmitter, GABA.

Regulation of the thalamic nuclei

Activity of a thalamic nucleus can be modulated by stimuli from different sources, which can also modulate output to the cortical regions. Inputs received in a thalamic nucleus are subject to several levels of processing:

- Local processing in the nucleus
- Modulation by inputs from the brain stem, particularly the adrenergic and serotoninergic systems
- Inhibitory feedback from the reticular nucleus
- Excitatory feedback from the neocortex.

The hypothalamus
Structure, location and function

The hypothalamus is located beneath the thalami and consists of a small mass of grey matter, on either side of the floor of the fourth ventricle. The hypothalamus is the major control of homoeostatic and autonomic systems in the body.

   The hypothalamus secretes hormones into the bloodstream. As a result, it is not protected from the vascular circulation by the blood–brain barrier.

Organisation of the hypothalamus

The hypothalamus is made up of many distinct clusters of cells each responsible for regulating discrete systems. The major nuclei and functions are defined below:

- The **anterior hypothalamus** is composed of the supraoptic, paraventricular and suprachiasmatic nuclei, and is involved in homoeostasis
  - the **suprachiasmatic nucleus** is the 'biological clock' responsible for regulating circadian rhythms and receives input directly from the retina
  - the **supraoptic nucleus** is responsible for producing antidiuretic hormone (ADH) which is involved in the regulation of fluid balance
  - the **paraventricular nucleus** produces oxytocin which is released from neurons that project to the posterior pituitary.
- The **periventricular cells** have a regulatory function through the release of peptides that act on the anterior pituitary.
- The **arcuate nucleus** is responsible for regulating prolactin release through the production of dopamine. It is also involved in the production of growth hormone-releasing hormone and gonadotrophin releasing hormone.
- The **mamillary bodies** are involved in memory, receiving input from the hippocampus, via the fornix, and projecting to the anterior thalamus.
- The **ventromedial nucleus** senses glucose levels and other signals that control appetite regulation.
- The **paraventricular nucleus** is made up of many different neural cell types, and appears to acts as the major site of integration of the different signals and stimuli processed by the hypothalamus.

Fibre tracts in the hypothalamus

Consistent with its role as a major regulator of homoeostasis, the hypothalamus receives and sends out large bundles to other regions of the brain. It also exerts an influence over the autonomic nervous system, as well as the emotional and higher centres of the nervous system:

- The **fornix** connects the hippocampus to the mamillary bodies of the hypothalamus.
- The **ventral amygdalofugal path** connects the hypothalamus and the amygdala, carrying inputs associated with emotion and stress.
- The **mamillothalamic tract** links the mamillary bodies with the anterior thalamus, and is a crucial part of the **Papez circuit**, involved in the laying down of memory.

- The **medial forebrain bundle** links the hypothalamus and thalamus, and is associated with the limbic system.
- The **hypothalamo-hypophyseal tract** contains the axons of the hypothalamic neurosecretory neurons, which release their hormones from the posterior pituitary gland.

Connections of the hypothalamus

The hypothalamus receives large numbers of fibres from other parts of the brain that do not form distinct tracts. These fibres make up reciprocal connections and are unmyelinated. The major inputs come from:

- Sensory systems:
  - the **retina** provides fibres to the suprachiasmatic nucleus, to regulate the biological clock
  - the **olfactory fibres** connect to the lateral hypothalamus and indirectly to the amygdala
  - **somatosensory fibres** provide an indirect input to the cutaneous system.
- Brain stem:
  - **pain fibres** from the periaqueductal grey send input to the hypothalamus
  - **sensory fibres** from the internal organs connect with the hypothalamus via the nucleus tractus solitarius
  - the **locus ceruleus** and **raphe nucleus** both provide inputs to regulate the function and activity of the hypothalamus.
- Higher centres: the **limbic system** provides many inputs to the hypothalamus

The pineal gland

The pineal gland is a small structure found in the posterior wall of the third ventricle. It is responsible for the production of melatonin, which regulates circadian rhythms. Melatonin secretion is promoted by darkness and inhibited by light. The pineal gland remains functional throughout life, though it becomes calcified with age.

The midbrain

The midbrain sits between the diencephalon and the hindbrain. It contains many white matter fibre tracts, as well as the most superior of the nuclei of the cranial nerves. The midbrain also contains the cerebral aqueduct.

The most prominent white matter structures are the colliculi, which act as a relay point for visual information from the optic nerve. On the posterior side, the cerebral peduncles link the cerebellum to the rest of the brain.

The midbrain contains grey matter nuclei that are responsible for many different functions:

- The **red nucleus** relays signals to the muscles in the rubrospinal tract.
- **Nuclei controlling the muscles of the oculomotor nerve** are present, as well as the Edinger–Westphal nucleus which controls the parasympathetic outflow to the eye.
- The **substantia nigra** makes up part of the basal ganglia pathways related to the initiation of movement.

The pons

The pons is located between the midbrain and the brain stem; the posterior surface of the pons makes up the wall of the fourth ventricle. The pons serves as a relay between the cerebrum and the cerebellum, and also contains many important regulatory nuclei, particularly:

- pontine nucleus of the trigeminal nerve
- the motor nucleus of the trigeminal nerve
- abducens nucleus
- facial nerve nucleus
- vestibulocochlear nerve nucleus.

The pons also contains the centres that regulate breathing:

- The **apneustic centre** in the lower pons inhibits inspiration.
- The **pneumotaxic centre** in the upper pons promotes inspiration.

Hindbrain

The hindbrain contains the cerebellum and the brain stem, which are involved in many 'unconscious' processes.

Cerebellum

The cerebellum is the largest part of the hindbrain and is connected to the brain stem by three sets of cerebellar peduncles. The cerebellum is entirely involved in the motor system, working to regulate and 'fine-tune' conscious and unconscious movement (Fig. 17.7).

Structure of the cerebellum

The cerebellum is made up of two hemispheres joined in the midline by a region known as the vermis. The organisation of the cerebellum follows

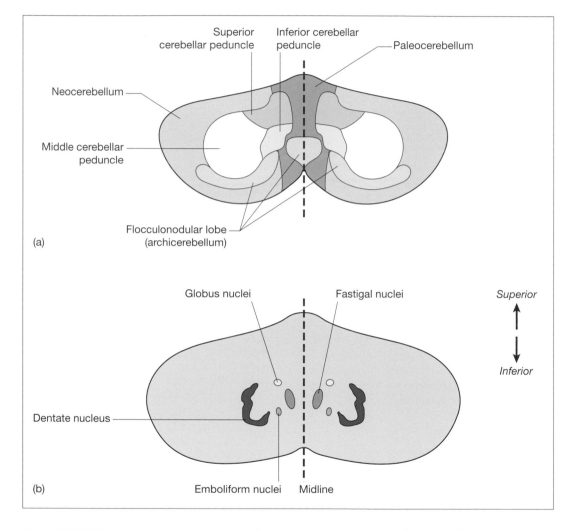

Figure 17.7 (a) The anterior aspect of the cerebellum (section taken at the level of the cerebellar peduncles). The cerebellum can be divided into functional regions. The flocculonodular lobe is evolutionarily the oldest part of the cerebellum, forming the archicerebellum. This is a highly folded structure so that much of the cortex is not apparent, but is folded into the anterior aspect of the cerebellum. The paleocerebellum occupies much of the midline cerebellar surface known as the vermis, whereas the more lateral portions make up the neocerebellum, the largest part of the cerebellum. Much of the anterior aspect of the cerebellum is taken up by the cerebellar peduncles, through which the nervous fibres to and from the cortex pass to the various structures in the rest of the central nervous system. (b) Deep within the cerebellum, the cerebellar nuclei can be found. These are the sites of synaptic connections and each group of nuclei is associated with a specific division of the cerebellum, the more lateral nuclei being associated with the more evolutionarily new regions of the cerebellum. The dentate nuclei are associated with the dentate nucleus, the globose and emboliform nuclei with the paleocerebellum and the fastigial nucleus with the archicerebellum.

a similar gross structure to the cerebral hemispheres. The surface of the cerebellum is very tightly folded grey matter, reflecting the huge number of cells found within it. The interior of the cerebellar hemispheres consists of white matter and grey matter nuclei.

The cerebellum can be divided into three lobes:

- The **anterior** and **posterior lobes** are separated by the primary fissure on the superior surface of the cerebellum.
- The **flocculonodular lobe** is made up of the vermis of the cerebellum, and the flocculus and nodule which are marked by the posterolateral fissure.

Cerebellar nuclei

There are four groups of grey matter nuclei on each side of the midline. These nuclei are made of many multipolar neurons which send outputs through the superior and inferior cerebellar peduncles. Lateral to medial, four nuclei groups can be identified:

1 The **dentate nucleus** is the largest and most lateral cerebellar nucleus and regulates voluntary movement. It is made up of a 'crumpled horseshoe-shaped' portion of grey matter, facing medially. Efferent fibres leave through the superior cerebellar peduncle.
2 The **emboliform nucleus** is a large ovoid nucleus located just medial to the dentate nucleus. Together with the globose nucleus, it receives fibres from the anterior lobe of the cerebellum and projects to the red nucleus.
3 The **globose nucleus** is made up of many cell groups.
4 The **fastigial nucleus** is the most medial nucleus close to the fourth ventricle. It projects to the vestibular nuclei and regulates the anti-gravity muscles involved in standing and locomotion.

The brain stem

The brain stem is made up of the medulla oblongata, pons and midbrain and is found in the posterior cranial fossa. The brain stem has three major functions:

- It carries the **ascending and descending tracts** that connect the spinal cord to the forebrain.
- It contains many **reflex centres** that control consciousness and autonomic function.
- It contains the **nuclei for cranial nerves III–XII.**

The medulla

The medulla is located between the pons and the spinal cord. It consists of white and grey matter, although in a different arrangement to the spinal cord due to the growth of the fourth ventricle in the brain stem.

The spinal cord

The spinal cord is part of the CNS that extends down the spinal canal to the level of L1–2 in adults. It is the major output of the brain below the neck, and provides the motor and sensory and sympathetic fibres to the entire body through the spinal nerves. The spinal cord contains both white and grey matter, with the grey matter located interiorly. The spinal cord is roughly cylindrical, although its diameter varies. In general its diameter increases as it ascends, reflecting the greater numbers of fibres present. There are two prominent enlargements associated with the large numbers of fibres that are received from or supply the limbs:

1 The **cervical enlargement** found at C3–T1 contributes to the brachial plexus.
2 The **lumbar enlargement** found at L1–S3 contributes to the lumbosacral plexus.

Coverings of the spinal cord

The spinal cord is covered by the meninges; it is much shorter than the spinal canal in an adult. As a result, the nerve fibres leave the cord at an angle and travel down to their site of exit. At the sacral region the fibres descend beyond the end of the cord, forming the **cauda equina**. The spinal cord terminates as the conus medullaris, and then the connective tissue extends downwards with the cauda equina as the filum terminale, which attaches to the dorsal part of the coccygeal vertebrae. The meninges cover the spinal nerves to the point at which the dorsal and ventral roots fuse.

Spinal nerves

Thirty-one pairs of roots arise along the spinal cord. These leave the spinal canal as dorsal and ventral nerve roots which leave through the intervertebral foramina and fuse to form the spinal nerve. The dorsal and ventral roots contain nerve fibres with different functions:

- **Dorsal nerve roots are made up of primary afferent fibres**. The sensory neurons are derived from the neural crest. There cell bodies are located outside the spinal cord, in dorsal root ganglia, which appear as small enlargements of the dorsal roots, close to the point where they fuse with the ventral root.
- **Ventral nerve roots contain the efferent nerve fibres** for the motor neurons and the preganglionic neurons of the autonomic nervous system at some segments. The cell bodies of the motor neurons are found in the grey matter of the spinal cord.

Internal structure of the spinal cord

The internal structure of the spinal cord is two symmetrical halves partially divided by the dorsal median sulcus and the ventral midline fissure. In the centre of the spinal cord is the spinal canal, which is a continuation of the ventricular system of the brain.

The central region of the spinal cord surrounding the spinal canal is made up of the grey matter and forms an H-shaped structure (Fig. 17.8):

- The **dorsal horns** of the spinal cord contain the synapses of the sensory fibres from the periphery.
- The **ventral horns** contain cell bodies of motor neurons.
- A small **lateral horn** is found in the thoracic segments. This contains cell bodies of preganglionic sympathetic neurons of the autonomic nervous system.

The white matter of the spinal cord surrounds the grey matter and contains the ascending and descending fibre tracts.

The dorsal horn

Afferent fibres entering the dorsal horn divide into ascending and descending tracts and rapidly terminate by synapsing in the grey matter. The location of termination depends on the type of fibre and this has led to the identification of distinct layers (Rexed's laminae) which receive different nervous inputs, and are grouped according to function:

- The **posteromarginal zone** (lamina I) is the dorsal-most tip of grey matter. It receives A

δ-sensory fibres and also interneurons from the substantia gelatinosa (laminae II and III). The efferents from the posteromarginal zone form the **anterolateral tracts**.
- The **substantia gelatinosa** (laminae II and III) and receives small Aδ- and unmyelinated C-fibres which are associated with transmission of pain signals. Efferent cells project to the **spinothalamic** and **spinoreticular** tracts. The substantia gelatinosa contains inputs from many descending tracts, which are thought to modulate the transmission of pain information.
- The **nucleus propria** (laminae IV and V) makes up of the major part of the dorsal horn and receives most of the fibres associated with somatosensation and proprioception. These fibres project to many of the ascending tracts in the white matter, as well as sending interneurons to other parts of the spinal cord.
- The **thoracic nucleus** is found between C8 and L3, and receives inputs from the fibres of many of the prioprioceptive organs. The efferent neurons ascend in the **posterior cerebellar tract**.

The ventral horn

The ventral horn of the grey matter is divided into three regions that innervate specific regions of the body:

1 The **medial group** of neurons is found in most segments of the spinal cord. Its efferent fibres innervate the muscles in the **axial skeleton**, including the intercostal muscles and the abdominal musculature.
2 The small **central group** is found in the cervical and lumbosacral regions. The central group provides innervation of the diaphragm at C3–5. Above this region, it is the origin of the spinal part of the accessory nerve.
3 The **lateral group** of neurons is found in the lumbosacral and cervical regions, and supplies the fibres innervating the limbs.

The lateral horn

The lateral horn is found in T1–L2, where it gives off preganglionic sympathetic fibres. The lateral horn is also present in the sacral region where it contributes preganglionic parasympathetic fibres.

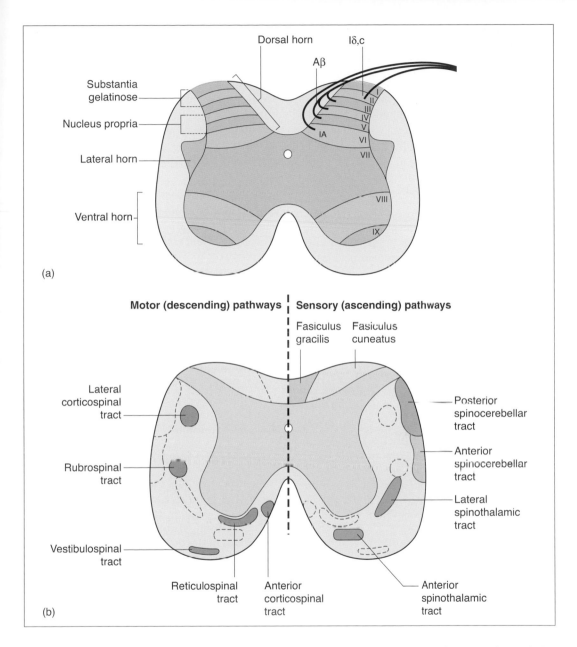

Figure 17.8 The **organisation of the spinal cord** is relatively well conserved. It consists of a series of tracts in the white matter of the spinal cord which surrounds the grey matter; this contains the cells that originate from, or project to, the periphery at that level. (a) Grey matter organisation: the grey matter of the spinal cord is made up of two main 'horns'. The dorsal horn receives sensory input from the spinal nerve at that level, whereas the ventral horn contains motor neurons. In the thoracic and lumbosacral regions there is also a small lateral horn that contains autonomic nerve fibres projecting at that level. The grey matter is grouped into a series of laminae (I–IX). In particular, within the dorsal horn, fibres of specific sizes enter the dorsal horn and form synapses within particular laminae. Although small A δ- and C-fibres are found in laminae I and II, larger fibres synapse in laminae III–VI. (b) The white matter of the spinal cord is organised into a series of tracts. Specific tracts project to particular regions of the brain and are associated with specific functions. Many tracts decussate at some point during their course, so that when they reach the brain they carry signals to or from the contralateral side of the brain. Evolutionarily older tracts, which do not project to higher areas, may not cross and run entirely ipsilaterally.

Organisation of the white matter of the spinal cord

The white matter of the spinal cord is arranged into a series of tracts that carry sensory and motor signals to and from the brain. Many of the tracts are associated with a specific type of signal and a specific region of the brain. The same organisation is seen at each level of the spinal cord.

The corticospinal tract

The corticospinal tract carries voluntary motor signals regulating skilled movements. The corticospinal tract neurons give off branches to inhibit other areas of cortex and the subcortical motor regions.

Fibres from the primary and secondary motor cortices and the parietal cortex converge at the posterior limb of the internal capsule. As the corticospinal tract passes through the midbrain, the fibres regulating lower body movement become located on the lateral part of the tract. The fibres form bundles as they pass through the pons and develop into the pyramids in the anterior surface of the medulla, where most of the fibres decussate:

- The **lateral corticospinal tract** is formed from those fibres that decussate and provides innervation to all spinal cord segments.
- The **anterior corticospinal tract** forms from the few fibres that do not decussate, and is present only in the cervical and upper thoracic regions.

The vestibulospinal tract

The vestibulospinal tract integrates signals that help maintain balance and posture through excitatory action on the extensor muscles and inhibitory action on the flexor muscles. The vestibulospinal tract arises from the lateral vestibular nucleus and projects down the length of the spinal column without decussating.

The reticulospinal tract

The reticulospinal tract is a descending tract that originates in the reticular formation. It modulates the function of motor neurons in the spinal column to regulate coarse voluntary movement and reflex activity.

The rubrospinal tract

The rubrospinal tract originates from the red nucleus and decussates to travel with the lateral corticospinal tract. The tract provides a major pathway for voluntary movement outside the corticospinal tract, often of the large muscles. It is important in regulating processes such as walking.

The dorsal columns

The dorsal columns contain the signals from large myelinated sensory fibres, which are concerned with proprioception and discriminative touch. These fibres are primary afferents originating in the periphery, and ascend in the dorsal columns to synapse in the medulla at the **nucleus gracilis** and **nucleus cuneatus**. Two divisions of the dorsal column can be identified:

1 The **fasiculus gracilis** is located medially and contains fibres from the lumbar and sacral parts of the body.
2 The **fasiculus cuneatus** is located laterally and contains fibres from the more thoracic and cervical roots.

The fibres of progressively higher spinal roots are added to the lateral aspect of the dorsal columns as they ascend towards the medulla.

The anterolateral columns

The sensory tracts are found ventral and lateral to the ventral horn and known collectively as the anterolateral column. The three structures found in the anterolateral column are named based on the regions of the brain, to which they project.

The spinothalamic tract

The spinothalamic tract carries pain and temperature stimuli, as well as non-discriminative touch and pressure signals. The tract contains neurons that originate in laminae I and V of the dorsal horn and decussate at the level of entry, ventral to the central canal, and ascend in the tract through the spinal cord, before running parallel to the **medial lemniscus**. The projections of the spinothalamic tract can be divided into two systems:

1 The **lateral tract** projects to central regions of the thalamus and reticular formation. It is thought to be involved in the processing of pain and temperature stimuli, as opposed to touch.

2 The **anterior tract** projects to the ventral posterolateral part of the thalamus and to nearby regions that are not directly associated with somatosensation.

The spinoreticular tract

Sensory neurons synapsing on laminae VII and VIII of the dorsal horn ascend in the spinoreticular tract. They project to the reticular formation and thalamus with sensory information that regulates the level of consciousness. Most fibres do not decussate.

The spinomesencephalic tract

The spinomesencephalic tract is involved in conveying the affective part of pain. It follows a similar course to the spinoreticular tract, although it is made up of fibres originating from laminae V and I, and terminates in the **periaqueductal grey** matter and mesencephalic reticular formation. It also projects to the amygdala.

The spinocerebellar tracts

The spinocerebellar tracts convey joint and proprioceptive information to the cerebellum, allowing feedback from movements. There are two major divisions:

1 The **posterolateral spinocerebellar tract** consists of neurons that originate in Clarke's column of the ipsilateral dorsal horn. These fibres receive afferents from muscle spindles, Golgi tendon fibres, and joint receptors of the trunk and lower limbs, providing information about movements and posture. They ascend up to the inferior cerebellar peduncle and enter the cerebellum, where they terminate.

2 The **anterior spinocerebellar tract** is made up of fibres that originate from Clarke's columns which, unlike the posterior spinocerebellar tract, decussate before ascending. These fibres ascend to the cerebellum via the superior cerebellar peduncle to provide information about the skin and fascia, in addition to the information provided by the joint receptors, muscle spindles and tendon organs.

Lissauer's tract

Lissauer's tract contains neurons that enter the tip of the dorsal horn, typically carrying information related to pain and temperature to **substantia gelatinosa**.

 CLINICAL Lesions of the spinal cord

Clinical syndromes caused by lesions of the spinal cord give characteristic patterns of sensory loss, reflecting the pathways and tracts that have been disrupted:

- **Brown–Séquard syndrome** is caused by a lesion of half the spinal cord. It is characterised by ipsilateral loss of touch perception and contralateral loss of pain and temperature sensation below the level of the lesion.
- **Syringomyelia** is caused by a cyst or cavity around the central canal, often in the cervical region, which compresses decussating secondary nociceptive afferents, causing a deficit in pain and temperature perception but leaving touch perception intact.
- **Anterior spinal artery syndrome** results from occlusion of the artery supplying the anterior two-thirds of the spinal cord. It is characterised by a deficit in pain and temperature perception, as a result of lesioning of the anterolateral tract, but touch perception is intact, because mechanoreceptor secondary afferents ascend in the dorsal columns.

The cranial nerves

There are 12 cranial nerves that have differing functions; other than the spinal nerve, these are the only means of nervous communication between the brain and the body. The cranial nerves are named sequentially in reference to the order in which they emerge from the brain. They provide all the sensory input from the special senses, much of the parasympathetic outflow, muscular control of the head and neck, and general sensory input from the head and neck.

The cranial nerves originate from nuclei that receive or provide signals associated with a specific function. The broad role and course of each cranial nerve are discussed below, although the mechanisms of the function related to them are discussed in more detail in the relevant motor or sensory section.

Cranial nerve I – the olfactory nerve

Function

The olfactory nerve is a special sensory nerve that conveys olfactory signals to the brain, allowing detection of substances and odours by olfactory receptors in the nose.

Course

The olfactory cells in the roof of the nasal cavity give off **central processes** that form around 20 bundles of fibres. These bundles make up the olfactory nerve. The fibres pierce the **cribriform plate** of the ethmoid bone and enter the olfactory bulb, where they synapse with mitral cells and form the olfactory tract; this divides into lateral and medial striae:

- The **lateral olfactory stria** terminates in the piriform cortex in the anterior part of the temporal lobe.
- The **medial olfactory stria** projects through the anterior commissure to the contralateral olfactory regions.

 CLINICAL Anosmia after skull fracture

In a severe head injury, the olfactory bulbs may be torn from the olfactory nerves, or the fibres may become torn if the cribriform plate is fractured. If all the fibres are torn, the sense of smell on that side may be lost; such damage is often associated with **CSF rhinorrhoea**, in which CSF leaks through the nose.

 CLINICAL Testing the sense of smell

Testing the sense of smell is relatively straightforward: the patient is blindfolded with one nostril occluded and then asked to identify a common odour. The test is then repeated for the other nostril.

Cranial nerve II: the optic nerve

Function

The optic nerve carries visual information from the retina to the brain.

Course

The optic nerve is formed from the axons of the retinal ganglion cells, which project from the eye and pass through the optic canal, to enter the middle cranial fossa. The medial portions of the nerves cross to form the optic chiasma, resulting in the formation of the optic tracts, which synapse in the **lateral geniculate bodies** of the thalamus.

 CLINICAL Optic neuritis

Optic neuritis defines lesions of the optic nerve that lead to a decrease in visual acuity, although with small changes to the peripheral fields of vision. There are many possible causes of optic neuritis, including inflammation, and degenerative and demyelinating conditions.

Cranial nerve III: the oculomotor nerve

Function

The oculomotor nerve innervates many of the muscles in the orbit that control eye movement. It controls the superior, medial and inferior rectus muscles of the eye and the inferior oblique muscle. It also controls the muscle of the upper eyelid – levator palpebrae superioris. The oculomotor nerve also transmits proprioceptive information from these muscles back to the brain. There is a parasympathetic component of CN III that controls dilatation of the pupil.

Nuclei

There are two nuclei of the oculomotor nerve:

1 The **somatic motor nucleus** which controls eye movements is found in the periaqueductal grey matter at the level of the **superior colliculus**.
2 The **parasympathetic nucleus** lies dorsal to the somatic motor nucleus 1. The **parasympathetic stimulus** from CN III is transmitted to the ciliary ganglion and then to the pupil, where it causes constriction of the pupil and ciliary muscles of the lens, which allows accommodation of the lens.

Course

The oculomotor nerve emerges in the midbrain and pierces the dura, running in the **cavernous sinus**. It leaves the cranial cavity through the superior orbital fissure and divides into two:

- The **superior division** innervates the superior rectus and levator palpebrae muscles.
- The **inferior division** innervates the inferior and medial rectus muscles and the inferior oblique, as well as carrying the parasympathetic fibres.

 CLINICAL Lesions of cranial nerve III

A lesion of CN III causes paralysis of almost all the muscles controlling eye movement. There is also paralysis of the sphincter pupillari, which control pupil size, and the ciliary muscle that regulates the lens. A complete lesion of CN III causes characteristic signs:

- Ptosis of the upper eyelid due to paralysis of the levator palpebrae superioris
- No pupillary reflex
- Dilatation of the pupil due to unopposed sympathetic stimulation
- Abduction of the eyeball slightly inferiorly, due to unopposed action of the muscles innervated by CN IV and CN VI
- The lens is unable to accommodate.

Lesions of CN III can be caused by the compression of the nerve as a result of an extradural haematoma pressing the nerve against the temporal bone, or an aneurysm of the posterior or superior cerebellar artery. The first signs are often a progressively dilating pupil and slowness in the pupillary response to light, as the parasympathetic fibres are the most superficial.

Cranial nerve IV: the trochlear nerve

Function

The trochlear nerve innervates the superior oblique muscle, which moves the eye inferomedially, and transmits proprioceptive information back to the brain.

Nucleus

The trochlear nucleus is located immediately inferior to the oculomotor nucleus in the periaqueductal grey matter, at the level of the inferior colliculus.

Course

The trochlear nerve is the only nerve to emerge from the dorsum of the midbrain and has the longest course of any cranial nerve. It travels around the brain stem and pierces the dura to travel along the lateral wall of the cavernous sinus, before entering the orbit through the superior orbital fissure.

 CLINICAL Lesions of cranial nerve IV

Trochlear nerve lesions cause paralysis of the superior oblique muscle, resulting in the eye being directed inferomedially. The CN IV may be torn in severe trauma due to its long intracranial course, although it is unusual for a lesion of CN IV to occur in isolation.

Cranial nerve V: the trigeminal nerve

Function

The trigeminal nerve is the main sensory nerve for the head, and also innervates the muscles of mastication.

Nuclei

The trigeminal nerve has two main nuclei:

- The **trigeminal sensory nucleus** receives branches from all three sensory divisions of CN V. The trigeminal sensory nucleus can be subdivided into three subnuclei:
  - **chief nucleus** which receives fibres conveying touch and pressure
  - **mesencephalic nucleus** which receives proprioceptive afferents from the muscles of mastication and the temporomandibular joint
  - **spinal nucleus** which receives fibres conveying pain and temperature.

- **Trigeminal motor nucleus** supplies the motor fibres that supply the muscles of mastication

Course

The trigeminal root emerges as a motor root, and a larger sensory root at the level of the pons. The roots pass to the trigeminal ganglion, where the **sensory route** splits into the three:

1 The ophthalmic
2 The maxillary
3 The mandibular.

The **motor branch of the trigeminal nerve** passes through the trigeminal ganglion to innervate the muscles of mastication.

Cranial nerve VI: the abducens nerve

Function

The abducens nerve innervates the lateral rectus muscle, responsible for abducting the eye.

Nuclei

The abducens nucleus is found in the floor of the fourth ventricle.

Course

CN VI exits the brain between the pons and the medulla, where it runs along the basilar artery before piercing the dura and travelling through the cavernous sinus. The abducens nerve enters the orbit through the superior orbital fissure.

Cranial nerve VII: the facial nerve

Function

The facial nerve includes sensory, motor and parasympathetic fibres:

- **Motor fibres** supply the muscles of facial expression, muscles in the throat and the stapedius muscle.
- **Sensory fibres** carry general sensation from the external ear, and taste information from the soft palate and anterior two-thirds of the tongue.
- **Parasympathetic fibres** innervate the submandibular and sublingual salivary glands, and the lacrimal glands.

Nuclei

Three modalities contribute to CN VII:

1 The **motor nucleus** of the facial nerve is found in the pons.
2 The **fibres carrying taste sensation** end in the rostral part of the nucleus of the tractus solitarius in the medulla.
3 The **general sensory information** from the external ear ends in the spinal nucleus of CN V.

Course

CN VII has two divisions – a larger motor root and a smaller intermediate root, which carries both sensory and parasympathetic fibres. CN VII emerges at the junction of the pons and the medulla, and travels through the posterior cranial fossa and the internal acoustic meatus, entering the facial canal in the temporal bone. The facial nerve exits the temporal bone through the stylomastoid foramen, and passes across the parotid gland.

The cell bodies of the sensory fibres of CN VII are located in the geniculate ganglion, which is situated on the medial aspect of the tympanic cavity. In the facial canal, CN VII gives off a number of branches:

- The nerve to the stapedius
- The greater petrosal nerve
- The chorda tympani nerve.

Around the parotid gland, CN VII forms a plexus of nerves which form six branches that innervate the corresponding areas of the face:

1 Posterior auricular
2 Temporal
3 Zygomatic
4 Buccal
5 Mandibular
6 Cervical.

 CLINICAL Facial nerve lesions

The facial nerve nucleus contributes to control of the upper facial muscles on both sides of the face, although it controls the lower facial muscles only on the same side of the face. As a result, an **upper motor neuron lesion** of the facial nerve results in only the lower part of the face on the opposite side being unaffected, whereas a **lower motor neuron lesion** results in motor weakness of the entire face on the same side as the lesion.

Cranial nerve VIII: the vestibulocochlear nerve

Function

The vestibulocochlear nerve carries special sensory information regarding both sound and balance from the organs in the ear.

Nuclei

Six nuclei are innervated by CN VIII:

- The **four vestibular nuclei** receive information concerning balance and movement from the vestibular system. They are located between the pons and medulla, on the lateral flood of the fourth ventricle.
- The **two cochlear nuclei** receive auditory signals from the cochlea.

Course

The nerve emerges from the junction between the pons and medulla and enters the internal acoustic meatus, where it separates into the vestibular and cochlear nerves:

- The **vestibular nerve** enters the maculae of the utricle and saccule, and the ampullae of the semicircular ducts, innervating the sensory cells there.
- The **cochlear nerve** transmits sound waves detected in the cochlea by synapsing with the **organ of Corti**. The cell bodies of the nerve fibres are found in the spiral ganglion.

Cranial nerve IX: the glossopharyngeal nerve

Function

The glossopharyngeal nerve innervates many structures in the head and the neck. It provides:

- **motor innervation** to stylopharyngeus
- **parasympathetic innervation** to the parotid gland
- **sensory innervation** to the posterior third of the tongue and the mucosa of the pharynx, eustachian tube and middle ear
- **taste information** from the posterior third of the tongue
- **information from chemoreceptors** in the carotid body and the **baroceptors** in the carotid sinus.

Nuclei

CN IX has three nuclei that are associated with different nerve fibres:

- The **nucleus ambiguus** is found in the superior part of the medulla and receives afferent visceral and taste fibres.
- The **inferior salivatory nucleus** is found in the inferior part of the pons and is the site of origin of the preganglionic parasympathetic neurons.
- The **nucleus tractus solitarius** is the site of termination of the visceral and taste fibres, and is found adjacent to the dorsal nucleus of the vagus.

Course

CN IX emerges from the medulla and leaves the skull through the jugular foramen. It follows stylopharyngeus before passing between the superior and middle constrictor muscles to the oropharynx and tongue.

Cranial nerve X: the vagus nerve

Function

The vagus nerve contains sensory motor and parasympathetic nerve branches:

- **Sensory input** is received from the pharynx, larynx, and organs of the thorax and abdomen.
- **Motor signals** are sent to the soft palate, pharynx, intrinsic laryngeal muscles (which control

speech and intonation) and the palatine muscle in the larynx.

- **Parasympathetic fibres** from the vagus nerve provide parasympathetic outflow to the abdominal and thoracic organs.

Course

The vagus nerve arises as a series of small rootlets on the side of the medulla. These unite and exit the cranial cavity with CN IX and CN XI through the **jugular foramen**. They travel down the carotid sheath before entering the chest to provide branches to the heart, bronchi and lung. The vagus nerves also provide branches to the oesophageal plexus and follow through the diaphragm into the abdomen. The anterior and posterior vagal trunks divide, innervating the gastrointestinal tract and supporting structures up to the left colic flexure.

Cranial nerve XI: the accessory nerve

Functions

The accessory nerve is a motor nerve that innervates the muscles of the soft palate and pharynx, as well as the sternocleidomastoid and trapezius muscles in the back.

Nuclei

The two roots of the accessory nerve are associated with different nuclei:

1 The **cranial root** originates in the medulla at the caudal end of the **nucleus ambiguus**, arising as a series of rootlets.
2 The **spinal root** arises from the spinal nucleus which is located in the anterior horn of the first five to six segments of the spinal cord.

Course

The cranial and spinal roots of CN XI unite to pass through the jugular foramen and then separate:

- The **cranial root** joins the vagus nerve and sends fibres to the striated muscles in the soft palate, pharynx, larynx and oesophagus.
- The **spinal root** descends down the internal carotid, innervating sternocleidomastoid. The remaining nerve fibres cross the posterior triangle of the neck, to innervate the superior part of trapezius.

Cranial nerve XII: the hypoglossal nerve

Function

The hypoglossal nerve is the motor nerve to all the muscles of the tongue except **palatoglossus**.

Course

The hypoglossal nerve arises as a series of rootlets in the medulla that exit the skull through the hypoglossal canal. In the neck, the nerve receives fibres from the cervical plexus and passes medial to the angle of the mandible before passing anteriorly to enter the tongue.

Synaptic transmission in the nervous system

There are junctions (synapses) between neurons across which action potentials must pass. Different cells at the same synapse may release neurotransmitters with different effects at the synapse to a single postsynaptic cell; this allows integration from the sum of excitatory and inhibitory electrical events, secondary to chemical transmission.

There are two main types of neurotransmitters that are used in the CNS:

1 **Classic amino acid or monoamine neurotransmitters** can cause both fast and slow neurotransmission, sometimes known as neuromodulation, depending on which receptors they act – ionotropic or metabotropic respectively. However, catecholamines are responsible only for slow neurotransmission.
2 **Peptide neurotransmitters** are responsible for slow neurotransmission (e.g. opioids).

Excitatory neurotransmission

Glutamate is the predominant excitatory neurotransmitter in the CNS. It is produced by glial cells from glutamine or glucose and taken up by nerve cells via a Na^+-dependent uptake mechanism. In addition to its role as the major excitatory transmitter, glutamate has some other significant effects:

- It is involved in the **laying down of memory**, through the function of its N-methyl-D-aspartate (NMDA) receptors.
- **Excitotoxicity** is associated with glutamate release due to ischaemia, which in turn activates NMDA receptors, resulting in cell death through excessive Ca^{2+} entry.

Membrane receptors

Glutamate receptors are mostly found in the cortex, basal ganglia and on neurons in the sensory pathway. Glutamate may bind to one of four different receptors, most of which take their names from pharmacological compounds that specifically activate them (Fig. 17.9):

1 AMPA (α-amino-3-hydroxy-5-methyl-4-isoxazolepropionic acid)
2 Kainate
3 NMDA
4 Metabotropic.

AMPA receptors

AMPA receptors are typically found postsynaptically and are responsible for the generation of fast excitatory action potentials; they can also be found on astrocytes. These channels have five subunits, and allow the flow of Na^+ channels and, to a limited extent, Ca^{2+} channels.

Kainate receptors

Kainate receptors are responsible for the generation of fast excitatory potentials; they have a much more limited distribution than AMPA or NMDA receptors and may be found post- or presynaptically. They are permeable to Na^+ and, to a lesser extent, to Ca^{2+}.

NMDA receptors

NMDA receptors are ion channels that are particularly permeable to Ca^{2+} and responsible for producing slow excitatory potentials. They are particularly associated with synaptic plasticity and laying down of memory. NMDA receptors are typically found co-localised with AMPA receptors. The opening of NMDA channels requires three simultaneous events:

1 **Binding of glutamate or aspartate** to the glutamate-binding site

2 **Binding of glycine** to a separate site; glycine is usually seen as an inhibitory neurotransmitter, although is found in the brain at relatively low concentrations that are sufficient to enable their binding to NMDA receptors
3 **Depolarisation of the cell membrane**: in the hyperpolarised membrane state the ion channel in the **NMD**A receptors is blocked by an Mg^{2+} ion, which must **be removed** to enable Ca^{2+} and other cations to flow through.

Metabotropic glutamate receptor

The metabotropic glutamate receptor is a G-protein-coupled receptor triggering an increase in Ca^{2+} through G_q. It also inhibits the action of **adenylyl cyclase**, and is thought to be involved in modulating the behaviour of a synapse:

- Postsynaptically through inhibition of K^+ channels
- Presynaptically through inhibition of Ca^{2+} channels.

Inhibitory transmission

The major inhibitor transmitter varies in the CNS:

- In the brain, **GABA** is the major inhibitory neurotransmitter, although it is found only in trace amounts outside the CNS.
- In the brain stem and spinal cord, **glycine** is the major inhibitory neurotransmitter.

GABA

GABA is the major inhibitory transmitter in the longer tracts running from the cerebellum and striatum. It is produced from glutamate by the enzyme glutamic acid decarboxylase (GAD), and can be converted back to glutamate through a transamination reaction. Major functions of GABA transmission include the following:

- **Regulation of muscle tone** through the inhibition of release of excitatory neurotransmitters
- **Movement control** as GABA is a major transmitter in the basal ganglia; in particular Huntington's disease is associated with loss of GABA-ergic neurons and leads to uncontrolled movements.

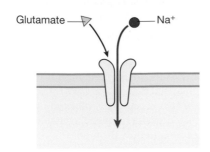

AMPA

The AMPA (α-amino-3-hydroxy-5-methyl-4-isoxazolepropionic acid) receptor is the most widely found of the glutamate receptors; upon binding it undergoes a conformation shift to allow the passage of Na^+ ions, through the pore into the cell.

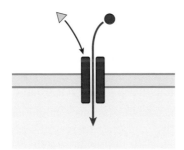

Kainate

Kainate receptors have a similar function to AMPA receptors, allowing the passage of Na^+ ions after their binding of glutamate; however, they have a much more limited distribution of sites where they are found.

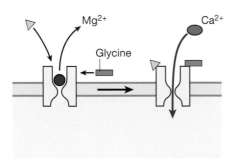

NMDA

The NMDA (N-methyl-D-aspartate) receptor is the third type of ion channel that responds to glutamate binding, although it is very different to AMPA and kainate receptors. The channels are selective for Ca^{2+} and require the binding not only of glutamate, but also of glycine in order to open. Furthermore, at resting cell membrane potential, the channel is blocked by Mg^{2+} ions, which prevent Ca^{2+} from entering the cell. To allow the flow of Ca^{2+}, the cell membrane must be depolarised at the same point as the NMDA channel is open, removing the Mg^{2+} ion to allow entry of Ca^{2+} into the cell.

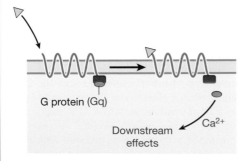

Metabotrophic

The metabotrophic glutamate receptor is a G-protein-coupled receptor, such that the binding of glutamate results in the activation of the Gq protein. This protein acts to increase intracellular calcium within the cell and activates a variety of downstream mechanisms.

Two major types of GABA receptor have been found:

1 **GABA$_A$-receptors** are ligand-gated ion channels with a pentameric structure. Binding of GABA to GABA$_A$-receptors causes the channel to open, allowing the influx of Cl$^-$ ions. This causes hyperpolarisation of the cell. Modulatory sites are also present. In particular, one binds benzodiazepines such as diazepam, to facilitate channel opening.

2 **GABA$_B$-receptors** are G-protein-coupled receptors that activate G$_i$ to decrease cAMP by inhibiting adenylyl cyclase. Presynaptically, this inhibition is mediated through decreased levels of Ca^{2+} in cells. Postsynaptically, inhibition is mediated through elevated intracellular K$^+$ levels.

Glycine

Glycine receptors resemble GABA$_A$-receptors and their activation causes hyperpolarisation. In addition to glycine, both taurine and β-alanine are agonists of the glycine receptor.

Monoamine transmission

Monoamine molecules are neurotransmitters for several key systems in the brain, especially those associated with behaviour and emotion. There are three particularly prominent monoamine neurotransmitters:

- Noradrenaline
- Dopamine
- Serotonin (5-HT).

Noradrenaline

The synthesis, release and reuptake of noradrenaline in the CNS are very similar to those in the periphery, as are the receptors. Noradrenergic neurons are located in discrete clusters, mainly in the pons and medulla – the locus ceruleus is a particularly important group of such neurons. They are also found in the median forebrain bundle and the descending spinal tracts. Noradrenaline has a predominantly inhibitory action through β-adrenoceptors, although it can also have an excitatory effect, acting through both α- and β-adrenoceptors.

Noradrenergic transmission is important in many processes, in particular:

- **Alertness**, through neurons in the locus ceruleus increasing the level of consciousness; this is reflected in the increased activity of these neurons to unfamiliar stimuli.
- **Blood pressure** regulation occurs through α$_2$-receptors in the regulatory centres in the medulla. The α$_2$-agonist **clonidine** may act at this site to lower blood pressure.
- **Control of mood** – a reduction in noradrenergic transmission is linked to depression.

Dopamine

Dopamine is a precursor to noradrenaline and is also a significant neurotransmitter. Five different types of dopamine receptor have been identified, all of which are coupled to G-proteins:

- D$_1$ and D$_5$ act through G$_s$ to increase levels of cAMP, causing an excitatory effect.
- D$_2$, D$_3$ and D$_4$ act through G$_i$ and decrease adenylyl cyclase activity, causing an inhibitory effect.

There are many different functions of dopamine. In particular it is involved in three important pathways:

- The **nigrostriatal system** is located in the basal ganglia and associated with the initiation of movement.
- The **mesolimbic/mesocortical pathway** in the limbic system is responsible for the regulation of reward response and emotion. As such many dopamine-based therapies are associated with mood effects.
- The **hypothalamus** releases dopamine to regulate pituitary hormones. It is the major inhibitory control of the release of prolactin and also stimulates (to a lesser extent) the release of growth hormone.

Dopamine neurons are a major target of drug therapies:

- The symptoms of **Parkinson's disease** can be treated by dopamine precursors (e.g. L-dopa) or

Figure 17.9 There are four different types of glutamate receptor found in the central nervous system. Three are ion channels, whereas the fourth is coupled to a G-protein. Each channel type has a different localisation and they have important roles in the propagation and regulation of synaptic transmission in the brain.

through receptor agonists (e.g. ropinerole, a D_2-receptor agonist).

- **Schizophrenia** is associated with excessive dopaminergic activity and may be treated by using D_2-receptor antagonists (e.g. haloperidol).

5-Hydroxytryptamine (serotonin)

5-HT is derived from tryptophan and synthesised in the CNS, because it does not pass the blood–brain barrier. 5-HT neurons are concentrated in the midline raphe nuclei of the pons and medulla. They project to many structures in the brain, in particular the cortex, limbic system, hypothalamus and spinal cord. 5-HT is degraded by monoamine oxidase and other enzymes (e.g. catechol-O-methyltransferase or COMT).

5-HT is associated with many different functions:

- Regulation of behavioural responses
- Control of mood and emotion
- Control of sleep and wakefulness
- Control of sensory pathways
- Vomiting
- Pain and analgesia.

5-HT receptor

5-HT can be found on the pre- and postsynaptic membranes of synapses, although the precise nature of the response is governed by the receptor type:

- 5-HT_1 receptors are G-protein-coupled receptors linked to G_i. Receptor activation has an **inhibitory effect**.
- 5-HT_2 receptors are G-protein-coupled receptors linked to G_q. Receptor activation has an **excitatory effect**.
- 5-HT_3 receptors are ligand-gated cation channels. Receptor activation has an **excitatory effect** on the generation of action potentials.

Many drugs act by modulating 5-HT:

- **5-HT uptake inhibitors** are used to treat depression (e.g. fluoxetine). These act by preventing the reuptake of 5-HT, increasing the effective concentration in the synapses.
- **5-HT_1-receptor agonists** are used to treat anxiety (e.g. buspirone).
- **5-HT_3-receptor antagonists** are used as antiemetics (e.g. odansetron).

Neurochemical disorders

Most psychiatric disorders are thought to have a neurochemical basis, although how a neurotransmitter imbalance leads to the symptoms of the disorder is often poorly understood.

Affective disorders: depression and bipolar affective disorder

Depression is characterised by feelings of sadness and apathy, low self-esteem, loss of motivation (including loss of libido and appetite), changes in sleep patterns and social withdrawal. In bipolar affective disorder, periods of depression alternate with periods of mania. Mania is characterised by euphoria, heightened mental activity and delusions of grandeur.

Causes of affective disorders

As affective disorders run in families, there is thought to be a genetic component. The success of drugs that increase the availability of monoamines, as well as some studies, suggest that a deficiency in monoamines might underlie affective disorders.

Treatments

Many pharmacological treatments of depression increase the availability of monoamines in the synapse:

- **Selective serotonin reuptake inhibitors** (SSRIs, e.g. fluoxetine) selectively inhibit serotonin reuptake.
- **Tricyclic antidepressants** (e.g. imipramine) inhibit reuptake of monoamines.
- **Monoamine oxidase inhibitors** (MAOIs, e.g. moclobemide) inhibit the breakdown of monoamines.
- **Lithium and sodium valproate** inhibit the formation of inositol trisphosphate as well as mimicking sodium ions. This modifies the membrane potential of neurons and ionic balance, although it is uncertain how this modulates mood.

Non-pharmacological treatments are also used in the treatment of depression. These include congnitive behavioural therapy psychotherapy and electroconvulsive shock therapy.

Schizophrenia

Schizophrenia is a psychotic disorder characterised by positive symptoms – hallucinations, paranoia and delusions; and negative symptoms – social withdrawal and emotional blunting.

Causes of schizophrenia

There is a very strong genetic component: individuals with both parents affected are 40 times more likely to develop schizophrenia. Reduced blood flow to the frontal cortex and dilatation of the ventricles in the brains of people with schizophrenia has led to the suggestion that schizophrenia is a neurodevelopmental disorder. The efficacy of dopamine receptor antagonists in treating the symptoms of schizophrenia suggests that schizophrenia may be due to excessive dopamine transmission in the mesolimbic reward system.

Treatment of schizophrenia

Dopamine receptor antagonists (e.g. chlorpromazine) are effective in the treatment of the schizophrenia. In particular, the efficacy of an antipsychotic drug best correlates with its affinity for the D_2 subtype of dopamine receptor. Dopamine receptor antagonists increase the release of prolactin, causing side effects of **galactorrhoea** and **gynaecomastia** in males. They can also cause a parkinsonian-like tremor.

Anxiety disorders

Anxiety is a normal psychological and physiological response to a threatening, or potentially threatening, situation.

Anxiety disorders are characterised by similar psychological and physiological reactions, but in disproportion to the stimulus, or in the absence of an overt stimulus. In generalised anxiety disorder, anxiety symptoms have a long duration and occur in response to a range of stimuli. In phobias, anxiety lasts only for the duration of the specific trigger stimulus. Panic attacks, periods in which the physiological symptoms of anxiety become very severe, can occur in either type of anxiety disorder. Physical symptoms, e.g. tremor, sweating, palpitations and chest tightness, result from increased sympathetic activity.

Causes of anxiety disorders

Anxiety disorders are thought to result from an imbalance in the GABA and serotonin neurotransmitter systems. It has also been suggested that an imbalance of several neuropeptides, e.g. corticotrophin-releasing hormone, substance P and cholecystokinin, contribute to anxiety disorders, because these neuropeptides cause anxiety symptoms when injected into the brains of animals.

Treatment of anxiety disorders

There are three common pharmacological treatments of anxiety disorders:

1 **Benzodiazepines** (e.g. diazepam) reduce neuron excitability, particularly in the raphe nucleus. They increase binding of the inhibitory neurotransmitter GABA to $GABA_A$-receptors. Benzodiazepines also have a sedative action, which is used therapeutically for insomnia, and an anticonvulsant action, which is used therapeutically for epilepsy. These other actions correspond to the unwanted side effects of sedation and motor ataxia when benzodiazepines are used to treat anxiety. More serious adverse long-term side effects include mild amnesia and dependence.
   – **Buspirone** reduces serotonin release by acting as a partial agonist at presynaptic 5-HT-inhibitory autoreceptors. The reduction in 5-HT release is thought to be responsible for buspirone's therapeutic effect.
   – β **Blockers** are given when the symptoms of the anxiety disorder are mainly physiological. Their actions are thought to be mainly peripheral because the effectiveness of β-antagonists is not linked to blood–brain barrier permeability.

There are also non-pharmacological treatments for anxiety disorders, e.g. cognitive–behavioural therapy (CBT).

 CLINICAL Cognitive–behavioural therapy

CBT aims to treat conditions by removing negative emotions associated with an event or state of mind, and reframing or re-evaluating an irrational belief. CBT is effective in treating conditions such as depression and obsessive–compulsive disorders. It may be used as a sole treatment or as an adjunct to drug therapy.

Recreational drugs, addiction and tolerance

Drugs that alter the user's state of mind are said to be **psychotropic**. Although most recreational drugs are illegal, some are licensed and used therapeutically.

Most recreational drugs are **addictive**: they give the user a compulsive urge to get hold of the drug and use it again. Addiction is caused by the following:

- **Positive reinforcement**: the drug induces pleasant feelings through its action on the dopamine **mesolimbic reward system**. Input of signals from the dopamine mesolimbic reward system to the ventral tegmental area (part of the limbic system) increases goal-oriented activity (i.e. actively seeking out the drug).
- **Negative reinforcement**: the patient experiences unpleasant psychological and physical symptoms (withdrawal) if he or she does not take the drug.

Environmental stresses and genetics contribute to the susceptibility of an individual to addiction.

Many recreational drugs induce *tolerance* so that increasing doses must be taken to have the same pharmacological effect. The drug induces homeostatic mechanisms that offset the drug's own effects.

Opioid analgesics: morphine and its derivatives

Morphine and its derivatives are used as recreational drugs because of their euphoria-inducing properties. Heroin (diamorphine) is the preferred form for recreational use because it is highly lipid soluble, crossing the blood–brain barrier very rapidly to give a fast 'hit'.

Some morphine derivatives are licensed for use as painkillers due to of their potent **analgesic properties**.

Mechanism of action

Morphine acts at opioid receptors, which are normally the target of the brain's endogenous analgesic neurotransmitters, e.g. the enkephalins and dynorphin. Activation of opioid receptors

triggers a G_i protein second-messenger cascade that decreases levels of cellular cAMP, causing K^+ channels to open and Ca^{2+} channels to shut. This hyperpolarises neurons and reduces neurotransmitter release, inhibiting some neural pathways but activating others (e.g. the dopamine mesolimbic pathway).

Euphoria is thought to be caused by morphine's action on μ opioid receptors in the frontal cortex. Analgesia is thought to be mediated by morphine's inhibition of ascending pain pathways, its activation of descending inhibitory pathways and its dulling of the affective component of pain, by its action on the limbic system.

Side-effects

Recreational abuse and therapeutic use of morphine and its derivatives can lead to respiratory depression: opioid analgesics decrease the sensitivity of chemoreceptors in the brain's respiratory centres to high arterial concentrations of carbon dioxide. Other side effects of the opioid analgesics include: pupillary constriction, nausea and vomiting.

Addiction and tolerance

Morphine and its derivatives are highly addictive:

- **Positive reinforcement** is due to morphine's ability to induce euphoria and its activation of the mesolimbic system.
- **Negative reinforcement** is due to unpleasant psychological and physiological withdrawal symptoms, including irritability, aggression, insomnia, fever, sweating and piloerection (goose bumps).

Tolerance rapidly develops to morphine, due to increases in the activity of **adenylyl cyclase**, offsetting the reduction in cAMP that it causes via the G_i protein second-messenger cascade.

CNS stimulants

CNS stimulants are used recreationally because they increase alertness and reduce fatigue. Amphetamines and cocaine, but not methylxanthines, also induce euphoria, by increasing activity in the dopamine mesolimbic pathway.

CNS stimulants also have some therapeutic applications. A licensed amphetamine derivative, methylphenidate, improves concentration in children with attention deficit hyperactivity disorder (ADHD). Cocaine derivatives are used as local anaesthetics because they block sodium channels, inhibiting conduction in primary afferent sensory neurons in the pain pathway.

Mechanism of action

CNS stimulants increase the availability or enhance the effects of catecholamines (noradrenaline, adrenaline and dopamine):

- **Amphetamines**, including MDMA (ecstasy), are substrates for the catecholamine reuptake transporters. By an exchange process, they increase catecholamine release from the presynaptic nerve terminal.
- **Cocaine** inhibits catecholamine reuptake.
- **Methylxanthines** (caffeine, found in tea and coffee, and theophylline, found in chocolate) prolong and enhance the actions of catecholamines by inhibiting the breakdown of the cAMP second-messenger cascade that is triggered by catecholamine receptor activation.

Side-effects

Side-effects are characteristic of overactivity in the sympathetic nervous system. These include a reduction in appetite, increased heart rate and blood pressure, and pupil dilatation.

Cocaine and amphetamine abuse can cause psychosis and hallucinations, stereotyped repetitive behaviour, pathological overheating (particularly with MDMA) and cardiac arrhthymias (irregular heart beat).

Addiction and tolerance

Cocaine and amphetamines are highly addictive:

- They trigger **positive reinforcement** through inducing **intense euphoria**.
- **Negative reinforcement** results from the side effects of drug withdrawal – depression and lethargy – which is thought to be due to catecholamine depletion.

Mild addiction to methylxanthines has been suggested in humans. Tolerance builds up to cocaine and amphetamines, causing the addict to binge on these drugs, with a risk of toxicity. Tolerance builds up to a lesser extent to methylxanthines.

Alcohol

Alcohol is used as a recreational drug because it increases self-confidence, decreases inhibitions and induces euphoria.

Mechanism of action

Alcohol inhibits neuron depolarisation, reducing activity in most of the neuronal pathways but increasing activity in a few (e.g. the dopamine mesolimbic system), by suppressing inhibitory interneurons. Alcohol hyperpolarises the membrane potential of neurons by:

- **increasing the affinity of GABA$_A$-receptors** for GABA
- **inhibiting voltage-gated Ca^{2+} channels**, reducing the release of excitatory neurotransmitters.
- **inhibiting NMDA receptors**, through which glutamate mediates an excitatory effect.

Side-effects

There are both short-term and long-term side effects due to overuse of alcohol:

- **Acute overuse** causes temporary deficits in cognition and motor coordination, and cutaneous vasodilatation, resulting in heat loss and risk of hypothermia.
- **Chronic overuse** causes permanent cognitive deficits and brain atrophy. It also causes dysfunction and cirrhosis of the liver. Chronic alcoholism can cause gastric ulcers (because of irritation of the gastric mucosa) and immunosuppression.

Addiction and tolerance

The addictive effects of alcohol are due to **positive reinforcement** by euphoria and **negative reinforcement** by the symptoms of alcohol withdrawal: sweating, tremor, anxiety and, in extreme cases, delirium tremens (confusion, hallucination and aggression).

Tolerance to alcohol builds up rapidly through two broad mechanisms:

- **Tissue tolerance** is mediated by a reduction in GABA$_A$-receptors and an increase in voltage-gated Ca^{2+} channels and NMDA receptors.
- Increased metabolism of alcohol in the liver results from increased expression of the enzymes

alcohol dehydrogenase and **acetaldehyde dehydrogenase**.

An inhibitor of acetaldehyde dehydrogenase, disulfiram, is sometimes given to individuals with alcohol problems. It causes unpleasant symptoms such as nausea, anxiety and palpitations, helping the patient to dissociate alcohol from pleasant feelings.

 CLINICAL Variations in alcohol metabolism

The kinetics of alcohol metabolism differs in different racial groups. This is associated with the expression of different alleles of acetaldehyde dehydrogenase. In the Asian population, there is a variant allele of the gene in which the resulting product metabolises alcohol less efficiently. This causes **alcohol intolerance** and affected individuals have mild, allergy-like syndromes on imbibing alcohol. These people rarely develop alcohol problems. Other variants of alcohol-metabolising genes have been identified that are associated with an increased risk of alcoholism.

Nicotine and tobacco

Nicotine induces either arousal or relaxation depending on the dose and mood of the smoker. Much of the pleasure of smoking derives from the satisfaction of an intense physical and psychological craving for nicotine.

Mechanism of action

Nicotine acts on nicotinic acetylcholine receptors in the CNS and PNS. Dose-dependent activation or desensitisation of these receptors in the cortex and hippocampus are responsible for mental arousal and relaxation, respectively. Nicotine's action at receptors on postsynaptic ganglion cells in the PNS is responsible for its side effects of increased heart rate and blood pressure.

Side-effects

- Nicotine and carbon monoxide increase the risk of cardiovascular disease and stroke.
- Smoking during pregnancy reduces birth weight.
- Tar in cigarettes increases the risk of lung, throat and bladder cancer, and of bronchitis.
- Smoking reduces appetite and food intake: smokers often put on weight when they try to give up the habit.

Addiction and tolerance

Nicotine is highly addictive:

- **Positive reinforcement** comes from activation of the dopamine mesolimbic system.
- **Negative reinforcement** results from mild withdrawal symptoms: irritability, impaired psychomotor performance, insomnia, increased aggression.

Some tolerance to the effects of nicotine develops in the CNS, although less than in the PNS. Although smokers actually express an increased number of nicotinic acetylcholine receptors, most are probably in the desensitised state.

Psychomimetics

Psychomimetic drugs distort sensory perception. These are a broad class and include potent hallucinogens (e.g. lysergic acid diethylamide or LSD) and mild hallucinogens (e.g. cannabis). Unlike most recreational drugs, psychomimetics appear to be only weakly addictive.

Cannabis

The active ingredient of cannabis is tetrahydrocannabinol (THC). Cannabis induces feelings of relaxation and well-being and increases the intensity of sensory stimuli.

Side-effects

In the short term, cannabis impairs memory, cognition and motor performance. It also increases heart rate, and causes dilatation of the blood vessels and bronchi. It has been suggested that, in the long term, it leads to schizophrenia as well as apathy and underachievement.

Cannabis also has analgesic properties and there have been some suggestions that it should be licensed for the therapeutic management of chronic pain syndromes and multiple sclerosis.

Mechanism of action

Cannabis inhibits depolarisation of neurons in the CNS. It acts on endogenous class I endocannabinoid receptors (CB1) in the hippocampus, cerebellum, substantia nigra, mesolimbic dopamine pathways and cortex. Activation of CB1 triggers a G_i protein second-messenger cascade to decrease levels of intracellular cAMP. This causes K^+ channels to open and Ca^{2+} channels to close, hyperpolarising neurons and reducing neurotransmitter release.

Cannabis withdrawal symptoms

Cannabis causes mild withdrawal symptoms in heavy users, including irritability, agitation, nausea, increased heart rate and sweating.

Principles of motor systems

The motor nervous system comprises neurons that initiate and control activity in the muscular system. Motor reflexes, coordinated gait and planned motor sequences are examples of movements that are regulated in different ways by the motor nervous system.

Regulation of motor function

In voluntary motor function, or motor responses to sensory input to the cortex, motor neurons at higher levels exert hierarchical control over those at lower levels. However, in reflex responses to a peripheral sensory input, lower motor neurons regulate movement independently.

The main components of the motor nervous system and the hierarchical relationship between them are briefly delineated below:

- The **supplementary motor area** and **premotor cortex** are involved in movement.
- The **primary motor cortex** receives input from the supplementary area and premotor cortex. The primary motor cortex is the main origin of motor neurons that descend the spinal cord in the descending motor tracts (often via subcortical nuclei), connecting the motor cortex with lower motor neurons and interneurons.
- The **basal ganglia** enhance or suppress activity in the motor cortex.
- The **cerebellum** compares activity in the motor cortex with sensory cues as to motor performance.

> **DEFINITION** **Upper and lower motor neurons**
>
> The motor neurons can be divided into two broad groups that relate to their origin and target, and affect the nature of lesions:
>
> 1 An **upper motor neuron** has a cell body in the brain and an axon that extends into the spinal cord, where it synapses. In upper motor neuron lesions, reflexes are increased below the level of the lesion. Spastic paralysis is also present.
> 2 A **lower motor neuron** has a cell body in the spinal cord or brain stem and an axon that extends outwards from the CNS to innervate an effector muscle. In lower motor neuron lesions, reflexes are reduced below the level of the lesion. There is also muscle wasting and weakness.

It sends output back to the motor cortex to correct discrepancies between motor intention and motor performance. When performing well-rehearsed motor skills, the cerebellum translates motor intention in the cortex into a series of motor commands, which it transmits directly to the descending motor tracts.

- **Interneurons** receive input from the descending motor tracts, in voluntary movement, and from peripheral sensory neurons, in a motor reflex. Interneurons are important in motor reflexes, in relaying input from the descending motor tracts to lower motor neurons and also in gait.
- **Lower motor neurons** arise from motor nuclei in the brain stem (cranial nerves) or ventral roots of the spinal cord (spinal nerves) and directly innervate muscles. They receive input from neurons in the descending motor tracts, interneurons and peripheral sensory neurons.

Functional units of the motor nervous system

Motor units

Lower motor neurons innervate muscle fibres. They are directly responsible for the initiation of any type of movement. The group of muscle fibres that a single lower motor neuron innervates is known as a **motor unit**. The number of muscle fibres that a lower motor neuron innervates varies from around six to several thousand. Smaller motor units enable more precise movements.

The force of contraction of a muscle depends on the following:

- The **frequency of action potentials** in the lower motor neuron. A single action potential causes a single contraction (**twitch**) in the muscle fibres that it innervates, whereas multiple action potentials arriving in rapid succession cause sustained contraction (**fused tetanus**).
- The **number of lower motor neurons recruited** (**spatial summation**). In general, the sequence in which motor neurons are recruited obeys the **size principle**:
  - Neurons with the **smallest diameter** are recruited first. They innervate type I muscle fibres which can generate low forces for long periods of time, because of the efficiency with which they perform aerobic respiration. This is a **slow twitch** motor unit.
  - Neurons with **intermediate diameter** are recruited next. They innervate type IIa muscle fibres which can generate large forces but become fatigued after about 5 min, because their metabolism is mainly (but not entirely) anaerobic. This is a **fatigue resistant** motor unit.
  - Neurons with the **largest diameter** are recruited last. They innervate type IIb muscle fibres which can generate very large forces but become fatigued after about 30 s, because their metabolism is entirely anaerobic. This is a **fast fatigue** motor unit.

Motor reflexes

In motor reflexes, lower motor neurons trigger muscle contraction or relaxation, in response to input from a peripheral sensory neuron. Unlike voluntary movement, initiation of electrical activity is independent of input from neurons in the descending motor tracts. Motor reflexes have the advantage over voluntary movements of speed, which can be a crucial factor in survival. There are two important types of motor reflex, which are regulated independently to maintain muscle tension:

- The **muscle spindle reflex** acts to rapidly oppose an increase in muscle length. It involves a

sensory afferent neuron that signals an increase in muscle length and a motor efferent that elicits muscle contraction. It is the only motor reflex in which no interneurons are involved.
- The **Golgi tendon organ reflex**, which opposes an increase in tension in the muscle.

The muscle spindle reflex and the Golgi tendon organ reflex often have opposing effects. This increases the tension in the muscle, so that the Golgi tendon organ reflex opposes contraction.

The muscle spindle reflex

Sensing of muscle stretch

Muscle stretch is detected by the muscle spindle, a 4–10 mm fluid-filled bag containing **nuclear bag fibres** and **nuclear chain fibres**. Nuclear bag fibres are of two types: B1 and B2 fibres. These two types of nuclear bag fibres, and nuclear chain fibres, vary according to the type of sensory neurons that innervate them (Fig. 17.10).

- **B1 fibres** are innervated at their centre by type Ia sensory neurons and signal the rate of change in the length of the fibre. The centre of the B1 fibre undergoes only a transient increase in length before contraction at its poles causes it to recoil to its initial length.
- **B2 fibres** are innervated not only by type Ia sensory neurons but also by type **II sensory neurons**. Type II sensory neurons are connected to the poles of the fibre. As the poles do not have the elastic properties of the centres of the fibre, sensory neurons that innervate B2 fibres signal the steady length of the fibre, as well as its rate of change.
- **Nuclear chain fibres** are innervated by type I and type II sensory neurons. Nuclear chain fibres signal the steady length of the fibre, as well as its rate of change.

Innervation and reflex

Afferent sensory neurons from the muscle spindles make an excitatory synapse in the ventral horns of the spinal cord with the α-motor neuron supplying the same muscle. Excitation of this motor neuron causes the muscle to contract.

The sensitivity of the muscle spindle fibres is optimised by the **servo-assist function**: γ-motor neurons innervate muscle spindle fibres, causing

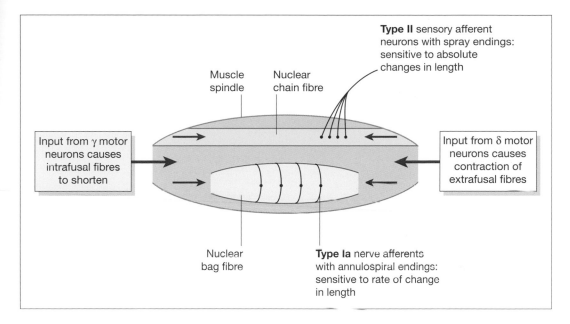

Muscle spindle

Nuclear chain fibre

Type II sensory afferent neurons with spray endings: sensitive to absolute changes in length

Input from γ motor neurons causes intrafusal fibres to shorten

Input from δ motor neurons causes contraction of extrafusal fibres

Nuclear bag fibre

Type Ia nerve afferents with annulospiral endings: sensitive to rate of change in length

Figure 17.10 Innervation of a muscle spindle.

them to shorten at the same time as α-motor neurons cause the muscle itself to shorten.

Excitation of afferent sensory neurons from muscle spindles not only triggers motor reflexes but also contributes to fine tuning of motor performance and proprioception (awareness of joint position), by sending branches to the cerebellum and motor cortex and to the somatosensory cortex, respectively.

> **CLINICAL Reflex testing**
>
> The myotactic stretch reflex is elicited clinically (e.g. by striking the patellar tendon which causes an increase in length in the muscle, quadriceps femoris) to test for intact function of the motor nervous system.

Golgi tendon organ reflex

Sensing of tension

Golgi tendon organs are arranged in series with the collagen fibres that connect a muscle to a tendon. When muscle tension increases, collagen fibres in the Golgi tendon organ are stretched. This distorts the terminals of type Ib sensory neurons, opening cation channels and depolarising the sensory afferent neuron.

Innervation and reflex

The Golgi tendon organ reflex involves a peripheral sensory neuron, a lower motor neuron and one inhibitory interneuron. It opposes the effects of the myotactic stretch reflex, to stimulate relaxation of the muscle. Type Ib afferent sensory neurons synapse on an inhibitory interneuron in the spinal cord which synapses with the α-motor neurons innervating the same muscle. Excitation of type Ib afferent sensory neurons dampens activity in α-motor neurons and inhibits muscle contraction.

Regulation of gait

The alternating flexion and extension of opposite limbs occurring in gait regulation is maintained (although not initiated) by clusters of interneurons acting as *central pattern generators* found in the spinal cord. These clusters of interneurons operate in *flexor and extensor half-centres* (Fig. 17.11):

- Release of glutamate from a descending motor neuron on to a flexor half-centre causes rapid depolarisation. This depolarisation is prolonged

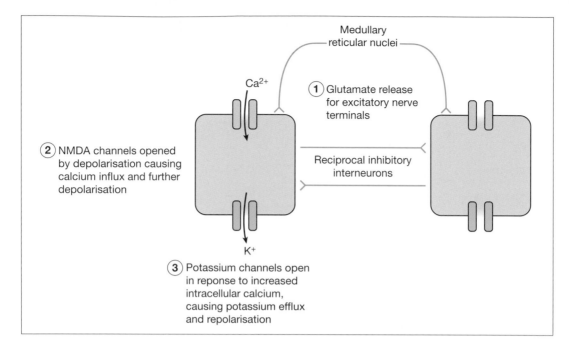

Figure 17.11 **Flexor and extensor half centres involved in locomotion**. The depolarisation of one half centre inhibits the depolarisation of the other half centre. This is followed by a hyperpolarisiation of one half centre, releasing its counterpart from inhibition and ensure that the half centres depolarise alternately.

by Ca^{2+} ion influx through NMDA channels. The firing of action potentials in the flexor half centre causes flexor muscles to contract.

- Ca^{2+} ions open Ca^{2+}-dependent potassium channels, so that the flexor half-centre eventually becomes hyperpolarised. This ends contraction of flexor muscles as well as removing excitatory input to inhibitory interneurons, which prevent depolarisation of the extensor half-centre.
- With this inhibition removed, the extensor half-centre depolarises and the cycle is repeated.

Descending motor tracts

Descending motor tracts convey signals from the motor cortex to motor neurons in the spinal cord. Descending motor tracts may be categorised, according to their relative position in the spinal cord (see Fig. 17.8):

- **Lateral spinal tracts** carry signals related to voluntary movements. The **corticospinal tract** operates when new movements are being learned whereas the **rubrospinal** tract executes learned, automated movements. Most fibres in the lateral spinal tracts cross the midline at the level of the

medulla and therefore innervate the contralateral musculature.
- **Ventromedial spinal tracts** include the vestibulospinal, reticulospinal and tectospinal tracts. The vestibular and reticular nuclei and tectum, from which these tracts originate, integrate vestibular, proprioceptive and visual cues, indicating a change in the centre of mass. These reflexes include the vestibulocolic and cerviocolic reflexes which keep the head upright and the vestibulospinal and cervicospinal reflexes which activate muscles in the limbs that oppose the force of gravity, so as to prevent, or brace against, a fall.

Motor cortex

The primary motor cortex is responsible for transmitting motor commands from the brain to the muscles. There is somatotopic mapping in the arrangement of neurons descending from M1. Neurons that transmit motor output to muscles in upper body regions originate inferiorly, whereas neurons that transmit motor output to lower body regions originate superiorly. The area of motor cortex that is involved in motor control of a particular body region is proportional to the density of that region's innervation by motor neurons. However, rather than a one-to-one relationship between activity in a particular cortical motor neuron and contraction of a specific muscle, electrical activity in an array of cortical motor neurons is thought to encode the force, velocity and direction of a movement.

M1 also receives sensory input from cortical sensory areas and the cortical branch of the muscle spindle stretch afferents. As sensory input corresponding to a particular part of the body is aligned with motor output to the same area in M1, motor function can be adjusted according to sensory stimuli that indicate joint position and posture.

Secondary motor cortex

The secondary motor cortex comprises the premotor cortex and the supplementary motor area. It is involved in planning complex movements and has both an indirect motor output via M1 and a direct output to the corticospinal tract. The supplementary area is particularly important in movement involving both sides of the body because it has a **bilateral somatotopic representation** (each hemisphere of the supplementary area exerts motor control over musculature on both sides of the body).

Cerebellum

The cerebellum regulates and refines movement. It can operate in two different ways:

1 In **feedback mode**, the cerebellum coordinates movement and corrects errors in motor function. The cerebellum computes a mismatch between motor intention, relayed from the motor cortex, and motor performance, relayed from peripheral sensory neurons, and sends out inhibitory output, which terminates the movement, accordingly.
2 In **feed-forward mode**, the cerebellum translates motor intention, relayed from the cortex, into a series of motor commands. A form of motor learning, long-term depression, enables the cerebellum to function in this way.

Functional subdivisions of the cerebellum

The precise arrangement of cerebellar cortical output to the deep cerebellar nuclei, and of cerebellar cortical input from parallel and climbing fibres, means that functional subdivisions of the cerebellum may be distinguished. The different regions of the cerebellar cortex send their output via deep nuclei. From medial to lateral, the names of these deep nuclei are: **fastigial**, **globose**, **emboliform** and **dentate**. The circuitry that connects the cerebellar cortical neurons and deep nuclei is repeated over the entire area of the cerebellar cortex. (Fig. 17.12)

Vestibulocerebellum

The vestibulocerebellum comprises the flocculonodular lobe, receives input from the vestibulocochlear nerve and sends output to the vestibular nuclei. It is involved in the maintenance of postural balance and in the vestibulo-ocular reflex. In the latter, the eyes move in an equal and opposite direction to the movement of the head.

Spinocerebellum

The spinocerebellum is divided into medial and intermediate areas. The medial area (consisting of the anterior lobe and the medial region of the posterior lobe) is important in maintaining posture. It receives input from the dorsal spinocerebellar tracts and sends output to the fastigial nuclei, which project to the medioventral descending motor tracts, involved in the control of axial musculature.

The intermediate area (consisting of the intermediate portion of the posterior lobe) is important in peripheral muscle control and fine motor movements. It receives input from the dorsal and ventral spinocerebellar tracts, as well as from the somatosensory and motor cortices via the corticopontine cerebellar tract, and sends output to the interpositus nuclei (subdivided into the globose and emboliform in humans). The interpositus nuclei send output, via the red nucleus and ventrolateral thalamus, to the lateral descending motor tracts, involved in the control of peripheral musculature.

Cerebrocerebellum

The cerebrocerebellum coordinates complex movements. It is made up of the lateral region of the posterior lobe and receives input, via the corticopontine cerebellar tract, from multiple areas of cortex. It sends output via the dentate nucleus and ventrobasal thalamus, to the motor and prefrontal cortices.

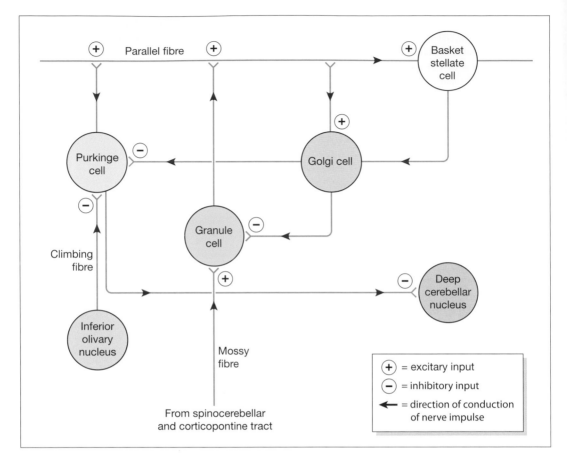

Figure 17.12 Circuitry of the cerebellum. The key process refining the movement programmes in the cerebellum is the longterm depression triggered in a purkinje cell by simultaneous signalling by a parallel fibre and a climbing fibre. This inhibits output by the purkinje fibress to the deep cerebellar nucleus, and is modulation and refinement of the movement programme.

 CLINICAL Lesions in the cerebellum

The effect of a lesion depends on its location:

- Lesions to the **vestibulocerebellum** cause a staggering gait and nystagmus (jerky eye movements) to the side of the lesion.
- Lesions to the **medial spinocerebellum** cause the individual to fall to the side of the lesion.
- Lesions to the **lateral spinocerebellum** result in **intention tremor** – large amplitude tremor in the limbs when reaching out for an object.
- Lesions to the **cerebrocerebellum** cause overshooting of movements involving single joints and gross impairments in multijointed movements, e.g. manipulations with the fingers.

Cerebellar circuitry

The cerebellum has a very large number of cortical neurons (about 11 million). These cortical neurons are of different types: Purkinje cells, granule cells, basket and stellate cells, and Golgi cells.

Purkinje cells

Purkinje neurons send inhibitory GABA-ergic output to the deep cerebellar and vestibular nuclei, which relay excitatory output from the cerebellum. Purkinje cells receive input from two types of fibres:

1 **Parallel fibres** originate from granule cells and make excitatory synapses with 2000–3000 longitudinally arranged Purkinje neurons.

However, each Purkinje neuron has only one synapse with each parallel fibre. Input from the parallel fibre elicits a **simple action** potential spike in the Purkinje neuron.

2 **Climbing fibres** wind around Purkinje neurons, making multiple excitatory synapses, in contrast with parallel fibres. Input from the climbing fibre elicits a **complex action potential** spike in the Purkinje neuron. Climbing fibres originate from the inferior olive in the midbrain.

Granule cells

The granule cells account for around half the cells in the CNS. These excitatory cells give off parallel fibres that form excitatory synapses with many Purkinje cells. The granules cells are themselves innervated by mossy fibres that reach the cerebellum in:

- **corticopontine cerebellar tracts** which project from the cortex, via the pontine nuclei
- **dorsal spinocerebellar tracts** which relay proprioceptive input (information about joint position) from spindle fibres and Golgi tendon organs
- **ventral spinocerebellar tracts** which relay sensory input from interneurons involved in gait.

Cerebellar inhibitory interneurons: basket, stellate and golgi cells

The three remaining classes of neuron in the cerebellum are inhibitory in nature:

- **Basket** and **stellate cells** are responsible for lateral inhibition between adjacent Purkinje cells. They receive input from parallel fibres and send inhibitory output to neighbouring Purkinje cells. As a single parallel fibre activates multiple Purkinje neurons, this focuses the cerebellar cortex output.
- **Golgi cells** terminate the generation of simple spikes in Purkinje cells after a period of time, so that Purkinje cells fire only for a brief duration. They receive input from parallel fibres and send inhibitory output back to granule cells.

Long-term depression

The cerebellum is responsible for improvement in the performance of a motor skill that comes from practice. Long-term depression (LTD) of parallel fibre activation of Purkinje cells is the mechanism underpinning this capacity of the cerebellum.

LTD is caused by simultaneous input from parallel fibres, which relay motor intention from the cortex and climbing fibres; this transmits error signals from the inferior olive. It reduces Purkinje cell inhibitory output to the deep cerebellar nuclei, enhancing excitatory output from these nuclei, which increases cerebellar regulation of the motor system and allows it to act in feed-forward mode, programming a sequence of movements.

The process of LTD correlates with improvements in motor function: when a new motor skill is first being learnt, a large number of errors are made and activity in climbing fibres is high. Eventually, when motor performance is perfected, activity in the climbing fibres falls to baseline. This implies that parallel fibre input to these Purkinje cells has been suppressed in the long term.

Molecular basis of LTD

The molecular processes underlying LTD occur as a series of continuous steps:

- **Simultaneous inputs from climbing and parallel fibres** of a single Purkinje cell result in depolarisation.
- Activation of **glutamate AMPA channels** and **G-protein-coupled receptors** (coupled with depolarisation of the cell membrane), in the Purkinje cell, triggers the opening of P-type voltage-gated calcium channels.
- Ca^{2+} **influx** induces the synthesis of protein kinase C, which phosphorylates AMPA receptors, desensitising them. This reduces subsequent depolarisation of Purkinje cells in response to glutamate release by parallel fibres (Fig. 17.13).

Repeated activation of this process leads to progressive increase in LTD and progressive refinement of the motor procedures.

Basal ganglia

The basal ganglia comprise various subcortical structures that form a closed loop with each other and with the motor cortex via the thalamus (the *basal ganglia–thalamocortical loop*). The basal ganglia facilitate intended movements and suppress unintended movements.

Components and circuitry of the basal ganglia

This section describes the components of the basal ganglia, their connections and influences over

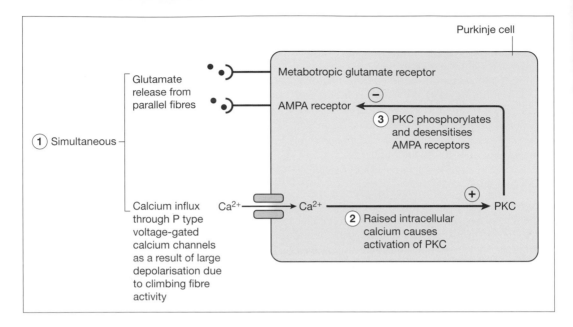

Figure 17.13 Molecular events in long-term depression in cerebellar motor learning.

each other. This facilitates understanding of the outcome of activity in basal ganglia–thalamocortical loops which is outlined in the next section (Fig. 17.14).

Caudate and putamen

The caudate and putamen make up a functionally coherent unit, the **dorsal striatum**. Medium spiny neurons in the dorsal striatum receive excitatory, glutamergic input from cortical neurons. All medium spiny neurons have a GABA-ergic, inhibitory output. However, two subgroups of medium spiny neurons may be distinguished according to their co-transmitters and their dopamine receptors:

- One type has **D_1-receptors**, through which dopamine exerts an excitatory effect (D_1-spiny neurons), and use substance P and dynorphin as co-transmitters.
- The other type has **D_2-receptors**, through which dopamine exerts a negative effect (D_2-spiny neurons), and use enkephalin as a co-transmitter.

Globus pallidus pars interna

The globus pallidus pars interna (GPi) receives inhibitory GABA-ergic input from D_1 neurons

and an excitatory, glutamergic input from the subthalamic nucleus (STN). The GPi sends an inhibitory GABA-ergic output to the cortex via the thalamus.

Globus pallidus pars externa

The globus pallidus pars externa (GPe) receives inhibitory, GABA-ergic input from D_2 neurons and sends an inhibitory GABA-ergic output to the STN.

Subthalamic nucleus

The STN receives inhibitory GABA-ergic input from the GPe and an excitatory input from the motor cortex. It also sends an excitatory, glutamergic output to the GPi and substantia nigra pars reticulata (SNpr).

Substantia nigra pars reticulata

The SNpr has a very similar role to the GPi, receiving inhibitory input from D_1-spiny neurons of the dorsal striatum, and excitatory input from the STN. It sends inhibitory output to the cortex, via the thalamus.

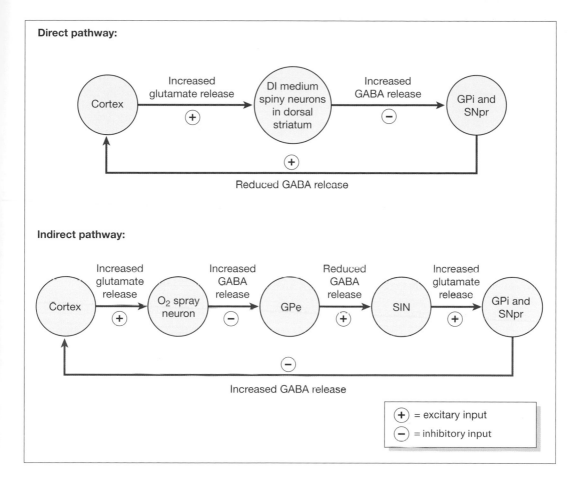

Figure 17.14 Direct and indirect pathways in the basal ganglia.

Substantia nigra pars compacta

The substantia nigra pars compacta (SNpc) receives a glutamergic input from the prefrontal cortex and limbic system.

SNpc sends a dopaminergic output to the dorsal striatum. This enhances cortical activation of D_1-medium spiny neurons but suppresses cortical activation of D_2-medium spiny neurons.

Basoganglia–thalamocortical loops

There are two main basoganglia–thalamocortical loops that are important in the control of movement.

The direct pathway enhances motor activity in the motor cortex

The cortex sends excitatory input to the D_1 neurons of the dorsal striatum. This enhances D_1 neuron GABA-ergic inhibitory output to the GPi and SNpr, which in turn reduces GABA-mediated inhibition of the cortex by GPi and SNpr. This increases activity in the motor cortex.

The indirect pathway suppresses motor activity

The cortex sends excitatory input to the D_2 neurons. This increases D_2 neuron GABA-ergic inhibitory input to the GPe, so decreasing GPe GABA-ergic inhibitory output to the STN, which in turn increases STN glutamergic excitatory output to the GPi and SNpr. This enhances inhibition of the cortex by GPi and SNpr.

CLINICAL Parkinson's disease

Parkinson's disease is an example of a **hypokinesia**. It is characterised by a triad of:

- **Bradykinesia:** difficulty in initiating movement; slow, shuffling gait with hunched posture and loss of arm swinging; difficulty in changing position; mask-like expression and slow, quiet speech.
- **Rigidity:** constant throughout range of movement – known as lead-pipe rigidity in contrast with clasp-knife rigidity caused by lesions of the pyramidal tract when the rigidity suddenly ceases.
- **Rest tremor:** usually in the hands (pill rolling) but sometimes also in the limbs, face, jaw or lips (not in the head and neck).

Cause

Parkinson's disease is caused by degradation of the dopaminergic neurons of the SNpc, indicated histologically by the inclusion of Lewy bodies (deposits of abnormally folded protein, α-synuclein, tagged with ubiquitin). This degradation is usually age related and idiopathic, but may result from anti-dopaminergic medication used to treat schizophrenia, head trauma resulting in injury to the midbrain or because of a genetic mutation in α-synuclein. Degradation of the dopaminergic neurons of the SNpc suppresses activity in the direct pathway, which allows movement, and enhances activity in the indirect pathway, which inhibits movement.

Treatment

A variety of treatments have been investigated for parkinsonism:

- **L-Dopa, a dopamine precursor,** is given to control the symptoms of Parkinson's disease. L-Dopa crosses the blood–brain barrier where it is taken up by the remaining dopaminergic neurons and converted to dopamine. Although L-dopa relieves symptoms in the short term, it typically causes motor fluctuations, e.g. abnormal writhing movements (tardive dsykinesia) and rigid muscle spasm (dystonias) after a period of 2–5 years.
- **Alternative pharmacological treatments** include dopamine agonists and monoamine oxidase inhibitors, which reduce dopamine catabolism.
- **Surgical treatments** have been introduced more recently, with limited success. Human fetal dopaminergic cells can be grafted. Lesioning of the globus pallidus, subthalamic nucleus or ventrolateral thalamus reduces tremor but not rigidity or bradykinesia.

 CLINICAL Huntington's disease

Huntington's disease is an example of a **hyperkinesia**. It is characterised by random twitch-like or writhing movements (choreoathetosis). Huntington's disease is a neurodegenerative, genetic disorder, caused by a mutation in a protein, Huntington. The function of this protein is unknown, but, in its mutated form, it is deposited in the nuclei of D_2-dorsal striatum medium spiny neurons, killing these cells. As a consequence, activity in the indirect pathway, which acts to block inappropriate movements, is reduced. At present treatment is symptomatic.

Eye movements

Eye movements are of two main types:

1. Gaze **stabilisation** (e.g. the **vestibulo-ocular reflex**): the eyes remain fixed on an object when the head is rotated.
2. Gaze **shifting** (e.g. **saccadic movements**): the gaze shifts to bring new objects on to the fovea, or to track a moving object.

Pathways involved in eye movement control

Movement of the eyes is controlled by three pairs of extraocular muscles:

1. The medial and lateral rectus
2. The superior and inferior rectus
3. The superior and inferior.

These extraocular muscles are innervated by motor neurons that emerge from the motor nuclei of the oculomotor (III), trochlea (IV) and abducens (VI) cranial nerves. Action potentials in the motor neurons encode both the speed at which the gaze is shifted and the static position of the eyes.

The motor nuclei receive input from neurons originating from the reticular and vestibular nuclei. Connection of the vestibular nuclei and the reticular nuclei on either side by the medial longitudinal fasiculus allows the two eyes to move in parallel (**conjugate gaze**).

The vestibular and reticular nuclei receive input from the cerebellum, the frontal eye fields (an area of cortex in front of the premotor cortex) and the superior colliculus.

Vestibulo-ocular reflex

The vestibulo-ocular reflex moves the eyes in the opposite direction when the head is rotated. Rotation of the head is detected by the semicircular canals of the inner ear, part of the vestibular system. This depolarises the vestibular nerve, causing it to send excitatory output to the vestibular nuclei. This action triggers eye movement in the opposite direction to that of head rotation. A connection of this reflex pathway with the cerebellum allows movement of the eyes to be exactly matched in magnitude (although in the opposite direction) to that of the head.

Optokinetic reflex

Movement of the eyes is triggered by the image 'slipping' on the retina. The magnitude of eye movement is equal and opposite to that of the head. The optokinetic reflex occurs in response to slower head rotations to those that trigger the vestibulo-ocular reflex. Slipping of the image on the retina is detected by large, movement-sensitive, retinal ganglion cells.

Saccades

Saccades are biphasic movements with a slow phase, which stabilises the retinal image, and a quick phase that resets it. By convention, the direction of the saccade is determined by the direction of the quick phase of the movement. Saccades may be reflex or voluntary:

- **Reflex saccades** are initiated by the superior colliculus. The **superior colliculus** has three layers: the superior layer receives a visual input; the deep layer receives an auditory and somatosensory input; and the intermediate layer sends a motor output to the reticular and vestibular nuclei. Somatotopic mapping in the three layers is in register, so that reflex saccades are oriented in the direction of sensory stimuli.
- **Voluntary saccades** are initiated by the frontal eye field area of the cortex. This area sends output to the reticular and vestibular nuclei, via the basal ganglia or the superior colliculus, and receives input from the posterior parietal cortex which integrates sensory information.

Smooth pursuit movements

Smooth pursuit movements are voluntary eye movements that allow tracking of an object moving across a limited area of the visual field. Smooth pursuit is initiated by detection of retinal slip in the primary visual cortex, as in the optokinetic reflex.

Vergence

Vergence allows for refocusing as an object moves closer or further away. Unlike in other eye movements, in vergence the two eyes move in *opposite* directions. Vergence is triggered by the perception of retinal blurring in the primary visual cortex due to a high degree of **retinal disparity** (the object is focused on very different parts of the retinas of the two eyes).

Sensory pathways

Sensory pathways are composed of a series of neurons that extend from the periphery to the cortex. Sensory pathways allow awareness and exploration of the external environment.

Sensory receptor transduction

Sensory receptors convert (**transduce**) a chemical, mechanical or thermal stimulus into an action potential. A sensory receptor may be the modified ending of the primary afferent neuron (somatosensory systems) or a specialised cell (all other systems). All sensory receptors can be described in terms of four properties:

- **Specificity** as to the type of stimulus that they will transduce into an electrical signal. Transduction occurs either by directly causing ion channels to open (e.g. somatosensation) or by triggering a G-protein-coupled, second-messenger cascade (e.g. vision), leading to a change in electrical potential across the receptor membrane. **Nociceptors** are an exception, responding to several different forms of stimuli.
- The **receptive field** refers to the restricted area where the receptor is responsive to its stimulus.
- The **threshold level** is the level that a stimulus must exceed to trigger transduction into a nervous signal. This determines the sensitivity of the sensory receptor.
- **Encoding of sensory information** by either spatial or temporal coding.

Encoding of different properties of a sensory stimulus

Afferent neurons synapse to specific cells in the primary sensory cortex in a precise manner. This gives rise to a 'map' of the stimulus, which encodes gradations in anatomical site or other attributes of the stimulus, e.g. the frequency of a sound. Different receptors are specialised to detect different aspects of a stimulus:

- **Rapidly adapting receptors** respond to changes in the intensity of stimulus input, but not to a continually applied stimulus. The frequency at which action potentials occur in the primary afferent neuron of a rapidly adapting receptor is therefore proportional to the intensity of the change in stimulus
- **Slowly adapting receptors** are responsive throughout the duration of a constantly applied stimulus. The rate of conduction of electrical impulses in a primary afferent neuron, which is associated with a slowly adapting receptor, is proportional to the intensity of the stimulus itself (**temporary summation**) and through recruitment of a greater number of sensory receptors (**spatial summation**).

Conduction from the periphery to the cerebral cortex

The signal generated by a sensory receptor is transmitted along a series of peripheral and central neurons, via the thalamus, to a specialised region of cerebral cortex (except in the olfactory pathway, which is not directed via the thalamus).

In general, central neurons have larger receptive fields because of the convergence of inputs from multiple peripheral neurons. Their **receptive fields** are also often more complex because they receive both stimulatory and inhibitory inputs, allowing **lateral inhibition**.

 DEFINITION Lateral inhibition

A stimulus applied to the centre of the receptive field of a central neuron is excitatory to the central neuron, but the same stimulus applied to the periphery (surround) is inhibitory. This is because peripheral neurons that correspond anatomically to the surround of the receptive field of a central neuron are inhibited by the stimulus, whereas peripheral neurons that correspond anatomically to the centre area of the receptive field are excited. Lateral inhibition permits more precise localisation (**spatial resolution**) of the stimulus

Areas of cerebral cortex receiving input from sensory neurons, **primary sensory cortex**, send out neuronal projections to **secondary sensory cortex**, which performs further sensory processing. Neurons from secondary sensory cortex project to **association cortex**, which integrates information about different sensory systems. In turn, association cortex sends out neural projects to the motor or limbic systems, which are responsible for the initiation of a response to a sensory stimulus.

Touch

Touch perception is the detection of contact with non-noxious stimuli. This permits grasping and tactile recognition of objects. It also facilitates limb-placing reactions that maintain posture (placing of the feet on a stable surface).

Stimulus

The stimulus input is deformation of the skin as an object exerts pressure on it.

Receptors

Touch receptors are the specialised endings of rapidly conducting, large-diameter, myelinated (Aα and Aβ), primary afferent neurons. Distinguishing two closely applied mechanical stimuli when they are applied to areas of skin requires touch receptors between the two points to be unstimulated – otherwise, it is impossible to distinguish two discrete stimuli from a single stimulus over a wide area. A high density of receptors in the fingertips and lips increases the accuracy of stimulus location and thus increases **acuity**.

Touch receptors vary according to their morphology, distribution, size of their receptive field and their adaptation properties:

- **Meissner's corpuscles** are located in superficial layers of skin and have small receptive fields. They are rapidly adapting, sensitive only to changes in skin displacement. Therefore, the rate of electrical conduction in the primary afferent neuron encodes the velocity of skin displacement.
- **Pacinian corpuscles** are located in deep layers of skin and have large receptive fields and adapt extremely rapidly. The force applied to a pacinian corpuscle is rapidly dissipated by surrounding concentric layers of connective tissue that

slide over each other. As a result, the rate of electrical conduction in the secondary afferent neuron encodes the acceleration of skin displacement

- **Ruffini endings** are also located in the deep layers of the skin, with large receptive fields. They adapt slowly and are sensitive throughout the duration of an applied stimulus. This means that the rate of electrical conduction in the primary afferent neuron is proportional to the extent of indentation of overlying skin.
- **Merkel's discs** are superficially situated, at the boundary of the epidermis and dermis. They have small receptive fields with well-defined boundaries and adapt slowly, allowing detection of changes in pressure and low vibrations.

Pathway

The touch perception pathway consists of a relay of three neurons, from periphery to cortex:

1 **Primary afferent axons** enter the spinal cord via the dorsal root, synapsing with interneurons and sending off branches that ascend in the dorsal columns of the spinal cord.
2 **Secondary afferent** axons project from the dorsal column nuclei to the ventroposterior nucleus (VPN) of the thalamus, **decussating** in the **medial lemniscus**. They are joined by fibres from the trigeminal sensory nerve, which detects touch sensation in the face.
3 **Tertiary afferent** neurons project from the VPN of the thalamus to the primary somatosensory cortex (S1).

S1 has somatotopic mapping in the form of an inverted homunculus. Lower body regions are represented superiorly and upper body regions inferiorly. The area of cortex corresponding to a particular body region is proportional to its density of receptors. S1 sends neuronal projections to secondary somatosensory cortex (S2), which is important in tactile recognition of objects.

 CLINICAL Lesions of somatosensory cortex

Lesions of the primary somatosensory cortex cause a loss of touch sensation down the contralateral side of the body, because of the decussation of secondary afferent neurons.

Pain

Pain is an unpleasant emotional experience relating to actual/potential tissue damage. A specific type of chronic pain, **neuropathic pain**, is caused by nerve damage. Pain has an objective, sensory component (**nociception**) and a subjective, affective component. The former is much easier to test experimentally and therefore more is known about it.

 DEFINITION Nociception and pain

Nociception and pain are closely related terms that describe aspects of damage to the body:

- **Nociception** is the physiological processing and sensation of a noxious stimulus
- **Pain** is the sensory and emotive feelings associated with potential or actual tissue damage.

Stimulus

There are various stimulus inputs for pain perception: high pressures, high temperatures (above approximately 42°C) and noxious chemicals. Mediators of inflammation, such as histamine, bradykinin and prostaglandins, are chemical mediators of nociception that can modulate the effects of the other stimuli, causing hyperalgesia.

Receptors

Pain receptors (**nociceptors**) are present in the skin, endothelium, viscera, skeletal and cardiac muscle, and all tissues except neural tissues. Different nociceptor types respond to different pain input stimuli:

- The termini of relatively rapidly conducting (10–45 m/s), large-diameter, myelinated Aδ-fibres respond to intense pressures. They have small receptive fields and high thresholds. Activation of these receptors gives rise to the sensation of sharp, well-localised pain.
- The termini of smaller, unmyelinated, slow-conducting (<2 m/s) C-fibres detect pressure, temperatures >42°C and noxious chemicals. They have large receptive fields. Activation of these nociceptors gives rise to the sensation of poorly localised, burning pain.

CLINICAL **Referred pain**

Pain signals from the viscera are transmitted via myelinated and unmyelinated autonomic nerve fibres that project to the dorsal horns of the spinal cord at the level corresponding to their origin in embryological development. As a result of the convergence of visceral and cutaneous nociceptor afferents on the dorsal horn cells, pain from the viscera may be referred to the skin.

Many painful stimuli are sensed by the capsaicin receptor, which is the best-understood nociceptor. This cation channel triggers depolarisation of the cell membrane when it is activated, in response to many different stimuli:

- **Mechanical deformation**
- **Heat** ($>42°C$)
- **Acidic conditions**
- **Capsaicin**, the active ingredient in chilli peppers.

There are many other channels that respond to painful stimuli (and have been implicated in nociception), and there are also receptors to other stimuli (such as inflammatory mediators) that can modulate a fibre's response to painful stimuli.

Gate mechanism

Pain perception may be reduced by the dorsal horn **gate mechanism**. Concurrent activity in large-diameter Aα and Aβ primary afferents of the touch pathway reduces transmission of electrical signals in secondary afferent neurons in the nociceptive pathway. This is because these large-diameter primary afferents activate interneurons in the substantia gelatinosa, which inhibit secondary afferents in the pain pathway.

Nociception transmission pathways

Primary afferent axons project to Rexed's laminae I and II (see Fig. 17.8a). There, they synapse with secondary afferent neurons that decussate several segments above their level of origin, passing ventral to the spinal cord before ascending the spinal cord in the spinothalamic, spinoreticulothalamic and spinomesencephalic tracts:

- The **spinothalamic tract** is involved in precise pain localisation. It projects to the ventroposterolateral thalamus. From here, tertiary neurons extend to multiple regions of the cortex, including the primary and secondary somatosensory cortex.

- The **spinoreticulothalamic tract** is involved in the affective components of pain. It projects via the reticular system of the medulla and pons to the intralaminar thalamic nuclei, and from there to the anterior cingulate cortex of the limbic system.

- The **spinomesencephalic tract** projects to the periaqueductal grey area (PAG). Activation of the spinomesencephalic tract reduces pain perception because the PAG activates inhibitory descending neurons that originate from the raphe nucleus and locus ceruleus. These descending neurons synapse on ascending secondary afferent neurons and decrease their transmission by releasing the inhibitory neurotransmitters, serotonin, noradrenaline and enkephalin.

 CLINICAL **Primary and secondary hyperalgesia**

Hyperalgesia is enhanced perception of a pain stimulus:

- **Primary hyperalgesia** occurs when inflammatory mediators increase the sensitivity of nociceptors to other noxious stimuli.
- **Secondary hyperalgesia** occurs in chronic pain syndromes (sustained and severe pain). It is due to enhanced synaptic transmission between primary and secondary afferent neurons in the pain pathway, as a result of long-term potentiation (see 'Higher cognitive functions' below).

Endorphins and enkephalins

In times of stress or activity, the body can stimulates the periaqeductal grey. This region of the brain has fibres that release enkephalin which binds to the presynaptic membrane of nociceptive fibres. The action of the enkephalin inhibits transmission in the postsynaptic pain fibre, and limits the body's response to pain, as in **emergency analgesia**; the presence of opioid receptors on the pain fibres accounts for the potent action of opiates as analgesics. The release of endorphins that

 CLINICAL **Emergency analgesia**

Descending inhibitory nociceptive pathways are activated by higher cortical centres. Emergency analgesia is thought to account for the ability of soldiers to ignore their wounds in battle.

occurs during exercise also acts on the pleasure centres in the brain and is responsible for the 'high' experienced during exercise.

Neuropathic pain

Neuropathic pain is caused by damage to a nerve rather than to tissues. Peripheral nerves are commonly damaged as they cross bony protuberances. Traumatic damage to nerves can result from:

- complete or partial section of the nerve
- neuroma formation
- involvement of the sympathetic nervous system, as occurs in regional pain syndrome.

The following are common sites at which neuropathic pain occurs:

- **Median nerve** passing under the carpal tunnel
- **Ulnar nerve** as it passes behind the olecranon process of the ulna
- **Common peroneal** nerve as it winds around the head of the fibula
- **Compression of nerve roots** emerging from the spinal cord by bony spurs on the vertebrae or by prolapsed intervertebral discs.

 CLINICAL **Phantom pain**

Phantom pain is a form of neuropathic pain perceived in a region of the body that no longer has sensory innervation. This is due to the loss of afferent input, or enhanced input from the remaining afferents, to the spinal cord and sensory cortex, as a result of limb or organ amputation or traumatic avulsion of the dorsal roots from the spinal cord. It can be explained by the fact that cortical neurons receiving pain signals from other parts of the body are rewired to the region that has lost its afferent input.

 CLINICAL **Complex regional pain syndrome**

This chronic condition is characterised by severe pain and swelling and changes to the skin. The syndrome is often associated with nerve damage. The mechanisms causing the syndrome are not clear but there is thought to be a contribution from 'physiological wind-up'. This system involves sensitisation of the NMDA receptors on CNS neurons in response to stimuli, including trauma, activation of the sympathetic nervous system and inflammation.

Pain management

Pain perception (Fig. 17.15) can be reduced by interference at multiple levels of the nociceptive conduction pathway:

- **Pharmacological suppressors** of local inflammatory mediators reduce activation of C-fibres and prevent primary hyperalgesia. These include antihistamines, which block the binding of histamine to its receptors on C-fibres, and cyclooxygenase inhibitors, which inhibit the synthesis of prostaglandins.
- **Local anaesthetics** (e.g. lidocaine) inhibit conduction in primary afferents by blocking voltage-gated sodium channels.
- **Opioid analgesics** (e.g. morphine) reduce synaptic transmission from primary to secondary afferents of the pain pathway in the dorsal horn, by hyperpolarising the neuronal membrane and reducing neurotransmitter release. The analgesic effect of opioids may also be mediated by an action on the frontal cortex, which modulates the affective component of pain.
- **Stimulation of the PAG** produces analgesia by activating descending inhibitory pathways.
- **Selective stimulation of large diameter primary afferents** in the touch pathway, by transcutaneous electrical stimulation (TENS), reduces transmission in secondary afferents in the pain pathway via the gate mechanism.

Proprioception

To allow the effective balance and movement of the body, the brain must be aware of the position and orientation of the skeleton. This is known as **proprioception** and is achieved through many different sensory processes. Posture and joint position are signalled by:

- the **vestibular system** which detects a change in head position
- the **touch pathway** which detects contact of the feet with a stable surface
- **muscle spindle fibres** and **Golgi tendon organs** in muscles, which detect muscle stretch and muscle, tension respectively.

All of these systems send inputs to the motor nervous system, allowing adjustment of posture to prevent, or brace against, a fall. The physiological importance of the system is highlighted by the rapidly conducting fibres that conduct impulses to the CNS. The feedback of this system is rapidly

Fibre type	Mean diameter (mm)	Mean speed of conduction (m/s)	Functions
Aα	15	100	Motor neurons
Aβ	8	50	Skin touch afferents
Aγ	5	20	Motor to muscle spindles
Aδ	4	15	Sharp pain and skin temperature afferents
B	3	7	Pain afferents
C	1	1	Poorly localised pain afferents

Figure 17.15 Properties of sensory fibres involved in touch and pain sensation.

relayed to the motor parts of the brain to allow rapid refinement of movement, which is reflected in the large size of the proprioceptive fibres, ensuring rapid nervous conduction.

Vision

Vision allows perception of colour, form and movement of objects in the environment. This facilitates object recognition and directional movement.

Sensory stimulus

The sensory stimulus for vision is light reflected off objects in the environment and focused on to the retina of the eye.

Visual receptors

Light is transduced into an electrical signal by rod and cone cells in the retina. They contain a photopigment substance that allows them to absorb light. To reach rod and cone cells, light reflected from an object in the environment must pass through structures in the eye (Fig. 17.16):

- Conjunctiva
- Cornea
- Aqueous humour
- Pupil
- Bioconvex lens
- The vitreous humour.

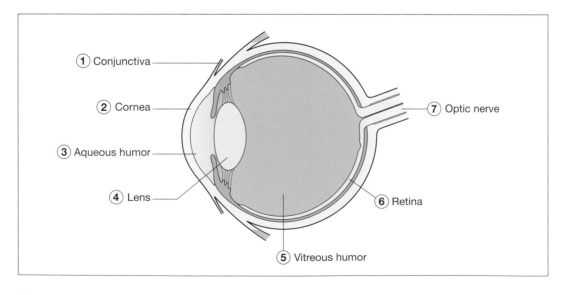

Figure 17.16 Structures in the eye through which light must pass to reach retina (numbered from front to back).

Cellular structure of the retina

Within the retina itself, light must pass through several layers of cells (Fig. 17.17). In sequential order, these include:

- optic ganglion cells
- amacrine cells
- bipolar and horizontal cells
- the rods and cones, which detect light.

Properties of rods and cones

Rods and cones have an outer region in which the plasma membrane is invaginated into discs, which contain the photopigment protein, and an inner region, which contains the nucleus and mitochondria and terminates in a synaptic process The rods and cones are located behind the neurons of the retina. As a result there is some distortion of the image as the light passes through the cells – this distortion is corrected for within the visual cortex. The photopigment of rods and cones differs and has different sensitivities to light.

- **Rhodopsin**, the photopigment in rods, contains a prosthetic group, retinal, derived from vitamin A in the diet by the enzyme retinol dehydrogenase.
- **Opsin**, the photopigment in cones, is of three types. Each opsin optimally absorbs light of a

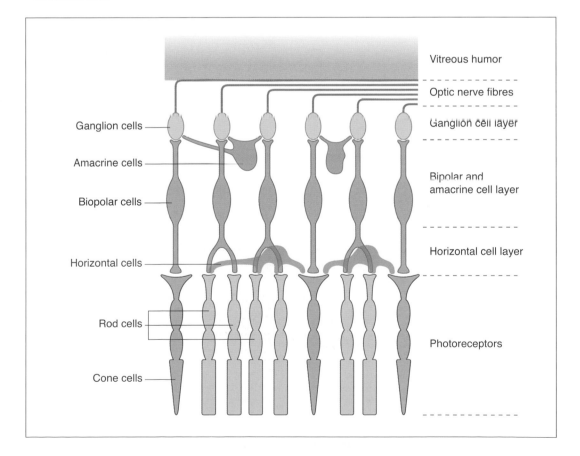

Figure 17.17 Cellular structure of the retina.

different wavelength. This allows colour vision as the brain compares input from three types of cone cell.

CLINICAL Colour blindness

Mutation in a gene encoding one or more cone opsins causes colour blindness. Red–green colour blindness, in which the person cannot distinguish red from green and either from grey, is most common, particularly in men because the mutation is X-linked and recessive.

CLINICAL Vitamin A deficiency and night blindness

Retinal is derived from vitamin A, which is obtained in the diet, by the enzyme retinol dehydrogenase. Vitamin A deficiency may therefore result in night blindness.

There are about 20-fold more rods than cones, although they have different distributions:

- **Rods are uniformly distributed across the retina**. They are much more sensitive to low-intensity lights than cones because they show spatial summation (input from multiple rods converges on to a single retinal ganglion cell) and temporal summation (electrical signals are integrated over about 100 ms). However, this reduces visual.
- **Cones are clustered in a small area of the retina**, known as the **fovea**. Clustering of cones means that there is high visual acuity for visual images that fall on the fovea.

Phototransduction

In the dark, calcium and sodium ion influx occurs through cGMP-controlled cation channels, depolarising photoreceptors to about $-40\,$mV. The opposite is true in the light when photoreceptors hyperpolarise. The molecular mechanism of hyperpolarisation of photoreceptors in the light is described below (Fig. 17.18):

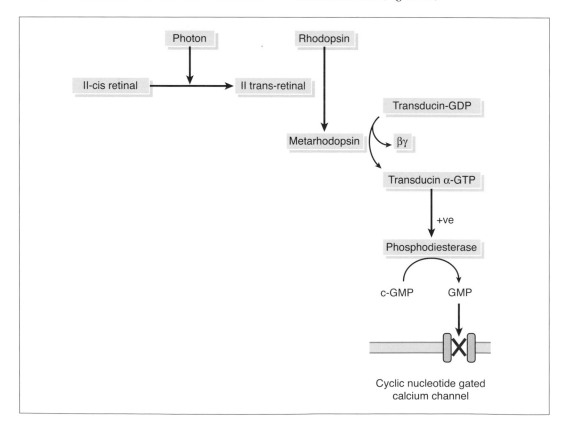

Figure 17.18 Sequence of events in phototransduction.

- Adsorption of photons isomerises the pigment, rhodopsin, in rod cells or iodopsin in cone cells to an un unstable intermediate
- This unstable intermediate binds a GTP-bound protein, transducin.
- The GTP-bound α-subunit of transducin dissociates and activates a phosphodiesterase, which hydrolyses cGMP to GMP, preventing cation influx and reversing depolarisation.

Adaptation to dim light

Exposure to bright light desensitises rod cells because 11-*trans*-retinal dissociates from rhodopsin, leaving it 'bleached'. In order for rod cells to regain their sensitivity, 11-*trans*-retinal must be converted to 11-*cis*-retinal by **retinal Isomerase**. This accounts for the delay in adjustment to dim light.

Adaptation to bright light

Cone cells also desensitise in response to continued exposure to bright light because a reduction in calcium ion influx in response to light activates **guanylyl cyclase**, which generates cGMP. An increase in cGMP re-establishes the influx of cations. This allows cone cells to distinguish light intensity over a wider range.

Processing in the retina

Photoreceptors synapse with two distinct types of bipolar cell:

1 **Flat bipolar cells** are hyperpolarised in the light, because they are depolarised by glutamate.
2 **Invaginating bipolar cells** are depolarised in the light, because they are hyperpolarised by glutamate.

This pattern of depolarisation and hyperpolarisation is transmitted to the retinal ganglion cells with which bipolar cells synapse, giving rise to 'on and off channels' and improving contrast within the image.

Contrast is enhanced by **lateral inhibition**. Illumination of the centre and surround of a visual field has the opposite effect, e.g. illumination of the centre of the receptive field of an invaginating bipolar cell will cause it to depolarise, whereas illumination of the surround will cause it to hyperpolarise. The cells mediating this differ between the photoreceptors:

- For **cone cell transmission**, this mechanism is mediated by horizontal cells. Glutamate is stimulatory to horizontal cells, causing them to secrete inhibitory GABA, which acts back on adjacent photoreceptors, reducing glutamate release.
- For **rod cell transmission**, this mechanism is mediated by amacrine cells. Amacrine cells also encode information about object movement.

Ganglion cells send out axons in the optic nerve; they are of two types:

1 **Magnocellular neurons** show transient responses in response to illumination and are sensitive to movement. They are not colour selective.
2 **Parvocellular neurons** show sustained responses to illumination, have small receptor fields, adapting them to high resolution form discrimination, and are wavelength selective. They exhibit **wavelength opponency** by which input from one type of cone cell is stimulatory but input from another is inhibitory. This opponency follows different patterns in simple concentric neurons and coextensive neurons (Fig. 17.19).

The different properties of parvocellular and magnocellular neurons represent the first stage of **parallel processing** in the visual system, in which different attributes of vision are processed simultaneously but separately.

> **DEFINITION Parallel processing**
>
> In many systems various features of the stimuli are extracted and processed simultaneously. This parallel processing allows distinct attributes to be analysed efficiently. In the visual system the parvocellular part processes colour, whereas the magnocellular part processes movement and edges.

Visual pathway

Axons of the parvocellular and magnocellular ganglion cells leave the eye in the optic nerve, at the **blind spot**, which lacks photoreceptors. The optic nerve is the primary afferent nerve in the visual pathway. Neurons in the optic nerve originating from the nasal half of the retina cross over at the **optic chiasma** to join the contralateral optic tract, whereas axons from the temporal half of the retina remain in the ipsilateral optic tract. The optic tracts convey neurons from the ipsilateral side of

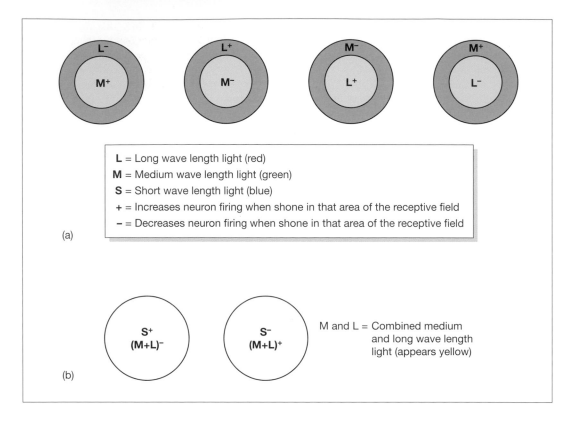

L = Long wave length light (red)
M = Medium wave length light (green)
S = Short wave length light (blue)
+ = Increases neuron firing when shone in that area of the receptive field
− = Decreases neuron firing when shone in that area of the receptive field

(a)

(b)

M and L = Combined medium and long wave length light (appears yellow)

Figure 17.19 Receptive fields of parvocellular retinal ganglion cells.

each eye, corresponding to the opposite sides of the visual field, i.e. the left optic tract carries signals from the left side of both retinas, which receive images from the right side of the visual field. The optic tract projects to the lateral geniculate nucleus of the thalamus in the optic radiation (Fig. 17.20).

 CLINICAL Visual impairments due to damage to the optic nerve or tract

Damage to the optic neural pathways produce different defects, depending on the location of the lesion:

- Lesions of the optic nerve cause monocular blindness, loss of site in one eye.
- The optic chiasma is situated above the pituitary fossa, making it vulnerable to compression by pituitary tumours. This results in bitemporal hemianopia (tunnel vision), because decussating axons from the nasal halves of the retina are damaged.
- Lesions of the optic tract beyond the optic chiasma give rise to specific sight deficits in the contralateral half of the visual field.

Organisation of neuronal input in the lateral geniculate nucleus of the thalamus

The lateral geniculate nucleus of the thalamus (LGN) has six layers:

- Magnocellular neurons project to the innermost two layers.
- Parvocellular neurons project to the outer four layers.
- Neurons originating in the eye on the same side as the LGN project to layers 2, 3 and 5.
- Neurons from the contralateral eye project to layers 1, 4 and 6.

Retinotopic mapping of input neurons to the LGN means that neighbouring sites in the eye's visual field are represented on adjacent vertical cross-sections through the LGN and the fovea is mapped to a disproportionately large area.

In the final part of the visual pathway, neurons pass from the LGN to the primary visual cortex (V1), in the calcarine sulcus of the occipital lobe.

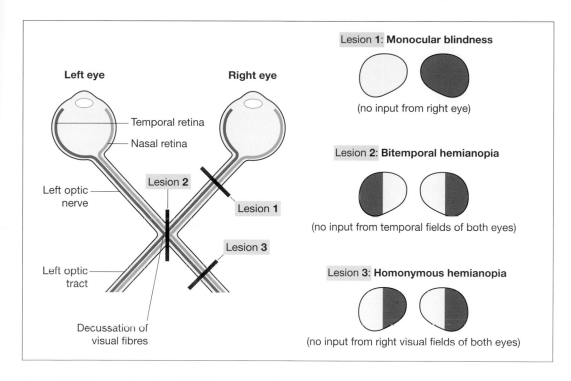

Figure 17.20 Decussation of nasal half of optic nerve and consequences of lesions at various sites in the optic nerve and optic tract.

Organisation of the visual cortex

The visual cortex is arranged into five areas, V1–V5, which progressively process visual information. Each region has a different role:

1 V1 is the primary visual cortex which receives the retinal signals from the LGN. It is located at the most rear part of the occipital lobe.
2 V2 is associated with the processing of visual stimuli and shares many features with V1, processing information on colour and orientation of an object. It is also has more complex processing and is thought to be involved in identifying whether a feature is part of a subject or part of the background of an image.
3 V3 can be divided effectively into two parts, the dorsal part being associated with the posterior parietal lobe, forming part of the 'where' stream, which processes spatial location and orientation. The ventral stream is associated with the inferior temporal lobe, and related to the identification of what a subject is. V3 is important in the recognition of form.
4 V4 is associated with the ventral stream and the recognition of something. It also shows

significant attention modulation, allowing selection of what stimuli reaching the region are processed.
5 V5 is associated with the dorsal stream processes of location and movement of an object. As a result it is also closely related to eye movement and integrating signals in the perception of movement.

Organisation of neuronal input in the primary visual cortex

The organisation of neuronal input to the primary visual cortex preserves retinotopic mapping. There is a convergence of input from the two eyes and also from multiple retinal cells with different receptor fields – signal information from the same visual axis, from simple cells to complex cells, and from complex cells to hypercomplex cells. Convergence of multiple inputs is responsible for two important aspects of the receptive field of hypercomplex cells:

1 Their **receptive field is defined by a given visual axis** as opposed to a discrete point in the visual field, as in simple cells.

2 They **receive input from both visual fields**, although this is normally biased towards either the ipsilateral or the contralateral side.

Hypercomplex cells are arranged into **hypercolumns** which comprise all cells representing a particular visual axis.

Neurons from the parvocellular pathway split into two distinct sub-pathways, which are labelled with cytochrome oxidase staining as blob and interblob regions:

- **Blob regions** show **colour opponency** (Fig. 17.21).
- **Interblob regions** show high-resolution definition of form but do not show colour opponency.

Properties of the primary visual cortex

The primary visual cortex, V1, is responsible for conscious perception of sight. V1 computes the depth of the visual field for distant objects by:

- **parallax**: closer objects appear to move relative to further ones
- **perspective**: convergence of parallel lines
- **visual occlusion**: closer objects obscure more distant ones.
- **shadows**.

V1 computes the depth of the visual field for nearby objects by the following:

- **Retinal disparity**: the same object falls in a slightly different visual axis on the left and right visual fields. This is known as binocular vision. The existence of internal visual pictures, intrinsic and learned, in V1 allows:
  - pattern completionobjects can be recognised even if the retinal image is incomplete

  - generalisationfamiliar objects can be recognised from multiple angles.
- Colour opponency in blob regions of V1 causes: **colour constancy**: objects appear the same colour irrespective of their illumination.
- Change in illumination wavelength causes equal but opposite effects on the centre and surround of double opponent cells.
- **Perceptual cancellation**: due to antagonism between light of different wavelengths, an object cannot appear reddish green but instead appears brown.

Accessory visual cortex

All types of primary visual field input to V1 have a corresponding output to the V2 region of the accessory visual cortex. These output regions are differentiated by their cytochrome oxidase staining pattern:

- **Regions in V1 with magnocellular input** send neuronal input to thick striped regions of V2.
- **Blob regions in V1** send neuronal input to thin striped regions in V2.
- **Inter-blob regions in V1** send neuronal input to interstripe regions in V2.

This parallel processing of different visual attributes is maintained in accessory areas of visual cortex:

- **Thick striped regions** send input to V5, which is important in **perception of motion**.
- **Thin striped regions** send input to V4, which is important in **colour recognition**.
- **Interstripe regions** send input to V3, which is important in **form recognition**.

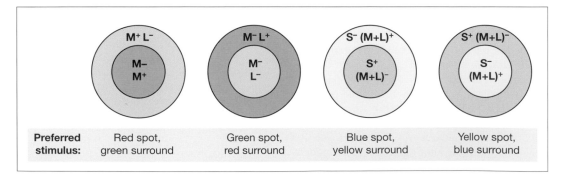

| Preferred stimulus: | Red spot, green surround | Green spot, red surround | Blue spot, yellow surround | Yellow spot, blue surround |

Figure 17.21 Double opponent cells in blob regions of the VI cerebral cortex. S, M and L refer to Short, Middle and Long wavelength light, respectively.

The different pathways are not entirely independent; there are reciprocal pathways between V3 and V4 and between V5 and V4.

 CLINICAL Blind sight

Patients with lesions to V1 can often localise an object with a high degree of accuracy, but deny awareness of its existence, a phenomenon known as blind sight. It is thought that this is because some neuronal projections from the LGN bypass V1, and connect directly to V2 and the accessory visual cortex.

Visual reflexes

Some neurons in the visual pathway project to subcortical motor nuclei, which are involved in motor reflexes of the eye in response to light. These reflexes enhance vision and protect the eye.

Consensual light reflex

Shining a bright light into one eye causes constriction of the pupil of both that eye and the contralateral eye. This **consensual light reflex** is important because variation in the diameter of the pupil can change the amount of light entering the eye by 30-fold. The neuronal pathway involved in this reflex is as follows:

- Neurons in the optic tract project to the pretectum.
- The pre-tectum sends output to the Edinger–Westphal nucleus in the brain stem.
- Preganglionic parasympathetic fibres in the Edinger–Westphal nucleus project to the ciliary ganglion in the oculomotor nerve.
- The ciliary ganglion sends postganglionic parasympathetic fibres to the pupil. Activity in these postganglionic nerve fibres causes constriction of the pupil.

Accommodation reflex

When an object gets closer, light reflecting off it diverges more as it enters the eye. Therefore, the lens must refract it to a greater extent, to focus the image on the fovea. This is achieved by **accommodation reflex**. The neural pathway involved in this reflex is as follows:

- **Blurring of the visual image** in V1, because of insufficient refraction by the lens, activates neurons that extend from V1 to the pre-tectum.
- The **pre-tectum stimulates the Edinger–Westphal nucleus**, which in turn stimulates the ciliary ganglion.
- **Activation of the parasympathetic fibres** emerging from the ciliary ganglion causes muscles in the ciliary body to contract.
- **Contraction of the ciliary body** reduces the tension in the suspensory ligaments and lens capsule, causing the lens to shorten and become more spherical, and so refract light rays more. Parasympathetic activity in the ciliary ganglion also causes the pupils to constrict, increasing the depth of the visual field.

Reflex eye movements

A projection of the optic tract to the superficial layer of the **superior colliculus** is involved in triggering movement of the eyes, so as to focus an object on to the fovea.

Hearing

Sound perception alerts an individual to noise coming from objects in the external environment and is important in aural language comprehension.

Sensory input in hearing

The sensory input in hearing is a pressure wave (sound wave) transmitted through a medium, e.g. air. Sound waves have **waveforms**: cycles of alternating compression and expansion. There are two important properties of sound waves in the context of hearing:

1 **Frequency**: the time taken for one complete waveform – the higher the frequency, the higher the pitch of the perceived sound. The unit of frequency is the hertz (Hz). Young people are sensitive to a frequency range of 20 Hz to 20 kHz. Maximum sensitivity is over the range 1–4 kHz and sensitivity to the upper end of the frequency spectrum decreases with age.

2 **Amplitude**: the maximum pressure that a sound wave causes in a medium. The amplitude of a sound wave corresponds to the loudness of the perceived sound: the greater the amplitude, the louder the perceived sound. The unit of amplitude is the decibel (dB). Speech is normally about 65 dB. Sounds over 120 dB damage hearing.

> 🔍 CLINICAL **Conductive deafness**
>
> Wax in the external meatus, overgrowth of bones in the middle ear (osteosclerosis) or infection of the middle ear (otitis media) can impair sound wave conduction, leading to **conductive deafness**.

Transmission of sound waves

Sound waves are funnelled into the external auditory meatus by the pinna. Sound waves pass through the external auditory meatus to the tympanic membrane, where a relay of three bones, the malleus, incus and stapes, connects the tympanic membrane to the oval window of the cochlea (Fig. 17.22):

- The **malleus** is closest to the tympanic membrane and moves in response to its vibrations.
- The **incus** articulates with the malleus and the stapes.
- The **stapes** is pushed inwards as a result of its articulation with the incus. This causes it to press against the oval window of the cochlea, to which it is attached by an annular ligament. The fact that the oval window has a 20-fold smaller area than the tympanic membrane causes a large increase in the pressure of the sound wave transmitted to the inner ear.

Structure of the cochlea

The cochlea is the structure in the inner ear responsible for the transduction of sound into nervous signals. The bony labyrinth of the cochlea winds around a central column, the modiolus. The cochlea is divided into three anatomical compartments, scalae, by the membranous cochlear duct (Fig. 17.23):

1 The **scala vestibuli** is adjacent to the oval window, via which pressure waves from the middle ear are transmitted.
2 The **scala vestibuli** is anatomically connected to the **scala tympani** via the helicotrema. At the end of the scala tympani there is a round window.
3 The **scala media** lies between the scala vestibuli and the scala tympani but is separated from them by the cochlear duct.

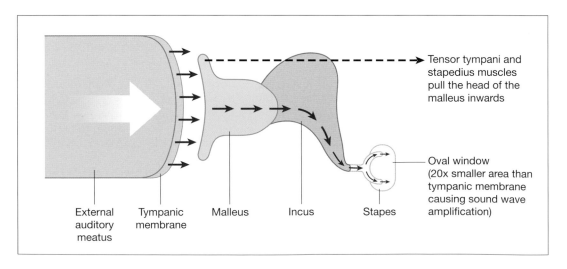

Figure 17.22 Bones of the middle ear transmit and amplify sound waves (arrows show the direction of transmission of sound waves).

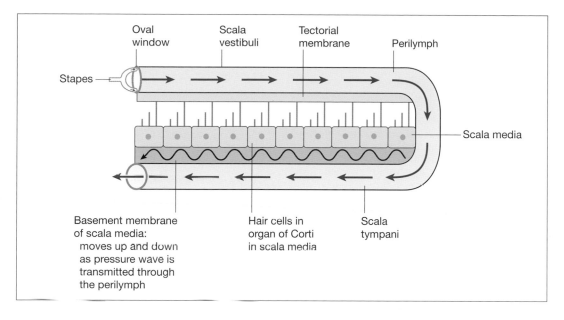

Figure 17.23 Inner ear (arrows show the direction of transmission of sound waves).

The organ of corti

The basement membrane of the scala media supports the **organ of Corti**, in which sensory transduction occurs. The organ of Corti contains hair cells from which projections (stereocilia) extend in ascending order of height. The tallest of these stereocilia contact the mucopolysaccharide tectorial membrane of the scala media above. Hair cells of two types can be found on the organ of Corti:

1 **Inner hair cells** are arranged in a single row. The inner hair cells send afferent output to the eighth cranial nerve and are responsible for sensing sound.
2 **Outer hair cells** are arranged in three rows and receive efferent input from CN VIII. The efferent output causes the outer hair cells to oscillate at a similar frequency to the sound wave, increasing the amplitude of the displacement of the basement membrane.

Transduction of sound waves to electrical impulses in the inner ear

Both the scala tympani and the scala vestibuli contain incompressible perilymph, which is secreted by the stria vascularis. Oscillation of the oval window causes conduction of a pressure wave from the scala vestibuli to the scala tympani, after which it is dissipated at the round window. Transmission of the pressure wave through the perilymph causes the basement membrane of the scala media to move up and down.

Oscillation of the basement membrane causes the tallest stereocilia of the hair cells in the organ of Corti to shear against the mucopolysaccharide tectorial membrane. As the stereocilia of the hair cells are joined to each other by tip links, bending of the tallest stereocilium creates tension on other stereocilia. This opens ion channels in membranes of the stereocilia. The scala media contains K^+-rich endolymph secreted by the stria vascularis. As a result of the high concentration of potassium ions and high positive charge of the endolymph relative to the intracellular fluid, potassium ions move into the hair cells, depolarising them.

Depolarisation causes the hair cells to release glutamate, triggering an action potential in the afferent neurons of the vestibulocochlear nerve with which they synapse.

 CLINICAL **Damage to outer hair cells**

Outer hair cells are selectively damaged by aminoglycoside antibiotics. This leads to **sensorineural deafness**, deafness due to impaired signal transduction in the inner ear, which should be differentiated from conductive deafness, deafness due to impaired conduction of the sound wave in the middle ear.

CLINICAL Conductive deafness versus sensorineural deafness

Conductive deafness can be distinguished clinically from sensorineural deafness by performing **Rinne's** and **Weber's tests**:

- In **Rinne's test**, a vibrating tuning fork is placed over the mastoid process and then over the external auditory meatus. People with normal hearing will hear a louder sound when the tuning fork is placed over the external auditory meatus, because sound waves are conducted better through air. However, in conductive deafness, the sound will be loudest when the tuning fork is held over the mastoid process.

- In **Weber's test**, the vibrating tuning fork is placed in the centre of the patient's forehead. A person with normal hearing will appreciate the sound as being equally loud in both ears. Someone with conductive deafness will hear the sound loudest in the affected ear. By contrast someone with sensorineural hearing loss will hear the sound loudest in the unaffected side.

Auditory pathway

Neurons of CN VIII have their cell bodies in the spiral ganglia in the cochlea. CN VIII projects to the vestibulocochlear nucleus of the pons (Fig. 17.24).

The ventral vestibulocochlear nuclei regulate reflex contraction of the tensor tympani and stapedius muscles in response to loud noises. These muscles pull the auditory bones away from the oval window, dampening sound conduction in the middle ear.

The dorsal vestibulocochlear nucleus carries sound signals to the auditory cortex projects to the contralateral nucleus of the lateral lemniscus via the dorsal acoustic striae. There are reciprocal connections between the nuclei of the lateral lemniscus on either side. From the nucleus of the lateral lemniscus, neurons project to the inferior colliculus and then on to the medial geniculate nucleus of the thalamus (MGN) and the primary auditory cortex (A1) in the superior temporal gyrus via the auditory radiation. A1 is responsible for conscious sound perception.

Encoding of sound frequency

The frequency of sound is encoded throughout the auditory system in different ways:

- **Place coding** occurs in the cochlear. As the basement membrane on which the organ of Corti rests becomes thicker and less rigid away from the stapedial end, the neurons at the stapedial end are more sensitive to high-frequency sounds and neurons at the apical end more sensitive to low-frequency sounds.

- Frequency coding for lower-frequency sounds also occurs by **phase locking**, by which different afferent neurons have the highest probability of firing at different phases of the waveform. Populations of neurons can together, therefore, encode frequency.

- Precise patterning of input from neurons originating from different points along the cochlear to the inferior colliculus, MGN and A1 gives rise to **tonotopic mapping**. The same frequency is represented in all layers of A1 along a vertical axis. High frequencies are represented inferiorly, low frequencies superiorly.

Sound localisation

The spatial origin of a sound is calculated by the superior olive:

- **Differences in the time** of input into the two ears are detected by bushy neurons in the left and right cochlear nuclei which are capable of phase locking. Bushy neurons in the left and right cochlear nuclei fire at slightly different times if there is a difference in the time the sound arrives between the two ears. Medial superior olive neurons fire maximally when input from the ipsilateral and contralateral cochlear nuclei arrives at the same time. Different populations of medial superior olivary neurons are wired to the two cochlear nuclei in different ways, so that, for a given time delay, only one population of these neurons will fire maximally. This mode of localisation is most efficient for low-frequency sounds, because high-frequency sounds may vary in the time of input to both ears by more than one phase.

- Neurons in the lateral superior olive detect differences in the **intensity of input** from stellate cells in the left and right cochlear nuclei. Input to the ear furthest from the sound is quieter, because passage of the sound wave through the head muffles it. Neurons in the lateral superior

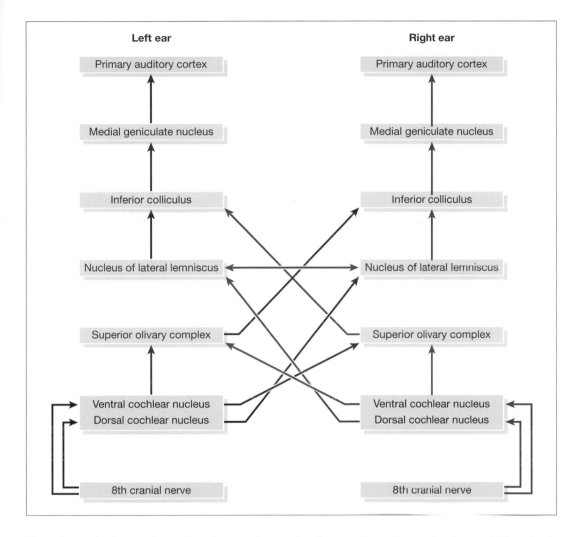

Figure 17.24 **Auditory pathway**. There is extensive crossings between the pathways of each ear, which assists in the localisation of sound, as well as aiding processing.

olive receive an excitatory input from stellate cells in the ipsilateral cochlear nucleus but an inhibitory input from stellate cells in the contralateral cochlear nucleus. Therefore, if the sound is closer to the contralateral ear, the lateral superior olive neuron is inhibited, whereas it is stimulated if the sound is closer to the ipsilateral ear.

Detection of the origin of a sound in the vertical axis

The capacity of bushy cells in the cochlear nuclei to phase lock also allows the origin of sound to be localised in the vertical axis. Sound waves enter the external auditory meatus by both a direct pathway and an indirect pathway, in which they are reflected off the bumpy surface of the pinna. Sound waves with different vertical origins show unique patterns of reflection off the surface of the pinna. This causes differences in the time of arrival at the ipsilateral cochlear nucleus for sound waves entering the ear by the indirect pathway, depending on the vertical origin of the sound wave; this causes different populations of bushy neurons to fire at different times. This phase-locked pattern of firing allows neurons in the medial superior olive to analyse the vertical origin of sounds.

No specific map has been identified in the primary or secondary auditory cortex.

Secondary auditory cortex

Secondary auditory cortex is involved in some of the higher processing of sound - it is involved in processing elements music and speech. It lacks clearly defined maps.

 CLINICAL Lesions of the secondary auditory cortex

One area of the secondary auditory cortex that is particularly important clinically is **Wernicke's area** which is important in speech comprehension. Lesions to this area result in **receptive aphasia**, an inability to understand language.

Vestibular system

The vestibular system is important in the maintenance of posture and balance; it also regulates reflexes related to eye movements.

Sensory input

The sensory input to the vestibular system is static position or acceleration of the head, either linear or rotational. The sensory transduction apparatus of the vestibular system comprises endolymph-containing components of the membranous labyrinth of the inner ear:

- **Otolith** organs, the utricle and saccule, detect static head position and linear acceleration in the horizontal and vertical axes, respectively
- **Semicircular ducts** – posterior, superior and horizontal – arranged 100° relative to each other, detect rotational acceleration.

Transduction in the otolith organs

The utricle and saccule contain endolymph. Within the utricle and saccule, transduction is performed by the macula. The macula comprises a sheet of sensory epithelial cells with stereocilia. The tallest stereocilia (konocilia) are embedded within a **gelatinous tectorial membrane** studded with calcium carbonate crystals, otoconia.

   Linear acceleration causes the tectorial membrane to be displaced relative to the hair cell, because of the otoconia's inertia. This bends the konocilia in the direction of movement. As the stereocilia are tethered to the konocilia, tension exerted on the connections between them and ion channels are opened in response to deformation of the cilia.

The electrical and chemical gradient between the intracellular fluid in the hair cells and the endolymph causes potassium ions to enter the hair cells through open ion channels, depolarising them and causing them to release glutamate. Glutamate depolarises the primary afferent neuron that synapses with the hair cells.

Transduction in the semicircular ducts

At the base of each semicircular duct is a dilatation, the ampulla. The ampulla contains hair cells embedded in a gelatinous matrix, the cupula.

   Rotational acceleration causes movement of the endolymph. However, inertia of the endolymph causes it to lag, exerting a force on the ampulla. This displaces the cupula relative to the hair cells, leading to transduction in a similar manner to that described for otolith organs.

Vestibular pathway

The primary afferent neurons project to the vestibular nuclei in the brain stem. These vestibular nuclei send neuronal output to:

- the **oculomotor nucleus**: involved in **vestibulo-ocular** reflexes in which the gaze is kept steady, despite rotation of the head
- the **cerebellum**, involved in **postural reflexes** which keep the position of the body constant
- the **contralateral ventroposterior lateral nucleus of the thalamus**: from here, an afferent projection is sent to areas of the cortex including the somatosensory cortex and posterior parietal cortex which contributes to conscious awareness of posture and balance.

 CLINICAL Ménière's disease

Ménière's disease is due to a failure to reabsorb endolymph in the cochlear duct of one ear. The increase in endolymph volume causes the membranous labyrinth to rupture and herniate. This causes loss of hearing and tinnitus in the affected ear, and episodes of vertigo and loss of balance accompanied by nausea or vomiting.

Smell

Smell is involved in taste preference and facilitates avoidance of potentially noxious objects.

Sensory stimulus in smell

Odorant receptors are present in olfactory cilia that project from the apical dendrites of bipolar olfactory receptor neurons. Olfactory cilia are found in the dorsal epithelial surface of the nose. Sniffing enhances smell, because odorant molecules are targeted by air currents to the back of the nose.

Olfactory transduction

There are approximately 1000 different odorant receptors. In all odorant receptor cells transduction is mediated by a G_s protein second-messenger cascade. This leads to an increase in the concentration of intracellular cAMP, causing cyclic nucleotide-gated cation channels to open, depolarising the neuron.

Each bipolar olfactory receptor neuron expresses one type of olfactory receptor. However, odorant molecules bind two to six different types of odorant receptor with different affinities. By comparing the range of odorant receptors that an odorant molecule binds, the brain is able to distinguish approximately 10 000 different odours.

Olfactory receptors become desensitised on prolonged exposure to the same odorant. This is because Ca^{2+} binds **calmodulin**, forming a complex that binds to the cyclic nucleotide-gated channels and reduces the efficacy of cyclic nucleotide binding.

Olfactory pathways

The axons of bipolar olfactory receptor neurons project from the nasal epithelium to the CNS in the olfactory nerve (CN I). The olfactory nerve enters the CNS at the top of the nose by piercing the cribriform plate of the ethmoid bone, where the olfactory nerve makes excitatory synapses with mitral and tufted cells in the glomeruli of the olfactory bulbs. Bipolar olfactory neurons responding to the same odour terminate in the same glomerulus.

Mitral and tufted cells send out axonal projections in the olfactory tract. Axons in the olfactory tract project to the:

- **contralateral olfactory bulb**
- **pyriform cortex and amygdala**: from here there is a projection to the hypothalamus, which controls behavioural responses to smell

- **hippocampus**: establishes olfactory components of episodic memories
- **mediodorsal nucleus of the thalamus** and from there to the prefrontal cortex: involved in conscious smell perception.

Taste

Taste perception permits selection of nutritionally valuable foods over noxious ones.

The sensory stimuli for taste are salt, sugar, acid, bitterness and unami (meat flavour). Olfactory pathways and smell also contribute heavily to our appreciation of taste.

Taste receptors

Transduction of taste stimuli into electrical signals occurs in epithelial cells in the tongue, pharynx and oesophagus; 50–150 taste receptor cells are typically clustered together to form a taste bud:

- **Taste receptor cells in the anterior two-thirds of the tongue** are most sensitive to sweet and salty tastes. They synapse with primary afferent nerves in CN VII.
- **Taste receptor cells in the posterior third of the tongue** are most sensitive to sour and bitter tastes. They synapse with primary afferent nerves in CN IX.
- **Taste receptor cells in the pharynx and oesophagus** detect differences in the ionic concentration of sodium and hydrogen ions. They synapse with primary afferent nerves in CN X.

Transduction in taste receptors

Transduction of taste signals occurs when a taste stimulus causes depolarisation of the taste receptor cell membrane, triggering calcium ion influx and neurotransmitter release. This activates the afferent neuron. The mechanism by which each taste stimulus causes depolarisation of the taste receptor cell membrane varies:

- **Salty tastes** directly cause depolarisation of taste receptor cells by the influx of Na^+.
- **Sour tastes** result from H^+ ions which depolarise taste receptor cells by blocking voltage-gated K^+ channels, responsible for maintaining the hyperpolarised resting membrane potential.

- **Sweet and unami tastes** cause depolarisation of taste receptor cells via a G_s protein second-messenger cascade, which leads to an increase in intracellular cAMP that closes voltage-gated K^+ channels.
- **Bitter tastes** depolarise taste receptor cells in multiple different ways, reflecting the diversity of molecules that are bitter flavoured.

Taste pathway

Primary afferent taste neurons in CN VII, IX and X project to the nucleus tractus solitarius (NTS) of the medulla. From the NTS, neurons project via the ipsilateral ventroposterior medial nucleus of the thalamus to an area of cortex adjacent to that mapping somatosensation from the tongue, which is involved in the conscious appreciation of taste. Neurons from the primary taste cortex project to the insula, which is involved in the emotional response to different tastes. The NTS is also thought to send a neuronal projection to the amygdala and lateral hypothalamus, which regulates behavioural responses to taste, i.e. feeding.

Association areas of cortex

Cortical association areas integrate signals from different sensory systems. This facilitates higher brain functions and motor planning.

Temporal cortex

The temporal cortex is involved in the complex processing of many stimuli, including the following:

- The **temporal auditory cortex** is responsible for the processing and comprehension of language.
- The **parahippocampal gyrus** is involved in the laying down of memory.
- The **inferior temporal cortex** processes visual information and is important in visual recognition. It receives neuronal input from V4 and V3 visual association cortex, which are involved in colour and form discrimination respectively. Connections from these areas of visual cortex to the temporal cortex are collectively termed the 'what stream'. Lesions of the inferior temporal

cortex cause an inability to recognise objects or faces.

Posterior parietal cortex

One part of the **posterior parietal cortex** receives input from the touch pathway and proprioceptive pathways. It is important in awareness of body position and recognition of objects through touch. Lesions to this area can lead to **neglect** of contralateral sensory input and, sometimes, denial of the existence of a limb, or to **astereogenesis,** an inability to recognise objects through touch.

Another part of the **posterior parietal cortex** receives input from the V5 area of visual association cortex, which is involved in perception of movement. The connection between V5 and the posterior parietal cortex is known as the 'where' **stream**. Lesions result in a difficulty in performing visuospatial tasks. Abnormalities in this area may cause **dyslexia** (difficulty in reading), **dyscalculia** (difficulty in performing mathematical calculations) and **dysgraphia** (difficulty in writing).

Prefrontal cortex

The prefrontal cortex is involved in planning motor responses to sensory stimuli. It is particularly developed in humans and plays a role in behavioural regulation and inhibition. Lesions to the prefrontal cortex result in a characteristic profile of clinical symptoms:

- Disinhibition with childish behaviour
- Emotional blunting or sometimes aggression
- Deficits in working memory
- A short attention span
- Reduction in spontaneous movement and speech
- An inability to formulate or pursue plans and goals.

 CLINICAL Broca's aphasia

Broca's region in the prefrontal cortex is responsible for speech. Lesions to this area result in **expressive aphasia**, an inability to form recognisable words. Broca's region has reciprocal connections with Wernicke's area in the temporal cortex via the arcuate fasiculus. Lesions to this arcuate fasiculus result in an inability to repeat words and phrases.

Neuroendocrine control of body systems

The hypothalamus can influence both the endocrine and neural homoeostatic systems in the body:

- **Endocrine regulation**: some hypothalamic nuclei release neurohormones that are transported via the hypothalamo-hypophyseal vessels to the anterior pituitary where they regulate pituitary hormone release, e.g. cortisol-releasing hormone (CRH). Other hypothalamic nuclei project to the posterior pituitary, directly secreting hormones into the bloodstream. ADH and oxytocin are secreted in this manner.
- **Neurological regulation**: both the sympathetic and parasympathetic nervous systems are regulated by pathways from the hypothalamus:
  - **Parasympathetic structures** that receive fibres from the hypothalamus include the pretectal and Edinger–Westphal nuclei and the parasympathetic neurons in the sacral part of the spinal cord (originate from the paraventricular nucleus of the hypothalamus)
  - **Sympathetic preganglionic neurons** located in the sympathetic chain receive signals from the hypothalamus.

Outputs to higher centres

The hypothalamus can modulate the function of the body as a result of signals received from the higher centres of the brain, reflecting perceived or anticipated stress on the body. Similarly, the state of the body is sensed by the hypothalamus and, in turn, may influence emotions and the higher centres of the brain. Finally, fibres within the tract project to the choroid plexus, where they may alter the production of CSF.

Higher cognitive functions

Higher cognitive functions are complex brain processes that entail more than the simple processing of sensory input and motor output. This section discusses the higher cognitive functions of memory, sleep and consciousness. Although appetite is regulated by similar pathways it is discussed elsewhere, in relation to the GI tract and endocrinology.

Memory

Memory is the storage of a fact, experience or skill as a neural circuit in the brain, allowing later recall. Memory requires **neuronal plasticity** (the potential of neurons to be rewired).

Memories can be categorised as short or long term. It is thought that distinct areas of the brain or different processes are involved in these two types of memory, because deficits in one type can occur independently of deficits in the other type.

Short-term memory

A finite number of items may be stored in short-term memory: seven plus or minus two items is the normal range. Short-term memories are temporary and require constant rehearsal if they are not to be displaced by new incoming information. Short-term memory has a phonological loop, involving the left cerebral hemisphere of the brain, which is required in sentence comprehension. It also has a visuospatial loop, involving the right hemisphere of the brain which is needed in navigation. Short-term memory is thought to be stored in the prefrontal cortex.

Long-term memory

The storage capacity of long-term memory is without obvious limits during an individual's lifetime. Long-term memories are retained without constant rehearsal. Long-term memory may be subcategorised into **procedural** and **declarative memory**:

- Formation of a **procedural memory** (knowing how to perform a skill) is slow and requires constant rehearsal. However, once formed, recall is unconscious and the memory is rarely lost. Procedural memories are stored in the cerebellum.
- **Declarative (factual) memory** is rapidly laid down, recalled consciously and easily lost. Declarative memories may be *episodic*, when a cluster of facts is memorised in relation to a specific time and place, or *semantic*, when facts are learned out of context.

Declarative memory is stored in structures in the medial temporal lobe: the hippocampus, parahippocampus, entorhinal cortex, amygdala, anterior

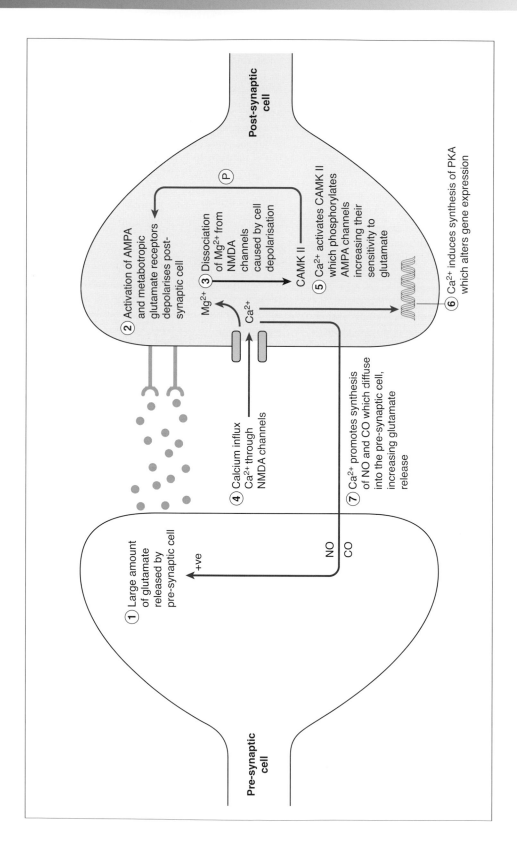

Figure 17.25 **Molecular pathways underlying long-term potentiation**. The numbers indicate the order of events occurring in Long-term potentiation.

cingulate cortex. The mamillary bodies and the anterior and dorsomedial nuclei of the thalamus are also thought to be involved. The amygdala plays a role in associative memory involving fear (when a non-noxious stimulus elicits physiological symptoms of fear, because it is normally closely followed by a noxious stimulus). Damage to the amygdala impairs the ability to learn new associations of this kind, and to recall those that have already been learnt.

> **CLINICAL Korsakoff's syndrome**
>
> Korsakoff's syndrome is characterised by an inability to form new memories. Long-term recall is unaffected and the person confabulates to compensate for deficits in short-term memory. The most common cause is thiamine deficiency, secondary to alcoholism. It is thought to be the structures in the midbrain involved in memory that are most affected by this deficiency.

Molecular basis of memory

Rewiring of neurons to form new memory circuitry is permitted by changes in the strength of synaptic connections. An increase in the strength of synaptic connections is called **long-term potentiation**. Long-term potentiation and long-term depression occur in the hippocampus, enabling the storage of declarative memories. Long-term depression alone occurs in the cerebellum, allowing the storage of procedural memories.

Long-term potentiation

Long-term potentiation (LTP) is caused by simultaneous excitation in the pre and postsynaptic neuron. As a result, subsequent inputs from the same presynaptic neuron cause a larger excitatory postsynaptic potential in the postsynaptic neuron. The molecular mechanism underlying this is as follows (Fig. 17.25):

- In response to a large excitation, presynaptic cells in the hippocampus release large amounts of glutamate which, by activating postsynaptic AMPA and metabotropic glutamate receptors, depolarise the postsynaptic neuron sufficiently so that Mg^{2+} ions dissociate from postsynaptic NMDA receptors.

- Once Mg^{2+} ions have dissociated, the action of glutamate on NMDA receptors causes an influx of Ca^{2+} ions into the postsynaptic cell.
- Ca^{2+} ion influx is crucial to the induction of LTP because it induces the changes responsible for increases in synaptic strength:
  - Ca^{2+} ions activate calcium–calmodulin-dependent protein kinase II (CAMKII), which phosphorylates AMPA channels, increasing their sensitivity to glutamate
  - Ca^{2+} ions promote the synthesis of molecules, such as NO and carbon monoxide, which diffuse into the presynaptic cell, increasing glutamate release.
- Ca^{2+} ions induce the synthesis of phosphokinase A, via a second-messenger cascade, which alters gene expression.

Sleep

Sleep is characterised by reduced responsiveness to external sensory stimuli, changes in the **electroencephalogram** (EEG), and changes in autonomic function.

> **DEFINITION EEG**
>
> In electroencephalography electrical activity across the cortex of the brain is measured by surface electrodes applied to the scalp and converted to a trace (the EEG), the pattern of which reflects the patient's state of consciousness. Its main applications are in the diagnosis and management of sleep disorders and epilepsy

Changes in the EEG during the different stages of sleep

High-frequency, low-amplitude, desynchronised β waves are recorded on the EEG of a person who is awake. On falling into a progressively deeper sleep (moving through stage 1 to stage 4 sleep), these EEG rhythms develop a lower frequency and higher amplitude, becoming α waves in stage 2 sleep and then δ waves in stage 3 and 4 sleep (Table 17.4).

Continuous electrical communication between the thalamus and cortex is recorded on the EEG of a person who is awake. In the early stages of deep sleep (also known as slow-wave or non- rapid eye movement</patentCit> [REM] sleep), there is still

Table 17.4 Changes during different stages of sleep

Stage of sleep	Type of wave form	Frequency (Hz)	Underlying thalamic activity	Muscle paralysis
Awake	β rhythm	8–12	Yes	No
REM sleep	β rhythm	8–12	Yes	Yes
Stage 1 and 2	α rhythm	3–7	Yes	No
Stage 3 and 4	δ rhythm	0.5–2	No	No

REM, rapid eye movement.

electrical communication between the thalamus and cortex. However, the thalamus becomes hyperpolarised, due to a loss of excitatory input from the hypothalamus, which causes it to fire repetitive and synchronised action potentials in rapid succession, known as sleep spindles. This characteristic pattern of electrical activity is transmitted to the cortex so that it also fires sleep spindles. These sleep spindles are responsible for the α rhythm recorded on an EEG. In the later stages of deep sleep, the thalamus becomes so hyperpolarised that it no longer fires action potentials and the cortex produces action potentials independently. This independent firing of action potentials by the cortex is responsible for the δ rhythm recorded on the EEG. During deep sleep, respiration rate, heart rate, blood pressure and GI activity decrease.

REM sleep

Approximately every 90 min (in adults), deep sleep is broken by a period of REM sleep (also known as paradoxical sleep or first-wave sleep), lasting 10–20 min. This is termed 'paradoxical sleep' because it is characterised by the same β rhythms as wakefulness, but the skeletal muscles are paralysed, apart from the extraocular muscles, which move the eyes back and forth, and the respiratory muscles, and the person is non-responsive. Autonomic function is also abnormal, with increases in respiration, heart rate, blood pressure and core temperature. People aroused from REM sleep report that they have been dreaming. Muscle paralysis prevents dreams being acted out.

Neuronal networks that regulate sleep cycles

The reticular activating system is active during wakefulness and REM sleep, but not during non-REM sleep. The reticular activating system comprises the following:

- **GABA- and glutamate-secreting, large-diameter neurons** that receive multiple sensory inputs and regulate postural and eye movement reflexes
- **Serotonin-, noradrenaline-** and **acetylcholine-** secreting, small-diameter neurons that project to the basal forebrain, and fire spontaneously according to levels of arousal.

Activity in acetylcholine-secreting neurons in the reticular activating system increases during REM sleep, but noradrenaline- and serotonin-secreting neurons are practically silent, compared with during wakefulness. There appears to be reciprocal inhibition between these two populations of cells, so that REM sleep and wakefulness are mutually exclusive. Acetylcholine-secreting neurons send projections to the vestibular and reticular nuclei which cause the features characteristic of REM sleep: excitation of oculomotor neurons; autonomic changes; an output to the LGN and visual cortex; and inhibition of sensory input and motor output.

The need to sleep

Sleep appears to be required for normal metabolic function because sleep-derived rats lose weight, become hypothermic, have a weakened immune system and eventually die.

Sleep may also be important in consolidation of 'experiences' because REM sleep is thought to promote LTP. This is supported by the observation that neonates (who experience many more 'new things' than older individuals) spend a disproportionate amount of time in REM sleep.

CLINICAL Abnormalities in sleep behaviour

Insomnia, an inability to get to sleep, may be caused by anxiety, depression and chronic pain.

Hypersomnia, sleeping more than is normal, may be caused by depression, obstructive sleep apnoea (see Chapter 7) or narcolepsy. Patients with narcolepsy have intermittent periods of extreme drowsiness during the day. This condition has a strong genetic component and is thought to be due to abnormalities in the brain-stem structures that control sleep.

Consciousness

Consciousness is characterised by an awareness of sensory stimuli, as well as an awareness of one's own physical and mental state.

Different degrees of consciousness

There are varying degrees of consciousness. This spectrum includes the following:

- **Being awake**.
- **Being asleep**.
- **Confusion** has many potential causes. The patient shows fluctuating consciousness. Sleep–wake cycles and reflexes are normal. Speech, audition and vision are also intact, although speech is disordered.
- **Anaesthesia**: in anaesthesia, the aim is to induce δ-wave activity (reminiscent of stage 3 and 4 deep sleep) in the patient's brain. Reflexes are also inhibited by a drug that blocks transmission at the neuromuscular junction.
- **Persistent vegetative state(PVS) and coma**: in both PVS and coma, the patient shows no sleep–wake cycles. Reflexes are reduced in PVS and very reduced in coma. There is no speech in either state. There is no evidence of audition or vision in a patient in a coma; patients in PVS show only a startle reflex. PVS and coma may be reversed only if the cause is eliminated.

Neurophysiological disorders

Neurophysiological disorders have a common underlying basis of abnormal electrical activity in the brain.

Epilepsy

Epilepsy is characterised by recurrent transient periods of abnormal electrical activity in the brain which give rise to seizures. Epilepsy may be primary, often with a genetic association, or secondary to another condition:

- If **abnormal electrical activity extends over the whole of the brain**, the epileptic seizure is said to be **general**. All general seizures involve a loss of consciousness; however, this is of variable duration, being much longer in tonic–clonic seizures (**grand mal**) than in absence seizures (**petit mal**). Tonic–clonic seizures are, in addition, characterised by muscle stiffness and spasm.
- If **abnormal electrical activity is restricted to part of the brain**, the epileptic seizure is said to be partial. The symptoms of a partial seizure vary according to the region of the brain affected, e.g. partial seizures of the parietal lobe cause abnormal sensations down the contralateral side of the body, whereas partial seizures of the occipital lobe cause visual hallucinations. Partial seizures do not necessarily entail a loss of consciousness. However, partial seizure activity may spread to affect the whole brain, in which case it is called a **complex partial seizure**.

Underlying basis of epilepsy

Seizures occur as a result of synchronisation of abnormal depolarisation spikes in multiple neurons. Individual prolonged depolarisation spikes are seen on the EEG of an individual with epilepsy between fits and are due to excessive neuronal excitation of neurons. This may result from reduced GABA-mediated inhibition or increased glutamate-mediated excitation.

Pharmacological management of epilepsy

Various drugs are available, all of which reduce neuron depolarisation and excitability, but by different mechanisms:

- **Sodium channel antagonists** (e.g. carbamazepine and phenytoin) suppress abnormal depolarisation spikes in hippocampal neurons by preventing the up-stroke of the action potential.
- **Calcium channel** antagonists (e.g. ethosuximide) prevent prolonged neuronal depolarisation, which can cause repetitive, burst firing.

- **Barbiturates and benzodiazepines** enhance GABA$_A$-channel function, so increasing GABA-mediated neuronal inhibition and opposing neuronal depolarisation. They are useful in terminating epileptic seizures.

Alzheimer's disease

Alzheimer's disease is the most common form of dementia, the clinical symptoms of which are deficits in memory, cognition, attention and motivation, and ultimately death.

Histopathology of alzheimer's disease

The histopathological characteristics are localised in the cortex, hippocampus and amygdala areas, crucial in memory.

- **Neuritic plaques** are made up of insoluble deposits of a peptide fragment, β-amyloid, deformed neuronal dendrites and inflammatory brain cells (microglia and astrocytes).
- **Neurofibrillary tangles** are made up of entwined helices of tau filaments (a normally soluble microtubule protein). They are commonly found in the deformed dendrites that surround neuritic plaques.
- **Ventricular enlargement** is indicative of atrophy and neuronal death in cortical and subcortical brain regions.

Molecular basis of neuronal death in alzheimer's disease

Neuronal death underlies Alzheimer's disease. Neuronal death is thought to be triggered when **β-amyloid deposits** promote massive calcium influx into neurons, which leads to formation of neurofibrillary tangles, disrupting the cytoskeleton, the integrity of which is crucial to neuronal survival.

Causes of alzheimer's disease

A minority of cases of (usually early onset) Alzheimer's disease are genetic in origin. Most cases are idiopathic. Genetic mutations predisposing to Alzheimer's disease development include:

- **Over-expression of the soluble precursor of β-amyloid**, amyloid precursor protein (APP)
- **Mutations in presenilin genes**: presenilin proteins are thought to increase the production of β-amyloid from APP, by altering the activity of two cleavage enzymes, β- and γ-secretase
- **Mutations in the genes encoding the tau protein**
- **Individuals with a common allele of the apolipoprotein E gene** may have a predisposition to the development of late-onset, idiopathic Alzheimer's disease. The protein product of this gene, ApoE4, is thought to enhance aggregation of β-amyloid into plaques.

Treatments for alzheimer's disease

Inhibitors of acetylcholinesterase (e.g. donepezil), the enzyme that breaks down acetylcholine, are the approved drugs in the treatment of Alzheimer's disease. They offset the death of cholinergic neurons in the prefrontal cortex, which is thought to make a particularly profound contribution to disease symptoms.

Stroke

Stroke is the leading cause of mental deficit in adults. Impairments in brain function after a stroke are caused by neuronal death following the formation of a blood clot or haemorrhage in an artery supplying the brain.

Treatment of stroke

Treatment focuses on reducing risk factors for future strokes (e.g. reducing blood pressure and lipid levels) and in rehabilitation of any impairment resulting from the stroke (e.g. physiotherapy, speech and language therapy). The exact course of the treatment is determined by the type of stroke and the region of the brain affected.

 RELATED CHAPTERS

18

Statistics

Statistics is the science of collecting, analysing and interpreting data. Statistics are used throughout medicine to identify significant differences underlying a condition or to determine effective treatments for conditions inherent in a population.

Key definitions

Hypotheses

In statistics the core aim is to test a hypothesis to determine whether the data support or refute them. For example, a hypothesis may be one such as 'drug X improves condition A'. As a result of making a hypothesis, it is essential to determine what is being tested and the precise conditions that are being used. The design of the experiment is likely to result in a more specific hypothesis: 'Drug X, at dose Y, reduces value B (which is a representative value of condition A).'

Much of statistics is interpreting whether the variable measured, and the differences between the samples, can or cannot be explained as a result of the random differences seen in the samples, unrelated to the intervention.

Populations and samples

When testing a theory, in most cases it is impossible to test everyone. As a result, a sample is taken from the population. This sample is unlikely to be completely representative of the entire population, and this **sampling variation** must be accounted for.

Data

In a study, data are collected for processing using statistics. The data collected consist of observations; these measurements are called variables. Variables can be divided into two types:

- **Qualitative variables** are not numerical, and usually refer to categories such as sex, type of drug or survival.
- **Quantitative variables** are numerical and can be further subdivided:
  - **discrete values** are usually whole numbers such as the number of cases of a condition, or number of offspring
  - **continuous values** can fall anywhere along a scale; examples include height and age.

Analysis

Data can be analysed by a variety of statistical tests, which depend on the type of data collected and the hypothesis that is being tested. The commonly used tests are described in more detail later in the chapter.

After testing, it is essential that the data are represented in an accurate and easily understandable form, which is not misleading. Again, the precise form used varies with the data and tests applied.

Biomedical Science Lecture Notes, First Edition. Ian Lyons.
© 2011 by Ian Lyons. Published 2011 by Blackwell Publishing Ltd.

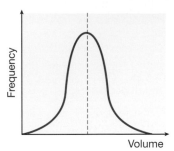

Symmetrical distribution

The data set is symmetrically distributed about its mean. The mean, median and mode of the data will be very similar. The distributions used to calculate significance are symmetrical (the normal, 't' and chi-squared distributions, for example). Additionally if a large sample is taken, the estimates of the means of the sample will be normally distributed around the true population mean - this is the **central limit theorem**.

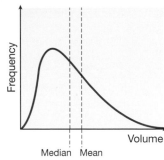

Median Mean

Positive skew

In positively skewed data the tail of the higher values is longer, which results in the mean value for the sample being greater than the median or modal values.

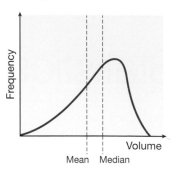

Mean Median

Negative skew

In this distribution, the tail of lower values is longer, which results in the opposite effects to a positive skewed distribution: the mean value for the sample is likely to be lower than either the median or the mode.

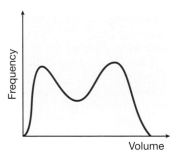

Bimodal distribution

In this distribution there are two 'peaks' in the data. This is likely to reflect two underlying distributions within the population. For example, in leukaemia there is an increased incidence in childhood and in old age, though fewer cases in the middle-aged, which will give rise to a bimodal distribution.

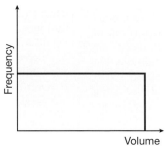

Uniform distribution

In a uniform distribution the frequency is the similar throughout the data set.

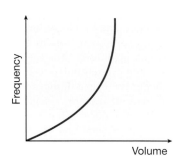

J-shaped distribution

This is an extremely asymmetrical distribution of data, where the frequency increases (or decreases) throughout the dataset.

Figure 18.1 The data in a sample can be distributed in a number of different ways. Although the precise distribution of the data depends on random sampling, various underlying distributions are commonly identified.

Frequency and frequency distribution

Having collected the data, it needs to be recorded on a form that is easily viewable and can allow trends to be identified. One of the first processes applied is to look at the frequency distribution of the data – how often a specific characteristic or range of values occurs.

Qualitative data

Analysing qualitative data is usually achieved by counting the number of observations in each category – determining the **frequency**. This can often be presented as a relative frequency, the percentage of the total number of observations in each category. Common representation of such data is by **pie chart** or **bar chart.**

Quantitative data – frequency distribution

A **frequency distribution** often provides a good starting point for the analysis of quantitative data. This involves determining the frequency of values, or ranges of values within the sample:

- For **discrete values**, the frequency of each value can be calculated.
- For **continuous values**, the frequency for a range of values must be determined. This approach can be applied to discrete values, if they occur over a particularly wide range of values.

To determine a frequency distribution the highest and lowest values must be determined and suitable groups should be defined. If too many groups are determined the data become difficult to process, whereas if too few groups are used, much of the detail of the distribution may be lost. When defining the groups, there should be no gaps between them.

Histograms are usually used to represent frequency distribution. In a histogram, the area of each bar is proportional to the frequency. For ease of representation, the widths of each group are usually the same, which ensures that the height of each bar becomes proportional to the frequency.

Frequency distribution curves

As the size of the sample grows, the groups can be made narrower to provide more detail. If this was taken to its limit (the whole population sampled and very narrow group ranges drawn), a smooth curve could be drawn for most variables. The typical distribution of a continuous value is one with the highest frequencies in the centre of the distribution, and with the frequencies decreasing at the extremes. Three variants of this **unimodal** distribution occur (Fig. 18.1):

- A **symmetrical distribution** is one where the highest frequency is located in the centre of the distribution, and the frequencies decrease evenly at both ends, resulting in a bell-shaped curve.
- A **positively skewed** distribution occurs when the upper tail of the distribution is longer than the lower tail.
- A **negatively skewed** distribution occurs when the lower tail is longer than the upper.

Other distributions of data can occur:

- **Bimodal** distribution occurs when there are two high-frequency peaks. Such a distribution is usually indicative of two separate distributions within the data-set.
- A **uniform** distribution occurs when the variable measured has no relationship with the outcome being tested. As such there are no discernable peaks and troughs in the distribution.
- A **J-shaped distribution**.

Means and variance

Although the frequency distribution can be used as a good starting point, it provides little indication for the comparison of data sets. Two measurements can usually accurately summarise a frequency distribution:

1 An **average value** of the data-set
2 A value indicating the **spread of values** in the data-set.

Averages

Three different averages are commonly used in analysing data, in a symmetrical unimodal data set; the values are likely to be very similar, although in other distributions there may be large differences between the three:

1 The **arithmetic mean** ($\bar{x}$) is the sum of all the values, divided by the number of values.
2 The **median** is simply the middle value of the distribution. If the distribution is ordered in an

increasing list, it would be the middle value. Median $= (n - 1)$th value in an ordered list of observations, where n is the number of observations.

3 The **mode** is the value that occurs most often.

Measurements of variation

The simplest assessment of the variation in a sample is simply to take the largest and smallest values in the sample – the **range**. However, it gives no indication of how the values are spread within the range. In addition, it is likely that the range will increase as the sample size increases.

The **variance** is commonly used to assess the spread of data. This assesses the spread of the data relative to the mean of the sample. This as expressed as the sum of the squares of the differences between the sample value and the mean, divided by the number of samples (n), minus 1.

The denominator $N - 1$ refers to the degrees of freedom within the sample. Within a sample, the sum of all the deviations must be 0, because only $N - 1$ values are unknown and the last value can be calculated because we know that the sum of the variances must equal 0.

Although the variance is a useful statistical tool, it takes the sum of the squares of the deviations, and, as such, provides a very large number; for many analyses, it is more convenient to express the standard deviation, which is the square root of the variance. In many distributions, the standard deviations can be used to assess how much of the sample is likely to be close to the mean. In a **normal distribution**, 70% of the values are likely to be within 1 standard deviation of the mean, and approximately 95% of observations are likely to lie within 2 standard deviations.

The standard deviation (SD) is sometimes expressed as a percentage of the sample mean. This is convenient when the size of variation relative to the sample mean is of interest. In addition it is a value that is independent of the units used. This value is referred to as the coefficient of variance.

The standard error

If many different samples are obtained from the same population, it is likely that each sample mean is closer to the mean of the population than any individual measurement. If a frequency distribution of these sample means is produced, the standard deviation of these sample meads is the **standard error of the sample mean**. As a measure of how closely the population mean is estimated by the sample mean, it is affected by two factors:

1 How much variation there is in the population
2 The size of the sample – the larger the sample the smaller the error.

Interpreting a sample mean is likely to be similar to that for a standard deviation. About 95% of the means obtained by repeated sampling of the same population are likely to lie within two standard errors of the population mean. This is used to construct a range of likely values for the population means, known as a **confidence interval** and is expressed as the observed sample mean and its standard errors.

Sampling from a finite population

When a large proportion of the total population is sampled, the sampling variation is likely to be considerably smaller than calculated by the standard error. For example, if the entire population is sampled, the variation between the sample mean and the population is 0, because they are one and the same. In samples where a large proportion of the population has been measured, a **finite population correction** can be applied:

$$FPC = \sqrt{\frac{N - n}{N - 1}}$$

where FPC is finite population correction, N is the number in population and n is the number in the sample.

This correction has little effect unless at least 10% of the population have been sampled.

The normal distribution

Many continuous values can be described by the **normal distribution**, which is a symmetrical, unimodal frequency distribution. The curve may be shorter and fatter for larger standard deviations, or taller and thinner for small deviations. The standard deviation is assumed for many statistical techniques applied and forms the basis of many tests of statistical significance. In practice, all normal distributions are transformed to the **standard normal distribution** for analysis. This is a normal distribution with a mean of 0 and with a standard deviation of 1. The relationship between the **standard normal distribution** and a curve with mean μ and standard deviation σ is.

This transformation allows a single table of probabilities (for the standard normal distribution) to be applied to all samples that are normally distributed.

Transforming a distribution to the standard normal

If the units or the base point of observations changes it affects the mean and the standard deviation in different ways:

- Adding or subtracting a constant affects the mean by the same amount, although the standard deviation is unaffected (the deviation from the mean of each value is unchanged).
- Multiplying or dividing alters both the mean and the standard deviation in the same way.

Probability density function

In the normal distribution the area under the curve represents the proportion of values that fall within the specified range of values, e.g. in a curve where the mean is $\bar{x}$ and the SD is σ, the proportion of people expressing a value greater than A can be demonstrated:

The number of standard deviations
from the mean $(Z) = \dfrac{\bar{x} - A}{\sigma}$.

The proportion of samples exceeding this value can be found by looking at a table of printed values (Table 18.1). This value is denoted as $\Phi(z)$.

Table 18.1 can be used the opposite way round, in that one can calculate at which value only 5% of the population exceed the value. This is done by finding the closest value to 0.05 (or 5%) and identifying the z value required (in this case 1.64). The corresponding value is found by inverting the definition of the **standard normal distribution**. This is denoted as $\Phi^{-1}(\Phi(z))$. In most statistical analyses, a 95% significance level is required, which is equivalent to 1.96 SD.

Percentage points in the normal distribution

Most statistical tests check whether the value found is within or outside specific limits. In most cases the level deemed statistically significant is 1.96 SD. At this level 5% of the distribution lay more than 2 SD (2.5% in each tail) from the mean.

Table 18.1 Standard Normal distribution

z	2-tailed P-value
0.0	1.000
0.1	0.920
0.2	0.841
0.3	0.764
0.4	0.689
0.5	0.617
0.6	0.549
0.7	0.484
0.8	0.424
0.9	0.368
1.0	0.317
1.1	0.271
1.2	0.230
1.3	0.194
1.4	0.162
1.5	0.134
1.6	0.110
1.7	0.089
1.8	0.072
1.9	0.057
2.0	0.046
2.1	0.036
2.2	0.028
2.3	0.021
2.4	0.016
2.5	0.012
2.6	0.009
2.7	0.007
2.8	0.005
2.9	0.004
3.0	0.003
3.1	0.002
3.2	0.001
3.3	0.001
3.4	0.001
3.5	0.000

Derived using Microsoft Excel Version 5.0

Confidence intervals

Confidence intervals are calculated to tell us the likely values of the population mean, and can be calculated using the sample mean and the standard error.

For a large sample ($>$60 observations), it is likely that the distribution of the sample means is normal and the sample SD is likely to reflect the population SD. From the normal distribution, we know that 95% of the sample means lie within 1.96 SD of the population mean. As a result, this can be used to calculate a range of values in which the population mean is likely to lie, based on the sample mean and its standard error. This is used to set confidence intervals, the upper and lower bounds at which the population mean is likely to lie. These are typically calculated as 95% confidence intervals (i.e. 1.96 standard errors); however, any values can be calculated by selecting an appropriate z from Table 18.1.

Calculation of confidence limits in small samples

If a sample is small (fewer than about 60 samples), two aspects may affect the use of the normal distribution

1 The sample SD, s, is subject to **sampling variation** and is not representative of the population SD, σ.
2 The distribution of the population is not normal, and the sample mean may also not be normal. This can be overcome by the **central limit theorem**.

 DEFINITION **The central limit theorem**

This states that, even for a non-normally distributed sample, the sample means will be normally distributed about the population mean. Provided that a sample is large enough (usually at least 15), the sample means will give a close approximation to a normal distribution.

As such by taking many samples from the population and then comparing the means of these samples, one can approximate the population mean. As a result for any population and hypothesis, provided that the experiment is well designed, a normal distribution (or a variant of it) can be used to test whether there is a statistically significant result.

The use of s as the normal distribution often invalidates the use of confidence intervals; instead the student's t-test distribution can be used in most cases, unless the population is extremely non-normal.

The t-test distribution

The frequency distribution in the t-test distribution is extremely similar to the normal; however it is more spread out at the tails. The shape is determined by the degrees of freedom ($n - 1$) of the sample SD – the fewer the degrees of freedom, the more spread out the sample is.

By accounting for the degrees of freedom, the t-test distribution can be used to calculate confidence intervals. For small numbers of degrees of freedom, a value generated by the t-test will be much larger than the corresponding value from a normal distribution; however, for larger sample sizes the t-test distribution approximates extremely closely to the normal distribution. When there is an infinite number of degrees of freedom, the normal and t-test distribution are identical.

Extremely non-normal distributions

Where data are not normal, the data are often transformed on to another scale so that a normal distribution can be applied. Alternatively, a **nonparametric** confidence interval can be calculated. This procedure is complex and beyond the scope of this text.

Significance tests

The simplest test that is regularly applied to data is to ask whether a sample mean is consistent with a hypothesised value for a population mean. This is usually achieved using a paired t-test, although it can also be achieved by the one-sample t-test and the normal test.

The paired t-test

This tests whether the difference between a pair of variables measured on each individual is 0, e.g. the effects of a drug on an individual compared with the administration of a placebo on the same individual at a different time. If the drug has no effect, the value measured should be no different from the placebo – differences seen should be down to chance variance. As the means measured are unlikely to be exactly the same, it is essential to determine whether any difference seen is due to this chance variance or whether there is a significant difference as a result of taking the drug.

The first step is to draw up a hypothesis 'that there is a difference between taking the drug and the placebo'. A **null hypothesis** is also produced that 'there is no real difference between taking the drugs and the placebo'. If the null hypothesis were true we would expect a mean difference of 0. The aim is to reject the null hypothesis (that any differences seen are due to chance variation), in favour of the hypothesis that there is a real effect.

We know that the difference in hours slept is likely to be normally distributed about the mean. The null hypothesis is that the population mean, μ, is 0. We apply the t-test as follows:

$$t = \frac{\bar{x} - \mu}{s/\sqrt{n}}$$

The resulting 't' value is compared against a series of printed values (Table 18.2). For this the number of degrees of freedom must be calculated, and is $(n - 1)$. Table 18.2 indicates within what p value a specific 't' is for a given number of degrees of freedom.

The smaller the significance level, the more significant a result – in practice a probability smaller than 5% is said to be significant. A probability greater than 5% is said to be non-significant, but there is no strong evidence against the null hypothesis being true.

Having established an effect, we can use a 95% confidence interval to calculate the range of values in which the true mean of the effect of the drug is likely to lie. Confidence intervals and significance tests are often closely linked:

- **Confidence intervals** give the range of values for a unknown population mean, which are consistent with the data gathered
- **Significance tests** assess whether data are consistent with one hypothesised value.

If a result is significantly different from the hypothesised value at a particular significance level, the corresponding confidence interval will not include this value.

One-sided and two-sided tests

In most tests discussed so far, the null hypothesis is that 'there is no difference between the populations'. The alternative hypothesis is that there is a

Table 18.2 t-distribution				
	Two-tailed p-value			
Degrees of freedom	**0.10**	**0.05**	**0.01**	**0.001**
1	6.314	12.706	63.656	636.58
2	2.920	4.303	9.925	31.600
3	2.353	3.182	5.841	12.924
4	2.132	2.776	4.604	8.610
5	2.015	2.571	4.032	6.869
6	1.943	2.447	3.707	5.959
7	1.895	2.365	3.499	5.408
8	1.860	2.306	3.355	5.041
9	1.833	2.262	3.250	4.781
10	1.812	2.228	3.169	4.587
11	1.796	2.201	3.106	4.437
12	1.782	2.179	3.055	4.318
13	1.771	2.160	3.012	4.221
14	1.761	2.145	2.977	4.140
15	1.753	2.131	2.947	4.073
16	1.746	2.120	2.921	4.015
17	1.740	2.110	2.898	3.965
18	1.734	2.101	2.878	3.922
19	1.729	2.093	2.861	3.883
20	1.725	2.086	2.845	3.850
21	1.721	2.080	2.831	3.819
22	1.717	2.074	2.819	3.792
23	1.714	2.069	2.807	3.768
24	1.711	2.064	2.797	3.745
25	1.708	2.060	2.787	3.725
26	1.706	2.056	2.779	3.707
27	1.703	2.052	2.771	3.689
28	1.701	2.048	2.763	3.674
29	1.699	2.045	2.756	3.660
30	1.697	2.042	2.750	3.646
40	1.684	2.021	2.704	3.551
50	1.676	2.009	2.678	3.496
100	1.660	1.984	2.626	3.390
200	1.653	1.972	2.601	3.340
5000	1.645	1.960	2.577	3.293

Derived using Microsoft Excel Version 5.0.

difference. As a result there is no direction of the difference hypothesised, so a two-sided test must be used, and the intervention may make the condition worse or better and the probabilities of both extremes must be included.

If we have strong reasons to believe that a drug would work one way or the other, a one-sided test can be applied. In this case, we would hypothesise that the intervention either improved or worsened the condition, but not both. If we hypothesised that a drug improved a condition, any decrease in the group would be attributed to chance. The significance would be based solely on the upper tail of the t-test distribution

A one-sided test may be tempting to use, because it is more likely to give a significant result; however, by the same token, it is also more likely to inappropriately reject the null hypothesis and invalidly accept the alternative hypothesis.

A one-sided test should be used with clear justifications, which are clearly stated and before the data are collected.

One-sample t-test

The one-sample t-test tests whether a sample mean is different from a specified value, which does not need to be 0. Its formula is:

$$t = \frac{(\bar{x} - \mu_1)}{s/\sqrt{n}}$$

Once again a range of p values can be calculated from the standard tables (Table 18.2), because it follows a t distribution with $(n-1)$ degrees of freedom. In effect, the paired t-test is a specific form of the one-sample t-test in that it is assumed that the mean tested is 0.

Normal test

When testing the mean of large samples, or when the population SD is known, the normal test can be applied instead of the t-test. The form is identical to that of the t-test, although different tables are used. This is commonly known as the z-test.

Errors in testing

Using statistics minimises the risk of an inaccurate interpretation of the data; although it is impossible to eliminate that due to sampling variation, a significant result is actually the result of chance, or when there is no significant difference in the sample mean, which is actually drawn from a significantly different population. These are known as the type I and type II errors (Fig. 18.2):

- Type I error occurs when the null hypothesis is incorrectly rejected. The probability of this occurring is the probability that is gained from the distribution tables, i.e. testing at a 5% significance level ($p = 0.05$) suggests that there is a 95% chance that a sample mean is different from a population mean. In the same way there is a 5% chance that the mean is in fact drawn from the same population.
- Type II errors occur when the null hypothesis is not rejected or when it is actually false. This is in effect the region of the sample distribution within which the range of the confidence intervals of the population mean falls. The lower the significance level, the greater the probability of rejecting the null hypothesis as a result of the lower likelihood of making a type II error. Conversely, if the significance level is increased, there is an increased likelihood of a type II error, although the potential for a type II error is reduced. The probability that a type II error is not made ($p = 1 - b\%$) is referred to as the power of the test.

Comparison of two means

Commonly we compare two distinct groups, such as the blood pressure of one group of individuals taking one form of blood pressure medication, with that of another group on a different medication. The calculations are similar for those used in one-sample tests; however, there is the additional assumption that the two population standard deviations are equal.

The sampling distribution of two means

The difference between two means of independent samples will be normally distributed if the means of each sample are normally distributed. As a result the null hypothesis is that $\mu_1 - \mu_2 = 0$, whereas the alternative hypothesis is that $\mu_1 - \mu_2 \neq 0$. The standard error is based on a combination of the standard errors of the individual means:

- The normal test is applied when large samples are known or if, rarely, the population standard deviations are known. Similarly the confidence interval for the samples can be calculated.
- The t-test is applied to small samples. In addition, the t-test requires that the standard

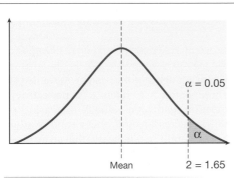 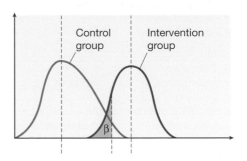

Type I error	Type II error
A Type I (α) error occurs when the null hypothesis is rejected when it is true. The size of the error is determined by the level of significance. For example, at p=0.05 this is the probability at which the null hypothesis is rejected.	A Type II (β) error occurs when we do not reject the null hypothesis when it is false. In a normally distributed group, this is the probability that the sample mean of the test group could fall below the significance level determined by test (this value is referred to as β). If such a result were to occur, the alternative hypothesis would be incorrectly rejected.

Figure 18.2 Type I and type II errors: various errors can occur during hypothesis testing. The most important ones are the type I and type II error which relate to when the null hypothesis is incorrectly rejected or accepted.

deviations of the two populations be the same. This can usually be assumed. In the case of the t-test, the degrees of freedom can be calculated as $n_1 + n_2 - 2$. Again, a 95% confidence interval can be calculated.

- If the samples are small and the standard deviations of the population unequal, a change of scale should be considered to overcome this. However, if this is not possible, a non-parametric test or a Fisher–Behrens or Welch test should be considered, all of which are beyond the scope of this book.

Analysis of variance – the comparison of several means

Many data-sets have more than two groups that need analysis. Although it is possible to perform many t-tests, each time comparing two groups, in practice this is not done because it is likely to yield inaccurate results – if a 5% significance level is used, 1 in 20 of the tests is likely to be significant even if there are no real differences.

Instead, an **analysis of variance (ANOVA)** test is used to compare many groups in one go – although the computations used are complex

and usually calculated by computer, a brief outline of the theory behind the test is illustrated below.

One-way analysis of variance

A one-way ANOVA can be used to test the means of several groups in which all the groups are classified by a single variable (e.g. the number of people). The basis of the test is comparison of whether the overall variation in the data are the result of differences between the means of the groups, and comparing this with the amount of variation that occurs due to differences between individuals in the same group.

The one-way ANOVA is in effect an extension of the two-sample t-test, when there are two groups with exactly the same results.

The starting point for an ANOVA is to determine the variance of all observations (irrespective of subgroup). The sum of the squared deviations from the overall mean divided by the degrees of freedom. This sum of squares is made up of two components:

1 The sum of squares due to difference between group means

2 The sum of squares due to difference between the observations within each group – the **residual** sum of squares.

The mean square is then calculated – this is the amount of variation per degree of freedom.

The significance (F test) compares the mean squares between groups with the mean squares within groups. If the observed differences were due to chance variation, the variation between group means would be similar to the variations between individuals in the same group. However, if there were real differences, the between-group variation would be far larger, because they are not drawn from the same underlying population. As a result the F test is often referred to as the variance ratio test.

There are two assumptions made in an F test:

1 The data are normally distributed.
2 The population value for the SD between individuals is the same for each group.

There are more complex forms of ANOVA, which are used to analyse data classified in two ways. They can be defined into several categories; the categories are summarised below, although they are not discussed in detail.

- Balanced design – there are equal numbers in each group. These are further divided to those experiments in which there is more than one observation per group (balanced design with replication) and those in which there is not (balanced design without replication).
- Unbalanced design – there are different numbers of observations in the groups.

Correlation and linear regression

Often two values are compared and it is important to determine the association between two variables, in two manners (Fig. 18.3):

1 Correlation determines how closely related the two values are to each other.
2 Linear regression gives the equation of the straight line that best describes the relationship between the two sets of values.

Correlation

Correlation is expressed as r, the correlation coefficient. It is calculated by comparing the change in each variable, related to the change in both. Mathematically, this can be expressed as:

$$r = \frac{\sum XY - \frac{\sum X \sum Y}{N}}{\sqrt{\left(\sum X^2 - \frac{(\sum X)^2}{N}\right)\left(\sum Y^2 - \frac{(\sum Y)^2}{N}\right)}}$$

The resulting value for r can be explained ideally in three states: -1, refers to a perfect negative correlation, with one value X increasing as the other, Y, decreases. At 0, there is no relationship between X and Y; $+1$ indicates that an increase in X sees a corresponding increase in Y. The correlation does not tell us anything about the underlying cause of the correlation (i.e. does X cause the change in Y or vice versa?), or they may both be different readouts of an underlying cause. In practice there is not a perfect relationship, and this results in a positive or negative value between -1 and $+1$, which implies a degree of correlation.

Significance of correlation

A t-test can be used to test where r is significantly different form 0 (no correlation). This significance is determined by both the correlation coefficient and the size of the sample used to calculate it – a large sample may produce a significant correlation even if this appears weak (i.e. close to 0), whereas a seemingly strong correlation based on very few observations may not be significant statistically.

Linear regression

Linear regression gives the equation of the line that best describes the correlation between the x and y axes. In a linear regression y is described in terms of x:

- x is termed the **independent**, or **explanatory**, **variable**.
- y is termed the **dependent variable**.

This is important in terms of the explanation, e.g. we would want to explain the dependence of heart rate on age as opposed to the dependence of age on heart rate.

A regression line has the form $y = a + bx$, where a is $y - bx$, and in which a is the value of y if $x = 0$, and b represents the proportionate increase of the value of y, for each increase in x. It will have the same sign as the correlation coefficient. As with other tests, the standard deviations of the sample points can be calculated because the values of a and b calculated from the samples are estimates of the population values.

Assumptions

The two major assumptions made during a regression analysis are:

Correlation

When comparing two sets of data from a sample, we would look to see if there is a correlation between the two – is a high value in one set of data likely to correlate with a high value for a different variable? The nature of this relationship can be defined by a regression line – this is a line of best fit which mathematically approximates the relationship between the two variables.

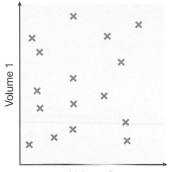

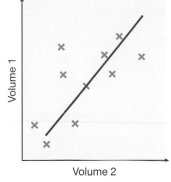

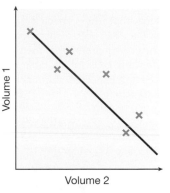

No correlation	**Positive correlation**	**Negative correlation**
If the two values are unrelated, then there is no correlation, and when plotted against each other, are unlikely to show any clear pattern. A regression line does not provide any additional information as there is not relationship that can be defined.	Here, a high value of one variable is likely to be related to a high value of another variable (e.g., blood pressure; likelihood of heart disease). The relationship between the two variables can be approximated by the regression line.	Here high values of one variable are likely to be related to low values for the other variable. Again, a regression line can be plotted.

Figure 18.3 Two variables taken from the same individuals can be plotted together to identify any relationship between the two – the correlation between the two variables (r^2) can be described between -1 (perfect negative correlation) and $+1$ (perfect positive correlation); if the correlation is 0, there is no relationship between the two variables.

1 that both variables are normally distributed
2 that the magnitude of the scatter of the points is the same throughout the line.

Non-linear regression (e.g. of the form $y = ax^2 + bx + c$) can also be calculated, although this is beyond the scope of this book.

Testing qualitative data – the chi-squared test

When qualitative variables need to be compared in two independent groups, we may need a statistical method to see if a similar proportion has a specific characteristic, e.g. in people who do or do not smoke we could look at the proportion who have had myocardial infarctions.

In this case we would use a chi-squared test. For this the data are obtained as frequencies (the numbers with or without the characteristic in each group) and they are entered into a contingency table that shows the observed (O) frequency:

Characteristic	Group 1	Group 2	Total
Present	A	B	A + B
Absent	C	D	C + D
Total	$N_1 = $ A + C	$N_2 = $ B + D	$N = $ A + B + C + D
Proportion with characteristic	$P_1 = \dfrac{A}{N_1}$	$P_2 = \dfrac{B}{N_2}$	$P = \dfrac{A+B}{N}$

This is then compared with the values that we would expect, i.e. what we would see if there is no difference between the groups. This is calculated from the overall proportion of the characteristic:

$$P = \frac{A+B}{N}$$

Such that the expected (E) frequencies are $N_1 \times P$ and $N_2 \times P$, respectively.

The chi-squared test is then performed on each of the four cells in the table comparing the observed and expected frequencies to obtain χ^2, the test statistic:

$$\chi^2 = \sum \frac{\left(|O - E| - \frac{1}{2}\right)^2}{E}$$

The χ^2 values are then compared against the probability distribution (Table 18.3) with 1 degree of freedom and the confidence intervals calculated. At 95% these are:

$$(p_1 - p_2) \pm 1.96 \sqrt{\frac{p_1(1 - p_1)}{n_1} + \frac{p_2(1 - p_2)}{n_2}}$$

Testing qualitative data for more than two groups

The chi-squared test can be applied to large numbers of independent groups for large numbers of characteristics. Once again a χ^2 value is calculated from the sum of the differences of the observed and expected values in each cell, although if the table is larger than 2×2 a slightly different formula is used:

$$\chi^2 = \sum \frac{(O - E)^2}{E}$$

The χ^2 value is then compared with the table, and the number of degrees of freedom is:

(Number of rows $- 1$) $\times$ (Number of columns $- 1$).

The p value is then calculated from Table 18.3, to show the known probability distribution.

Assumptions

For a chi-squared test to be valid the following assumptions are made:

- Each individual can be represented in only one row and one column (i.e. all the categories are mutually exclusive).
- Most (>80% of the frequencies) are ≥ 5. In a 2×2 table **all** frequencies must be ≥ 5.

Table 18.3 Chi-squared distribution

Degrees of freedom	Two-tailed P-value			
	0.10	0.05	0.01	0.001
1	2.706	3.841	6.635	10.827
2	4.605	5.991	9.210	13.815
3	6.251	7.815	11.345	16.266
4	7.779	9.488	13.277	18.466
5	9.236	11.070	15.086	20.515
6	10.645	12.592	16.812	22.457
7	12.017	14.067	18.475	24.321
8	13.362	15.507	20.090	26.124
9	14.684	16.919	21.666	27.877
10	15.987	18.307	23.209	29.588
11	17.275	19.675	24.725	31.264
12	18.549	21.026	26.217	32.909
13	19.812	22.362	27.688	34.527
14	21.064	23.685	29.141	36.124
15	22.307	24.996	30.578	37.698
16	23.542	26.296	32.000	39.252
17	24.769	27.587	33.409	40.791
18	25.989	28.869	34.805	42.312
19	27.204	30.144	36.191	43.819
20	28.412	31.410	37.566	45.314
21	29.615	32.671	38.932	46.796
22	30.813	33.924	40.289	48.268
23	32.007	35.172	41.638	49.728
24	33.196	36.415	42.980	51.179
25	34.382	37.652	44.314	52.619
26	35.563	38.885	45.642	54.051
27	36.741	40.113	46.963	55.475
28	37.916	41.337	48.278	56.892
29	39.087	42.557	49.588	58.301
30	40.256	43.773	50.892	59.702
40	51.805	55.758	63.691	73.403
50	63.167	67.505	76.154	86.660
60	74.397	79.082	88.379	99.608
70	85.527	90.531	100.43	112.32
80	96.578	101.88	112.33	124.84
90	107.57	113.15	124.12	137.21
100	118.50	124.34	135.81	149.45

Derived using Microsoft Excel Version 5.0.

Cohort and case–control studies

Many medical studies use either a case–control or a cohort study. These are often used interchangeably with prospective and retrospective, but the terms are not equivalent.

A cohort study

In a cohort study a sample of individuals, some of whom may be exposed to the risk factor(s) of interest, are followed over a period of time and the subsequent rates of disease occurrence compared. For example, in a hypothetical example, a cohort study may follow smokers and non-smokers as to their likelihood of developing a condition, x, over a defined period of time. The occurrence of the condition is assessed for both smokers and non-smokers and is found to be 6.0 and 0.2 per 1000 respectively.

Relative risk

The relative risk (RR) gives an indication of the strength of association between a risk factor and an outcome. A RR is calculated by:

$$RR = \frac{Incidence\ among\ exposed}{Incidence\ among\ non\text{-}exposed}$$

Using the examples above:

$$RR = \frac{60}{0.2} = 300.$$

An RR of 1.0 suggests that there is no association between exposure and outcome. A risk of >1 suggests that risk of disease is higher among those who have been exposed. A risk of <1 suggests that exposure is protective towards the outcome. In this case someone exposed would be 300 times more likely to develop the condition.

The significance of the RR can be tested using a 2×2 chi-squared test, and the confidence intervals for the result can be calculated from the chi-squared test.

Attributable risk

This gives an indication of the magnitude of the risk in absolute terms by an individual who is exposed to the stimulus in question.

$$AR = Incidence\ among\ exposed\ -$$
$$Incidence\ among\ non\text{-}exposed.$$

Attributable risk is sometimes given as a proportion:

$$PAR = \frac{RR - 1}{RR}$$

Population-attributable risk

The impact of a risk factor on the population depends on the prevalence of exposure; a risk factor with a strong association is unlikely to be serious to a general population if the number of people exposed is very small. However, a risk factor experienced by a large proportion of a population may be far more serious, even if the relative risk is far lower. The resulting measure is the population-attributable risk:

Population-attributable risk =
Overall incidence – Incidence among non-exposed.

Incidence rates and odds ratios

In a cohort study there is typically a gradual accumulation of cases as the study progresses; as a result a good measure of the rate of the disease can be expressed as an odds ratio – the ratio of the odds of getting the disease within the exposed sample to the odds of acquiring the disease in the non-exposed sample.

Case–control studies

In a case–control study, sampling is based on the disease rather than exposure status. The **cases** that have the disease are compared with **controls** that do not have the disease, and the study seeks to identify risk factors that are associated.

No information from the case–control study directly informs about incidence of exposed and non-exposed populations; however, the cross-product ratio of the case–control table estimates the odds ratio:

- In rare disorders, this will be equivalent to the RR.
- In a common disease $0 < |RR| < |OR|$.

Addendum: Reference table of symbols and formulae

Null hypothesis	H_0
Alternative hypothesis	H_1
Sample mean	$\bar{x}$
Population mean	μ
Variance (Var(X) or σ^2)	$Var(X) = \sum (X - \mu)^2 = \sum X^2 - \sum x^2$
Standard deviation (σ)	$\sigma = \sqrt{\dfrac{1}{N}\left(\left(\sum x^2\right) - Nx^2\right)} = \sqrt{\dfrac{1}{N}\left(\sum x^2\right) - \bar{x}^2}$
Standard deviation of sample (s)	$s = \sqrt{\dfrac{1}{N-1}\sum (x - \bar{x})^2}$
Standard error of the mean (SEM or $SE_{\bar{x}}$)	$SE_{\bar{x}} = \dfrac{s}{\sqrt{n}}$
Standard normal distribution (Z) where ($\bar{x} = 0$, $\sigma^2 = 1$)	$Z = \dfrac{X - \mu}{\sigma}$
Finite population correction	$FPC = \sqrt{\dfrac{N-n}{N-1}}$
Confidence intervals – *in this example a significance level of 0.05 is used* ($\alpha = 0.05$)	$\Phi(z) = P(Z \leq z) = 1 - \dfrac{\alpha}{2} = 0.975,$ $\Phi^{-1}(\Phi(z)) = \Phi^{-1}(0.975) = 1.96$ $0.95 = 1 - \alpha = P(-z \leq Z \leq z) = P\left(-1.96 \leq \dfrac{\bar{X}-\mu}{\sigma/\sqrt{n}} \leq 1.96\right)$ $P = \left(\bar{X} - 1.96\dfrac{\sigma}{\sqrt{n}} \leq \mu \leq \bar{X} + 1.96\dfrac{\sigma}{\sqrt{n}}\right)$
One variable independent student's *t* test	$t = \dfrac{\bar{x}-\mu}{s/\sqrt{n}},$ where there are $n - 1$ degrees of freedom
Dependent *t*-test for paired samples	$t = \dfrac{\bar{X}_D - \mu_0}{s_D/\sqrt{n}},$ where there are $n - 1$ degrees of freedom
Type 1 error (α)	Level of significance $= z$
Type 2 error (β)	
Linear regression	$y = a + bx$ where, $a = \dfrac{\sum Y - b(\sum X)}{N}, \quad b = \dfrac{\sum XY - (\sum X)(\sum Y)}{N\sum X^2 - (\sum X)^2}$ where a = the intercept point of the regression line and the y axis, b = the slope of the regression line, X = first score, Y = second score, $\sum X$ = sum of the first scores, $\sum Y$ = sum of the second scores and $\sum XY$ = sum of the product of the first and second scores
Correlation coefficient	$r = \dfrac{\sum XY - \dfrac{\sum X \sum Y}{N}}{\sqrt{\left(\sum X^2 - \dfrac{(\sum X)^2}{N}\right)\left(\sum Y^2 - \dfrac{(\sum Y)^2}{N}\right)}}$ x and y are the two variables being analysed, for N samples. R should be $-1 < r < 1$, where -1 is a perfect negative correlation and $+1$ is a perfect positive correlation.
Chi-squared (χ^2) for 2×2 table	$\chi^2 = \sum \dfrac{(\lvert O - E\rvert - \frac{1}{2})^2}{E}$
Chi-squared (χ^2) for table larger than 2×2	$\chi^2 = \sum \dfrac{(O - E)^2}{E}$
Confidence interval for χ^2test, 2×2 table at a 5% significance level	$(p_1 - p_2) \pm 1.96\sqrt{\dfrac{p_1(1 - p_1)}{n_1} + \dfrac{p_2(1 - p_2)}{n_2}}$

Index

Page numbers in *italics* denote figures, those in **bold** denote tables.

Biomedical Science Lecture Notes, First Edition. Ian Lyons.
© 2011 by Ian Lyons. Published 2011 by Blackwell Publishing Ltd.